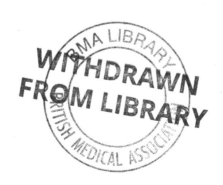

Urological Cancers

Jonathan Waxman (Ed)

Urological Cancers

With 45 Illustrations

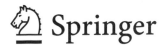 Springer

Jonathan Waxman, BSc, MD, FRCP
Professor of Oncology
Faculty of Medicine
Hammersmith Campus
Imperial College London
London, UK

Library of Congress Control Number: 2005923575

ISBN-10: 1-85233-911-X   e-ISBN: 1-84628-015-X   Printed on acid-free paper.
ISBN-13: 978-1-85233-911-1

Printed in Singapore.   (BS/KYO)

9 8 7 6 5 4 3 2 1   SPIN 10945964

Springer Science+Business Media

springeronline.com

I would like to acknowledge the amazing competence and considerable help given by Sandie Coward in the preparation of this book.

Preface

Urological cancer constitutes approximately 30% of all cancer occurring in the Third and Second Worlds. In the main, these diseases are caused by environmental factors, such as diet and smoking, and it is hoped that action to regulate the influence of these environmental pathogens will lead to a decreased incidence over the next two or three decades.

In the meantime, our understanding of the scientific basis for urothelial malignancy has broadened significantly. For example, studies in prostate cancer, which were few and far between 20 years ago, have increased, and the degree of government intervention, both in Europe and the United States, to support work in this field has grown significantly as a result of patient pressure. Interest too has increased from the pharmaceutical industry, and this has led to the development of new treatment options for all of the urological malignancies and real improvements in remission rates and durations.

This book summarizes developments in all areas of urological cancer, including clinical and molecular advances.

Jonathan Waxman, BSc, MD, FRCP
London, UK

Contents

Preface vii
Contributors xiii

I—Prostate Cancer

1 The Molecular Biology of Prostate Cancer
  Sarah Ngan and Jonathan Waxman 3

2 Familial Prostate Cancer
  Sashi S. Kommu and Rosalind A. Eeles 17

3 Screening for Prostate Cancer
  Joshua Phillips and Freddie C. Hamdy 31

4 Diet and Prostate Cancer
  Danish Mazhar 41

5 Radical Radiotherapy for Prostate Cancer
  Mererid Evans and Malcolm D. Mason 48

6 Prostate Cancer: Immediate vs. Deferred Treatment
  Mark A. Underwood and David Kirk 60

7 Surgical Treatment of Prostate Cancer
  Mark R. Feneley and Roger S. Kirby 69

8 Hormone Therapy for Prostate Cancer
  Gairin J. Dancey and Jonathan Waxman 77

9 Chemotherapy in Prostate Cancer
  Srikala S. Sridhar and Malcolm J. Moore 83

10 Proteomic Approaches to Problem Solving in Prostate Cancer
   Simon C. Gamble 95

11 Gene Therapy for Prostate Cancer
   Danish Mazhar and Roopinder Gillmore 104

II—Bladder Cancer

12 Molecular Biology of Bladder Cancer
    Margaret A. Knowles 115

13 Treatment Options in Superficial (pTA/pT1/CIS)
    Bladder Cancer
    Jeremy L. Ockrim and Paul D. Abel 131

14 Chemotherapy for Bladder Cancer
    Matthew D. Galsky and Dean F. Bajorin 145

15 Gene Therapy of Urothelial Malignancy
    Sunjay Jain and J. Kilian Mellon 156

III—Kidney Cancer

16 Molecular Biology of Kidney Cancer
    Jeffrey M. Holzbeierlein and J. Brantley Thrasher 169

17 Cytokine and Angiogenesis Inhibitors
    Simon Chowdhury, Timothy G. Eisen, and Martin Gore 184

18 Novel Therapies for Renal Cell Cancer
    Mayer N. Fishman 204

IV—Testicular Cancer

19 Genetics and Biology of Adult Male Germ Cell Tumors
    Jane Houldsworth, George J. Bosl, and R.S.K. Chaganti 221

20 Chemotherapy for Testicular Cancer
    Thomas R. Geldart and Graham M. Mead 230

21 Surgery for Testicular Cancer
    Gillian L. Smith and Timothy J. Christmas 243

22 Pathobiological Basis of Treatment Strategies of
    Germ Cell Tumors
    J. Wolter Oosterhuis, Friedemann Honecker, Frank Mayer,
    Carsten Bokemeyer, and L.H.J. Looijenga 252

V—Penile Cancer

23 A Scientific Understanding of the Development of
    Penile Tumors
    T.R. Leyshon Griffiths and J. Kilian Mellon 275

24 The Clinical Management of Penile Cancer
    Rajiv Sarin, Hemant B. Tongaonkar, and Reena Engineer 283

VI—Unusual Urological Tumors

25 Oncocytomas and Rare Renal Tumors
      Holger Moch   301

26 Small Cell Tumors, Lymphomas, and Sertoli Cell and Leydig Cell
      Tumors of the Bladder, Prostate, and Testis
      Chris M. Bacon and Alex Freeman   309

Index   333

Contributors

Paul D. Abel, ChM, FRCS
Department of Surgery
Faculty of Medicine
Hammersmith Hospital Campus
Imperial College London
London, UK

Chris M. Bacon, MB ChB, PhD,
BMedSci
Department of Histopathology
Royal Free and University College
Medical School
London, UK

Dean F. Bajorin, MD
Division of Solid Tumor Oncology
Department of Medicine
Memorial Hospital for Cancer and
Allied Diseases
Memorial Sloan-Kettering Cancer Center
New York, NY, USA

Carsten Bokemeyer, MD
Department of Hematology/Oncology
University of Tübingen, Germany

George J. Bosl, MD
Department of Medicine
Memorial Sloan-Kettering Cancer
Center
New York, NY, USA

R.S.K. Chaganti, PhD
Cell Biology Program and Department
of Medicine
Memorial Sloan-Kettering Cancer
Center
New York, NY, USA

Simon Chowdhury, MB BS
Department of Medicine
Royal Marsden Hospital
London, UK

Timothy J. Christmas, MD, FRCS(Urol)
Department of Urology
Royal Marsden NHS Foundation Trust
London, UK

Gairin J. Dancey, MRCP
Department of Clinical Oncology
Hammersmith Hospital
London, UK

Rosalind A. Eeles, MA, PhD, FRCP,
FRCR
Cancer Genetics Unit
Institute of Cancer Research
Sutton, UK

Timothy G. Eisen, PhD, FRCP
Renal, Melanoma and Lung Units
Department of Medicine
Royal Marsden Hospital
London, UK

Reena Engineer, DNB
Department of Radiation Oncology
Tata Memorial Hospital
Mumbai, India

Mererid Evans, MB BCh, BSc, PhD,
MRCP
Department of Radiotherapy
Velindre Hospital
Cardiff, UK

Mark R. Feneley, MD, FRCS
Institute of Urology and Nephrology
University College London and UCLH
Foundation Trust
London, UK

Mayer N. Fishman, MD, PhD
Department of Interdisciplinary
Oncology
H. Lee Moffitt Cancer Center and
Research Institute
University of South Florida
Tampa, FL, USA

Alex Freeman, MB BS, MD, BSc
Department of Histopathology
Royal Free and University College
Medical School
London, UK

Matthew D. Galsky, MD
Genitourinary Medical Oncology
Service
Department of Medicine
Memorial Sloan-Kettering Cancer
Center
New York, NY, USA

Simon C. Gamble, BSc, PhD
Cancer Cell Biology
Imperial College London
London, UK

Thomas R. Geldart, MB BS, BSc, MRCP
Wessex Medical Oncology Unit
Southampton University Hospital NHS
Trust
Southampton, UK

Roopinder Gillmore, MA, MRCP
Department of Immunology
Imperial College London
London, UK

Martin Gore, MB BS, PhD, FRCP
Department of Medicine
Royal Marsden Hospital
London, UK

T.R. Leyshon Griffiths, BSc, MD, FRCS
Department of Cancer Studies and
Molecular Medicine
University of Leicester
Clinical Sciences Unit
Leicester General Hospital
Leicester, UK

Freddie C. Hamdy, MB ChB, MD, FRCS
Academic Urology Unit
Division of Clinical Sciences (South)
School of Medicine & Biomedical Sciences
University of Sheffield
Royal Hallamshire Hospital
Sheffield, UK

Jeffrey M. Holzbeierlein, MD
Department of Urology
University of Kansas Medical Center
Kansas City, KS, USA

Friedemann Honecker, MD
Department of Pathology
Josephine Nefkens Institute
Erasmus MC-University Medical Center
Rotterdam
Daniel den Hoed Cancer Center
Rotterdam
The Netherlands
and
Department of Hematology/Oncology
University of Tübingen, Germany

Jane Houldsworth, PhD
Cell Biology Program and Department
of Medicine
Memorial Sloan-Kettering Cancer
Center
New York, NY, USA

Sunjay Jain, BSc, MB BS, FRCS
Urology Group
Department of Cancer Studies and
Molecular Medicine
University of Leicester
Clinical Sciences Unit
Leicester General Hospital
Leicester, UK

Roger S. Kirby, MA, MD, FRCS
Department of Urology
St George's Hospital
London, UK

David Kirk, BM BCh, MA, DM, FRCS
Department of Urology
Gartnavel General Hospital
Glasgow, UK

Margaret A. Knowles, PhD
Cancer Research UK Clinical Centre
St James's University Hospital
Leeds, UK

Sashi S. Kommu, MB BS, BSc, MRCS
Cancer Genetics Unit
Institute of Cancer Research
Sutton, UK

L.H.J. Looijenga, MD
Department of Pathology
Josephine Nefkens Institute
Erasmus MC-University Medical Center
Rotterdam
Daniel den Hoed Cancer Center
Rotterdam, The Netherlands

Malcolm D. Mason, MD, FRCP, FRCR
Section of Clinical Oncology and
Palliative Medicine
Velindre Hospital
Cardiff, UK

Frank Mayer, MD
Department of Hematology/Oncology
University of Tübingen, Germany

Danish Mazhar, MA, MBBS, MRCP
Cancer Centre
Division of Medicine
Faculty of Medicine
Hammersmith Campus
Imperial College
London, UK

Graham M. Mead, DM, FRCP, FRCR
Wessex Medical Oncology Unit
Southampton University Hospital NHS
Trust
Southampton, UK

J. Kilian Mellon, MD, FRCS
Department of Cancer Studies and
Molecular Medicine
University of Leicester
Clinical Sciences Unit
Leicester General Hospital
Leicester, UK

Holger Moch, MD
Institute for Surgical Pathology
Department Pathology
University Hospital
Zürich, Switzerland

Malcolm J. Moore, MD
Department of Medical Oncology and
Hematology
Princess Margaret Hospital
University Health Network
Toronto, ON, Canada

Sarah Ngan, BMedSci, MBBS, MRCP
Department of Medical Oncology
Hammersmith Hospital NHS Trust
London, UK

Jeremy L. Ockrim, MD, BSc, FRCS
Department of Urology
Institute of Urology
The Middlessex Hospital
London, UK

J. Wolter Oosterhuis, MD, PhD
Department of Pathology
Erasmus MC-University Medical Center
Rotterdam
Josephine Nefkens Institute
Rotterdam, The Netherlands

Joshua Phillips, MBChB, MRCS
Academic Urology Unit
Division of Clinical Sciences (South)
School of Medicine & Biomedical
Sciences
University of Sheffield
Royal Hallamshire Hospital
Sheffield, UK

Rajiv Sarin, MD, FRCR
Department of Radiation Oncology
Tata Memorial Hospital
Mumbai, India

Gillian L. Smith, MD, FRCS
Department of Urology
Charing Cross Hospital
London, UK

Srikala S. Sridhar, MD, MSc
Department of Medical Oncology and
Hematology
Princess Margaret Hospital
University Health Network
Toronto, ON, Canada

J. Brantley Thrasher, MD
Section of Urology/Department of
Surgery
University of Kansas Medical Center
Kansas City, KS, USA

Hemant B. Tongaonkar, MS
Urologic Oncology Service
Tata Memorial Hospital
Mumbai, India

Mark A. Underwood, MB ChB, MD,
FRCS
University Department of Urology
Glasgow Royal Infirmary, UK

Jonathan Waxman, BSc, MD, FRCP
Professor of Oncology
Faculty of Medicine
Hammersmith Campus
Imperial College London
London, UK

Part I

Prostate Cancer

1

The Molecular Biology of Prostate Cancer

Sarah Ngan and Jonathan Waxman

Prostate cancer is the most frequently diagnosed malignancy among men in industrialized countries. In the United States, one in eight men will develop prostate cancer during their lifetime [1], and in 1999 approximately 37,000 died from the disease [2]. In England and Wales, 17,000 cases are diagnosed and there are nearly 9000 deaths annually from prostate cancer [3].

Advances in our understanding of the molecular basis of cancer have led to the characterization of critical pathways regulating tumor growth, which should provide the potential for the development of more effective and less toxic targeted therapies. In 1941 Huggins and Hodges first demonstrated that malignant tumors arising from the prostate were responsive to androgen withdrawal. Since then, hormonal therapy has been established as the principal treatment modality for advanced disease. Over time, however, resistance to treatment occurs. As a result, there has been much interest not only in the molecular changes associated with prostate cancer but also in the molecular mechanisms of tumor resistance. This chapter describes the current status of research into the molecular biology of prostate cancer, with emphasis on recent progress.

Epidemiology of Prostate Cancer

The epidemiology of prostate cancer has provided a number of clues to the etiology of the disease. The incidence of prostate cancer increases with age. However, there is a discrepancy between the clinical incidence of prostate cancer and prevalence of the disease at autopsy [4]. The frequency of autopsy-detected cancer has been reported to be 30% to 40% in men over the age of 50. The incidence also varies markedly throughout the world, with the United States, Canada, Sweden, Australia, and France having the highest rates and Asian populations the lowest [5]. These differences may be due to genetic factors, but environmental factors may also be at play. Japanese male immigrants in the United States have a higher mortality rate compared with those in Japan [6]; dietary changes are thought to be a significant environmental factor [4,7] (Table 1.1).

Prostate cancer risk, particularly that of early-onset disease, is affected by family history. The association, however, is not as marked as in breast and colon cancer. The relative risk of prostate cancer increases markedly when the age of the index case decreases and when the number of affected family members increases [8]. The importance of an inherited predisposition is also supported by the finding that monozygotic twins have a fourfold increased concordance of prostate cancer compared with dizygotic twins [8]. Epidemiological studies suggest that dominantly inherited susceptibility genes with high penetrance account for only 5% to 10% of all prostate cases but as many as 30% to 40% of cases with early-onset disease [9].

3

Table 1.1. Proposed risk factors for prostate cancer

Possible/likely risk factors
Age
Race
Premalignant lesions (prostatic intraepithelial
  neoplasia)
Affected relatives
Carnivorous diet
Dietary fat
Vitamin D
Sexual habits

Controversial/disproved risk factors
Benign prostatic hypertrophy
Sexually transmitted diseases
Cigarette smoking
Alcohol intake
Cadmium exposure

From Morton [7].

Inherited Genetic Changes

Unlike in breast and colon cancer, no major predisposition genes for prostate cancer have been detected. However, a number of susceptibility loci have been identified. As yet the susceptibility genes for most of these regions remain unknown [10]. This suggests that the predisposition to prostate cancer is heterogeneous and may involve multiple genes.

Seven prostate cancer susceptibility loci have thus far been described and tested on independent data sets [5,11]: *HPC1* (hereditary prostate cancer) at 1q24, *PCaP* (predisposing for prostate cancer) at 1q42, *HPCX* at Xq27, *CAPB* (cancer, prostate, and brain) at 1q36, *HPC20* at 20q13, *HPC2/ELAC2* at 17p11, and a new locus at 8p22-23 and at 16q23.2 [10]. Candidate genes, which have been identified from a small number of families, include *HPC2/ELAC2*, *RNASEL*, and *MSR1* [9]. As well as being involved in the pathogenesis of prostate cancer, *MSR1* and *RNASEL* are also involved in the host response to infectious agents [9]. It therefore has been hypothesized that mutations in these genes might reduce the ability to eradicate certain infectious agents within the prostate, resulting in a chronic inflammatory response.

As well as breast and ovarian cancer, *BRCA1* mutation carriers have been found to have an increased risk of prostate cancer [12]. The relative risk of prostate cancer in *BRCA1* carriers was 2.95 compared with the general population. A later study from the Breast Cancer Linkage Consortium also found that in breast/ovarian cancer families with a deleterious *BRCA2* mutation, the relative risk for prostate cancer was 4.65 [13]. Furthermore, this risk was even higher before age 65. Subsequent analysis of 38 prostate cancer familial clusters found no germline mutations in *BRCA1*; however, two novel deletions were found in *BRAC2* [14]. The authors of this report proposed that *BRAC2* germline mutations might account for up to 5% of prostate cancers in familial clusters.

Other germline mutations and common sequence variant alleles in the population, which may play a part in modifying prostate cancer risk, include those encoding key proteins involved in androgen biosynthesis and action. These are discussed later in this chapter.

Somatic Genetic Changes

Although the molecular genetic changes responsible for prostate cancer development and progression is poorly understood, as with other solid tumors the number of changes increases with the stage of disease [9], suggesting that the disease progresses as the result of an accumulation of genetic changes (Fig. 1.1). This may involve activation of dominant oncogenes–by amplification, translocations or point mutations, or inactivation of recessive tumor suppressor genes–loss of an allele (known as loss of heterozygosity, LOH), allele inactivation by mutation, promoter hypermethylation, and haploinsufficiency.

Chromosomal Alterations

Up to 54% of primary cancers and 100% of metastatic tumors have LOH occurring in at least one chromosome. The technique of comparative genomic hybridization (CGH) has helped to identify the most commonly altered chromosomal regions in prostate cancer. Chromosomal losses are far more common that gains in primary tumors; however, they are found at equal frequencies in hormone-refractory tumors [10]. This suggests that tumor suppressor inactivation may be an early event in prostate cancer

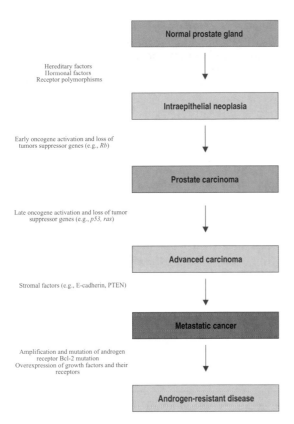

Fig. 1.1. A possible pathway for the pathogenesis and progression of prostate cancer.

development with the activation of oncogenes occurring later.

The commonly deleted regions are 8p, 10q, 13q, and 16p, and the regions that most commonly show gain are 7p, 7q, 8p, and Xq [15]. Unfortunately, target genes for these regions have not yet been identified.

Tumor Suppressors

p53

The *p53* gene encodes a 53-kd phosphoprotein, which is crucial in regulating cell proliferation and apoptosis. Mutations of *p53* occur in up to 50% of most cancers, and LOH occurs in 80% of breast, lung, and colon cancers. In prostate cancer, *p53* mutations are rarely seen in benign prostatic hypertrophy [16], and the incidence in localized untreated specimens is approximately 20%. In metastatic or treatment-resistant disease, however, the incidence reaches 50% to 75% [17]. This suggests that mutations of the *p53* gene are a late development in prostate cancer progression.

Rb

The retinoblastoma gene *Rb* is located at 13p and encodes a protein involved in the cell-cycle pathway. As with *p53* and the other classic tumor suppressor gene *CDKN2A*, genetic inactivation is rarely seen in primary cancers but occurs at higher frequencies in metastatic and hormone refractory lesions [9].

The PTEN/PI₃K/Akt Pathway

PTEN is located on 10q23 and is mutated in up to a third of hormone refractory prostate cancer [9]. Homozygous deletions and mutations have also been identified in a subset of primary prostate cancers [18]. The loss of *PTEN* expression in primary prostate cancer has been found to correlate with a high Gleason score and an advanced stage [19].

PTEN phosphatase functions as a tumor suppressor, via its ability to indirectly reverse phosphatidylinositol-3 kinase (PI₃K)-mediated phosphorylation and activation of the serine-threonine kinase and survival factor Akt. Akt signaling leads to the inhibition of apoptosis and to increased cell proliferation [9]. Therapeutic strategies involving the inhibition of signaling through PI₃K and Akt are currently being explored.

KLF6

Kruppel-like factor-6 (*KLF6*) has been mapped to chromosome 10p, and LOH analysis has found allele deletion in 17 (77%) of 22 primary tumors [20]. However, confirmation of its role as a tumor suppressor gene is awaited.

NKX3-1

Two separate sites on chromosome 8 (8p23 and 8p12-22) have shown chromosomal deletions or allelic loss most frequently in prostate cancer [9]. *Nkx3-1* maps to 8p21 and has been proposed as a tumor suppressor. *NFK3-1* is expressed in normal prostate epithelium and is decrease in prostate tumor cells [21]. In addition, Bhatia-Gaur et al. [21] have suggested that loss of a single allele may be linked to a predisposition to prostate cancer.

CpG Island Promoter Methylation

The most common genomic change in prostate cancer is silencing of the gene encoding the pi class of glutathione-S transferase (GSTP1) by hypermethylation of the promoter region. This change has been found in 90% to 95% of prostate cancers and 70% of high-grade prostatic intraepithelial neoplasia lesions [9]. The GSTP1 enzyme has a cell-detoxifying function, and therefore may protect cells from environmental carcinogens and DNA damage. Detection of the methylated GSTP1 promoter in urine and semen is being investigated as a possible biomarker for prostate cancer diagnosis [9].

Other genes that have been found to have selective promoter methylation in prostate cancer include CD44–, a cell adhesion molecule that may have a role in metastasis; EDNRB, which encodes the endothelin B receptor; and ER-$\alpha\beta$, which encodes the estrogen receptors α and β.

Oncogenes

ras

Mutations in the ras oncogene family are common in human solid tumors. The ras oncogene family encodes for cell membrane proteins that are involved in signal transduction via guanosine triphosphate (GTP)/guanosine diphosphate (GDP) binding and thus promote cell growth. Point mutations have been found at codons 12, 13, and 61 of the Ha-, Ki-, and N-ras genes, in prostate cancer specimens, but the overall frequency of ras gene mutations is low [22]. The expression of the mutated ras oncogene protein, however, is correlated with grade [23].

myc

Amplification of regions on chromosome 8q correlates with aggressiveness of prostate cancer tumors [9]. A candidate gene located on 8p is the myc gene because amplification of myc in prostate cancer correlates with a poor prognosis [9]. The myc proto-oncogene family encodes for nuclear phosphoproteins, which control DNA replication, cell cycle regulation, and differentiation. C-myc expression in the hormone sensitive LNCaP cell line is inhibited by androgens [24]. The level of c-myc transcripts in prostate cancer tissues was also found to be higher than in normal tissues or benign hypertrophy [25]. In situ hybridization, however, failed to demonstrate a relationship between c-myc expression and prostate cancer biology [26].

Other genes on chromosome 8q also have been investigated as potential targets of amplification including the elongin c gene [10] and EIF3S3 [9].

Inhibitors of Apoptosis

bcl-2

The BCL2 protein is an antiapoptotic factor. Changes in the bcl-2 proto-oncogene were initially described in association with the t (14:18) translocation found in follicular lymphoma. The BCL2 protein is expressed mostly in basal cells in healthy prostate tissue. It is overexpressed within the luminal epithelium in a subset of high-grade prostatic intraepithelial neoplasia lesions and in many androgen-independent prostate cancers; however, it is absent in most low- to intermediate-grade carcinomas [9,27]. Androgen resistance might also involve the bcl-2 oncogene induced through androgen deprivation [27]. The use of BCL2 as a therapeutic target is currently being investigated; the BCL2 antisense oligonucleotide G3139 is being assessed in clinical trails in patients with metastatic prostate cancer [28].

Other antiapoptotic proteins that may be important in the survival of resistant prostate cancer cells include survivin and the caspase group of proteins. Survivin messenger RNA (mRNA) is virtually undetectable in normal adult tissues but is highly expressed in most human cancers and prostate cell lines [28]. Neuroendocrine cells in the normal and malignant prostate have also been found to overexpress survivin [29].

Telomere Length

Telomeres are found at the ends of all eukaryotic chromosomes and protect chromosome ends from being recognized as double-strand breaks and erroneous recombination. Because they cannot be fully replicated during cell division, they are subject to progressive shortening, which limits the life span of the cell. The telomeres from prostate cancer tissue and high-grade prostatic intraepithelial neoplasia have been found to be significantly shorter than those from normal cells and benign prostatic tissue [30]. The relationship between telomerase length and malignancy is paradoxical and the reason unclear. However, it may prove useful as a prognostic marker because reduced telomere DNA content is associated with survival and disease recurrence [30].

Other Amplified Genes with Clinical Potential

α-Methylacyl–coenzyme A (CoA) racemase (AMACR) is an enzyme involved in the β oxidation of dietary branched-chain fatty acids. It is overexpressed in prostate cancer at both the RNA and protein level [9]. Recent work has identified AMACR as a new diagnostic marker for prostate cancer needle biopsies [9]. It is also an androgen-independent growth modifier and so has the potential to be a complementary target with androgen ablation in prostate cancer treatment [31].

Another gene product that is overexpressed in prostate cancer is fatty acid synthetase (FAS). Inhibitors to FAS are therefore also being investigated as a therapeutic target in the disease [9].

The Androgen Receptor

The action of androgens in prostate cancer, as in the normal prostate, is mediated through the androgen receptor. Androgen deprivation is the accepted treatment for advanced prostate cancer and results in responses in 50% to 80% of patients. Unfortunately, despite initial responses to such treatment, prostate cancer inevitably progresses to an androgen–independent state within 13 months from starting treatment. As a result, much research has focused on androgen signaling in prostate cancers.

The Androgen Receptor and Androgen Synthesis

Testosterone is the main circulating androgen and is primarily produced by the Leydig cells in the testes. Its release is influenced by the pituitary hormones, luteinizing hormone (LH) and follicle-stimulating hormone (FSH) (Fig. 1.2). Once reaching the prostate, 90% of the testosterone is converted intracellularly by the enzyme 5α-reductase to dihydrotestosterone (DHT). Both DHT and testosterone bind to the androgen receptor (AR) and DHT has 100 times more relative androgenicity than testosterone.

The AR is a member of the steroid receptor hormone superfamily, and its gene is located on chromosome Xq11–12 [32]. The entry of ligand into the cell results in receptor binding, causing a conformational change that releases heat shock proteins and allows receptor dimerization. The ARs then bind to specific DNA binding sequences, known as AR response elements, which are located in the promoter regions of target genes. This is the first step in the assembly of a protein complex on the DNA, which under the influence of coactivators initiate RNA polymerase activity and thus transcription. In this way the AR acts as a transcription factor (Fig. 1.2).

There are a number of target genes that are regulated in this way including those encoding prostate-specific antigen (PSA), insulin-like growth factor-1 (IGF-1), vascular endothelial growth factor (VEGF), and keratinocyte growth factor (KGF). These have been found to have an important role in prostate cancer angiogenesis, metastases, and differentiation.

In addition to coactivators and co-repressors, a number of hormones and cytokines have been shown to interact with the AR and influence transcription. These include peptide growth factors such as KGF, IGF-1, and epidermal growth factor (EGF), which may play a part in activating the AR in an androgen-deprived environment [33].

Treatment Resistance

Androgen deprivation using luteinizing hormone–releasing hormone (LHRH) agonists is

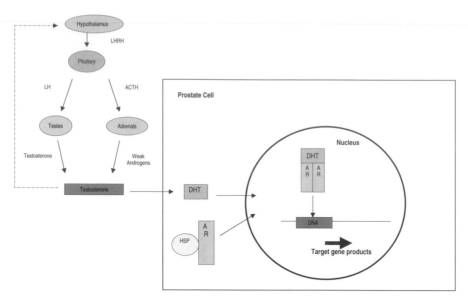

Fig. 1.2. The hypothalamic-pituitary gonadal axis and the intracellular action of the androgen receptor (AR). ACTH, adreno-corticotropic hormone; AR, androgen receptor; DHT, dihydrotestosterone; HSP, heat shock protein; LH, luteinizing hormone; LHRH, luteinizing hormone–releasing hormone.

used now not only in the treatment of metastatic prostate cancer, but also in patients with locally advanced disease as an adjunct to irradiation [34]. Luteinizing hormone-releasing hormone agonists exert their effect by inhibiting LH and FSH secretion from the pituitary, thereby inhibiting testicular androgen production. They may also have a direct local affect in the prostate [35].

Androgen-independent progression of metastatic disease occurs at a median of 13 months from the initiation of treatment. A number of possible mechanisms that lead to hormone independence have been proposed, including clonal selection of preexisting androgen-independent cells, and adaptive processes, particularly changes in the AR itself.

In vitro studies using the AR-positive human prostate cancer cell line LNCaP provided the first evidence of structural alterations of the AR in prostate cancer [36]. This cell line, which was isolated from a lymph node deposit of a hormone-refractory prostate cancer, was found to be growth stimulated by androgens, estrogen, progesterone, and the antiandrogen flutamide, despite expression of AR but not estrogen or progesterone receptors. Sequencing of AR complementary DNA (cDNA) revealed a single point mutation in the ligand-binding domain of the receptor. This mutation has subsequently been found in human cancer specimens [37].

A number of other point mutations have now been elucidated, which have been found to have effects on AR function [32]. For example, a point mutation in codon 730 was found to result in the induction of AR transcriptional activity by the antiandrogen hydroxyflutamide [38], and a point mutation in codon 715 led to AR activation by lower concentrations of adrenal androgens and progesterone compared with the wild-type receptor [38]. These mutations are rare in patients with primary prostate cancer and are found in higher frequency in patients with advanced disease, suggesting that mutations occur before hormonal treatments and play a role in prostate tumor progression [39,40].

Further evidence of abnormal AR function has been provided by reports of clinical improvement of patients with hormone-refractory disease following withdrawal of antiandrogen treatment [41,42]. It has been postulated that this may be due to receptor mutation, leading to activation or stabilization of the receptor by the antiandrogen itself as an adaptation to long-term androgen ablation [43,44].

Amplification of the androgen receptor gene, leading to overexpression of the receptor, is another postulated mechanism for the development of androgen-independent disease, by increasing the sensitivity of prostate cancer cells to low circulating levels of androgen. A number of studies have reported no AR gene amplification in pretreatment tissue specimens from which AR gene amplification developed [45–47]. This suggests that gene amplification may be an adaptive response. This is consistent with the finding that patients with AR amplification at the time of recurrence on hormone ablative treatment have a higher chance of responding to second-line hormonal treatment than those without amplification [48,49]. In addition, these patients with receptor amplification have a better prognosis than those with receptor mutation [49].

Other mechanisms at the molecular level, for the development of androgen insensitivity, include the expression of AR coactivators and co-repressors and activation of ligand-independent androgen receptor signaling pathways such as the overexpression and loss of control of growth factors.

Interleukin-6

Interleukin-6 (IL-6) is a multifunctional cytokine, and there has been much interest in its role in the regulation of growth in a number of malignant tumors. It has also been found to be one of the most important nonsteroidal regulators of AR activity. Serum levels of IL-6 are elevated in patients with hormone-resistant disease [50]. In prostate cancer cells, IL-6 can induce divergent proliferative responses. In DU-145 cells, IL-6 causes ligand-independent and synergistic activation of the AR [50]. In LNCaP cell lines, however, cell growth is initially inhibited IL-6, but long-term treatment renders the cells resistant to such inhibition and confers a growth advantage [50]. This cytokine therefore may have an important role in progression of prostate cancer toward resistance to endocrine treatment.

Trinucleotide Repeats

The first exon of the AR gene contains several regions of repetitive DNA sequences. Of interest is a CAG triplet repeat, the length of which is highly polymorphic, ranging from 14 to 35 repeats, and its length may affect AR activity and prostate cancer risk. The number of X- chromosome–associated CAG and GGC trinucleotide repeats has been shown to correlate with the severity of a number of neuromuscular degenerative disorders, such as Kennedy's disease. Of interest, this condition is also accompanied by androgen insensitivity caused by attenuated activity of the AR [51]. A shorter glutamide repeat coded by the CAG sequence has also been shown to increase AR activity. This has subsequently been found to predict for a higher grade and more advanced disease at diagnosis [52]. Racial differences have also been noted, with a significantly reduced number of CAG repeats in African-American men and elevated number in Asian-American men compared with Caucasian men [53]. This may be associated with the observed frequency of prostate cancer in different population groups.

Erb-B2/HER-2/neu

This oncogene codes for a transmembrane tyrosine kinase growth factor, similar to the EGF receptor. HER-2 is overexpressed in up to 50% of prostate cancers [54] and is more commonly seen in patients treated with androgen-ablation and in androgen-dependent disease [55]. HER-2/neu has been implicated in the activation of the androgen receptor and in inducing hormone-independent cell growth [56].

Androgen Receptor and Prostate Cancer Etiology

The reason for the varying incidence of prostate cancer between racial groups is undoubtedly multifactorial, with the contribution of both genetic and environmental factors. African-American men have the highest risk of prostate cancer and Asian populations have the lowest [38].

5α-Reductase, which converts testosterone into the more active androgen DHT activity, correlates with race, with low levels of activity in Japanese men and higher levels in African Americans and Caucasian [57]. Racial variations have also been found in the gene encoding 3β-hydroxysteroid dehydrogenase 2, which is involved in the breakdown of DHT, suggesting it may play a role in prostate cancer predisposition [58]. There has been much interest in possible racial differences in male testosterone levels; however, studies have shown conflicting results [59,60].

Interestingly, although the incidence of clinical prostate cancer is high in the United States and low in Asian countries, the frequency of subclinical prostate cancer identified at autopsy is similar in the two populations [38]. In one study, AR mutations were found in 22% of Japanese men, with no AR gene mutations in latent or clinical prostate cancers of American men or clinical prostate cancers of Japanese men [61]. A number of mutations were identified, which, based on studies of AR in inherited androgen insensitivity syndromes, would result in reduced receptor activity. Such findings suggest that these inactivating AR gene mutations may prevent malignant progression.

Tumor–Environment Interactions

The prostate gland is composed of epithelial cells, which form two cell layers, and stromal cells. The basal epithelial cells are androgen independent, lack AR, and are thought to be stem cells for secretory epithelial cells. The stroma of the prostate is composed of fibroblasts, smooth muscle cells, lymphocytes, and neuromuscular tissue embedded in an extracellular matrix.

During early prostate cancer development, the AR is initially expressed in mesenchymal tissue [62]. Later it is found in both mesenchymal and epithelial cells. This epithelial–stromal interaction plays an important role in normal prostatic morphogenesis and remains significant in the adult prostate. Growth factors are thought to maintain homeostasis between these cell types in a paracrine fashion. It may be that imbalances of these factors lead to benign prostatic hypertrophy and prostate cancer development, and in androgen-independent prostate tumors replace androgen as the primary-stimulatory growth signal.

The role of growth factors may also explain the pattern of tumor spread, which is unique to prostate cancer. Tumor dissemination to bone causes sclerotic lesions, suggesting that the bone stroma is fertile ground for prostate cancer cell growth, which may be due to a similar pattern of growth factor production as in the prostate itself.

Growth Factors

A number of growth factor families have now been found to be involved in normal and cancerous growth of the prostate and are summarized in Table 1.2.

Epidermal growth factor and transforming growth factor-α (TGF-α) are two related peptide growth factors that signal through the same EGF receptor (EGFR), a transmembrane tyrosine kinase. They are found in normal and cancerous prostate cells. In the nondiseased prostate, EGF appears to be an important regulator of growth [63]. Its expression is regulated by androgen; castrated mice and rats have reduced EGF expression that can be restored by the administration of testosterone [64,65] The EGFR, however, is negatively regulated by androgen [66]. In prostate cancer cell lines, EGFR expression is upregulated with progression; however, results from immunohistochemistry of human tumors have been inconclusive. Upregulation of EGF and TGF-α has been observed in prostate cancer specimens [65], which correlates with tissue testosterone levels, suggesting they may be significant in pathogenesis. Increased EGF expression may also be associated with the invasive ability of prostate cancer cells [67].

The TGFs are a family of peptides that are expressed during prostate development, and in both normal and cancerous prostate cells. The role of TGF-β is complex. In the nondiseased prostate, TGF-β is believed to play a role in regulating growth by counterbalancing the mitogenic effects of other growth factors such as EGF/TGF-α on epithelial cells [68] and basic fibroblast growth factors (bFGFs) on stromal cells [69]. Its expression is negatively regulated by androgens in the prostate [70] and is associated with castration-induced cell apoptosis. Increasing levels of TGF-β appear to be important in prostate cancer expression, but its precise role is yet to be elucidated [33]. Transforming growth factor-β has also been found to modulate extracellular matrix proteins and stimulate cell adhesion to bone matrix proteins, suggesting a role in prostate cancer cell metastasis [71,72].

The fibroblast growth factors (FGP) are another family of structurally related peptides, a number of which have been implicated in prostate cancer. FGF-2 (bFGF) is synthesized by prostatic stromal and epithelial cells [73]. In the normal prostate, only the stromal cells express the bFGF receptor and respond to the growth factor; in cancerous cells the opposite is observed [74]. With cancer progression the production of bFGF becomes independent of androgen [33]. Because its biological functions include a role in angiogenesis and tissue differentiation

Table 1.2. The possible role of growth factors in normal prostate development and in prostate cancer

Growth factor	Activities reported	Expression in normal/ benign tissues	Expression in prostate cancer
EGF	Stimulates replication of epithelial/fibroblast cell lines	Present in prostatic fluid/ epithelial cells	Increased by epithelial cells
		Stimulated by androgens	Increased further in androgen-dependent cell lines
	Stimulates invasion of cells	EGFR on epithelial cells	EGFR expression increased
TGF-α	Binds to EGFR?	Produced usually in stroma	Produced by epithelial cells
	Similar function	Stimulated by androgens	Increased in androgen-independent cell lines
		Receptor, EGFr on epithelial cells	c-*erb*-b2, EGFR expression increased
TGF-β	Inhibits epithelial growth in vitro	Expression by epithelium and stroma	Increased with tumor progression
	Stimulates angiogenesis, stromal growth, cell adhesion	Downregulated by androgens	Change in receptor responsiveness with loss of inhibitory effect
aFGF	Not defined	Produced by stroma in developing rat prostate, not in humans	Produced by rat epithelial tumor cells in aggressive lines
		Receptor present in stroma/ epithelium	
bFGF	Strongly angiogenic	Produced by epithelium/ stroma	Production independent of androgens
	Regulates matrix enzymes	Increased by androgens bFGF receptor only in stroma	Receptor produced by epithelial cells
KGF (FGF-7)	Mitogen for normal and tumor	Produced by stroma, stimulated cells by androgens	Produced by epithelial cells in a androgen-independent tumors
		Receptor, bFGFR2 in epithelial cells	Increased receptor levels, lost in androgen-independent
IGF-1/2	Mitogenic for epithelial cells	Produced by stroma IGFRs and IGFBP present in epithelial cells	IGFBP expression altered in cell lines
			May affect release of stored IGF from epithelial cells

aFGF, fibroblast growth factor; IGFBP, insulin-like growth factor binding protein; for explanation of abbreviations, see text.

[33], there is much interest in further investigations into the role of the bFGF pathway in prostate cancer.

Keratinocyte growth factor is another member of the FGF family. It is thought to act as a paracrine mediator of androgen action [75,76]; KGF and its receptor BEK/FGFR-2 are expressed in the stromal and epithelial cells of the prostate. In vitro it acts as a potent mitogen for nondiseased human prostatic epithelial cells [77]. In situ hybridization studies have shown increased expression of the KGF gene and receptor in epithelial cells of high-grade carcinomas but not in benign prostatic hyperplasia. This implies a change from paracrine to autocrine activity [78].

Fibroblast growth factor-7 is synthesized by fibroblasts in normal prostate tissue, and acts as a mitogen for epithelial cells via its receptor FGFR2/IIIb. This suggests FGF-7 has a paracrine role in normal prostate tissue [79]. It is thought to be a mediator of androgen function, inducing growth and differentiation. In advanced prostate cancers, there is a loss of FGRF2/IIIb expression [74]. This suggests that the loss of this pathway may contribute to the development of hormone-resistance.

Fibroblast growth factor-8 acts as a potent mitogenic and transforming protein in prostate cancer cells. Interestingly its expression appears to be induced by androgen. A negative correlation between tumor grade and FGF-8 expression has been found in human prostate specimens, indicating that a loss of FGF-8 may be a factor involved in the development of prostate cancer [80].

The role of the IGF-1 and IGF-2 in prostate cancer development and progression has also been investigated. In the normal prostate IGFs are produced by stromal cells, with epithelial cells expressing IGF-1 receptors and also IGF-binding proteins [81]. These binding proteins are important because they are in part regulated by androgen, and differing concentrations have been note in normal versus cancerous cells [33]. Insulin-like growth factors are mitogenic for prostate epithelial cells [82]. In some prostate cancer cell lines an autocrine production of IGF-1 has been observed [83].

Figure 1.3 summarizes the interaction among various growth factors, prostate cancer cells, and their surrounding stroma.

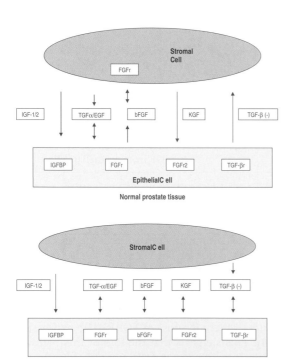

Fig. 1.3. Possible epithelial–stromal interactions in the normal prostate gland and in prostate cancer. For explanation of abbreviations, see text.

Nuclear Factor κB

Nuclear factor κB (NF-κB) is a proinflammatory transcription factor and is an important survival factor in many cancer cell types [9]. Hormone-resistant prostate cancer cell lines produce multiple cytokines including IL-6, IL-1α, and granulocyte colony-stimulating factor, which are thought to be critical in tumor growth and progression [84]. These cytokines are also thought to enhance the malignant potential of hormone-refractory tumors. Nuclear factor κB is one of the most critical regulators of cytokine-inducible gene expression [84]. Constitutive activation of NF-κB is seen in androgen-insensitive prostate cancer cell lines PC-3 and DU145 but not in the androgen-sensitive LNCaP cell line [84]. This constitutive activation may increase the expression of antiapoptosis proteins, thus reducing the effectiveness of anti-cancer treatment and promoting the development of chemotherapy resistance [84]. There is also evidence suggesting that NF-κB itself has a central role in prostate cancer metastasis to bone [85].

A number of strategies are being developed to inhibit NF-κB, which may have therapeutic potential. A novel inhibitor, dehydroxymethyle-poxyquinomicin (DHMEQ) has been found to inhibit growth and induce apoptosis in three hormone refractory cell lines. Furthermore, administration of DHMEQ inhibited pre-established JCA-1 tumor growth in nude mice [85]. Pharmacological inhibition of NF-κB can also be achieved by overexpression of IκBα. Glucocorticoids and the proteasome inhibitor PS341 have been found to increase the concentration of IκB and tumor necrosis factor-α (TNF-α) in cellular models [9]. Glucocorticoids have been found to show palliative benefit in patients with advanced prostate cancer.

Other Cellular–Matrix Interactions

The cadherins are a class of cell-adhesion molecules that are involved with cell-to-cell recognition, and thus help maintain epithelial tissue differentiation and structural integrity. Reduced expression of E-cadherin is associated with advanced stage and grade [54] of prostate cancers and also poor clinical outcome [9]. In a cellular model, inhibition of E-cadherin leads to disruption of normal contact inhibition of growth and an invasive phenotype [86]. α-Catenin associates with E-cadherin and can also be altered in prostate cancer [9].

CD44 is part of the CD family of transmembrane glycoproteins principally involved in cell–extracellular matrix interactions and is encoded on chromosome 11. In a rat model of prostate cancer CD44 behaves as a metastases suppressor gene [87]. Downregulation of CD44 expression also occurs in high-grade prostate cancer [9]. A proposed mechanism for CD44 downregulation is hypermethylation of the CpG island promoter [88]. Another gene located on chromosome 11, which is thought to affect cell-matrix interactions is *KA11*. It is thought to code for a transmembrane protein of uncertain function. Transfection of the *KA11* gene in a prostate cancer rat model inhibits metastases, and its underexpression has been noted in a significant proportion of primary and metastatic cancer specimens [89].

The matrix metalloproteinases (MMPs) are a group of enzymes that are also thought to be involved in tumor invasion and metastasis. As prostate tumor cells grow and divide they secrete MMPs, which break down the basement membrane and stroma. Concurrently, tissue inhibitors of MMPs are downregulated, which amplify the process [90]. Serum levels of both metalloproteinases and tissue inhibitors of metalloproteinases distinguish those patients who have metastases from those who do not and are predictive of relapse.

A number of other peptide growth and survival factors have been identified that may promote survival of prostate epithelial cells in bone. These include osteocalcin, osteopontin and endothelin-1 (ET-1) [9]. Clinical trials are currently underway to evaluate a selective ET-1 inhibitor in patients with advanced prostate cancer. The initial results suggest that the drug may palliate pain and delay progression of disease [91].

Conclusion

Over the last two decades, research into prostate cancer has accelerated at a great pace. Prostate cancer development and progression is an evolving process, involving complex interactions among cancer cells, their microenvironment, and genes affecting growth and metastasis.

Much research has been based on the androgen receptor and cell survival pathways associated with hormone resistance. Several molecular abnormalities have been identified, leading the way for the development of new combination targeted treatments. The development of microarray expression analysis should hasten the identification of further diagnostic and prognostic markers and therapeutic targets. A better understanding of the biology of prostate cancer will also enable us to improve hormonal and chemotherapy options.

References

1. Hsing AW, Tsao L, Devesa SS. International trends and patterns of prostate cancer incidence and mortality. Int J Cancer 2000;85(1):60–67.
2. Landis SH, et al. Cancer statistics 1999. CA Cancer J Clin 1999;49(1):8–31.
3. Chamberlain J, et al. The diagnosis, management, treatment and costs of prostate cancer in England and Wales. Health Technol Assess 1997;1(3):i–vi, 1–53.
4. Holund B. Latent prostatic cancer in a consecutive autopsy series. Scand J Urol Nephrol 1980; 14(1):29–35.
5. Simard J, et al. Perspective: prostate cancer susceptibility genes. Endocrinology 2002;143(6): 2029–2040.
6. Haenszel W, Kurihara M. Studies of Japanese migrants. I. Mortality from cancer and other diseases among Japanese in the United States. J Natl Cancer Inst 1968;40(1):43–68.
7. Morton RA Jr. Racial differences in adenocarcinoma of the prostate in North American men. Urology 1994;44(5):637–645.
8. Carter BS, et al. Mendelian inheritance of familial prostate cancer. Proc Natl Acad Sci USA 1992; 89(8):3367–3371.
9. DeMarzo AM, et al. Pathological and molecular aspects of prostate cancer. Lancet 2003;361(9361): 955–964.
10. Visakorpi T. The molecular genetics of prostate cancer. Urology 2003;62(5 suppl 1):3–10.
11. Cunningham JM, et al. Genome linkage screen for prostate cancer susceptibility loci: results from the Mayo Clinic Familial Prostate Cancer Study. Prostate 2003;57(4):335–346.
12. Ford D, et al. Risks of cancer in BRCA1–mutation carriers. Breast Cancer Linkage Consortium. Lancet 1994;343(8899):692–695.

13. Cancer risks in BRCA2 mutation carriers. The Breast Cancer Linkage Consortium. J Natl Cancer Inst 1999;91(15):1310–1316.

14. Gayther SA, et al. The frequency of germ-line mutations in the breast cancer predisposition genes BRCA1 and BRCA2 in familial prostate cancer. The Cancer Research Campaign/British Prostate Group United Kingdom Familial Prostate Cancer Study Collaborators. Cancer Res 2000;60(16):4513–4518.

15. Bova GS, Isaacs WB. Review of allelic loss and gain in prostate cancer. World J Urol 1996;14(5):338–346.

16. Mellon K, et al. p53, c-erbB-2 and the epidermal growth factor receptor in the benign and malignant prostate. J Urol 1992;147(2):496–499.

17. Heidenberg HB, et al. Alteration of the tumor suppressor gene p53 in a high fraction of hormone refractory prostate cancer. J Urol 1995;154(2 pt 1):414–421.

18. Wang SI, Parsons R, Ittmann M. Homozygous deletion of the PTEN tumor suppressor gene in a subset of prostate adenocarcinomas. Clin Cancer Res 1998;4(3):811–815.

19. McMenamin ME, et al. Loss of PTEN expression in paraffin-embedded primary prostate cancer correlates with high Gleason score and advanced stage. Cancer Res 1999;59(17):4291–4296.

20. Narla G, et al. KLF6, a candidate tumor suppressor gene mutated in prostate cancer. Science 2001;294(5551):2563–2566.

21. Bhatia-Gaur R, et al. Roles for Nkx3.1 in prostate development and cancer. Genes Dev 1999;13(8):966–977.

22. Carter BS, Epstein JI, Isaacs WB. Ras gene mutations in human prostate cancer. Cancer Res 1990;50(21):6830–6832.

23. Viola MV, et al. Expression of ras oncogene p21 in prostate cancer. N Engl J Med 1986;314(3):133–137.

24. Wolf DA, et al. Transcriptional down-regulation of c-myc in human prostate carcinoma cells by the synthetic androgen mibolerone. Br J Cancer 1992;65(3):376–382.

25. Fleming WH, et al. Expression of the c-myc protooncogene in human prostatic carcinoma and benign prostatic hyperplasia. Cancer Res 1986;46(3):1535–1538.

26. Funa K, Nordgren H, Nilsson S. In situ expression of mRNA for proto-oncogenes in benign prostatic hyperplasia and in prostatic carcinoma. Scand J Urol Nephrol 1991;25(2):95–100.

27. Furuya Y, et al. Expression of bcl-2 and the progression of human and rodent prostatic cancers. Clin Cancer Res 1996;2(2):389–398.

28. Shaffer DR, Scher HI. Prostate cancer: a dynamic illness with shifting targets. Lancet Oncol 2003;4(7):407–414.

29. Xing N, et al. Neuroendocrine cells in human prostate over-express the anti-apoptosis protein survivin. Prostate 2001;48(1):7–15.

30. De Marzo AM, et al. Human prostate cancer precursors and pathobiology. Urology 2003;62(5 suppl 1):55–62.

31. Zha S, et al. Alpha-methylacyl-CoA racemase as an androgen-independent growth modifier in prostate cancer. Cancer Res 2003;63(21):7365–7376.

32. Gelmann EP. Molecular biology of the androgen receptor. J Clin Oncol 2002;20(13):3001–3015.

33. Russell PJ, Bennett S, Stricker P. Growth factor involvement in progression of prostate cancer. Clin Chem 1998;44(4):705–723.

34. Bolla M, et al. Improved survival in patients with locally advanced prostate cancer treated with radiotherapy and goserelin. N Engl J Med 1997;337(5):295–300.

35. Culig Z, et al. Synergistic activation of androgen receptor by androgen and luteinizing hormone-releasing hormone in prostatic carcinoma cells. Prostate 1997;32(2):106–114.

36. Veldscholte J, et al. A mutation in the ligand binding domain of the androgen receptor of human LNCaP cells affects steroid binding characteristics and response to anti-androgens. Biochem Biophys Res Commun 1990;173(2):534–540.

37. Gaddipati JP, et al. Frequent detection of codon 877 mutation in the androgen receptor gene in advanced prostate cancers. Cancer Res 1994;54(11):2861–2864.

38. Bentel JM, Tilley WD. Androgen receptors in prostate cancer. J Endocrinol 1996;151(1):1–11.

39. Marcelli M, et al. Androgen receptor mutations in prostate cancer. Cancer Res 2000;60(4):944–949.

40. Tilley WD, et al. Mutations in the androgen receptor gene are associated with progression of human prostate cancer to androgen independence. Clin Cancer Res 1996;2(2):277–285.

41. Scher HI, Kelly WK. Flutamide withdrawal syndrome: its impact on clinical trials in hormone-refractory prostate cancer. J Clin Oncol 1993;11(8):1566–1572.

42. Kelly WK, Scher HI. Prostate specific antigen decline after antiandrogen withdrawal: the flutamide withdrawal syndrome. J Urol 1993;149(3):607–609.

43. Kemppainen JA, Wilson EM. Agonist and antagonist activities of hydroxyflutamide and Casodex relate to androgen receptor stabilization. Urology 1996;48(1):157–163.

44. Culig Z, et al. Switch from antagonist to agonist of the androgen receptor bicalutamide is associated with prostate tumour progression in a new model system. Br J Cancer 1999;81(2):242–251.

45. Visakorpi T, et al. In vivo amplification of the androgen receptor gene and progression of human prostate cancer. Nat Genet 1995;9(4): 401–406.

46. Koivisto P, Visakorpi T, Kallioniemi OP. Androgen receptor gene amplification: a novel molecular mechanism for endocrine therapy resistance in human prostate cancer. Scand J Clin Lab Invest Suppl 1996;226:57–63.

47. Miyoshi Y, et al. Fluorescence in situ hybridization evaluation of c-myc and androgen receptor gene amplification and chromosomal anomalies in prostate cancer in Japanese patients. Prostate 2000;43(3):225–232.

48. Palmberg C, et al. Androgen receptor gene amplification at primary progression predicts response to combined androgen blockade as second line therapy for advanced prostate cancer. J Urol 2000;164(6):1992–1995.

49. Koivisto P, et al. Androgen receptor gene amplification: a possible molecular mechanism for androgen deprivation therapy failure in prostate cancer. Cancer Res 1997;57(2):314–319.

50. Culig Z, Bartsch G, Hobisch A. Interleukin-6 regulates androgen receptor activity and prostate cancer cell growth. Mol Cell Endocrinol 2002; 197(1–2):231–238.

51. La Spada AR, et al. Androgen receptor gene mutations in X-linked spinal and bulbar muscular atrophy. Nature 1991;352(6330):77–79.

52. Kantoff P, Giovannucci E, Brown M. The androgen receptor CAG repeat polymorphism and its relationship to prostate cancer. Biochim Biophys Acta 1998;1378(3):C1–5.

53. Irvine RA, et al. The CAG and GGC microsatellites of the androgen receptor gene are in linkage disequilibrium in men with prostate cancer. Cancer Res 1995;55(9):1937–1940.

54. Solit DB, Scher HI, Rosen N. Hsp90 as a therapeutic target in prostate cancer. Semin Oncol 2003;30(5):709–716.

55. Signoretti S, et al. Her-2–neu expression and progression toward androgen independence in human prostate cancer. J Natl Cancer Inst 2000; 92(23):1918–1925.

56. Craft N, et al. A mechanism for hormone-independent prostate cancer through modulation of androgen receptor signaling by the HER-2/neu tyrosine kinase. Nat Med 1999;5(3): 280–285.

57. Ross RK, et al. 5–alpha-reductase activity and risk of prostate cancer among Japanese and US white and black males. Lancet 1992;339(8798):887–889.

58. Devgan SA, et al. Genetic variation of 3 beta-hydroxysteroid dehydrogenase type II in three racial/ethnic groups: implications for prostate cancer risk. Prostate 1997;33(1):9–12.

59. Ellis L, Nyborg H. Racial/ethnic variations in male testosterone levels: a probable contributor to group differences in health. Steroids 1992;57(2): 72–75.

60. Ross R, et al. Serum testosterone levels in healthy young black and white men. J Natl Cancer Inst 1986;76(1):45–48.

61. Takahashi H, et al. Prevalence of androgen receptor gene mutations in latent prostatic carcinomas from Japanese men. Cancer Res 1995;55(8): 1621–1624.

62. Cooke PS, Young P, Cunha GR. Androgen receptor expression in developing male reproductive organs. Endocrinology 1991;128(6):2867–2873.

63. Culig Z, et al. Regulation of prostatic growth and function by peptide growth factors. Prostate 1996;28(6):392–405.

64. Fowler JE Jr, et al. Epidermal growth factor and prostatic carcinoma: an immunohistochemical study. J Urol 1988;139(4):857–861.

65. Yang Y, Chisholm GD, Habib FK. Epidermal growth factor and transforming growth factor alpha concentrations in BPH and cancer of the prostate: their relationships with tissue androgen levels. Br J Cancer 1993;67(1):152–155.

66. Fiorelli G, et al. Growth factors in the human prostate. J Steroid Biochem Mol Biol 1991; 40(1–3):199–205.

67. Jarrard DF, et al. Effect of epidermal growth factor on prostate cancer cell line PC3 growth and invasion. Prostate 1994;24(1):46–53.

68. Schuurmans AL, Bolt J, Mulder E. Androgens and transforming growth factor beta modulate the growth response to epidermal growth factor in human prostatic tumor cells (LNCaP). Mol Cell Endocrinol 1988;60(1):101–104.

69. Story MT, Hopp KA, Meier DA. Regulation of basic fibroblast growth factor expression by transforming growth factor beta in cultured human prostate stromal cells. Prostate 1996;28(4):219–226.

70. Landstrom M, et al. Estrogen induces apoptosis in a rat prostatic adenocarcinoma: association with an increased expression of TGF-beta 1 and its type-I and type-II receptors. Int J Cancer 1996;67(4):573–579.

71. Sehgal I, Baley PA, Thompson TC. Transforming growth factor beta1 stimulates contrasting responses in metastatic versus primary mouse prostate cancer-derived cell lines in vitro. Cancer Res 1996;56(14):3359–3365.

72. Kostenuik PJ, Singh G, Orr FW. Transforming growth factor beta upregulates the integrin-mediated adhesion of human prostatic carcinoma cells to type I collagen. Clin Exp Metastasis 1997; 15(1):41–52.

73. Sherwood ER, et al. Basic fibroblast growth factor: a potential mediator of stromal growth in the

human prostate. Endocrinology 1992;130(5): 2955–2963.

74. Matsubara A, et al. Inhibition of growth of malignant rat prostate tumor cells by restoration of fibroblast growth factor receptor 2. Cancer Res 1998;58(7):1509–1514.

75. Sugimura Y, et al. Keratinocyte growth factor (KGF) can replace testosterone in the ductal branching morphogenesis of the rat ventral prostate. Int J Dev Biol 1996;40(5):941–951.

76. Yan G, et al. Heparin-binding keratinocyte growth factor is a candidate stromal-to-epithelial-cell andromedin. Mol Endocrinol 1992;6(12):2123–2128.

77. Finch PW, et al. Human KGF is FGF-related with properties of a paracrine effector of epithelial cell growth. Science 1989;245(4919):752–755.

78. McGarvey TW, Stearns ME. Keratinocyte growth factor and receptor mRNA expression in benign and malignant human prostate. Exp Mol Pathol 1995;63(1):52–62.

79. Story MT. Regulation of prostate growth by fibroblast growth factors. World J Urol 1995; 13(5):297–305.

80. Wang Q, et al. Correlation between androgen receptor expression and FGF8 mRNA levels in patients with prostate cancer and benign prostatic hypertrophy. J Clin Pathol 1999;52(1): 29–34.

81. Cohen P, et al. Insulin-like growth factors (IGFs), IGF receptors, and IGF-binding proteins in primary cultures of prostate epithelial cells. J Clin Endocrinol Metab 1991;73(2):401–407.

82. Iwamura M, et al. Insulin-like growth factor I: action and receptor characterization in human prostate cancer cell lines. Prostate 1993;22(3): 243–252.

83. Pietrzkowski Z, et al. Inhibition of growth of prostatic cancer cell lines by peptide analogues of insulin-like growth factor 1. Cancer Res 1993; 53(5):1102–1106.

84. Kikuchi E, et al. Suppression of hormone-refractory prostate cancer by a novel nuclear factor kappaB inhibitor in nude mice. Cancer Res 2003;63(1):107–110.

85. Andela VB, et al. NFkappaB: a pivotal transcription factor in prostate cancer metastasis to bone. Clin Orthop 2003(415 suppl):S75–85.

86. Behrens J, et al. Dissecting tumor cell invasion: epithelial cells acquire invasive properties after the loss of uvomorulin-mediated cell-cell adhesion. J Cell Biol 1989;108(6):2435–2447.

87. Gunthert U, et al. A new variant of glycoprotein CD44 confers metastatic potential to rat carcinoma cells. Cell 1991;65(1):13–24.

88. Kito H, et al. Hypermethylation of the CD44 gene is associated with progression and metastasis of human prostate cancer. Prostate 2001;49(2):110–115.

89. Dong JT, et al. Down-regulation of the KAI1 metastasis suppressor gene during the progression of human prostatic cancer infrequently involves gene mutation or allelic loss. Cancer Res 1996;56(19):4387–4390.

90. Cooper CR, et al. Stromal factors involved in prostate carcinoma metastasis to bone. Cancer 2003;97(3 suppl):739–747.

91. Lassiter LK, Carducci MA. Endothelin receptor antagonists in the treatment of prostate cancer. Semin Oncol 2003;30(5):678–688.

2

Familial Prostate Cancer

Sashi S. Kommu and Rosalind A. Eeles

Prostate cancer (PCa) is the most common cancer diagnosed in North American men, excluding skin cancers. It is estimated that, in 2004, approximately 230,110 new cases and 29,900 prostate cancer-related deaths will occur in the United States [1]. In Australia, one in 11 men will develop the disease during their lifetime [2]. The annual number of new cases registered in England and Wales increased by over threefold between 1971 and 2004, from 6174 to over 21,000 [3] (www.icr.ac.uk/Everyman). Prostate cancer remains a major public health problem.

Several risk factors for the disease have been suggested, including diet, sexually transmitted agents, and endocrine factors [4]. However, none of these environmental factors has been confirmed to have a significant causative effect on PCa. Current known risk factors include race [5,6] and a positive family history of the disease. The degree to which the differences in these cohorts can be attributable to environmental factors is unclear.

Over the last 45 years, prostate cancer has been observed to run in families. Familial aggregation (at least two cases in the family) has been observed in around 20% of cases and a hereditary form of PCa in approximately 5% [7]. Epidemiological evidence shows familial clustering of PCa, and it is currently established that a positive family history is a strong risk factor.

One of the major issues surrounding familial prostate cancer (FPC) includes identifying gene(s) predisposing to PCa in families at high risk. If a predisposition gene(s) could be characterized, then those at increased risk of PCa can be potentially identified and offered modes of prevention and targeted screening. The other major issue is the clinical management of patients who are known to have a family history of prostate cancer.

Evidence for the Genetic Etiology of Prostate Cancer

Evidence for familial aggregation of prostate cancer dates as far back as 1956 [8]. Significant linkage in familial prostate cancer was first published in 1996 by a group from Johns Hopkins University, Baltimore, Maryland [9]. This group reported linkage at a locus on chromosome 1q24-25, which was named hereditary prostate cancer 1 (*HPC1*). Several large linkage studies have since been conducted, and the results revealed new loci and challenged others [summarized in refs. 10–13].

So far, genotyping data have been reported in over 1600 families. There are numerous conflicting reports supporting or refuting linkage within many areas in the genome. This challenges our understanding of the genetic basis of this disease. This search is distinct from the search for a familial breast cancer predisposition gene, in which analysis of linkage in select regions revealed a site where the *BRCA1* gene was situated [14]. This work shows that the genetic predisposition to PCa is highly complex, probably involving numerous predisposition genes, and that a high proportion of high-risk families may not be due to a single high-risk gene.

Epidemiological Evidence

It was observed in the 1950s and 1960s that the risk of PCa in relatives of sufferers was higher [15,16]. Early observations were made in large families in Utah [17,18] in which PCa seemed to cluster. To appreciate the evidence of a familial component, case control, cohort and twin studies, must be explored.

Case-Control Studies

Case-control studies can be grouped into two main types. The first type compares PCa incidence in first-degree relatives of affected patients (cases) with the incidence in the relatives of cancer free men (controls). The second type compares the fraction of PCa cases vs. controls with a positive family history of the disease [15–17,19–34]. These studies are summarized in Table 2.1.

These studies indicate that the relative risks (RR) in first-degree relatives of PCa patients range from 0.64 to 11.00-fold [summarized in refs. 35–37]. With the single exception of the RR of 0.64 [19], in a study that was done on a small sample set of 39 families, 15 of these 16 studies reported an RR of 1.76 or higher. Furthermore, the RR has been observed to increase when more than one relative is affected. Steinberg et al. [23] in 1990 showed that the RR with an affected first-degree relative was 2.0 and with a second-degree relative was 1.7, but with both first- and second-degree relatives combined the RR rose considerably, to 8.8. It was also observed that the RR increased as the number of family members increased, with RRs of 2.2, 4.9, and 10.9 for one,

Table 2.1. A comparison of case-control studies

| Reference | No. of cases | No. of cases in first-degree relatives of: | | Relative risk |
		Cases	Controls	
Morganti et al., 1959* [8]	183	11	1	11.0
Woolf, 1960† [16]	228	15	5	3.0
Krain, 1974* [20]	221	12	2	6.0
Fincham et al., 1990* [24]	382	58	31	3.2
Cannon et al., 1982† [17]	2824	‡	‡	2.4
Meikle et al., 1985† [22]	150	11	1	4.0
				(at age 80)
		Brothers only		16.6
				(at age <49)
Isaacs et al., 1995* [29]	690	119	55	1.76
Keetch et al., 1995† [30]	1084	273§	85	3.40
% with positive family history		%	%	
Steele et al., 1971* [19]	39	12.8	20.0	0.64
Schuman et al., 1977* [21]	40	16.7	7.3	2.30
Steinberg et al., 1990* [23]	691	15.0	8.0	1.90
Spitz et al., 1991* [25]	378	13.0	5.7	2.30
Ghadirian et al., 1991* [26]	140	15.0	2.0	7.50
Ghadirian et al., 1997† [32]	640	15.0	5.0	3.32

* Information from patient/control questionnaire only.
† Diagnosis verified by hospital records, cancer registration or death certificate.
‡ Measured genealogical index; see Neuhausen, et al. (Br J Urol 1997;79).
§ First- and second-degree relatives.

Table 2.2. Relative odds for prostate cancer in brothers of prostate cancer cases by age

Age of affected case	Age of brother (years)		80+
	<65	65–79	
<65	5.97**	2.77*	2.29
65–79	2.77*	2.04**	2.52*
80+	2.29	2.52*	1.14

* $p < .01$; ** $p < .001$.
Reprinted from Cannon L, Bishop DT, Skolnick M, Hunt S, Lyon JL, Smart CR. Genetic epidemiology of prostate cancer in the Utah Mormon Geneology. Cancer Survey. 1982;1:47–69.

two, and three additional affected relatives besides the proband, respectively. This is strong evidence for at least a genetic *component* in predisposition to familial disease. The observed increases in RR are too large to be explained by an environmental effect alone.

Another interesting observation is that the RR to family members increases as the age of the proband decreases [17,38], rendering further support to a genetic role. This pattern, in which the relative risk markedly increases as the age of the proband decreases, offers some of the best evidence that there is a genetic role (Table 2.2). This table is helpful in risk assessment for genetic counseling. A brother of a proband with prostate cancer at age 50 has a 1.9-fold higher risk of developing prostate cancer compared with a brother of a man diagnosed with the disease at age 70 [38]. As the closeness and number of affected members in the family increases (Tables 2.3 and 2.4), and when both factors are taken together, there is a marked increase in the level of RR (Table 2.5).

Table 2.3. Relative risks for prostate cancer in relatives of prostate cancer cases by degree of relationship

Affected relatives	Relative risk (95% confidence interval [CI])
First-degree	2.0 (1.2–3.3)
Second-degree	1.7 (1.0–2.9)
Both first- and second-degree	8.8 (2.8–28.1)

Steinberg GD, Carter BS, Beaty TH, et al. Family history and the risk of prostate cancer. Prostate 1990;17(4):337–3347. Copyright © 1990 John Wiley & Sons, Inc. Reprinted with permission of Wiley-Liss, Inc., a subsidiary of John Wiley & Sons, Inc.

Table 2.4. Age-adjusted relative risk estimates for prostate cancer by number of additional affected family members

Affected relatives (besides proband)	Odds ratio (95% CI)
1	2.2 (1.4–3.5)
2	4.9 (2.0–12.3)
3	10.9 (2.7–43.1)

Steinberg GD, Carter BS, Beaty TH, et al. Family history and the risk of prostate cancer. Prostate 1990;17(4):337–47. Copyright © 1990 John Wiley & Sons, Inc. Reprinted with permission of Wiley-Liss, Inc., a subsidiary of John Wiley & Sons, Inc.

Cohort Studies

One of the potential pitfalls in the studies conducted is the potential bias introduced by focusing on an unselected population. Cohort studies attempt to avoid this bias. Goldgar et al. [39] showed a familial PCa RR of 2.21 in first-degree relatives of 6350 probands from an unselected PCa population from the Utah Population Database. In another study involving 5496 sons of Swedish men from Cancer Registry data, Gronberg et al. [40] found a RR of 1.70.

Twin Studies

Several twin studies show an increased RR in mono- compared with dizygotic twins of just over three- to sixfold [41]. In a study by Page et al. [42] on 15,924 male twin pairs, they found that pair-wise concordance (twins where both men had PCa) rates among monozygotic twins was 15.7%, while that of dizygotic twins was 3.7% ($p = < .001$). Proband-wise concordance (number of concordant affected twins divided by total number of affected twins) was 27.1%

Table 2.5. Estimated risk ratios for prostate cancer in first-degree relatives of probands, by age at onset in proband and additional family members

Age at onset of proband	No. of additional relatives affected	One or more additional first-degree relatives affected
50	1.9 (1.2–2.8)	7.1 (3.7–13.6)
60	1.4 (1.1–1.7)	5.2 (3.1–8.7)
70	1.0*	3.8 (2.4–6.0)

* Reference group.
Carter BS, Beaty TH, Steinberg GD, Childs B, Walsh PC. Mendelian inheritance of familial prostate cancer. Proc Natl Acad Sci USA. 1992 Apr 15;89(8):3367–3371.

for monozygotic twins and 7.1% for dizygotic twins, which gives a risk ratio of 3.8. These results were supported by another study in Finland [43]. Lichtenstein et al. [44] showed in another study that up to 42% of PCa risk could be attributable to heritable factors. The absolute risk of PCa for twins diagnosed up to age 75 was sixfold higher for mono- versus dizygotic twins (18% vs. 3%). The time interval between age at diagnosis for monozygotic twins compared with that for dizygotic twins (5.7 years vs. 8.8 years; p = 0.04) was shorter, and this was statistically significant. These data all support a genetic component for PCa, possibly from multiple interacting genes.

Segregation Analyses

Despite the fact that the case-control studies described support the significance of genetic factors in the development of PCa, the genetic mode of transmission is still debated. Segregation analyses study the structure of familial clusters and describe the mode of inheritance, age-specific cumulative risk (penetrance), and allele frequency of genetic predisposition to a disease. Carter et al. [38], using such analyses, observed that PCa diagnosed at < 55 years might be caused by a rare autosomal-dominant, highly penetrant allele, which could account for up to 43% of disease in this age group and up to 9% of PCa in men aged up to 85 years. Alleles were predicted to exist at a frequency of 0.003 and to cause a cumulative risk of PCa of 88% by age 85 years versus 5% for noncarriers. Similar conclusions have been reached by other reports, but with a higher allele frequency and lower penetrance of about 67% (Gronberg et al. [40], allele frequency 0.0167; Schaid et al. [45], allele frequency 0.006). Some studies noted higher risks to brothers of prostate cancer cases compared with fathers [46,47], suggesting a recessive or X-linked model. Ewis et al. [48] reported an odds ratio of 2.04 (p = .02) for allele C of dYs19 in Japanese PCa patients, whereas other alleles of this region were protective [allele D, odds ratio (OR) 0.26, p = .002]. Thus the Y chromosome (father to son transmission) also seems to be implicated. It is possible that several models coexist, giving rise to the observed age-linked risks [49]. Dominantly inherited risk allele(s) could partially explain early-onset PCa, and a recessive or X-linked model could account for its later onset [50].

Molecular Analysis Evidence: Linkage Studies

In contrast to other common cancers such as breast and colon cancer, in which a small number of high-risk genes account for a percentage of the high-risk multiple case families, familial PCa is likely to be caused by numerous different genes. Linkage analysis is performed by using a gene-hunting technique that identifies co-segregation of the disease in large, high-risk families, with disease-causing genetic mutations. Linkage analysis has been used to map many familial cancer loci, for example, colorectal cancer, breast/ovarian cancer, and melanoma [reviewed in ref. 51]. By analyzing co-inheritance of polymorphic stretches of DNA, linkage analysis focuses on the region within which a disease-causing locus may lie. Having identified a region of linkage, candidate gene mutation analysis within the region is undertaken to identify the disease-causing mutation.

Candidate Gene Analysis Evidence: *BRCA2*, *NBS*, and *CHEK2* Genes

The candidate gene approach is used to search for genetic markers of disease susceptibility, where a gene is targeted based on the characteristics of its protein product. PCa cases were noted, in the early 1990s, to be clustered within breast cancer families [52,53]. The RR of PCa in male carriers of mutations in the breast cancer predisposition genes *BRCA1* and *BRCA2* is increased. The RR with respect to *BRCA1* was found to be 3.33 [54] and 1.82 in a further study by the Breast Cancer Linkage Consortium (BCLC) [55].

For *BRCA2*, the RR was found to be 4.65 in the BCLC series. The RR is higher in men with PCa diagnosed before 65 years (RR 7.33), with an estimated cumulative incidence by age 70 of 7.5% to 33.0%.

A founder mutation in *BRCA2* mutation is reported to confer a cumulative PCa risk to carriers of 7.6% by age 70 [56]; 67% of men who had the mutation developed advanced PCa with a high mortality [57]. This raised the possibility that *BRCA2* predisposes to more aggressive disease. A report in a Swedish family carrying a deleterious *BRCA2* mutation [58] supports the evidence that such mutations could be pathogenic. Gayther et al. [59], in a set of 38 United Kingdom families, conducted a mutation screen of *BRCA1* and *BRCA2* genes. Two germline deleterious *BRCA2* mutations were observed. A further study was conducted by Edwards et al. [60] on 263 men aged ≤55 at diagnosis, and they found six pathogenic mutations. Interestingly, these were downstream of the ovarian cancer cluster region, which is central in the gene, implying a genotype/phenotype correlation. The mutations accounted for 2% of PCa diagnosed at this young age. This equated to a RR of 23-fold by 60 years of age and an absolute risk of PCa of 1.3% by age 55 and 10% by age 65. This seems to support claims that *BRCA2* is a high-risk PCa gene. More recently, studies reported an increased risk of PCa in conjunction with the Ashkenazi founder mutations in the *BRCA1* and *BRCA2* genes [61,62].

Following these initial observations, germline mutations have been found in the *NBS* gene at a higher frequency in PCa cases than controls [63], albeit only in a founder Slavic population to date, and in the *CHEK2* gene [64]. This raises the possibility that PCa predisposition in a proportion of cases might be caused by mutations in the DNA repair pathway genes. It is thought that these gene mutations in the homozygous form may give rise to a severe phenotype (in the case of *NBS* this would be the Nijmegen breakage syndrome and in the case of *BRCA2* this would be Fanconi anemia D2). However, in the heterozygous form, there would be a risk of getting PCa.

Genome Searches in Prostate Cancer

A genome-wide search (GWS) involves the process of running a large (typically in the region of 400) number of microsatellite markers throughout the genome to locate disease-predisposing genes by looking for co-segregation of markers with the disease in families. The attempt to identify prostate cancer susceptibility loci has been undertaken across the genome by numerous groups. The Anglo-Canadian-Texan-Australian-Norwegian–European Union Biomed (ACTANE) group has defined age at onset and number of cases and focused on the collection of clinically significant PCa, because the disease manifests 10 years later on average than prostate-specific antigen (PSA)-detected disease, and hence men with clinically detected early-onset PCa could have had a raised PSA level at an earlier age [36].

Thus far, several GWSs have been reported for prostate cancer [9,11,13,65–80]. The significant results are summarized as follows:

1q23-24: *HPC1* and the *RNASEL* Data

A group from Johns Hopkins University, Baltimore, Maryland, conducted a study in 91 North American and Swedish families, and its report suggested that 34% of families might be linked to this locus [9]. This GWS identified a locus named *HPC1* (hereditary prostate cancer 1) at 1q24-25. Various groups have since either confirmed [81–84], or challenged [65,66, 68,72,85,86] the Hopkins' observation. Goode et al. [72], and Goddard et al. [87] identified evidence of linkage in families with more aggressive PCa.

Xu [88], in a meta-analysis, found that approximately 6% of all PCa families were linked to 1q24–25. A further analysis concluded that *HPC1* might play a role in a subset of families with several young-onset cases especially in African-American men. Carpten et al. [89] subsequently found mutations in the cell proliferation and apoptosis regulating gene *RNASEL*. Some reports have shown *RNASEL* mutations to be associated with PCa, but with a much lower RR than would be extrapolated by the linkage evidence. Rokman et al. [90] showed that the Glu265X in *RNASEL* was present 4.5-fold more often in affected family members compared with controls. *RNASEL* was found by other groups to confer much smaller PCa risks or have found no mutations in this gene in PCa families. *RNASEL* seems not to be a highly penetrant prostate cancer gene, which seems to conflict with current linkage evidence [91,92].

Other Loci and Candidates from GWS

Other loci have been identified that have significant logarithm of odds (LOD) scores or whose risks fall on further detailed scrutiny [93,94].

Other Significant Loci

PCaP (1q42.2–43 [65]) was a locus identified in the German/French population, but not confirmed by other groups. *CAPB* (1p36 [67]) is a locus associated with primary brain tumor and PCa, which on further analysis was probably more associated with young-onset PCa rather than brain tumor [95]. Suarez et al. [66] described a locus on chromosome 16q in sibling pairs. Berry et al. [71] described another one on 20q (*HPC20*). These are still to be confirmed. It is likely that the *HPC20* locus is not real, as recent analyses from multiple groups in the International Consortium for Prostate Cancer Genetics (ICPCG) have failed to confirm linkage to this locus in a meta-analysis (Schaid and the ICPCG, in press, 2004). A further locus has been described on the long arm of chromosome X (*HPCX;* Xq27–28) by Xu et al. [96]. Some loci, for example, 7q, 19q [97–99], have been found to be associated with more aggressive PCa. Eight GWSs have been published recently in one issue of *The Prostate* (ACTANE Consortium [80]; Lange et al. [73]; Schleutker et al. [74]; Cunningham et al [75]. Xu et al. [76]; Wiklund et al. [77]; Janer et al. [78]; Witte et al. [79]). This work was summarized in an accompanying review by Easton et al. [13]. The conclusion of these GWSs to date is that there is considerable genetic heterogeneity.

Low-Penetrance Genes

Some of the genetically acquired risks of inheritance of PCa could be due to common low-penetrance genes. A significant association between a susceptibility to PCa and common genetic variants, for example, the androgen receptor (AR) genes, has been observed. Although the AR has been excluded as a site for a highly penetrant dominant PCa susceptibility locus, it is a candidate for a lower penetrance PCa susceptibility gene. The most consistent polymorphisms to date that confer a moderately increased risk are in the *SRD5A2, GSTP1* and *AR* genes [100–110].

Clinical Management

About 10% of PCa cases are thought to be due primarily to *high-risk* inherited genetic factors or PCa susceptibility genes. Men with a father or brother with PCa are twice as likely to develop PCa as men with no affected relatives. The risk increases with increasing number of relatives that are affected, for example, men with two or three first-degree relatives affected have a fivefold and 11-fold increased risk of PCa, respectively (see Tables 2.1 to 2.5).

With the increase in PCa awareness among patients and health care professionals, an increasing number of people are querying the optimal management of individuals with a family history of PCa. The clinical management of FPC remains a challenge. Due to the significant number of men with a family history of PCa, the appreciation and understanding of key management issues is critical.

The current clinical management issues surrounding FPC involves several components: (1) biological aggressiveness, (2) outcomes following definitive treatment, (3) survival curve differences between FPC and sporadic cases, (4) treatment vs. observation in screen-detected patients, (5) role of chemoprevention, (6) role of targeted screening, and (7) genetic counseling.

Biological Aggressiveness

The biologic aggressiveness of FPC has been the focus of interest of several investigators. Walsh [111] first noted that there was no significant difference between phenotypes of hereditary, familial, and sporadic prostate cancer among those who underwent radical prostatectomy with respect to preoperative PSA, PSA density, Gleason score, tumor histology, pathological stage, or clinical stage. Kupelian et al. [112] later observed that men with localized PCa with a positive family history may have a worse outcome at 3 and 5 years following either radiation therapy or surgery than those with sporadic cases. Three further studies found no difference in the aggressiveness of the disease in familial compared with sporadic cases [113–115].

These seemingly equivocal results can partially be explained by the heterogeneous nature of the various target groups studied, bias in the self-reporting of family history, and the different subgroups of family history, for example, single first-degree versus multiple relatives with PCa. Recently, *E2F3* expression was found to be a potential independent factor in predicting overall survival of patients with PCa [116]. Such prognostic markers, if replicated in FPC, would be useful in identifying a subset of FPC that has a poorer prognosis.

Outcomes Following Definitive Treatment in Familial Prostate Cancer

Kupelian et al. [117] conducted a study to determine if FPC patients have a less favorable prognosis than patients with sporadic PCa after treatment for localized disease with definitive treatment, that is, either radical prostatectomy or radiotherapy. The 5-year biochemical relapse-free survival rates for patients with negative and positive family histories were 52% and 29%, respectively ($p < .001$). This is the first study that demonstrated that the presence of a family history of PCa correlates with treatment outcome and suggests that FPC may have a more aggressive course than nonfamilial PCa. Further studies are currently underway to validate this finding.

In patients not stratified as having FPC, biochemical failure rates were shown to be similar irrespective of whether radical prostatectomy or radiotherapy was the monotherapy undertaken for clinically localized PCa [118]. Eight-year biochemical failure rates were found to be identical in men treated with either radical prostatectomy or radiotherapy [119]. With respect to FPC, the key question is whether the outcomes are different between those offered different modes of monotherapy. Hanlon and Hanks [120], in an attempt to evaluate biochemical outcome after definitive radiotherapy as a function of family history groupings, found no significant difference in biochemical failure rates between carefully matched men with and without FPC. The findings of this study support others that failed to show an increased risk of failure after definitive therapy for clinically localized PCa in men with familial disease.

Azzouzi et al. [121] compared the biological and clinical features of sporadic and familial clinically localized PCa treated with radical prostatectomy, and found that the outcome is similar in those with and without a family history.

Large-scale prospective family history data collection and outcome analyses, therefore, need to be done to see whether a genetic change influencing PCa etiology correlates with factors altering treatment response.

At present the comparative roles of radiotherapy versus radical prostatectomy in the management of men with FPC are not ratified by robust studies; however, preliminary studies seem to suggest that outcome in FPC is not influenced by the mode of definitive therapy.

Sporadic and Familial Prostate Cancer: Biochemical Failure and Differences in Survival

Gronberg et al. [122] tried to estimate the survival of men with FPC and compare them with prostate cancer cases unselected for family history. No significant differences in either overall or prostate cancer-specific survival between familial and sporadic cases were found.

Tumor grade at diagnosis in familial cases did not differ from that in a population with prostate cancer unselected for family history. The conclusion, based on the result from this study, was that no differences in treatment between men with and without a positive family history of prostate cancer are justified.

However, Kupelian et al. [123], in an analysis of the outcome after radical prostatectomy of patients with familial versus sporadic prostate cancer, observed that the former group has a higher likelihood of biochemical failure after radical prostatectomy. They concluded that this effect was independent of pretreatment or pathological factors. Currently, it may be reasonable to recommend that treatment plans should not be altered based on presence or absence of FPC, but further large-scale studies are needed.

Treatment Versus Observation in Screen-Detected Patients

If highly penetrant genes responsible for PCa, such as the results of risk due to germline mutations in *BRCA2*, were replicated, there would be a rationale for offering genetic counseling and testing for this disease. At present, these results should be replicated on a further sample set of blood samples from PCa cases diagnosed at young age prior to offering clinical diagnostic *BRCA2* genetic counseling and testing, and this is in progress in the U.K. Familial Prostate Cancer Study [10].

The American Urological Association currently recommends that men at high risk of developing PCa, that is, those with a family history of the disease or men of African-American descent, begin receiving routine prostate cancer screening at age 40 [124]. Its recommendation is that such men receive PSA testing and digital rectal examination (DRE) annually starting at age 50. This is recommended earlier if there is a family history of the disease or if one is of African-American descent, as above [125].

However, the exact age for initiation of screening has yet to be clearly defined. A targeted screening study using PSA alone in first-degree relatives of men diagnosed at <65 years or relative pairs with an average age of onset of 70 years or three or more relatives diagnosed at any age is underway in South Thames (the Cancer Research U.K. TAPS study, principal investigator Dr. Melia). The age of screening in different ethnic groups is currently under debate and further adds to the complexity of defining an optimal age for screening. Those men, however, found to be positive for PCa following the screen should be treated as documented in current clinical guidelines irrespective of family history.

The main recent area of controversy is the utility of the PSA value, particularly at low levels (see below) [126]. In the finasteride chemoprevention study, all men were offered biopsy, and 15% of those with a PSA of <1.5 had histological prostate cancer. The dilemma is that these diagnoses may not be clinically significant, and better progression markers are needed both in sporadic and familial disease.

Role of Chemoprevention

The chemoprevention of PCa involves the delivery of agents that could potentially inhibit the crucial carcinogenic steps in its development. The characterization of genetic susceptibility loci could enable men at high risk of developing PCa to be identified and to serve as subjects for chemoprevention trials. Provided these trials yield positive results, they could potentially lead to a recommendation for preventative therapy in genetic carriers.

The key components of chemoprevention include specific agents and their biochemical targets, intermediate end-point biomarkers, with their critical pathways and cohorts identified by both genetic and acquired risk factors [127]. Several putative chemopreventive agents are currently under investigation. Results of a population-based, randomized phase III trial demonstrate that finasteride may prevent PCa. However, the study was slightly disappointing in that only low-grade tumors seem to have been prevented, and in fact the number of high-grade tumors was greater in the finasteride group [126].

Clarke et al. [128], in their study of the role of selenium, found that although selenium shows no protective effect against the primary end point of squamous and basal cell carcinomas of the skin, the selenium-treated group in their series had substantial reductions in the incidence of PCa as a secondary end point. Preliminary data seem to indicate that there may be some benefit with the use of other agents as potential preventatives in addition to selenium. These include vitamin E, vitamin D, other 5α-reductase inhibitors, cyclooxygenase-2 inhibitors, lycopene, and green tea. Some of these agents are being tested in new large-scale phase III clinical trials [129].

The Selenium and Vitamin E Cancer Prevention Trial (SELECT) is a phase III clinical trial designed to test the efficacy of selenium and vitamin E alone and in combination in the prevention of prostate cancer [130]. Refinements in new powerful tools such as proteomic analysis of tissue-based and secreted proteins [131] and gene chip complementary DNA (cDNA) microarrays for multiplex gene expression profiling could help optimize the identification of new molecular targets, cohorts at risk, and the design of suitable combination trials.

The patient with FPC may benefit from the use of chemopreventive agents, and the results of further large-scale trials will define its putative role in the future. The prospect of recommending surgical prophylactic therapy in genetic mutation carriers would be extremely controversial.

Targeted Screening

Targeted screening studies have shown a greater proportion of raised PSA levels in relatives of patients as compared to sporadic cases of prostate cancer. In a screening study of prostate cancer in high-risk families performed by McWhorter et al. [132], it was shown that previously unsuspected and clinically relevant cancers were found in 24% of a total of 34 first-degree relatives, compared to the approximately one expected ($p < .01$). This emphasizes the importance of PSA screening in first-degree relatives of prostate cancer patients. Targeted screening can be done by checking serum PSA levels in relatives of young- or early-onset PCa patients or families with multiple cases. It is reasonable to start screening either at age 40 or 5 years younger than the youngest age at diagnosis of a relative (whichever is the higher).

The first targeted screening study based on *BRCA1/2* genotype will start later this year (the Identification of Men with Genetic Predisposition to Prostate Cancer and Its Clinical Treatment [IMPACT] study [133]). Several large units have already started targeted screening programs with the objective of identifying markers of disease aggression. The programs have been initiated despite the established general setbacks of PSA screening, including lack of clearly defined optimal intervals between individual screens, increased false-negative biopsy rates, and diagnosis and subsequent management of incidentally found prostatic intraepithelial neoplasia.

Genetic Counseling and Testing/Research

Currently, genetic analysis (e.g., *BRCA2* mutation analysis) should be performed only within the context of a research study that will determine penetrance and genotype-phenotype correlation of specific mutations. The criteria for the Cancer Research U.K./British Prostate Group/British Association of Urological Surgeons' Section of Oncology Familial Prostate Cancer Study (principal investigator Dr. Eeles) are as follows:

- Men with PCa diagnosed at <60 years
- Affected relative pairs with PCa where one is <65 years at diagnosis
- PCa families with three or more members diagnosed at any age

Even in the absence of genetic testing, African-American men and men with a strong family history of prostate cancer (as defined in the TAPS study, see above), may opt to initiate screening by PSA and DRE from as early as 40 years.

Conclusion

Prostate cancer is one of the common cancers where there is good evidence for a larger genetic component to its etiology, but the genetic models are complex. It is highly likely that the PCa predisposition genes will be polygenic and may be interacting within families. Some PCa predisposition genes are likely to be DNA repair genes (e.g., *BRCA2*) but these may account for only a small proportion of young cases. However, the discovery of high-risk *BRCA2* mutations has led to the first clinical targeted screening trial based on genotype in this disease (the IMPACT study, discussed above), and this trial will serve as a basis for further targeted screening and chemoprevention trials based on genotype as further genes are identified. The lessons learned in IMPACT will be screening uptake in a high-risk male population, the psychological issues of screening men at higher risk of PCa, the utility of PSA in a higher risk population, the identification of new and better biomarkers and the clinical parameters of PCa so identified.

References

1. American Cancer Society. Cancer Facts and Figures 2004. Atlanta: American Cancer Society, 2004.
2. AIHW and AACR. AIHW National Mortality Database, Australia's Health 2004, AIHW.
3. Majeed A, Babb P, Jones J, Quinn M. Trends in prostate cancer incidence, mortality and survival in England and Wales 1971–1998. BJU Int 2000;85(9):1058–1062.
4. Dijkman GA, Debruyne FM. Epidemiology of prostate cancer. Eur Urol 1996;30(3):281–295.

5. Parkin DM, Pisani P, Ferlay J. Estimates of the worldwide incidence of eighteen major cancers in 1985. Int J Cancer 1993;54(4):594–606.

6. Whittemore AS, Wu AH, Kolonel LN, et al. Family history and prostate cancer risk in black, white, and Asian men in the United States and Canada. Am J Epidemiol 1995;141(8):732–740.

7. Cussenot O, Cancel-Tassin G. Genetic susceptibility to prostate cancer. Med Sci (Paris) 2004; 20(5):562–568 (French).

8. Morganti G, et al. Recherches clinico-statistiques et génétiques sur les néopasies de la prostate. Acta Genet Statist 1959;6:304–305.

9. Smith JR, Freije D, Carpten JD, et al. Major susceptibility locus for prostate cancer on chromosome 1 suggested by a genome-wide search. Science 1996;274(5291):1371–1374.

10. Eeles RA, the UK Familial Prostate Study Coordinating Group and the CRC/BPG UK Familial Prostate Cancer Study Collaborators. Genetic predisposition to prostate cancer. Prostate Cancer Prostatic Dis 1999;2(1):9–15.

11. Ostrander EA, Stanford JL. Genetics of prostate cancer: too many loci, too few genes. Am J Hum Genet 2000;67(6):1367–1375.

12. Simard J, Dumont M, Labuda D, et al. Prostate cancer susceptibility genes: lessons learned and challenges posed. Endocr Relat Cancer 2003; 10(2):225–259.

13. Easton DF, Schaid DJ, Whittemore AS, Isaacs WJ. International Consortium for Prostate Cancer Genetics. Where are the prostate cancer genes? A summary of eight genome wide searches. Prostate 2003;57(4):261–269.

14. Hall JM, Lee MK, Newman B, et al. Linkage of early-onset familial breast cancer to chromosome 17q21. Science 1990;250(4988):1684–1689.

15. Morganti G, Gianferrari L, Cresseri A, Arrigoni G, Lovati G. [Clinico-statistical and genetic research on neoplasms of the prostate]. Acta Genet Stat Med 1956–1957;6(2):304–305.

16. Woolf CM. An investigation of the familial aspects of carcinoma of the prostate. Cancer 1960;13:739–744.

17. Cannon L, Bishop DT, Skolnick M, Hunt S, Lyon JL, Smart CR. Genetic epidemiology of prostate cancer in the Utah Mormon Genealogy. Cancer Surv 1982;1:47–69.

18. Cannon-Albright L, Eeles RA. Progress in prostate cancer. Nat Genet 1995;9(4):336–338.

19. Steele R, Lees RE, Kraus AS, Rao C. Sexual factors in the epidemiology of cancer of the prostate. J Chronic Dis 1971;24(1):29–37.

20. Krain LS. Some epidemiologic variables in prostatic carcinoma in California. Prev Med 1974;3(1):154–159.

21. Schuman LM, Mandel J, Blackard C, Bauer H, Scarlett J, McHugh R. Epidemiologic study of prostatic cancer: preliminary report. Cancer Treat Rep 1977;61(2):181–186.

22. Meikle AW, Smith JA, West DW. Familial factors affecting prostatic cancer risk and plasma sex-steroid levels. Prostate 1985;6(2):121–128.

23. Steinberg GD, Carter BS, Beaty TH, Childs B, Walsh PC. Family history and the risk of prostate cancer. Prostate 1990;17(4):337–347.

24. Fincham SM, Hill GB, Hanson J, Wijayasinghe C. Epidemiology of prostatic cancer: a case-control study. Prostate 1990;17(3):189–206.

25. Spitz MR, Currier RD, Fueger JJ, Babaian RJ, Newell GR. Familial patterns of prostate cancer: a case-control analysis. J Urol 1991;146(5):1305–1307.

26. Ghadirian P, Cadotte M, Lacroix A, Perret C. Family aggregation of cancer of the prostate in Quebec: the tip of the iceberg. Prostate 1991; 19(1):43–52.

27. Whittemore AS, Wu AH, Kolonel LN, et al. Family history and prostate cancer risk in black, white, and Asian men in the United States and Canada. Am J Epidemiol 1995;141(8):732–740.

28. Hayes RB, Liff JM, Pottern LM, et al. Prostate cancer risk in U.S. blacks and whites with a family history of cancer. Int J Cancer 1995; 60(3):361–364.

29. Isaacs SD, Kiemeney LA, Baffoe-Bonnie A, Beaty TH, Walsh PC. Risk of cancer in relatives of prostate cancer probands. J Natl Cancer Inst 1995; 87(13):991–996.

30. Keetch DW, Rice JP, Suarez BK, Catalona WJ. Familial aspects of prostate cancer: a case control study. J Urol 1995;154(6):2100–2102.

31. Lesko SM, Rosenberg L, Shapiro S. Family history and prostate cancer risk. Am J Epidemiol 1996; 144(11):1041–1047.

32. Ghadirian P, Howe GR, Hislop TG, Maisonneuve P. Family history of prostate cancer: a multi-center case-control study in Canada. Int J Cancer 1997;70(6):679–681.

33. Glover FE Jr, Coffey DS, Douglas LL, et al. Familial study of prostate cancer in Jamaica. Urology 1998;52(3):441–443.

34. Bratt O, Kristoffersson U, Lundgren R, Olsson H. Familial and hereditary prostate cancer in southern Sweden. A population-based case-control study. Eur J Cancer 1999;35(2):272–277.

35. Eeles RA, Dearnaley DP, Ardern-Jones A, et al. Familial prostate cancer: the evidence and the Cancer Research Campaign/British Prostate Group (CRC/BPG) UK Familial Prostate Cancer Study. Br J Urol 1997;79(suppl 1):8–14.

36. Singh R, Eeles RA, Durocher F, et al. High risk genes predisposing to prostate cancer development-do they exist? Prostate Cancer Prostatic Dis 2000;3(4):241–247.

37. Johns LE, Houlston RS. A systematic review and meta-analysis of familial prostate cancer risk. BJU Int 2003;91(9):789–794.

38. Carter BS, Beaty TH, Steinberg GD, Childs B, Walsh PC. Mendelian inheritance of familial prostate cancer. Proc Natl Acad Sci USA 1992; 89(8):3367–3371.

39. Goldgar DE, Easton DF, Cannon-Albright LA, Skolnick MH. Systematic population-based assessment of cancer risk in first-degree relatives of cancer probands. J Natl Cancer Inst 1994; 86(21):1600–1608.

40. Gronberg H, Damber L, Damber JE. Familial prostate cancer in Sweden. A nationwide register cohort study. Cancer 1996;77(1):138–143.

41. Ahlbom A, Lichtenstein P, Malmstrom H, Feychting M, Hemminki K, Pedersen NL. Cancer in twins: genetic and nongenetic familial risk factors. J Natl Cancer Inst 1997;89(4):287–293.

42. Page WF, Braun MM, Partin AW, Caporaso N, Walsh P. Heredity and prostate cancer: a study of World War II veteran twins. Prostate 1997; 33(4):240–245.

43. Verkasalo PK, Kaprio J, Koskenvuo M, Pukkala E. Genetic predisposition, environment and cancer incidence: a nationwide twin study in Finland, 1976–1995. Int J Cancer 1999;83(6):743–749.

44. Lichtenstein P, Holm NV, Verkasalo PK, et al. Environmental and heritable factors in the causation of cancer-analyses of cohorts of twins from Sweden, Denmark, and Finland. N Engl J Med 2000;343(2):78–85.

45. Schaid DJ, McDonnell SK, Blute ML, Thibodeau SN. Evidence for autosomal dominant inheritance of prostate cancer. Am J Hum Genet 1998; 62(6):1425–1438.

46. Narod SA, Dupont A, Cusan L, et al. The impact of family history on early detection of prostate cancer. Nat Med 1995;1(2):99–101.

47. Monroe KR, Yu MC, Kolonel LN, et al. Evidence of an X-linked or recessive genetic component to prostate cancer risk. Nat Med 1995;1(8):827–829.

48. Ewis AA, Lee J, Naroda T, et al. Linkage between prostate cancer incidence and different alleles of the human Y-linked tetranucleotide polymorphism DYS19. J Med Invest 2002;49(1–2):56–60.

49. Cui J, Staples MP, Hopper JL, English DR, McCredie MR, Giles GG. Segregation analyses of 1,476 population-based Australian families affected by prostate cancer. Am J Hum Genet 2001;68(5):1207–1218.

50. Conlon EM, Goode EL, Gibbs M, et al. Oligogenic segregation analysis of hereditary prostate cancer pedigrees: evidence for multiple loci affecting age at onset. Int J Cancer 2003;105(5): 630–635.

51. Eeles RAPB, Easton DF, Ponder BAJ, Eng C, eds. Genetic Predisposition to Cancer, 2nd ed. London: Arnold, 2004.

52. Tulinius H, Olafsdottir GH, Sigvaldason H, Tryggvadottir L, Bjarnadottir K. Neoplastic diseases in families of breast cancer patients. J Med Genet 1994;31(8):618–621.

53. Anderson DE, Badzioch MD. Familial breast cancer risks. Effects of prostate and other cancers. Cancer 72:114–119.

54. Ford D, Easton DF, Bishop DT, Narod SA, Goldgar DE. Risks of cancer in BRCA1–mutation carriers. Breast Cancer Linkage Consortium. Lancet 1994; 343:692–695.

55. Thompson D, Easton DF, and the Breast Cancer Linkage Consortium. Cancer Incidence in BRCA1 Mutation Carriers. J Natl Cancer Inst 94:1358–1365.

56. Thorlacius S, Struewing JP, Hartge P, et al. Population-based study of risk of breast cancer in carriers of BRCA2 mutation. Lancet 1998;352: 1337–1339.

57. Sigurdsson S, Thorlacius S, Tomasson J, et al. BRCA2 mutation in Icelandic prostate cancer patients. J Mol Med 1997;75:758–761.

58. Gronberg H, Ahman AK, Emanuelsson M, Bergh A, Damber JE, Borg A. BRCA2 mutation in a family with hereditary prostate cancer. Genes Chromosomes Cancer 2001;30:299–301.

59. Gayther SA, de Foy KA, Harrington P, et al. The frequency of germ-line mutations in the breast cancer predisposition genes BRCA1 and BRCA2 in familial prostate cancer. The Cancer Research Campaign/British Prostate Group United Kingdom Familial Prostate Cancer Study Collaborators. Cancer Res 2000;60:4513–4518.

60. Edwards SM, Kote-Jarai Z, Meitz J, et al. Cancer Research UK/British Prostate Group UK Familial Prostate Cancer Study Collaborators, British Association of Urological Surgeons Section of Oncology. Two percent of men with early-onset prostate cancer harbor germline mutations in the BRCA2 gene. Am J Hum Genet 2003;72(1): 1–12.

61. Kirchhoff T, Kauff ND, Mitra N, et al. BRCA mutations and risk of prostate cancer in Ashkenazi Jews. Clin Cancer Res 2004;10(9):2918–2921.

62. Giusti RM, Rutter JL, Duray PH, et al. A twofold increase in BRCA mutation related prostate cancer among Ashkenazi Israelis is not associated with distinctive histopathology. J Med Genet 2003;40(10):787–792.

63. Cybulski C, Gorski B, Debniak T, et al. NBS1 is a prostate cancer susceptibility gene. Cancer Res 2004;64(4):1215–1219.

64. Dong X, Wang L, Taniguchi K, et al. Mutations in CHEK2 associated with prostate cancer risk. Am J Hum Genet 2003;72(2):270–280.

65. Berthon P, Valerie A, Cohen-Akenine A, et al. Predisposing gene for early-onset prostate cancer, localized on chromosome 1q42.2–43. Am J Hum Genet 1998;62(6):1416–1424.

66. Suarez BK, Lin J, Burmester JK, et al. A genome screen of multiplex sibships with prostate cancer. 66(3):933–944.

67. Gibbs M, Stanford JL, McIndoe RA, et al. Evidence for a rare prostate cancer prostate cancer-susceptibility locus at chromosome 1p36. Hum Genet 1999;64(3):776–787.

68. Berry R, Schaid DJ, Smith JR, et al. Linkage analyses at the chromosome 1 loci 1q24–25 (HPC1), 1q42.2–43 (PCAP), and 1p36 (CAPB) in families with hereditary prostate cancer. Am J Hum Genet 2000;66(2):539–546.

69. Tavtigian SV, Simrad J, Teng DH, et al. A candidate prostate cancer susceptibility gene at chromosome 17p. Nat Genet 2001;27(2):172–180.

70. Hsieh CL, Oakley-Girvan I, Gallagher RP, et al. Re: prostate cancer susceptibility locus on chromosome 1q: a confirmatory study. J Natl Cancer Inst 1997;89(24):1893–1894.

71. Berry R, Schroeder JJ, French AJ, et al. Evidence for a prostate cancer- susceptibility locus on chromosome 20. Am J Hum Genet 2000;67(1):82–91.

72. Goode EL, Stanford JL, Chakrabarti L, et al. Linkage analysis of 150 high-risk prostate cancer families at 1q24–25. Genet Epidemiol 2000; 18(3):251–275.

73. Lange EM, Gillanders EM, Davis CC, et al. Genome-wide scan for prostate cancer susceptibility genes using families from the University of Michigan prostate cancer genetics project finds evidence for linkage on chromosome 17 near BRCA1. Prostate 2003;57(4):326–334.

74. Schleutker J, Baffoe-Bonnie AB, et al. Genome-wide scan for linkage in Finnish Hereditary Prostate Cancer (HPC) families identifies novel susceptibility loci at 11q14 and 3p25–26. Prostate 2003;57(4):280–289.

75. Cunningham JM, McDonnell SK, Marks A, et al. Mayo Clinic, Rochester, Minnesota. Genome linkage screen for prostate cancer susceptibility loci: results from the Mayo Clinic Familial Prostate Cancer Study. Prostate 2003;57(4):335–346.

76. Xu J, Gillanders EM, Isaacs SD, et al. Genome-wide scan for prostate cancer susceptibility genes in the Johns Hopkins hereditary prostate cancer families. Prostate 2003;57(4):320–325.

77. Wiklund F, Gillanders EM, Albertus JA, et al. Genome-wide scan of Swedish families with hereditary prostate cancer: suggestive evidence of linkage at 5q11.2 and 19p13.3. Prostate 2003; 57(4):290–297.

78. Janer MFD, Stanford JL, Badzioch MD, et al. Genomic scan of 254 hereditary prostate cancer families. Prostate 2003;57(4):309–319.

79. Witte JSSB, Thiel B, Lin J, et al. Genome-wide scan of brothers: replication and fine mapping of prostate cancer susceptibility and aggressiveness loci. Prostate 2003;57(4):298–308.

80. The International ACTANE Consortium. Results of a genome-wide linkage analysis in prostate cancer families ascertained through the ACTANE consortium. Prostate 2003;57(4):270–279.

81. Gronberg H, Smith J, Emanuelsson M, et al. In Swedish families with hereditary prostate cancer, linkage to the HPC1 locus on chromosome 1q24–25 is restricted to families with early-onset prostate cancer. Am J Hum Genet 1999;65(1):134–140.

82. Cooney KA, McCarthy JD, Lange E, et al. Prostate cancer susceptibility locus on chromosome 1q: a confirmatory study. J Natl Cancer Inst 1997; 89(13):955–959.

83. Neuhausen SL, Farnham JH, Kort E, Tavtigian SV, Skolnick MH, Cannon-Albright LA. Prostate cancer susceptibility locus HPC1 in Utah high-risk pedigrees. Hum Mol Genet 1999;8(13):2437–2442.

84. Xu J, Zheng SL, Chang B, et al. Linkage of prostate cancer susceptibility loci to chromosome 1. Hum Genet 2001;108(4):335–345.

85. McIndoe RA, Stanford JL, Gibbs M, et al. Linkage analysis of 49 high-risk families does not support a common familial prostate cancer-susceptibility gene at 1q24–25. Am J Hum Genet 1997;61(2):347–353.

86. Eeles RA, Durocher F, Edwards S, et al. Linkage analysis of chromosome 1q markers in 136 prostate cancer families. The Cancer Research Campaign/British Prostate Group U.K. Familial Prostate Cancer Study Collaborators. Am J Hum Genet 1998;62(3):653–658.

87. Goddard KA, Witte JS, Suarez BK, Catalona WJ, Olson JM. Model-free linkage analysis with covariates confirms linkage of prostate cancer to chromosomes 1 and 4. Am J Hum Genet 2001;68(5):1197–1206.

88. Xu J. Combined analysis of hereditary prostate cancer linkage to 1q24–25: results from 772 hereditary prostate cancer families from the International Consortium for Prostate Cancer Genetics. Am J Hum Genet 2000;66(3):945–957; erratum in Am J Hum Genet 2000;67(2):541–542.

89. Carpten J, Nupponen N, Isaacs S, et al. Germline mutations in the ribonuclease L gene in families showing linkage with HPC1. Nat Genet 2002; 30(2):181–184.

90. Rokman A, Ikonen T, Seppala EH, et al. Germline alterations of the RNASEL gene, a candidate

HPC1 gene at 1q25, in patients and families with prostate cancer. Am J Hum Genet 2002;70(5): 1299–1304; erratum in Am J Hum Genet 2002; 71(1):215.

91. Casey G, Neville PJ, Plummer SJ, et al. *RNASEL* Arg462Gln variant is implicated in up to 13% of prostate cancer cases. Nat Genet 2002;32(4): 581–583.

92. Chen H, Griffen AR, Wu YQ, et al. *RNASEL* mutations in hereditary prostate cancer. J Med Genet 2003;40(3):e21.

93. Wang L, McDonnel SK, Cunningham JM, et al. No association of germline alteration of *MSR1* with prostate cancer risk. Nat Genet 2003;35(2): 128–129.

94. Meitz JC, Edwards SM, Easton DF, et al. Cancer Research UK/BPG UK Familial Prostate Cancer Study Collaborators. *HPC2/ELAC2* polymorphisms and prostate cancer risk: analysis by age of onset of disease. Br J Cancer 2002;87(8): 905–908.

95. Badzioch M, Eeles R, Leblanc G, et al. Suggestive evidence for a site specific prostate cancer gene on chromosome 1p36. The CRC/BPG UK Familial Prostate Cancer Study Coordinators and Collaborators. The EU Biomed Collaborators. J Med Genet 2000;37(12):947–949.

96. Xu J, Meyers D, Freije D, et al. Evidence for a prostate cancer susceptibility locus on the X chromosome. Nat Genet 1998;20(2):175–179.

97. Witte JS, Goddard KA, Conti DV, et al. Genomewide scan for prostate cancer-aggressiveness loci. Am J Hum Genet 2000; 67(1):92–99.

98. Slager SL, Schaid DJ, Cunningham JM, et al. Confirmation of linkage of prostate cancer aggressiveness with chromosome 19q. Am J Hum Genet 2003;72(3):759–762.

99. Neville PJ, Conti DV, Krumroy LM, et al. Prostate cancer aggressiveness locus on chromosome segment 19q12–q13.1 identified by linkage and allelic imbalance studies. Genes Chromosomes Cancer 2003;36(4):332–339.

100. Irvine RA, Yu MC, Ross RK, Coetzee GA. The CAG and GGC microsatellites of the androgen receptor gene are in linkage disequilibrium in men with prostate cancer. Cancer Res 1995;55: 1937–1940.

101. Hardy DO, Scher HI, Bogenreider T, et al. Androgen receptor CAG repeat lengths in prostate cancer: correlation with age of onset. J Clin Endocrinol Metab 1996;81:4400–4405.

102. Ingles SA, Ross RK, Yu MC, et al. Association of prostate cancer risk with genetic polymorphisms in vitamin D receptor and androgen receptor. J Natl Cancer Inst 1997;89:166–170.

103. Stanford JL, Just JJ, Gibbs M, et al. Polymorphic repeats in the androgen receptor gene: molecu-lar markers of prostate cancer risk. Cancer Res 1997;57:1194–1198.

104. Giovannucci E, Stampfer MJ, Krithivas K, et al. The CAG repeat within the androgen receptor gene and its relationship to prostate cancer. Proc Natl Acad Sci USA 1997;94:3320–3323.

105. Hakimi JM, Schoenberg MP, Rondinelli RH, Piantadosi S, Barrack ER. Androgen receptor variants with short glutamine or glycine repeats may identify unique subpopulations of men with prostate cancer. Clin Cancer Res 1997;3: 1599–1608.

106. Miller EA, Stanford JL, Hsu L, Noonan E, Ostrander EA. Polymorphic repeats in the androgen receptor gene in high-risk sibships. Prostate 2001;48:200–205.

107. Hsing AW, Gao YT, Wu G, et al. Polymorphic CAG and GGN repeat lengths in the androgen receptor gene and prostate cancer risk: a population-based case-control study in China. Cancer Res 2000;60:5111–5116.

108. Edwards SM, Badzioch MD, Minter R, et al. Androgen receptor polymorphisms: association with prostate cancer risk, relapse and overall survival. Int J Cancer 1999;84:458–465.

109. Makridakis NM, Ross RK, Pike MC, et al. Association of mis-sense substitution in *SRD5A2* gene with prostate cancer in African-American and Hispanic men in Los Angeles, USA. Lancet 1999;354:975–978.

110. Kote-Jarai Z, Easton D, Edwards SM, et al. CRC/BPG UK Familial Prostate Cancer Study Collaborators. Relationship between glutathione S-transferase M1, P1 and T1 polymorphisms and early onset prostate cancer. Pharmacogenetics 2001;11:325–330.

111. Walsh PC. Hereditary Prostate Cancer, podium talk at the annual meeting of the American Society of Clinical Oncology, 1996.

112. Kupelian PA, Kupelian VA, Witte JS, Macklis R, Klein EA. Family history of prostate cancer in patients with localized prostate cancer: an independent predictor of treatment outcome. J Clin Oncol 1997;15(4):1478–1480.

113. Valeri A, Azzouzi R, Drelon E, et al. Early-onset hereditary prostate cancer is not associated with clinical and biological features. Prostate 2000; 45(1):66–71.

114. Klein EA, Kupelian PA, Witte JS. Does a family history of prostate cancer result in more aggressive disease? Prostate Cancer Prostatic Dis 1998; 1(6):297–300.

115. Bova GS, Partin AW, Isaacs SD, et al. Biological aggressiveness of hereditary prostate cancer: long-term evaluation following radical prostatectomy. 1998;160(3 pt 1):660–663.

116. Foster CS, Falconer A, Dodson AR, et al. Transcription factor E2F3 overexpressed in prostate

cancer independently predicts clinical outcome. Oncogene 2004;23(35):5871–5879.

117. Kupelian PA, Kupelian VA, Witte JS, Macklis R, Klein EA. Family history of prostate cancer in patients with localized prostate cancer: an independent predictor of treatment outcome. J Clin Oncol 1997;15(4):1478–1480.

118. Potters L, Klein EA, Kattan MW, et al. Monotherapy for stage T1–T2 prostate cancer: radical prostatectomy, external beam radiotherapy, or permanent seed implantation. Radiother Oncol 2004;71(1):29–33.

119. Kupelian PA, Elshaikh M, Reddy CA, Zippe C, Klein EA. Comparison of the efficacy of local therapies for localized prostate cancer in the prostate-specific antigen era: a large single-institution experience with radical prostatectomy and external-beam radiotherapy. J Clin Oncol 2002;20(16):3376–3385.

120. Hanlon AL, Hanks GE. Patterns of inheritance and outcome in patients treated with external beam radiation for prostate cancer. Urology 1998;52(5):735–738.

121. Azzouzi AR, Valeri A, Cormier L, Fournier G, Mangin P, Cussenot O. Familial prostate cancer cases before and after radical prostatectomy do not show any aggressiveness compared with sporadic cases. Urology 2003;61(6):1193–1197.

122. Gronberg H, Damber L, Damber JE. Familial prostate cancer in Sweden. A nationwide register cohort study. Cancer 1996;77(1):138–143.

123. Kupelian PA, Klein EA, Witte JS, Kupelian VA, Suh JH. Familial prostate cancer: a different disease? J Urol 1997;158(6):2197–2201.

124. American Urological Association. Prostate Cancer Awareness For Men: A Doctor's Guide for Patients. AUA, 2001:4–5.

125. Cancer Reference Information: Can Prostate Cancer Be Found Early? American Cancer Society. October 3, 2001.

126. Thompson IM, Goodman PJ, Tangen CM, et al. The influence of finasteride on the development of prostate cancer. N Engl J Med 2003;349(3): 215–224.

127. Lieberman R. Chemoprevention of prostate cancer: current status and future directions. Cancer Metastasis Rev 2002;21(3–4):297–309.

128. Clark LC, Dalkin B, Krongrad A, et al. Decreased incidence of prostate cancer with selenium supplementation: results of a double-blind cancer prevention trial. Br J Urol 1998;81(5):730–734.

129. Klein EA, Thompson IM. Update on chemoprevention of prostate cancer. Curr Opin Urol 2004; 14(3):143–149.

130. Klein EA. Clinical models for testing chemopreventative agents in prostate cancer and overview of SELECT: the Selenium and Vitamin E Cancer Prevention Trial. Recent Results Cancer Res 2003;163:212–225; discussion 264–266.

131. Kommu S, Sharifi R, Edwards S, Eeles R. Proteomics and urine analysis-a potential promising new tool in urology. BJU Int 2004;93(9): 1172–1173.

132. McWhorter WP, Hernandez AD, Meikle AW, et al. A screening study of prostate cancer in high risk families. J Urol 1992;148(3):826–828.

133. Tischkowitz M, Eeles R, IMPACT study: Identification of Men with genetic predisposition to Prostate Cancer and its Clinical Treatment collaborators. Mutations in BRCA1 and BRCA2 and predisposition to prostate cancer. Lancet 2003;362(9377):80; author reply 80.

3

Screening for Prostate Cancer

Joshua Phillips and Freddie C. Hamdy

Prostate cancer screening is one of the most controversial public health issues in urology. The natural aging of the population and the continued and widespread use of improved diagnostic tests, such as serum prostate-specific antigen (PSA), are resulting in an increase in the numbers of men diagnosed with localized prostate cancer. The issue of screening to identify organ-confined prostate cancer has provoked much public and scientific attention, and there is intense debate about its role in improving men's health. Despite constant pressure from strong advocates of screening, including the general public, special-interest groups, and certain aspects of the media, the findings from most reviews of the scientific evidence conclude that it is insufficient, at present, to recommend routine population screening because of the lack of evidence that this would improve either survival or the quality of men's lives. Particular concerns in these reviews relate to the lack of knowledge about the natural history of screen-detected prostate cancer, and the lack of evidence about the effectiveness of treatments.

Evidence from many studies shows that with the use of PSA testing, prostate cancer can be diagnosed in a clinically locally confined state in 70% to 80% of cases. This fact, together with the widely accepted evidence that prostate cancer can be cured only as long as it is locally confined, provides simple and convincing logic that drives opportunistic screening. To date, however, no survival advantage has been shown

in screen-detected cases for any of the major treatments (radical prostatectomy, radical radiotherapy including brachytherapy, and "watchful waiting," otherwise known as active monitoring or surveillance) and each can result in damaging iatrogenic complications and outcomes, including various levels of incontinence and impotence for radical interventions and anxiety relating to the presence of cancer in "watchful waiting." The problem is compounded because many of the published studies contain flawed analyses and unsubstantiated conclusions. The same evidence has resulted in different approaches to screening on either side of the Atlantic, and even among states in the United States.

General Criteria for Establishing a Screening Program

In 1968 Wilson and Jungner [1] established key principles that a disease should satisfy before introducing screening as a public health policy. Despite further refinements, more recent guidelines for screening programs continue to adhere to the merits of Wilson and Jungner's original criteria, the most important of which will be used below as the framework for discussing the issues involved in screening for prostate cancer.

The Disease Should Be an Important Health Problem

As the most common male cancer in Europe and the United States, and second only to lung cancer in terms of male cancer deaths, there is little doubt that prostate cancer represents a significant public health burden in Western countries [2]. In the U.S. alone, an estimated 220,900 new prostate cancer cases were diagnosed in 2003, with 28,900 deaths attributable to the disease [3]. Although a dramatic increase has been observed in the number of men diagnosed with localized disease as a consequence of PSA testing, those with advanced prostate cancer continue to present a significant burden to the community, developing metastatic disease at a rate of 8% per year, and reaching 40% at 5 years. These metastases predominately affect the skeleton, causing high levels of morbidity and hospitalization, and necessitating expensive palliation. In addition, the use of hormone manipulation in the form of androgen suppression to treat advanced disease causes iatrogenic morbidity by reducing bone density and inducing osteoporosis, again leading to skeletal-related events requiring possible prophylaxis by using agents such as bisphosphonates, or treatment to correct the complications [4,5].

There Should Be a Preclinical State More Amenable to Successful Treatment than Clinical Disease

This criterion remains unclear in prostate cancer, largely because of the rather loose definition of "clinically significant" disease. Despite the fact that with increasing age most men will develop microscopic foci of prostate cancer, only a small percentage of these slow-growing tumors will develop into invasive prostate cancer, and an even smaller proportion will cause premature death. It is hoped that the epidemiological investigation of prostate cancer will identify factors—ideally amenable to intervention—that cause the common microscopic form of the disease to progress to invasive disease. However, to date, the etiology of prostate cancer remains virtually unknown and continues to pose a major challenge to epidemiologists. Although both genetics and environment are

likely to play a role in the evolution of the disease, the role of genetic factors in prostate cancer susceptibility has stimulated significant interest following a number of genetic linkage analyses based on families in which several men have prostate cancer, most of whom have early-onset disease. Genetic factors will undoubtedly prove important in prostate cancer, although major susceptibility genes account for only 5% to 10% of prostate cancer cases. Whether high-risk genetic mutations or common low-risk genetic polymorphisms (variants) produce familial aggregation remains unclear, although several common polymorphisms are associated with a modest increase in disease risk. Many published studies lack sufficient sample size and statistical power to be conclusive, and even if confirmed, the magnitude of effect would not justify the inclusion of genotyping for these polymorphisms in a screening program. The findings for other potential factors such as diet and sexual lifestyle fall short of the evidence required for public health recommendations [6].

Prostatic Intraepithelial Neoplasia

Prostatic intraepithelial neoplasia (PIN) is believed to be the preinvasive end of a morphological continuum of cellular proliferation affecting prostatic ducts, ductules, and acini. It tends to be multifocal and occurs in the peripheral zone, as does prostate cancer. It is divided into two grades: low and high. The continuum from normal prostatic epithelium through low- and high-grade PIN to invasive cancer is characterized by increased epithelial dysplasia within the luminal secretory cell layer. The dysplastic changes with increasing grade of PIN include nuclear enlargement, hyperchromatism, prominent nucleoli, cellular crowding with overlapping nuclei, and epithelial hyperplasia. The basal cell layer remains intact, although there may be some disruption in high-grade PIN. There is strong clinical, histological, and molecular evidence linking high-grade PIN with prostate cancer. High-grade PIN is seen in up to 16% of needle biopsies in men over 50 years of age. In malignant prostates, PIN is more frequent and of higher grade than in glands without cancer. The incidence of PIN increases with age, with low-grade PIN occurring in men in their third and fourth decade and high-grade PIN occurring in their fifth decade [7,8].

Chemoprevention

Chemoprevention is an area that shows potential promise as an adjunct or alternative to screening. Potential agents include vitamin E, selenium, zinc, and lycopene as dietary supplements. Other epidemiological associations may also prove appropriate for pharmaceutical development, including inhibitors of cyclooxygenase-2 (COX-2) and insulin-like growth factor-1 (IGF-1) activity. More recently, chemoprevention using the 5α-reductase inhibitor finasteride was tested in the context of a large randomized controlled trial (Prostate Cancer Prevention Trial, PCPT) in the U.S. [9]. In this trial, 18,882 men with serum PSA of 3 ng/mL or lower from the age of 55 years were randomized to finasteride or placebo treatment for 7 years. End-of-study biopsies were performed on the majority of men. There was a reduction in the incidence of prostate cancer by 24.8% in the finasteride compared with the placebo group, although high-grade prostate cancer (Gleason score 7 to 10) was more common in the treatment group. From the screening point of view, one of the important observations in the study was the overall high rate of prostate cancer detection in this cohort of men in comparison with previously published studies of screening. This raises questions as to the real incidence of clinically significant prostate cancer in the general population of men in this age group, the true value of serum PSA measurements, the various thresholds used in detection of the disease, and the possible effect of 5α-reductase inhibition on the biology of prostate cancer. Further analyses of data from this study are awaited.

The Natural History of the Disease Should Be Known

The natural history of prostate cancer in the PSA era is uncertain, because men are far more likely to die *with*, rather than *from*, the disease. The lifetime risk of having microscopic prostate cancer for a man aged 50 years is 42%, although his risk of dying from the disease is about 3% [10]. There is little published long-term outcome data for prostate cancer in the PSA era, which

makes any previous data difficult to translate in contemporary terms. In clinical practice, it has become customary to state that unless a man has a minimum of 10-year life expectancy, conservative therapy is indicated. This appears to stem from the work by Barnes [11] in the late 1960s, who investigated the long-term survival of patients with clinically localized prostate cancer who were treated conservatively. Barnes noted that over two thirds of these patients died from competing medical hazards rather than from their prostate cancer.

Between 1989 and 1997, Johansson et al. [12] carried out a prospective study of the natural history of prostate cancer among 648 men with newly diagnosed prostate cancer from a large county in Sweden. Diagnosis was made by several methods (aspiration cytology of palpable nodules, prostate chips from transurethral resection of the prostate [TURP] or prostate specimens from open surgery for benign prostatic hypertrophy [BPH]), for which the study received criticism. The patients were followed for an average of 14 years, at the end of which the data demonstrated that the higher the stage and grade of the disease, the more likely were the patients to die of prostate cancer, with many men who had well- and moderately differentiated low-volume disease showing a favorable outcome. Johansson et al. concluded that men with early-stage disease were unlikely to benefit from aggressive intervention in the majority of cases. A further multicenter and international analysis by Chodak et al. [13] looked at outcomes in patients receiving no active treatment, and showed similar findings, with poorly differentiated cancers being particularly fatal.

In 1997 Lu-Yao and Yao [14] published data from the Surveillance, Epidemiology, and End Results (SEER) database, evaluating the outcomes of 59,876 patients diagnosed with prostate cancer over a 10-year period. Their results demonstrated that men with poorly differentiated prostate cancer had a 10-fold greater risk of dying from their disease compared to men with well-differentiated tumors, again confirming previous findings.

Albertsen et al. [15,16], using the Connecticut Tumor Registry to identify men diagnosed with localized prostate cancer who had been managed conservatively, explored the impact that coexisting medical problems had on the patients' risk of dying from their cancer. The authors' analysis concluded that men with well-differentiated disease experienced little if any loss of life, whereas patients with moderately to poorly differentiated disease lost between 4 and 8 years of life compared to age-matched controls. Retrospective analysis to look at the impact of comorbidity in this same cohort of patients showed that those men whose competing medical problems placed them in the highest risk categories rarely died of prostate cancer. Among all the men diagnosed with clinically localized disease and treated conservatively, 40% died of competing medical hazards rather than from their prostate cancer within 10 years of diagnosis. Interpreting these studies in the present-day context is difficult, because they do not provide information on PSA-detected tumors.

The PSA testing era is likely to revolutionize these previous observations. Since its introduction in the late 1980s, there has been a dramatic increase in the incidence of prostate cancer. Most men detected through PSA testing having T1c disease, and contemporary lead times are long (6 to 8 years). In 1995 Gann et al. [17] published an analysis of the potential lead time introduced by PSA testing. From among 14,916 male participants in the Physicians' Health Study of trial beta-carotene, they identified 366 men who were diagnosed with prostate cancer within 10 years of follow-up. From the analysis of patient records and histology reports, and using a PSA cutoff value of 4 ng/mL, the authors calculated the diagnostic lead time for all prostate cancer diagnoses to be 5.4 years, and the diagnostic lead time for fatal prostate cancer cases to be 3.6 years. Whereby traditionally, 5-year and 10-year survival statistics (i.e., the proportion of individuals with cancer who are alive 5 or 10 years after diagnosis, respectively) are quoted to demonstrate improvements in cancer management, the introduction of PSA testing has accelerated the date of diagnosis of prostate cancer for many patients. Consequently, this lead-time bias has influenced the perception that contemporary men, with prostate cancer detected through screening, are surviving longer. Welch et al. [18] analyzed 5-year survival outcomes between 1950 and 1995 for 20 common tumors using data from the National Cancer Institute's SEER program. When the results were correlated with the incidence rates

for each cancer, they showed an absolute increase in 5-year survival for each of the tumor types studied, ranging from 3% for pancreatic cancer to 50% for prostate cancer. Over the same period, however, mortality rates declined for 12 tumor types, but increased for the remaining eight. The data showed a positive correlation between increase in 5-year survival for a specific tumor and increase in that tumor's incidence, but little correlation between increase in 5-year survival and change in tumor-related mortality.

There Should Be an Acceptable Screening Instrument for the Disease

The advent of PSA testing in the late 1980s as a simple blood test to indicate the possibility of prostate cancer has revolutionized its diagnosis. Although the triad of PSA, digital rectal examination (DRE), and transrectal ultrasound (TRUS) and biopsies remain conventional in confirming the diagnosis and staging the disease [19], it is now accepted that neither DRE nor TRUS should be included in a screening context for prostate cancer. In the absence of the disease, serum PSA concentrations are known to vary in relation to age and prostate gland volume, and can be raised after ejaculation, prostate biopsy, surgery that involves the prostate, or during prostatitis. Despite these limitations, the acceptability of screening by PSA test has been widely demonstrated. A raised PSA alone, however, is not diagnostic of prostate cancer, as the diagnosis can only be made after biopsy, which itself can be uncomfortable and carries the risks of bleeding and sepsis. PSA cutoff points remain controversial. Using the initial widely accepted serum PSA cutoff level of 4 ng/mL, up to two thirds of cancers can be missed [20]. In a community-based study of serial PSA testing, Catalona et al. [21] found that 22% of men older than 50 years with PSA concentrations between 2.6 and 4.0 µg/mL had prostate cancer. In the European Randomized Study of Screening for Prostate Cancer (ERSPC), 36.5% of detectable prostate cancers were identified in the 87.5% of men who had PSA concentrations lower than 4 ng/mL [22], leading to the reduction of the PSA threshold in the study to 3 ng/mL, and abandonment of DRE as a screening tool [23]. The same protocol was adopted by the U.K. Protect trial, discussed later in this chapter [24].

There Should Be an Accepted and Effective Treatment

Until recently, there was a significant lack of first-degree evidence through large randomized controlled trials that aggressive treatment of localized prostate cancer improves survival or quality of life. Outcomes for different treatment options in men with localized prostate cancer are difficult to interpret, because many of the published studies are observational, contain too small numbers, and are otherwise insufficiently robust. For example, men treated by watchful waiting may have been selected because they are older, with lower grade tumors, whereas those treated by radiotherapy may have been more likely to have more advanced tumors. Therefore, only data from well-conducted large randomized controlled trials can confidently be used to compare treatment options. Such a trial has been performed in Scandinavia, the results of which were published recently [25,26]. The trial randomized 695 men with early prostate cancer to either watchful waiting or radical prostatectomy, with a median follow-up of 6.2 years. The most important findings were a 50% reduction in disease-specific mortality following radical prostatectomy, and a 14% increased risk of progression to metastatic disease as well as a 40% increase in local progression in patients receiving watchful waiting. There was no significant difference in overall mortality between the two groups, but morbidity from the surgery was significant, with 49% of patients experiencing varying degrees of urinary leakage, and 100% erectile dysfunction—results that are incompatible with current standard surgical practice in institutions dealing with large numbers of patients [27]. Further limitations of the study include the following: (1) it essentially preceded the PSA era, since only 5% of cases were detected through screening; (2) more than 50% of men were symptomatic, and 76% had palpable stage T2 tumors, findings that have become unusual in contemporary practice, where most men detected by PSA testing have T1c disease with low PSA levels; (3) the criteria for local pro-

gression in the watchful waiting arm were unreliable, defined by the subjective parameters of DRE and symptoms of bladder outflow obstruction, which may have been related to symptomatic benign enlargement of the prostate; (4) the length of follow-up to date may be insufficient to assess the true impact of the chosen therapy. In addition, 23 patients randomized to radical prostatectomy were found to have positive lymph nodes at surgery, and it is not known whether these patients were subsequently given early hormone manipulation, which may have partly influenced the apparent benefit of surgery. Furthermore, the authors did not present detailed pathological staging of patients receiving radical prostatectomy (i.e., rates of positive margins and upstaging), who may have also received early hormonal ablation. On the basis of the results from this study alone, therefore, one may conclude that the effectiveness of treatment in screen-detected prostate cancer remains so far unproven. In the U.S., the Prostate Cancer Intervention Versus Observation Trial (PIVOT) has been recruiting and randomizing men aged 75 years or younger to a trial of treatment, comparing radical prostatectomy with expectant management, with all-cause mortality as a primary end point. The trial has closed recently, having recruited 731 men, and the results are awaited [28].

In the United Kingdom, the Protect (Prostate Testing for Cancer and Treatment) study is a randomized controlled trial of treatment effectiveness in men with clinically localized prostate cancer initiated in 1999 as a feasibility phase that proved successful [24,29]. The main trial started in 2001, and aims to test 130,000 asymptomatic men aged 50 to 70 years over a period of 5 years. Of those, 1800 patients with clinically localized prostate cancer will be randomized to active monitoring, radical prostatectomy, or radiotherapy. The primary end point will be survival at 10 years, with a number of secondary end points, including detailed quality of life analyses. The study, funded by the Health Technology Assessment panel of the National Health Service (NHS) research and development program, has been extended recently through further support from Cancer Research UK and the Department of Health to include the evaluation of case finding. This effectively converts the Protect study into the intervention arm of a clustered randomized trial of screening. Results will become available within the next decade, at the same time as the other much-awaited screening studies in Europe and the U.S.

Does Screening for Prostate Cancer Reduce Mortality from the Disease?

Since the introduction of the PSA test, screening for early prostate cancer has become prevalent in the United States, with, as expected, a sharp rise in the incidence of the disease in the early 1990s. This was contrasted by a static incidence rate in countries where screening was not widely practiced, such as the United Kingdom. However, by 1996 the U.S. started to experience a slow but constant decrease in the prostate cancer mortality rate, which was advocated by some as resulting from early aggressive intervention with the intensive screening program. This conclusion is flawed by a number of problems. First, in view of the protracted natural history of the disease, it is unlikely that early treatment could have caused this reduction in mortality within such a short time period. Second, similar reductions in mortality rates were observed in countries where screening had not been adopted, such as England and Wales, and the Netherlands, suggesting that other factors, including diet and environmental factors yet to be determined, must have been involved in this continuing reduction in mortality from the disease [30,31]. A similar trend to that observed in the U.S. was seen in the Tyrol region of Austria, where in 1993 PSA testing was made freely available to all male inhabitants of ages 45 to 75 years. The effects of this intensive screening, and treatment of early disease, has been associated with a significant reduction in mortality from prostate cancer between 1993 and 1999, which was in contrast to the modest downward trend in prostate cancer death rates observed throughout the rest of Austria [32]. Again, this cause-and-effect association has yet to be confirmed, but it is clear that current reduction in mortality in Tyrol cannot be attributed to screening alone.

More recently, Lu-Yao et al. [33] analyzed mortality data between two areas of the U.S. with substantially different rates of screening and treatment. Several studies had previously docu-

mented that the frequency of PSA testing, prostate biopsy, and radical prostatectomy among men in the Seattle–Puget Sound area was initially higher than in Connecticut. Using the SEER database, Lu-Yao et al. analyzed data from 94,000 men in Seattle and 120,621 men in Connecticut over an 11-year follow-up period, with the conclusion that in Seattle, intensive PSA screening (5.39-fold compared with Connecticut), and treatment (5.9-fold for radical prostatectomy and 2.3-fold for radiotherapy) did not lead to an improved disease-specific survival rate from prostate cancer, compared with the Connecticut practice.

How Can We Study Screening?

As mentioned above, screening for prostate cancer can be studied by randomized controlled trials such as the ones currently underway in Europe and the U.S. These involve randomizing a population of men at risk of harboring the disease, with good life expectancy, to either an intensive screening program or to no screening. The outcome is measured by analyzing differences in mortality between the two groups, on the assumption that the screened group would have received early aggressive intervention, compared with the nonscreened group. The ERSPC trial, and the Prostate, Lung, Colon, and Ovary (PLCO) cancer trial in the U.S. represent such examples [34]. The ERSPC trial is a large international cooperative study that was initiated in 1994 involving the Netherlands, Belgium, Finland, Italy, Sweden, Spain, and Switzerland, and was planned with a total sample of 190,000 men aged 55 to 74 years. However, over time, targets have changed, and it is now estimated that 120,000 and 140,000 men will be required in the intervention and control arms, respectively. These changes were implemented to take into account the variability of the countries involved, increased knowledge about compliance within the study, and the increasing rate of contamination (i.e., men in the control arm seeking PSA screening for prostate cancer and potentially receiving subsequent treatment), which was ranging from 10% to 30%. Randomization to the large PLCO study was initiated in 1993. The aim of both studies was originally to detect a 20% mortality reduction in the screened population, with a statistical power of 90%. Data from the prostate arm of the PLCO trial will be merged with ERSPC trial data, and results are expected by approximately 2008. However, treatments are not defined in these studies, and a significant proportion of men may opt for watchful waiting. This is compounded by the uncertainty of treatment effectiveness, and ever-increasingly sensitive methods of detection, which may not allow the screening studies to show differences sufficient to have an impact on public health policies. Despite these reservations, results are eagerly awaited, and will represent a phenomenal milestone in determining the value of PSA-driven screening in reducing mortality from prostate cancer, complemented by the U.K. Protect study.

What Do Men with Prostate Cancer Think of Screening for the Disease?

Public perception of screening for the disease varies. There is widespread pressure for the establishment of national screening programs, with resistance to this pressure often misinterpreted as attempts to save money, deceive the public, or even as sex discrimination. A recent interesting and elegant qualitative research study by Chapple et al. [35] highlighted these feelings, interviewing 52 men with prostate cancer from various geographical areas of the U.K. Although some factual conceptions were revealed, there were also many misconceptions, such as early diagnosis brings better chances of cure, 5-year survival figures in the U.S. are higher than in Britain because of PSA screening programs, PSA testing is not taking place because of lack of resources in the NHS, men should be tested for prostate cancer as women are for breast cancer, men with urinary tract symptoms should all be tested for prostate cancer, and the government is not spending enough money on prostate cancer treatment. These examples of arguments from men with the disease can be mostly refuted, and reflect a profound lack of knowledge about prostate cancer in the general population, compounded by misleading information in the media. However, as eloquently stated in a recent editorial by Thornton and Dixon-Woods [36], these arguments convey "the

irresistible logic of finding the cancer early, the drive to avoid regretting later the decision not to have the test, the right to obtain information about oneself by testing, and a perceived right to parity with women's access to screening, which may all be important arguments." The study also showed clearly how ill prepared men are to suffer the consequences of screening, and the controversies surrounding treatment issues. The public does not appear to perceive an important aspect and consequence of screening, as again highlighted by Thornton and Dixon-Woods: "that screening is about changing identities, and becoming a patient, which is no trivial matter." It is therefore our duty not only to inform and educate men about these difficult issues, but also to engage them firmly into decision and policy making in the management of prostate cancer.

Screening Policies Worldwide

Because of the uncertainties described above, it is not surprising to find that screening policies for prostate cancer differ considerably among countries where prevalence is high. A recent survey of large numbers of countries requested three specific pieces of information [37]: (1) Does the country have a mass screening program? (2) Does the country encourage and allow early detection? and (3) Is the PSA test reimbursable? Interestingly, the only country that appears to have a mass screening program for prostate cancer is one of the smallest, Luxembourg. A large proportion of countries allow early detection, and a few reimburse the cost of PSA tests, but opinions and practices are divided. For instance in the U.S., the American Cancer Society and American Urological Association recommend prostate screening for all men aged 50 years and older, whereas the U.S. Preventative Services Task Force, American Academy of Family Physicians, and American College of Physicians recommend not screening for prostate cancer [38–41].

In the U.K., opinions are divided. Some clinicians and a large part of the public, driven by patient support groups and the media, advocate screening for prostate cancer as a public health policy. Others promote joining ongoing trials of screening in Europe, or advocate testing treatment effectiveness before screening. In the early

1990s, a pilot study of screening was undertaken in the southwest, suggesting that British men would be amenable to a mass screening program [42]. In 1996 the British government commissioned two key systematic reviews of the literature [43,44]. These reviews led to the recommendation by health ministers that there was currently insufficient evidence to establish screening as a public health policy in the U.K., and that PSA measurement in asymptomatic men should be discouraged. In the year 2000, however, further recommendations were made, allowing men who request a PSA test to receive it, providing that adequate counseling is delivered regarding the uncertainties about the detection and treatment of prostate cancer [45]. Furthermore, in an attempt to generally improve delivery of cancer services in the U.K., the Department of Health requested that all men whose PSA is elevated over 4 ng/mL should be seen by a urological surgeon within 2 weeks for further management. The intellectual incompatibility between these rules and existing evidence about screening and the treatment of prostate cancer is flagrant, adding confusion to the existing uncertainties for physicians and patients alike.

Conclusion

The dilemmas surrounding the value of screening and treatment in clinically localized prostate cancer remain unresolved. Recently published work from Scandinavia sheds some light into potential benefits of radical prostatectomy in preventing patients from dying from prostate cancer, although aggressive treatment did not improve overall survival compared with watchful waiting. Results from the now-merged ERSPC in Europe and PLCO in the U.S., the Protect study in the U.K., and the PIVOT study in the U.S. are awaited eagerly. It is reassuring for the medical community and prostate cancer patients worldwide that these long-standing dilemmas in the management of prostate are being resolved through large and robust randomized controlled trials supported by governments and funding institutions in Europe and the U.S.

References

1. Wilson JMG, Jungner G. Principles and Practice of Screening for Disease. Public health paper No. 34. Geneva: World Health Organization, 1968.
2. Jenson OM, Esteve J, Renhard H. Cancer in the European Community and its member states. Eur J Cancer 1990;26:1167–1256.
3. Greenlee RT, Hill-Harmon MB, Murray T, et al. Cancer statistics 2001. CA Cancer J Clin 2001;5: 15–36.
4. Diamond TH, Higano CS, Smith MR, Guise TA, Singer FR. Osteoporosis in men with prostate carcinoma receiving androgen-deprivation therapy: recommendations for diagnosis and therapies. Cancer 2004;100(5):892–899.
5. Smith MR, Eastham J, Gleason DM, Shasha D, Tchekmedyian S, Zinner N. Randomized controlled trial of zoledronic acid to prevent bone loss in men receiving androgen deprivation therapy for nonmetastatic prostate cancer. J Urol 2003;169(6):2008–2012.
6. Schaid DJ. The complex genetic epidemiology of prostate cancer. Hum Mol Genet 2004;13(special No. 1):R103–121.
7. Sakr WA. Haas GP, Cassin BF, Pontes JE, Crissman JD. The frequency of carcinoma and intraepithelial neoplasia of the prostate in young male patients. J Urol 1993;150:379–385.
8. Häggman MJ, Macoska JA, Wojna KJ, Oesterling JE. The relationship between prostatic intraepithelial neoplasia and prostate cancer: critical issues. J Urol 1997;158:12–22.
9. Thompson IM, Goodman PJ, Tangen CM, et al. The influence of finasteride on the development of prostate cancer. N Engl J Med 2003;349(3): 215–224.
10. Whitmore WF Jr. Localised prostate cancer: management and detection issues 1994. Lancet 1994; 343:1263–1267.
11. Barnes RW. Survival with conservative therapy. JAMA 1969;210:331–332.
12. Johansson J, Holmberg L, Johansson S, et al. Fifteen-year survival in prostate cancer. A prospective population based study in Sweden. JAMA 1997;227:467–471.
13. Chodak GW, Thisted RA, Gerber GS, et al. Results of conservative management of clinically localized prostate cancer. N Engl J Med 1994;330: 242–248.
14. Lu-Yao GL, Yao SL. Population based study of long-term survival in patients with clinically localised prostate cancer. Lancet 1997;349:906–910.
15. Albertsen PC, Frybeck DG, Storer BE, et al. Long-term survival among men with conservatively

treated localized prostate cancer. JAMA 1995;274: 626–631.

16. Albertsen PC, Hanley JA, Gleson DF, et al. A competing risk analysis of men aged 55–74 years at diagnosis managed conservatively for clinically localized prostate cancer. JAMA 1998;280:975–980.

17. Gann PH, Hennekens CH, Sampfer MJ. A prospective evaluation of plasma prostate specific antigen for detection of prostatic cancer. JAMA 1992;273:289–294.

18. Welch HG, Schwartz LM, Woloshin S. Are increasing 5-year survival rates evidence for success against cancer? JAMA 2000;283(2):2975–2978.

19. Wilkinson BA, Hamdy FC. State-of-the-art staging in prostate cancer. BJU Int 2001;87(5):423–430.

20. Kranse R, Beemsterboer P, Rietbergen J, et al. Predictors for biopsy outcome in the European Randomized Study of Screening for Prostate Cancer (Rotterdam Region). Prostate 1999;39: 316–322.

21. Catalona WJ, Smith DS, Ornstein DK. Prostate cancer detection in men with serum PSA concentrations of 2.6 to 4.0 ng/mL and benign prostate examination: enhancement of specificity with free PSA measurements. JAMA 1997;277:1452–1455.

22. Schröder FH, van der Cruijsen-Koeter I, Koning HJ, et al. Prostate cancer detection at low prostate specific antigen. J Urol 2000;163:806–812.

23. Schröder FH, van der Maas P, Beemsterboer P, et al. Evaluation of the digital rectal examination as a screening test for prostate cancer. Rotterdam section of the European Randomized Study of Screening for Prostate Cancer. J Natl Cancer Inst 1998;90(23):1817–1823.

24. Donovan JL, Hamdy FC, Neal DE, et al. Prostate testing for cancer and treatment (Protect) feasibility study. Health Technol Assess 2003;7(14).

25. Holmberg L, Bill-Axelson A, Helgesen F, et al. A randomised trial comparing radical prostatectomy with watchful waiting in early prostate cancer: Scandinavian Prostatic Cancer Group Study Number 4. N Engl J Med 2002;347:781–789.

26. Steineck G, Helgesen F, Adolfsson J, et al. Quality of life after radical prostatectomy or watchful waiting. Scandinavian Prostatic Cancer Group Study Number 4. N Engl J Med 2002;347:790–796.

27. Begg CB, Riedel CR, Bach PB, et al. Variations in morbidity after radical prostatectomy. N Engl J Med 2002;346:1138–1144.

28. Wilt TJ, Brawer MK. The prostate Cancer Intervention Versus Observation Trial (PIVOT). Oncology (Huntington) 1997;11(8):1133–1139.

29. Donovan J, Mills N, Smith M, et al. Improving design and conduct of randomised trials by embedding them in qualitative research: Protect (Prostate Testing for Cancer and Treatment) study. BMJ 2002;325:766–770.

30. Oliver SE, Gunnell D, Donovan JL. Comparison of trends in prostate cancer mortality in England and Wales and the USA. Lancet 2000;355:1788–1789.

31. Schröder FH, Wildhagen MF. Screening for prostate cancer: evidence and perspectives. BJU Int 2001;88:811–817.

32. Bartsch G, Horninger W, Klocker H, et al. Prostate cancer mortality after introduction of prostate specific antigen mass screening in the Federal State of Tyrol, Austria. Urology 2001;58:417–424.

33. Lu-Yao G, Albertsen PC, Stanford JL, et al. Natural experiment examining impact of aggressive screening and treatment on prostate cancer mortality in two fixed cohorts from Seattle area and Connecticut. BMJ 2002;325:740–745.

34. de Koning HJ, Auvinen A, Berenguer Sanchez A, et al. European Randomized Screening for Prostate Cancer (ERSPC) Trial; International Prostate Cancer Screening Trials Evaluation Group. Large-scale randomised prostate cancer screening trials: program performances in the European Randomized Screening for Prostate Cancer trial and the Prostate, Lung, Colorectal and Ovary Cancer trial. Int J Cancer 2002;97:237–244.

35. Chapple A, Ziebland S, Sheppard S, et al. Why men with prostate cancer want wider access to prostate specific antigen testing: qualitative study. BMJ 2002;325:737–739.

36. Thornton H, Dixon-Woods M. Prostate specific antigen testing for prostate cancer. BMJ 2002;325: 725–726.

37. Perrin P. Personal communication, 2002.

38. Mettlin C, Jones G, Avetett H, et al. Defining and updating the American Cancer Society guidelines for the cancer-related check-up: prostate and endometrial cancers. Cancer J Clin 1993;43:42–46.

39. American Urological Association. Early detection of prostate and cancer use of transrectal ultrasound. In: AUA, ed. American Urological Association 1992 Policy Statement Book. Baltimore: American Urological Association, 1992:4–20.

40. U.S. Preventative Service Task Force. Screening for Prostate Cancer: Guide to Clinical Preventative Services, 2nd ed. Baltimore: Williams & Wilkins, 1996:119.

41. American College of Physicians. Screening for prostate cancer. Ann Intern Med 1997;126: 480–484.

42. Chadwick DJ, Kemple T, Astley JP, et al. Pilot study of screening for prostate cancer in general practice. Lancet 1991;338:613–616.

43. Selley S, Donovan J, Faulkner A, et al. Diagnosis, management and screening of early localised prostate cancer. Health Technol Assess 1997;1(2): i, 1–96.

44. Cheamberlain J, Melia J, Moss S, et al. The diagnosis, management, treatment and costs of prostate cancer in England and Wales. Health Technol Assess 1997;1(3):i–iv, 1–53.

45. Milburn A. http://www.doh.gov.uk/cancer, 2000.

4

Diet and Prostate Cancer

Danish Mazhar

Prostate cancer is the most commonly diagnosed malignancy in men in industrialized countries and the second leading cause of male cancer-related death. Given the trebling of death rates in the last 30 years and the relative lack of a survival benefit from the treatment of advanced disease, it is critical that we look at preventative stratagems to reduce death rates. Although aging is the most significant risk factor for prostate cancer with a virtually exponential increase in age-related incidence and mortality, prostate cancer is also characterized by a marked variation in its worldwide incidence. Superficially, it would seem to be difficult to separate environmental factors from racial factors in explaining this difference in the incidence of this tumor, but studies of migrant populations suggest that environment is overwhelmingly more significant than genetics in the origins of this cancer. For example, when migrants from a low-risk country such as Japan move to the United States, a high-risk nation, their prostate cancer incidence and mortality become severalfold higher than native Japanese counterparts [1]. Moreover, a positive correlation exists between the number of years since migration to the United States and cancer risk [2]. Diet is one of the environmental factors suspected to play a role in the etiology of prostate cancer. High dietary intakes of diary products, meat, and fat, and low consumption of tomatoes, selenium, and vitamins D and E have all been associated with higher prostate cancer risk.

Is the current balance of laboratory, epidemiological and clinical data strong enough to prove a direct relation between diet and prostate cancer? Does it already warrant dietary modifications or the use of nutritional supplements? Are we currently in a position to advise men about how they can minimize their risk of developing prostate cancer by manipulating what they eat?

Diet and Prostate Cancer Biology

Although prostate cancer is primarily a disease of older men, neoplastic changes may occur in the prostatic epithelium as early as in the third decade. The time required for some of these early neoplastic transformations is likely to be long. Some dietary compounds display antioxidant properties, thus preventing peroxidation and generation of free radicals with potential DNA-damaging effects. Others are inhibitors of cell proliferation, apoptosis inducers, or enhancers of cellular differentiation. Some may act at a hormonal level, as the prostate is an androgen-regulated organ. In many cases, though, the precise pathways modulated by these compounds and mechanisms of DNA damage induced by carcinogenic agents are still poorly understood.

Fat

Laboratory Studies

There is conflicting preclinical evidence of a possible association between fat and prostate cancer. Studies in several animal models have shown increased tumor growth with high fat intake and inhibition of growth with low levels of fat intake [3,4]. Wang et al. [3] injected androgen-dependent LNCaP human prostate cancer cells into mice and placed them on a diet containing 40% fat. In 3 weeks, prostate cancer growth was noted. The animals were then divided into subgroups receiving diets containing approximately 40%, 30%, 20%, 10%, and 2% of calories as fat. Tumor progression ceased or was reversed in some animals placed on 10% and 20% fat diets. This was in contrast to continued tumor growth in groups ingesting higher amounts of fat. Levels of prostate-specific antigen (PSA) were also lower in mice on the 2% fat diet as compared to those on the 40% fat diet [3].

Other reported studies that have controlled for isonutrient intake have not shown relationships between transplanted prostate carcinoma growth or the induction of prostate cancer by varying dietary fat [5–7]. However, an investigation examining the relation between prostate cancer and fat and energy intakes is instructive [8]. Androgen-sensitive prostate tumors from donor rats were transplanted into rats that were then fed either fat-restricted or carbohydrate-restricted diets. In a parallel experiment, severe combined immunodeficient mice were injected with LNCaP cells to produce tumors and were fed similar diets. The subsequent tumor shrinkage was found to be independent of the percentage of fat in the diet, as long as the total energy was restricted. The reduction in tumor growth was similar in both types of energy-restricted laboratory animal. These experiments suggest that a reduction in energy intake, and not just fat, is needed to reduce prostate cancer growth.

Epidemiologic and Clinical Studies

Most of the available clinical evidence regarding the effect of dietary fat intake on prostate cancer comes from observational rather than interventional studies. A close correlation exists between average per capita fat intake and prostate cancer mortality in numerous countries round the world [9]. Japanese and Chinese men who migrate to the United States experience dramatic increases in prostate cancer risk within one generation compared to their Caucasian neighbors [10]. Numerous case-control studies over the past 25 years have demonstrated a positive correlation between prostate cancer and increased fat or fat-type food consumption. Such studies include an analysis of 384 men diagnosed with prostate cancer between 1990 and 1992 in Quebec, Canada [11]. On average, after controlling for age, grade, clinical stage, initial treatment, and total energy intake, saturated fat consumption was significantly associated with disease-specific survival. Compared with men in the lower tercile of saturated fat intake, those in the upper tercile had three times the risk of dying from prostate cancer. Another study has reported an attributable risk of 13% for saturated fat intake in excess of 26 g per day as compared to diets with less than 13 g per day [12].

However, other studies have failed to show an association between prostate cancer and total fat or total saturated fat. A prospective study of 6763 white male Seventh-Day Adventists observed for 21 years failed to find a significant relation between prostate cancer risk and fat-associated food—meat or poultry, milk, cheese, and eggs. There was a suggested positive association that was stronger when an individual consumed all four of these dietary items, but overall there was no significant relation between diet and prostate cancer [13]. A further finding of this study was that overweight men had a significantly higher risk of dying from prostate cancer compared with nonobese men (relative risk 2.5). Another cohort study of 7999 men of Japanese ancestry living in Hawaii also found no association between fat and prostate cancer risk [14].

The largest cohort study examining the relation between fat and prostate cancer risk was the Netherlands Cohort Study [15]. For over 6 years, approximately 58,000 men were observed and 642 cases of prostate cancer were documented. An extensive 150-item food frequency questionnaire was used. No significant association was found between total fat or subtypes of fat and prostate cancer risk. The average intake of fat as a percentage of total calories in this study was high (40%), so any influence of extremely low levels of fat or reduced calorie intake and prostate cancer risk was not mentioned. Another large cohort study involved 47,855 men who were sent biannually an expanded food frequency questionnaire with 131 items. There was a positive association of fat but no statistically significant difference was found [16]. Linoleic acid, which is the major polyunsaturated fat in most diets, has been associated with an increased risk of prostate carcinoma in some studies [17,18]. It is difficult, though, for adequate conclusions to be drawn from these investigations because of the potential for recall bias and confounding. Omega-3 fatty acids, obtained mainly from fatty fish, have been shown to inhibit prostate cancer cell lines in laboratory experiments [19]. The Netherlands Cohort Study found a potential protective effect of omega-3 fatty acids, but this was not statistically significant [15].

Only one large prospective study has demonstrated a statistically significant finding between high-fat foods and prostate cancer [20]. This study involved a cohort of 20,316 men of multiethnic backgrounds living in Hawaii. There were 198 cases of prostate cancer documented during follow-up that ranged from 9 to 14 years. The relative risks for consuming beef, milk, and high-fat foods were 1.6, 1.4, and 1.6, respectively. However, a closer look at the study showed that the food questionnaire assessed only 13 dietary items. In addition, height was demonstrated as being the largest risk factor for prostate cancer with the most significance ($p < .01$), compared with food associations with fat ($p < .05$). Furthermore, high intakes of milk and beef were not found for this cohort, so these could not be compared with the lowest intakes to determine whether there was a consistent trend with these dietary variables. Another cohort study, the Physicians' Health Study, also found an association between red meat consumption and prostate cancer risk, but this association was not statistically significant [21].

Vitamins

Vitamin E is thought to prevent oxidation and peroxidation of membrane phospholipids. It has been shown in one study to inhibit growth of established prostate LNCaP tumors in nude mice [22]. Long-term supplementation with α-tocopherol, a form of vitamin E, was found to significantly reduce prostate cancer incidence and mortality in smokers [23]. In the U.S. Health Professional Study, supplemental vitamin E was not associated with prostate cancer risk [24]. However, an inverse association between supplemental vitamin E and the risk of metastatic or fatal prostate cancer among smokers was suggested. Caution, though, should be exercised in interpreting these data because of the possible bias in end-point assessment and the use of different types of vitamin E. Whether the inclusion of smokers affected the result also requires consideration.

Laboratory studies have shown decreased proliferation activity and increased differentiation activity of vitamin D on malignant prostate cells. Moreover, epidemiological evidence shows an inverse relationship between prostate cancer risk and ultraviolet radiation, the primary source of endogenous vitamin D synthesis [25]. Cohort studies have suggested that vitamin D is an important determinant of prostate cancer risk. Inherited polymorphisms in the vitamin D receptor gene are associated with the risk and progression of prostate cancer [26]. Clinical studies looking at a possible protective role of vitamin D in prostate cancer are generally lacking. However, one trial in patients with advanced refractory prostate cancer treated with $1,25(OH_2)D_3$ showed a rapid drop in the levels of PSA [27].

Dietary calcium suppresses the formation of $1,25(OH_2)D_3$. It is hypothesized that dietary and supplemental calcium intake or diets high in milk are associated with prostate cancer risk by lowering the serum levels of bioactive metabolites of vitamin D. A clinical study of 47,781 men found a higher consumption of calcium to be related to a risk of advanced prostate cancer (relative risk 2.97) and metastatic cancer (relative risk 4.57) [28]. Milk and calcium intake have been found in cohort studies in five countries to be associated with increased risk of prostate cancer [29].

Carotenoids have been shown to display antioxidant potential. Some carotenoids, such as β-carotene, are precursors of vitamin A, but others such as lycopene, found in tomatoes, are not convertible to vitamin A. In case-control studies, lycopene has been associated with a protective effect on various cancers including prostate cancer [30]. In a cohort study of approximately 14,000 Adventist men over a 6-year period, consumption of tomato products was associated with lower prostate cancer risk [31]. β-carotene, however, has been found in epidemiological studies not to be associated with prostate cancer risk or even associated with an increased risk [32]. To add to the confusion, some studies have suggested that vitamin A may have a protective role in prostate cancer development [33].

Trace Elements

Selenium is a trace element, entering the food chain through plants, and it is present in bread, cereals, fish, chicken, and meat. It is a key component of a number of functional proteins required for normal health, including glutathione peroxidase enzymes, antioxidants that remove hydrogen peroxide, and lipid hydroperoxidases generated in vivo by free radicals. The products of lipid peroxidases have carcinogenic properties. Studies in human prostate cancer cell lines have shown that selenium inhibits cell proliferation at physiological doses and that its protective effect may be mediated through an androgen-sensitive gene that encodes a selenium-binding protein [34,35].

A clinical double-blind study in the United States showed that selenium reduced the overall cancer incidence by 37% and that of prostate cancer by 50% [36]. However, the inclusion criteria were narrow. Similar findings were demonstrated in a nested case-control trial of the Health Professionals' Follow-Up Study. The investigators found that higher selenium intake, as reflected in nail selenium levels, was significantly protective [37].

Plant Steroids

One of the major differences in the diet between Asian and Western countries is the consumption of soy-derived products. A limited amount of clinical evidence points to a beneficial role of soy in reducing the level of androgenic steroids, the biological driving factor for prostate cancer. The beneficial effects of a soy diet have been attributed to isoflavonoids, which are plant pigments found in vegetables, with the soya bean a major source. Genistein and daidzein are the principal soya-derived isoflavones. Davis et al. [38] showed that genistein inhibits prostate cancer cell growth in culture and induces apoptosis in a dose-dependent manner. Others have demonstrated that genistein is an inhibitor of tyrosine kinase and suggest that genistein may act through inhibition of upregulated tyrosine kinases in proliferative cancerous states [39]. Animal studies have also suggested that isoflavones may suppress the development of invasive prostate cancers [40]. There is just one large-scale epidemiological study of the effects of soy-derived products on prostate cancer development. This cross-national study in 59 countries showed that soy products were found to be significantly protective ($p = .0001$), with an effect size per kilocalorie (kcal) at least four times as large as that of any other dietary factor [41].

A protective role for green tea, a beverage consumed in high quantities in Asia, has been suggested by some investigators. In vitro studies by Yang et al. [42] showed that polyphenol extracts from tea inhibited growth of cancer cell lines and induced apoptosis in a dose-dependent manner. Furthermore, studies have demonstrated that tea polyphenols can inhibit ornithine decarboxylase, a testosterone-induced enzyme that is upregulated in prostate cancer [43,44].

Prostate Cancer Risk Reduction by Dietary Modification

Preventive medicine is currently a topical issue. Cardiovascular disease is a well-known example. The identification of atherosclerosis as one of the causative mechanisms of cardiovascular disease has resulted in important lifestyle modifications in diet, tobacco use, and exercise. This has led to a significant decrease in the incidence of heart disease in many countries. Prostate cancer potentially represents an ideal target for chemoprevention because of its long latency. Although the use of new biological strategies is being examined in the context of primary prevention and progression of prostate cancer, it has been suggested that nutrition may also have a role. However, does the weight of current scientific and clinical data support a relation between diet and prostate cancer? Is there enough evidence for us to be able to advise dietary modifications, such as reduced fat and increased soy protein consumption, and the use of nutritional supplements, for example vitamin E and selenium, to reduce the risk of developing or improve outcomes in prostate cancer?

Some of the data are conflicting. In the case of the suggested link between dietary fat and prostate cancer, the balance of the prospective data is at odds with laboratory investigations, international comparisons, and case-control studies. The value of case-control studies is limited because of the potential for recall bias and confounding. Moreover, these studies have been conducted in different populations, have often had different inclusion criteria, and included questionnaires varying substantially from one study to another. Cohort studies have also been subject to bias depending on the methods used. Large randomized trials would provide the most meaningful data, but these are extremely difficult to carry out in this context because of the lengthy follow-up needed with a disease that may take decades to reveal itself.

Though we are not at a stage where we can justifiably advise patients to, say, cut their fat intake to reduce the chances of their developing prostate cancer, we should not ignore what is already known about the benefits of dietary manipulation. So reducing animal fat and consuming more oily fish may or may not prevent prostate cancer, but we know these measures will reduce the risk of cardiovascular disease. Practical and simple dietary changes should always be encouraged by health professionals because they could improve the overall quality and longevity of the lives of their patients. Although controlled enthusiasm about diets and their effect on specific diseases is appropriate, we must not let ourselves get carried away with the hype that is borne of our politically correct times.

References

1. Shimizu H, Ross RK, Bernstein L, Yatani R, Henderson BE, Mack TM. Cancers of the prostate and breast among Japanese and white immigrants in Los Angeles County. Br J Cancer 1991;63:963–966.
2. Whittemore AS, Kolonel LN, Wu AH, et al. Prostate cancer in relation to diet, physical activity and body size in blacks, whites, and Asians in the United States and Canada. J Natl Cancer Inst 1995;87:652–661.
3. Wang Y, Corr JG, Thaler HT, Tao Y, Fair WR, Heston WD. Decreased growth of established human prostate LNCap tumors in nude mice fed a low fat diet. J Natl Cancer Inst 1995;87:1456–1462.
4. Pollard M, Luckert PH. Promotional effects of testosterone and high fat diet on the development of autochthonous prostate cancer in rats. Cancer Lett 1986;32:223–227.
5. Bosland MC, Dreef van der Meulen HC, Scherrehberg PM. Effect of dietary fat on rat prostate carcinogenesis induced by N-methyl-N-nitrosurea and testosterone. Proc Am Assoc Cancer Res 1990;31:144.
6. Pour PM, Groot K, Kazakoff K, Anderson K, Schally AV. Effects of high-fat diet on the patterns of prostate cancer induced in rats by N-nitrosobis (2-oxopropyl)amine and testosterone. Cancer Res 1991;51:4757–4761.
7. Clinton SK, Palmer SS, Spriggs CE, Visek WJ. Growth of Dunning transplantable prostate adenocarcinomas in rats fed diets with venous fat content. J Nutr 1988;118:908–914.
8. Mukherjee P, Sotnikov AV, Mangian HJ, Zhou JR, Visek WJ, Clinton SK. Energy intake and prostate tumour growth, angiogenesis, and vascular endothelial growth factor expression. J Natl Cancer Inst 1999;91:512–523.
9. Rose DP, Boyar AP, Wynder EL. International comparisons of mortality rates for cancer of the breast, ovary, prostate and colon, and per capita food consumption. Cancer 1986;58:2363–2371.
10. Muir CS, Nectoux J, Staszewski J. The epidemiology of prostatic cancer: geographical distribution and time trends. Acta Oncol 1991;30:133–140.
11. Bairati I, Meyer F, Fradet Y, Moore L. Dietary fat and advanced prostate cancer. J Urol 1998;159:1271–1275.
12. Hankin JH, Zhao LP, Wilkens LR, Kolonel LN. Attributable risk of breast, prostate, and lung cancer in Hawaii due to saturated fat. Cancer Causes Control 1992;3:17–23.
13. Snowdon DA, Phillips RL, Choi W. Diet, obesity and risk of fatal prostate cancer. Am J Epidemiol 1984;120:244–250.
14. Severson RK, Nomura AM, Grove JS, Stemmermann GN. A prospective study of demographics, diet and prostate cancer among men of Japanese ancestry in Hawaii. Cancer Res 1989;49:1857–1860.

15. Schuurman AG, van den Brandt PA, Dorant E, Brants HA, Goldbohm RA. Association of energy and fat intake with prostate cancer risk: results from the Netherlands Cohort Study. Cancer 1999;86:1019–1027.

16. Giovannucci E, Rimm EB, Colditz GA, et al. A prospective study of dietary fat and risk of prostate cancer. J Natl Cancer Inst 1993;85:1571–1579.

17. Godley PA, Campbell MK, Gallagher P, Martinson FE, Mohler JL, Sander RS. Biomarkers of essential fatty acid consumption and risk of prostatic carcinoma. Cancer Epidemiol Biomarkers Prev 1996; 5:889–895.

18. Ramon JM, Bou R, Romea S, et al. Dietary fat intake and prostate cancer risk: a case-control study in Spain. Cancer Causes Control 2000;11: 679–685.

19. Pandalai PK, Pilat MJ, Yamazaki K, Naik H, Pienta KJ. The effects of omega-3 and omega-6 fatty acids on in vitro prostate cancer growth. Anticancer Res 1996;16:815–820.

20. Le Marchand L, Kolonel LN, Wilkens LR, Myers BC, Hirohata T. Animal fat consumption and prostate cancer: a prospective study in Hawaii. Epidemiology 1994;5:276–282.

21. Gann PH, Hennekens CH, Sacks FM, Grodstein F, Giovannucci EL, Stampfer MJ. Prospective study of plasma fatty acids and risk of prostate cancer. J Natl Cancer Inst 1994;89:281–286.

22. Fleshner N, Fair WR, Huryk R, Heston WD. Vitamin E inhibits the high-fat promoted growth of established human prostate LNCaP tumours in nude mice. J Urol 1999;161:1651–1654.

23. Heinonen OP, Albanes D, Virtamo J, et al. Prostate cancer and supplementation with alpha-tocopherol and beta-carotene: incidence and mortality in a controlled trial. J Natl Cancer Inst 1990;90:440–446.

24. Chan JM, Stampfer MJ, Ma J, Rimm EB, Willett WC, Giovannucci EL. Supplemental vitamin E intake and prostate cancer risk in a large cohort of men in the United States. Cancer Epidemiol Biomarkers Prev 1999;8:893–899.

25. Hanchette CL, Schwartz GG. Geographic patterns of prostate cancer mortality. Evidence for a protective effect of ultraviolet radiation. Cancer 1992;70:2861–2869.

26. Habuchi T, Suzuki T, Sasaki R et al. Association of vitamin D receptor gene polymorphism with prostate cancer and benign prostatic hyperplasia in a Japanese population. Cancer Res 2000;60: 305–308.

27. Konety BR, Johnson CS, Trump DL, Getzenberg RH. Vitamin D in the prevention and treatment of prostate cancer. Semin Urol Oncol 1999;17:77–84.

28. Giovannucci E, Rimm EB, Wolk A, et al. Calcium and fructose intake in relation to risk of prostate cancer. Cancer Res 1998;58:442–447.

29. Grant WB. An ecological study of dietary links to prostate cancer. Altern Med Rev 1999;4:162–169.

30. Giovannucci E. Tomatoes, tomato-based products, lycopene, and cancer: review of the epidemiological literature. J Natl Cancer Inst 1999;91:317–331.

31. Mills PK, Beeson WL, Phillips RL, Fraser GE. Cohort study of diet, lifestyle, and prostate cancer in Adventist men. Cancer 1989;64:598–604.

32. Schulman CC, Ekane S, Zlotta AR. Nutrition and prostate cancer: evidence or suspicion? Urology 2001;58:318–334.

33. Hirayama T. Epidemiology of prostate cancer with special reference to the role of diet. Natl Cancer Inst Monogr 1979;53:149–155.

34. Webber MM, Perez-Ripoll EA, James GT. Inhibitory effects of selenium on the growth of DU-145 human prostate carcinoma cells in vitro. Biochem Biophys Res Commun 1985;130:603–609.

35. Yang M, Sytkowski AJ. Differential expression and androgen regulation of the human selenium-binding protein gene hSP56 in prostate cancer cells. Cancer Res 1998;58:3150–3153.

36. Clark LC, Dalkin B, Krongrad A, et al. Decreased incidence of prostate cancer with selenium supplementation: results of a double-blind cancer prevention trial. Br J Urol 1998;81:730–734.

37. Yoshizawa K, Willett WC, Morris SJ, et al. Study of prediagnostic selenium level in toe nails and risk of advanced prostate cancer. J Natl Cancer Inst 1998;90:1219–1224.

38. Davis JN, Singh B, Bhuiyan M, Sarkar FH. Genistein-induced upregulation of p21WAF 1, downregulation of cyclin B, and induction of apoptosis in prostate cancer cells. Nutr Cancer 1998;32:123–131.

39. Akiyama T, Ishida J, Nakagawa S, et al. Genistein, a specific inhibitor of tyrosine–specific protein kinases. J Biol Chem 1987;262:5592–5595.

40. Aronson WJ, Tymchuk CN, Elashoff RM, et al. Decreased growth of human prostate LNCaP tumours in SCID mice fed to a low-fat, soy protein diet with isoflavones. Nutr Cancer 1999;35:130–136.

41. Hebert JR, Hurley TG, Olendzki BC, Teas J, Ma Y, Hampl JS. Nutritional and socioeconomic factors in relation to prostate cancer mortality: a cross-national study. J Natl Cancer Inst 1998;90:1637–1647.

42. Yang GY, Liao J, Kim K, Yurkow EJ, Yang CS. Inhibition of growth and induction of apoptosis in

human cancer cells by tea polyphenols. Carcino-genesis 1998;19:611–616.

43. Mohan RR, Challa A, Gupta S, et al. Overexpression of ornithine decarboxylase in prostate cancer and prostatic fluid in humans. Clin Cancer Res 1999;5:143–147.

44. Gupta S, Ahmad N, Mohan RR, Husain MM, Mukhtar H. Prostate cancer chemoprevention by green tea: in vitro and in vivo inhibition of testosterone-mediated induction of ornithine decarboxylase. Cancer Res 1999;59:2115–2120.

5

Radical Radiotherapy for Prostate Cancer

Mererid Evans and Malcolm D. Mason

The incidence of prostate cancer is rising worldwide due to the ageing of the population and the increasing availability of prostate-specific antigen (PSA) screening. Prostate-specific antigen testing has led specifically to an increase in the proportion of patients diagnosed with early-stage (localized) prostate cancer. Radical radiotherapy is one of the curative treatment options for localized prostate cancer and it also has a role to play in locally advanced and even metastatic disease. This chapter reviews the relative merits of radiotherapy in comparison to the other management options for early prostate cancer and summarizes the staggering technological advances that have occurred in prostate radiotherapy over the last decade.

Treatment of Early (Localized) Prostate Cancer

The Role of Radical Radiotherapy

The optimum management of patients with localized prostate cancer remains controversial. Three major treatment options are available: radical prostatectomy, radical radiotherapy (external beam radiotherapy [EBRT] or brachytherapy), and active surveillance (also known as active monitoring and watchful waiting). Each treatment involves its own risk. Radical treatments can cause harmful side effects including incontinence, erectile dysfunc-

tion, and even death, whereas watchful waiting causes anxiety relating to the presence of cancer and carries a risk of disease progression. However, outcomes in terms of overall survival appear similar with each of the three modalities.

There is relatively little randomized evidence concerning the effectiveness of the different management options for early prostate cancer. In a Scandinavian study [1], men with early prostate cancer (stages T1b-c or T2) were randomly assigned to radical prostatectomy or watchful waiting. After a median follow-up of 6.2 years, there was a significant reduction in disease-specific mortality in the radical prostatectomy group compared with the watchful waiting group (4.6% vs. 8.9%, $P = .02$), but there was no significant difference in overall survival between the two groups. A randomized trial comparing surgery with radiotherapy published in 1982 showed better survival outcomes in the surgery group [2]. However, this was a small (97 patients), single-center trial conducted in the pre-PSA era, and it is unlikely to be relevant to contemporary practice. Unfortunately, a United Kingdom Medical Research Council (MRC) trial (PR06) randomizing patients to radical prostatectomy, radical radiotherapy, and watchful waiting was closed in 1997 because of poor recruitment, which was attributed to an unwillingness among participants and clinicians to accept randomization.

A number of nonrandomized, retrospective studies have compared the outcomes of the different treatment modalities for early prostate cancer. A study from Boston compared outcomes in 2254 men treated with radical prostatectomy and 381 men treated with conventional dose (66 Gy) radiotherapy [3]. There was a possible advantage for surgery in low-risk patients, but no difference between treatment modalities in intermediate or high-risk cases. Another study from the Cleveland Clinic compared outcomes in 1054 men who underwent radical prostatectomy and 628 treated with radiotherapy [4]. When stratified by prognostic risk groups, there was no difference in biochemical control between patients undergoing prostatectomy and patients having radiotherapy to dose levels ≥72 Gy; however, the outcome of patients who received lower-dose radiotherapy was less favorable. There are many problems with retrospective comparisons like these, including differences in case selection and length of follow-up, and the inherent disadvantages of analyzing past rather than contemporary practice.

At least two large randomized trials are currently in progress, although their results are not yet available. The United States Prostate Cancer Intervention Versus Observation Trial (PIVOT) is comparing radical prostatectomy and watchful waiting for localized prostate cancer [5]; it opened in 1994 and has now closed to recruitment. The U.K. Protect study (*Prostate Testing for Cancer and Treatment*) combines the identification of men with prostate cancer detected by PSA screening with a randomized trial comparing radical prostatectomy, radical EBRT, and watchful waiting. The issue of randomization to the various treatment options was successfully addressed in a feasibility study, which has aided recruitment into this study, and has shown that with careful management, it is possible to randomize prostate cancer patients into trials such as this.

While the results of these studies are awaited, clinical decision making in early prostate cancer should be tailored to the individual patient and take account of tumor prognosis (Gleason grade, stage, and PSA), background health, life expectancy, and patient preference. It is common to offer curative treatment to men who have a life expectancy of 10 years or more and to consider treatment for men with a life expectancy of 5 years or more if the tumor is poorly differentiated. Treatment-related morbidity and quality-of-life issues are important considerations and

patients should be counseled appropriately. Prostatectomy patients are significantly more likely than radiotherapy patients to experience urinary incontinence (39% to 49% vs. 6% to 7%) and erectile dysfunction (80% to 91% vs. 41% to 55%), whereas radiotherapy patients are more likely to experience bowel urgency (30% to 35% vs. 6% to 7%) [6].

Standard External Beam Radiotherapy (EBRT)

Radical EBRT is an alternative to radical prostatectomy for patients with early, organ-confined prostate cancer (T1-2, N0, M0) and can also be used for patients with nonmetastatic locally advanced disease (T3-T4) where surgery is inappropriate.

Pretreatment Assessment

The primary tumor is assessed by digital rectal examination, cystoscopy, and transrectal ultrasound (TRUS). Staging of systemic disease usually comprises bone scanning and pelvic lymph node imaging (with computed tomography [CT] or magnetic resonance imaging [MRI]), although these investigations are sometimes omitted in patients with particularly "good risk" features. Magnetic resonance imaging scanning is particularly useful in assessing capsular invasion, seminal vesicle involvement, and periapical extension, and can aid treatment planning.

Treatment Planning

Computed tomography planning is now standard practice in most U.K. centers. Prior to the advent of CT planning, the size and position of the prostate was indirectly visualized using a cystourethrogram, putting barium in the rectum and taking orthogonal films, upon which the target volume could be drawn. The target volume is usually defined as the prostate plus all/base of the seminal vesicles, or any grossly visible tumor, with a margin of 1 to 1.5 cm to allow for microscopic spread and for variations in treatment setup (Fig. 5.1). A smaller margin is often allowed at the rectal–prostate interface if there is too much rectum in the high-dose volume. In the absence of macroscopic disease in the seminal vesicles, there is some debate as to whether they

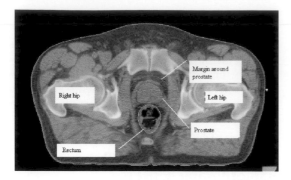

Fig. 5.1. Computed tomography (CT) scan through the center of the target volume showing the rectum, femoral heads, prostate (or clinical target volume, CTV), and a margin around the prostate to be treated to high dose (the planning target volume, PTV).

should be included in the treatment volume or not. Simple formulas for predicting the probability of microscopic seminal vesicle involvement based on the T stage, Gleason score, and pretreatment PSA level can be helpful.

Inconsistencies in treatment volume definition occur among clinicians [7], especially in outlining the prostatic apex, superior aspect of the prostate projecting into the bladder, seminal vesicles, the base of the seminal vesicles, and superior rectum. These should be considered when designing and comparing trials of radiotherapy.

Technique

Patients are treated in the supine position with a full bladder (this helps push bowel out of the high-dose area), once daily, 5 days a week. Skin tattoos are placed anteriorly over the pubic symphysis and laterally over the iliac crests to aid treatment setup. Three-field techniques using an anterior and two posterior oblique fields are commonly used, although four- and even six-field techniques are used in some centers (Fig. 5.2).

Dose and Fractionation

The optimum dose and fractionation schedule for EBRT is unclear. Until recently, standard treatment schedules in many centers delivered daily fractions of 1.8 to 2 Gy per day, to a total dose upwards of 64 Gy.

There is evidence that the α/β ratio for prostate cancer may be as low as 1.5, comparable to late-responding normal tissues, probably because of the slow turnover rate of prostate tumors [8]. This suggests that prostate cancers may be particularly sensitive to hypofractionation and that using larger fraction sizes could result in greater cell kill. In addition to the possible radiobiological gains, other benefits to hypofractionation include shorter overall treatment times and a smaller number of hospital visits, which increases patient convenience and reduces resource utilization.

The outcome of 705 men with T1-4 prostate cancer treated in Manchester with conformal, hypofractionated radiotherapy (50 Gy in 16 daily fractions) has been analyzed [9]. The 5-year biochemical-free survival rates for good, intermediate, and poor prognostic groups were 82%, 56%, and 39%, respectively, which are comparable to published results using conventional fractionation, and normal tissue toxicity rates were not increased. The results of the first randomized study of hypofractionated radiotherapy for localized prostate cancer were presented at the 45th annual meeting of the American Society for Therapeutic Radiology and Oncology (ASTRO) [10]; 936 patients with T1/T2 prostate cancer were randomized at 16 Canadian centers to receive either 66 Gy in 33 fractions over $6^1/_2$ weeks or 52.5 Gy in 20 fractions over 4 weeks. After a median follow-up of 59 months, the treatment failure rate appeared to be slightly higher in the hypofractionated arm than

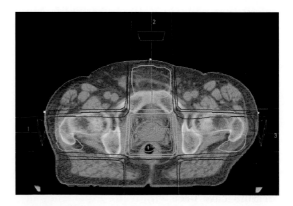

Fig. 5.2. Three-field technique for prostate radiotherapy showing the 10, 20, 50, 70, 90, 95, 100, and 102 isodoses. The CTV, PTV, and rectum are outlined.

in the conventional arm, but there was no significant difference between the two groups in biopsy positivity 2 years after radiotherapy or in overall survival (with a trend for both in favor of the hypofractionated arm). Also, although acute toxicity was higher in the hypofractionated group, late toxicity was similar in both groups.

The development of conformal radiotherapy has led to a surge of interest in dose escalation (above 70 Gy), which is discussed later in the chapter.

Toxicity

The side effects of EBRT can be divided into acute and late reactions. Acute reactions start about halfway through a course of treatment and principally involve the bladder (cystitis) and bowel (proctitis, occasional enteritis). These effects normally settle with conservative management within 4 to 6 weeks of the end of treatment. Rarely, severe acute side effects may necessitate a break in treatment, but it is unusual for acute effects to be dose limiting in practice. It is rare for patients to experience significant skin toxicity with EBRT, though a reaction is not infrequently seen superior to the natal cleft due to the exit dose from the anterior beam in a three-field arrangement.

Late side effects are generally more "dose-limiting" than acute effects because they can have a significant impact on quality of life and are often permanent. They may appear between 6 months and 2 years after radiotherapy, although sometimes acute effects do not settle and can continue as late effects. Late urogenital toxicity manifests as chronic cystitis, urinary incontinence (2% to 11%) and erectile dysfunction (10% to 40%). Late damage to the rectum results in late radiation proctitis, rectal ulceration, or stricture; severe damage occasionally necessitates a defunctioning colostomy (risk <1%).

Efficacy

The outcome of patients treated with modern, high-dose radiotherapy is comparable to surgery, at least over a 5-year period. Five-year actuarial biochemical relapse-free survival rates of 90% have been reported for favorable risk patients treated with >75 Gy [11]. Pretreatment PSA level, Gleason score, tumor stage, radiation dose (<70 Gy or ≥70 Gy), and treatment year are all significant prognostic factors. The posttreatment PSA nadir has been found to be highly predictive of outcome; in one study, 75% of patients with a PSA nadir of <0.5 ng/mL had PSA disease-free survival (DFS) at 8 years compared to only 12% of patients with a PSA nadir >4 ng/mL [12].

Three-Dimensional Conformal Radiotherapy (3D-CRT)

Conventional radiotherapy is delivered using rectangular-shaped treatment fields, which inevitably encompass large volumes of normal tissues as well as the required target volume. The major focus over the last decade has been the development of conformal radiotherapy techniques, which allow delivery of irregularly shaped fields that conform more closely to the tumor target while reducing the radiation to the dose-limiting normal tissues. Shaping of fields can be achieved in one of two ways: by putting a custom-made lead shield in front of the beam, or by making the beam itself irregular in shape by using multileaf collimators (MLCs) (Fig. 5.3).

Does Conformal Radiotherapy Reduce Toxicity?

A randomized study comparing conventional and conformal radiotherapy at a standard dose of 64 Gy [13] showed a significant reduction in late (>3 months after treatment) radiation-induced proctitis and bleeding in the conformal group compared with the conventional group (5% vs. 15%, Radiation Therapy Oncology Group [RTOG] grade 2 or higher, $p = .01$). There were no differences between groups in bladder function after treatment. After a median follow-up of 3.6 years, there was no significant difference between groups in local tumor control: conformal 78% (95% confidence interval [CI] 66–86); conventional 83% (95% CI 69–90). These results have provided the basis for dose-escalation studies in an attempt to improve local tumor control with acceptable toxicity.

Dose Escalation

In a randomized dose-escalation trial conducted at the M.D. Anderson Cancer Center, 305 men with localized (T1 to T3) prostate cancer were randomized to receive either conventional-dose

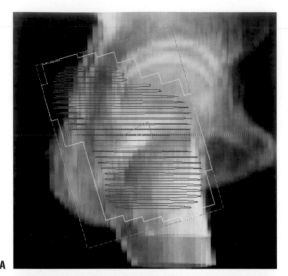

A

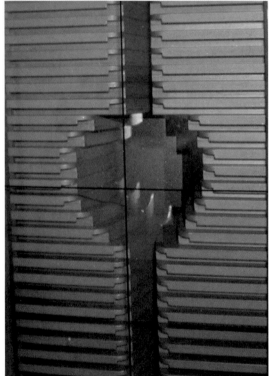

B

Fig. 5.3. (a) Beam's-eye view of right lateral treatment field for conformal prostate radiotherapy. Field shaping has been achieved by the use of multileaf collimators (MLCs) (shown in yellow). The collimator angle has been optimized to conform to the posterior edge of the PTV (shown in red) to protect the rectum. (b) The multileaf collimator.

(70 Gy) or high-dose (78 Gy) conformal radiotherapy to the prostate and seminal vesicles [14]. With a median follow-up of 60 months, the biochemical control rates at 6 years were significantly higher in the 78-Gy arm compared to the 70-Gy arm (70% vs. 64%, $p = .03$). Subgroup analysis suggested that the benefit of dose escalation was limited to patients with a pretreatment PSA of $\geq$10 ng/mL (biochemical control rate, 62% vs. 43%, $p = .01$) but that there was no significant dose response in patients who had a pretreatment PSA of ≤10 ng/mL. The trial did not show a significant effect of dose escalation on overall survival, although there was a trend toward a higher freedom from distant metastasis rate at 6 years in patients with PSA levels >10 ng/mL who were treated with 78 Gy (98% vs. 88%, $p = .056$). Rectal side effects were significantly greater in the 78-Gy group (grade 2 rectal toxicity rates at 6 years, 26% vs. 12%, $p = .001$), whereas the rate of bladder complications was similar in both arms. The risk of rectal toxicity correlated highly with the proportion of the rectum treated to >70 Gy, and it was suggested by the authors that the rectal volume receiving ≥70 Gy should be limited to <25% in future dose escalation trials. The ongoing RTOG 94-06 trial is attempting to establish the maximum tolerated dose that can be delivered to the prostate using 3D-CRT. Interim results for patients treated to 79.2 Gy using 1.8-Gy fractions have demonstrated low levels of toxicity [15], and the study has continued using 2-Gy fractions to dose levels of 74 and 78 Gy.

The M.D. Anderson data are supported by data from a number of retrospective and prospective PSA-era trials that have provided evidence for a dose response in prostate cancer. However, more studies are required to define the groups of patients who may benefit from dose escalation and to assess whether there is any benefit in terms of survival. It is possible that conventional doses are sufficient in low-risk patients and that dose escalation may just increase toxicity with no benefit in terms of disease control in these patients. The results of several randomized trials of dose escalation in the UK, the Netherlands, France, and North America are awaited. The UK MRC RT01 trial, which randomized men to standard-dose (64 Gy) or high-dose (74 Gy) conformal radiotherapy in addition to neoadjuvant androgen suppression, closed to accrual in 2001 with around 800 patients randomized.

Intensity-Modulated Radiotherapy

Intensity-modulated radiotherapy (IMRT) is an advanced form of 3D-CRT that allows tighter conformation to the target volume and sparing of normal tissues in the vicinity of and even within the target volume to an extent that was not previously possible. In general, IMRT uses inverse treatment planning systems that work backward from a desired dose distribution to generate treatment fields with varying intensities across the cross section of the beam. Treatment delivery utilizes MLCs where each set of opposing leaves travel across the beam under computer control during radiation delivery according to a prescribed scheme, to produce the required intensity pattern across the beam.

Early toxicity and biochemical outcomes have been reported for 772 patients with localized prostate cancer treated with high-dose IMRT (81 to 86.4 Gy, 1.8 Gy/fraction) at the Memorial Sloan-Kettering Cancer Center [16]. Intensity-modulated radiotherapy was associated with decreased rectal toxicity, and the actuarial rate of grade ≥2 proctitis at 3 years was only 4% compared to the rate of 14% previously reported at the same center for patients receiving 81 Gy with 3D-CRT [11]. The 3-year actuarial PSA relapse-free survival rates were comparable to published results using 3D-CRT; however, median follow-up was only 24 months and longer follow-up is required to substantiate these results. Preliminary results using hypofractionated IMRT (70 Gy at 2.5 Gy/fraction) show similar rates of late toxicity and biochemical outcome to high-dose 3D-CRT [17], although again, longer follow-up is required.

Although prophylactic pelvic lymph node radiotherapy is not routine practice in the U.K., there is evidence from the RTOG 9413 study that it may be beneficial in carefully selected patients [18]. The potential of IMRT to irradiate pelvic lymph nodes while sparing critical pelvic organs has been investigated [19]. Conventional radiotherapy plans were compared to 3D-CRT and IMRT plans for 10 patients. The mean percentage volume of small bowel receiving >45 Gy for the conventional radiotherapy, 3D-CRT, and IMRT plans were 21%, 18%, and 5%,

respectively, ($p < .001$). The rectal and bladder volumes irradiated with doses ≥45 Gy were also reduced by IMRT. The reduction in critical pelvic organ irradiation seen with IMRT may reduce side effects and allow modest dose escalation. A phase I dose-escalation trial has been initiated to assess the tolerance of radiotherapy to the pelvic lymph nodes of 50 to 60 Gy using IMRT.

Concerns have been raised that reducing treatment volumes to such an extent carries a risk of incurring a geographical miss of the target, which would inevitably result in reduced tumour control. However, results so far suggest that PSA outcomes after IMRT are comparable to conventional 3D-CRT, although mature data are not yet available. Other potential drawbacks to IMRT include the added workload on physicians, physicists, and radiotherapists, the risk of errors due to the complexity of planning and delivery, and the complexity of quality assurance. An additional concern is that IMRT may lead to an increase in the incidence of second malignancies. There are two reasons for this: (1) IMRT involves the use of more fields than conventional radiotherapy and, as a consequence, a larger volume of normal tissues is exposed to low radiation doses; (2) IMRT usually requires more time to deliver a specified dose than conventional radiotherapy (hence more monitor units needed) thus increasing the total body exposure, due to leakage radiation. Careful long-term follow-up of patients treated with IMRT is necessary to address this issue.

Prostate Brachytherapy

Prostate brachytherapy involves placement of radioactive sources directly into the parenchyma of the prostate. It is a highly conformal form of therapy, permitting dose escalation to the target volume far exceeding that of other radiation modalities. The surrounding normal tissues are spared because of the rapid dose falloff with distance from the source (inverse square law). The evolution of TRUS imaging, a closed transperineal approach, and the increasing sophistication of computerized planning have resulted in a worldwide resurgence of interest in this treatment technique. Its appeal lies in its speed and convenience (it can be done as an outpatient procedure) and the low long-term risk of proctitis; impotence is also less likely than after radical prostatectomy. Brachytherapy to the prostate can be delivered either with permanent seed implants or with removable implants, which are often delivered at a high dose rate with iridium wire.

Permanent Implants

Permanent implants may be used alone as monotherapy for localized prostate cancer or, less commonly, as a boost in combination with EBRT. Patient selection is extremely important for two reasons: (1) to identify patients who are likely to have a good outcome in terms of biochemical disease free survival, and (2) to identify patients who will have a good functional outcome. Patients who are likely to have a good outcome from brachytherapy alone have an initial PSA level <10 ng/mL, Gleason score ≤6, and low-volume disease with a low risk of extracapsular spread (stage T1/T2). If the prostate is large (>50 cm^3), the pubic rami may shield part of the gland that cannot be adequately implanted; these patients also need a large number of seeds and are at increased risk of morbidity. If otherwise suitable, neoadjuvant hormone treatment with a luteinizing hormone–releasing hormone (LHRH) analogue for 3 months can lead to a reduction in prostate volume of >30%. Brachytherapy should be avoided in men with a history of transurethral resection of the prostate (TURP) because it increases the risk of long-term urinary incontinence following brachytherapy from 1% to ~12.5%. An alternative procedure may also be preferable in patients with significant pretreatment lower urinary tract obstructive symptoms who are more likely to develop urinary retention after brachytherapy.

Two isotopes are used as the radioactive seed source, iodine (^{125}I) and palladium (^{103}Pd), although only ^{125}I is readily obtainable in the U.K. Both isotopes have low energy but different half-lives (59.4 days for ^{125}I, 16.97 days for ^{103}Pd) and initial dose rate. ^{103}Pd has the higher dose rate and is biologically more active; therefore, equivalent prescribed doses are lower. For patients treated by brachytherapy alone, typical doses are 145 Gy with ^{125}I and 100 Gy with ^{103}Pd, which is the minimum peripheral dose to the margin of the target volume. If brachytherapy is used in conjunction with EBRT, typically prescribed doses are 45 Gy in 25 fractions given by EBRT followed by 110 Gy via an ^{125}I-brachytherapy implant [20].

A two-stage technique is most commonly used for permanent implantation in the U.K. The initial stage requires a preplanning TRUS examination performed with the patient in the lithotomy position, done either as an outpatient or day-hospital procedure under general anesthesia. The TRUS images are digitized to produce a 3D model of the prostate on the planning computer, which can be used to determine the number and position of seeds required. The implant is performed a few weeks later in an identical lithotomy position. Thin needles are inserted percutaneously into the prostate through a perineal template to a precalculated depth guided by an ultrasound probe in the rectum. The needles may either be preloaded with the appropriate number of seeds or the seeds can be inserted individually. Between 20 and 30 needles containing 60 to 120 seeds are implanted depending on the volume and seed activity. The needles are then removed, leaving the seeds permanently in place. A CT scan is performed after implantation to identify the seeds and prostatic outline, and this information is used to calculate the actual dose delivered to the prostate.

Almost all patients develop urethritis of variable intensity which may last for ~3 months. Symptoms may be helped by alpha-blockers and nonsteroidal antiinflammatory drugs. A minority of patients (15%) develop acute retention either immediately or in the few days following implantation. This is usually due to postimplant edema and requires catheterization. In most patients, micturition resumes within 2 weeks as edema resolves, although recovery may occasionally take longer. Long-term effects include persistent cystitis and prostatitis (3%), proctitis (2%), and impotence (25%). The risk of urinary incontinence is small (~1%) unless patients have had a previous TURP.

There have been no randomized trials comparing brachytherapy with other interventions for early prostate cancer (though a trial randomizing patients to brachytherapy or radical prostatectomy is now open, under the auspices of the American College of Surgeons). Most results come from single centers reporting retrospective series [e.g., 21]. These results are extremely promising, but what is difficult to gauge is the extent to which such results reflect the benefit of brachytherapy per se, and to what extent they reflect patient selection factors. Some workers advocate EBRT in conjunction with brachytherapy for patients with intermediate and high risk factors, but it is not yet proven whether this improves outcome.

High Dose Rate Brachytherapy

Remote afterloading systems can also be used with TRUS and template guidance to deliver temporary, high dose rate (HDR) brachytherapy to the prostate. The isotope used is iridium (^{192}Ir), which has higher emission energies than ^{125}I and ^{103}Pd. The greater range may be more suitable for the treatment of patients with bulkier tumors and the possibility of extracapsular extension. Treatment is hypofractionated (with the potential benefits of hypofractionation previously discussed) and treatment times are a few minutes only. Most trials investigating the usefulness of HDR to date have given it as a boost (8 to 10 Gy × 2) prior to, during, or after EBRT (45 to 50 Gy) with good results even in patients with unfavorable prostate cancer [22]. More recently, a number of HDR monotherapy trials [e.g., 23] have shown that the treatment is feasible and well tolerated, but longer follow-up is required for outcome.

Combined Radiotherapy and Hormone Therapy

The use of combined modality treatment, with hormone therapy and radiotherapy, for the treatment of prostate cancer may be beneficial for two reasons. First, by combining two effective modalities, there is hope that the anticancer effects will be additive. Second, the use of hormone therapy to shrink a large prostate before irradiation may improve efficacy by reducing the tumor burden and also may reduce rectal toxicity by reducing the volume irradiated to high dose [24]. The LHRH agonists (e.g., goserelin) are usually used, but antiandrogens (e.g., bicalutamide) may be useful in men who wish to retain their potency, although they result in less prostate shrinkage [25].

The combination of hormone therapy and radiotherapy has been tested in a number of clinical trials with some variation in the way in which hormone therapy was administered (Table 5.1). Based on these findings, there do appear to be several subsets of prostate cancer patients who benefit from hormone therapy plus radiotherapy over radiotherapy alone:

1. Patients with bulky tumors without evidence of distant metastases and Gleason score ≤6 benefit from short-course neoadjuvant hormone therapy for 4 months (2 months before and 2 months during radiotherapy). It is not known if an LHRH agonist alone would produce the same benefit as the combination of LHRH agonist and antiandrogen used in RTOG 86-10.

2. Patients with any T stage and no evidence of distant metastases with Gleason score 8 to 10 tumors benefit from long-term hormone therapy (2 to 3 years). Periods of 2 to 3 years have been chosen empirically in most trials, but it is possible that a shorter course may be equally effective; the European Organization for Research and Treatment of Cancer (EORTC) trial 22961 is investigating this possibility.

3. At least some patients with T3 tumors and lower Gleason grade also appear to benefit from long-term hormone therapy, based on a meta-analysis of the RTOG protocols [33], and the EORTC study [29].

The potential benefits of androgen deprivation have to be balanced against toxicity. Most patients experience hot flushes, fatigue, and impotence of varying degrees, which can impact significantly on quality of life. Other toxicities include loss of libido, weight gain, muscle wasting, and changes in texture of hair and skin. Longer-term concerns include the development of osteoporosis and the possibility that low testosterone levels may predispose to cardiovascular disease. There is no evidence yet that long-term hormone therapy increases non–prostate cancer mortality, but this is being investigated; in the meantime, it is sensible to restrict the use of long-term hormone therapy to patient groups in which it has been shown to have an overall survival benefit.

None of the trials in Table 5.1 included a hormone therapy alone arm. Because of this, it is not possible to say with certainty whether the benefits that appear in the patients treated with combined modality therapy are due to the com-

Table 5.1. Randomized trials of hormone therapy plus radiotherapy

Study	Patient numbers	Patient characteristics	Timing	Outcome
RTOG 85–31 [26,27]	977	T3 or LN positive	Adjuvant goserelin, last week of RT until progression	↑ LC, ↓ DM but OS NS except in Gleason 8 to 10
EORTC [28,29]	415	T1–2 grade 3 or T3–4, any grade (LN negative)	Adjuvant goserelin, first week of RT for 3 years	↑ DFS and OS at 5 years
RTOG 86–10 [30]	471	Bulky T2–4 (+/− LN positive)	Neoadjuvant CAS, 2 months before and 2 months during RT	Overall, ↑ LC, ↓ DM but not in Gleason 7 to 10; OS NS except in Gleason 2 to 6
RTOG 92–02 [31]	1554	T2C–T4, PSA <150 ng/mL	Neoadjuvant CAS for 2 months before +2 months during RT for all patients, then adjuvant goserelin for 2 years or no further treatment	↑ LC, ↑ DFS, ↓ DM but OS NS except in Gleason 8 to 10
RTOG 94–13 [18,32]	1323	T1–4 with risk LN positive >15% or T2C–T4 Gleason ≥6 even if risk LN positive <15%	2 × 2 design: whole pelvic vs. prostate RT; neoadjuvant CAS for 2 months before +2 months during RT or adjuvant CAS for 4 months after RT.	↑ PFS for whole pelvic + neoadjuvant hormones but OS NS

CAS, combined androgen suppression (goserelin + flutamide); DFS, disease-free survival; DM, distant metastases; EORTC, European Organization for Research and Treatment of Cancer; LC, local control; LN, lymph node; NS, nonsignificant; OS, overall survival; PFS, progression free survival; RT, radiotherapy; RTOG, Radiation Therapy Oncology Group.

bination of radiotherapy and androgen ablation or the androgen ablation *per se*. The MRC PR02 study [34] did include a hormones-alone arm and randomized 277 patients with T2 to T4 prostate cancer and no bone metastases to orchidectomy alone, radiotherapy alone, or a combination of the two. The study was too small to detect a statistically significant difference in overall survival between the groups, but there was a delay in time to metastasis in patients treated with hormone therapy (with or without radiotherapy). A randomized Medical Research Council study (MRC Prof) is investigating whether radiotherapy contributes anything to long-term hormone therapy in patients with nonmetastatic locally advanced or poor prognosis organ-confined prostate cancer.

Adjuvant or Salvage Radiotherapy After Surgery

Following radical prostatectomy, patients with positive resection margins, extraprostatic exten-

sion (pT3 disease), or seminal vesicle invasion are at increased risk of disease recurrence. There is increasing interest in the role of postoperative radiotherapy in these patients. Radiotherapy (RT) can be administered immediately following prostatectomy (adjuvant RT) or may be postponed until the PSA has risen to a level that is indicative of residual or recurrent prostate cancer (salvage RT). There are no published randomized clinical trials of postprostatectomy radiotherapy, and it is not known whether the results of immediate adjuvant radiotherapy and early salvage radiotherapy are equivalent. Most retrospective studies, however, show that both are generally well tolerated.

Adjuvant radiotherapy is given postoperatively to eradicate possible microscopic residual disease in the periprostatic tissues or adjacent pelvic lymph nodes. It may be considered in men with positive resection margins, extraprostatic extension, or an elevated PSA after surgery. Retrospective studies show that it reduces the local and biochemical recurrence rates in high-risk patients after radical prostatectomy, but there is no evidence yet that it improves survival [35]. Seminal vesicle invasion predicts biochemical failure (rise in PSA) after adjuvant radiotherapy, presumably because it is associated with a high risk of distant metastases. The results of two completed, but yet to be reported, randomized trials of postoperative radiotherapy are awaited in the near future. The Southwest Oncology Group (SWOG) 8794 trial and EORTC 22911 trial have randomized a combined total of over 1300 patients with unfavorable prostate cancer to receive either adjuvant radiotherapy or observation (with salvage radiation on recurrence) following radical prostatectomy.

Salvage radiotherapy is given for patients with biochemical or clinical evidence of recurrent disease following prostatectomy. This approach spares ~40% of patients with high-risk features postprostatectomy who may never have a recurrence. Only patients with disease recurrence confined to the prostatic bed are likely to benefit, and it is therefore important to determine whether a rising PSA represents local recurrence or whether it is an indicator of metastatic disease. Even with local-only recurrence, salvage radiation may not be necessary if life expectancy is short and the risk of symptomatic prostate cancer is low. This is supported by a study of patients with biochemical failure following prostatectomy from Johns Hopkins University, in which the median time from biochemical failure to detection of metastases was 8 years, and the median time from detection of metastases to death was 5 years [36].

Response rates after salvage radiotherapy vary between 10% and 76%, with different patient selection criteria being the most likely explanation for the enormous difference between studies. Factors that predict a favorable outcome after salvage radiotherapy include low preradiation PSA level, low Gleason grade, absence of seminal vesicle involvement, and biochemical failure to be consistent >1 year after prostatectomy [37]. Presalvage PSA appears to be the most consistently reported prognostic variable, and salvage rates are low for patients with pre-RT PSA >2 ng/mL. The increasing sensitivity of PSA testing means that salvage radiotherapy can now be started at much lower PSA levels (0.01 to 0.1 ng/mL) with the expectation that this will yield better results. Consequently, trials using salvage radiotherapy for men with higher PSA levels (including SWOG 8794 and EORTC 22911) may

therefore underestimate the efficacy of early salvage radiotherapy compared to adjuvant radiotherapy, and this needs to be considered in their interpretation.

The role of hormone therapy in combination with postoperative radiotherapy is currently unknown. Two RTOG studies currently in progress are addressing this issue: RTOG P-0011 is comparing adjuvant radiotherapy alone versus adjuvant combined modality therapy in high-risk postprostatectomy patients, whereas RTOG 9601 is comparing salvage radiotherapy alone versus combined modality therapy in patients with a rising PSA (>0.2 ng/mL and <4 ng/mL) after radical prostatectomy.

Conclusion

Current evidence suggests that radiotherapy is as effective as other curative modalities for prostate cancer. As well as the need for more mature data from high-dose, conformal studies, the ongoing randomized trials will better define its role. The optimum duration of hormone therapy is still unclear, and the patient population that most benefits from combined hormone therapy plus radiotherapy needs to be better defined. The next 5 to 10 years will yield some important data in clarifying these and other issues.

References

1. Holmberg L, Bill-Axelson A, Helgesen F, et al. A randomised trial comparing radical prostatectomy with watchful waiting in early prostate cancer. N Engl J Med 2002;347:781–789.
2. Paulson DF, Lin GH, Hinshaw W, et al. Radical surgery versus radiotherapy for adenocarcinoma of the prostate. J Urol 1982;128:502–504.
3. D'Amico AV, Whittington R, Malcowicz SB, et al. Biochemical outcome after radical prostatectomy or external beam radiation therapy for patients with clinically localised prostate carcinoma in the prostate specific antigen era. Cancer 2002;95: 281–286.
4. Kupelian PA, Elshaikh M, Reddy CA, et al. Comparison of the efficacy of local therapies for localised prostate cancer in the prostate-specific antigen era: a large single-institution experience with radical prostatectomy and external-beam radiotherapy. J Clin Oncol 2002;20:3376–3385.

5. Wilt TJ, Brawer MK. The prostate cancer intervention versus observation trial; a randomised trial comparing radical prostatectomy versus expectant management for the treatment of clinically localised prostate cancer. J Urol 1994;152: 1910–1914.

6. Madalinska JB, Essink-Bot M-L, de Koning HJ, et al. Health-related quality-of-life effects of radical prostatectomy and primary radiotherapy for screen-detected or clinically diagnosed localised prostate cancer. J Clin Oncol 2001;19: 1619–1628.

7. Seddon B, Bidmead M, Wilson J, et al. Target volume definition in conformal radiotherapy for prostate cancer: quality assurance in the MRC RT-01 trial. Radiother Oncol 2000;56:73–83.

8. Brenner DJ, Hall EJ. Fractionation and protraction for radiotherapy of prostate carcinoma. Int J Radiat Oncol Biol Phys 1999;43:1095–1101.

9. Livsey JE, Cowan RA, Wylie JP, et al. Hypofractionated conformal radiotherapy in carcinoma of the prostate: five-year outcome analysis. Int J Radiat Oncol Biol Phys 2003;57:1254–1259.

10. Lukka H, Hayter C, Warde P, et al. A randomised trial comparing two fractionation schedules for patients with localised prostate cancer. Int J Radiat Oncol Biol Phys 2003;57(suppl).

11. Zelefsky MJ, Fuks Z, Hunt M, et al. High dose radiation delivered by intensity modulated conformal radiotherapy improves the outcome of localised prostate cancer. J Urol 2001;166:876–881.

12. Kuban DA, Thames HD, Levy LB, et al. Long-term multi-institutional analysis of stage T1-T2 prostate cancer treated with radiotherapy in the PSA era. Int J Radiat Oncol Biol Phys 2003;57: 915–928.

13. Dearnaley DP, Khoo VS, Norman AR, et al. Comparison of radiation side-effects of conformal and conventional radiotherapy in prostate cancer: a randomised trial. Lancet 1999;353:267–272.

14. Pollack A, Zagars GK, Starkschall G, et al. Prostate cancer radiation dose response: results of the M.D. Anderson Phase III randomised trial. Int J Radiat Oncol Biol Phys 2002;53:1097–1105.

15. Ryu JK, Winter K, Michalski JM. Interim report of toxicity from 3D conformal radiation therapy (3D-CRT) for prostate cancer on 3DOG/RTOG 9406, level III (79.2 Gy). Int J Radiat Oncol Biol Phys 2002;54:1036–1046.

16. Zelefsky MJ, Fuks Z, Hunt M, et al. High-dose intensity modulated radiation therapy for prostate cancer: early toxicity and biochemical outcome in 772 patients. Int J Radiat Oncol Biol Phys 2002;53:1111–1116.

17. Kupelian PA, Reddy CA, Carlson TP, et al. Preliminary observations on biochemical relapse-free survival rates after short-course intensity-modulated radiotherapy (70 Gy at 2.5 Gy/fraction) for localised prostate cancer. Int J Radiat Oncol Biol Phys 2002;53:904–912.

18. Roach M III, DeSilvio M, Lawton C, et al. Phase III trial comparing whole-pelvic versus prostate-only radiotherapy and neoadjuvant versus adjuvant combined androgen suppression: Radiation Therapy Oncology Group 9413. J Clin Oncol 2003;21:1904–1911.

19. Nutting CM, Convery DJ, Cosgrove VP, et al. Reduction of small and large bowel irradiation using an optimised intensity-modulated pelvic radiotherapy technique in patients with prostate cancer. Int J Radiat Oncol Biol Phys 2000;48:649–656.

20. Merrick GS, Butler WM, Galbreath RW, et al. Five-year biochemical outcome following permanent interstitial brachytherapy for clinical T1-T3 prostate cancer. Int J Radiat Oncol Biol Phys 2001;51:41–48.

21. Grimm PD, Blasko JC, Sylvester JE, et al. 10-year biochemical (prostate-specific antigen) control of prostate cancer with ^{125}I brachytherapy. Int J Radiat Oncol Biol Phys 2001;51:31–40.

22. Martinez AA, Gustafson G, Gonzalez J, et al. Dose escalation using conformal high-dose-rate brachytherapy improves outcome in unfavourable prostate cancer. Int J Radiat Oncol Biol Phys 2002;53:316–327.

23. Yoshioka Y, Nose T, Yoshida K, et al. High-dose-rate brachytherapy as monotherapy for localised prostate cancer: a retrospective analysis with special focus on tolerance and chronic toxicity. Int J Radiat Oncol Biol Phys 2003;56:213–220.

24. Zelefsky MJ, Leibel SA, Burman CM, et al. Neoadjuvant hormonal therapy improves the therapeutic ratio in patients with bulky prostatic cancer treated with three-dimensional conformal radiation therapy. Int J Radiat Oncol Biol Phys 1994; 29:755–761.

25. Henderson A, Langley SEM, Laing RW. Is bicalutamide equivalent to goserelin for prostate volume reduction before radiation therapy? A prospective, observational study. Clin Oncol 2003;15: 318–321.

26. Pilepich MV, Caplan R, Byhardt RW, et al. Phase III trial of androgen suppression using goserelin in unfavourable-prognosis carcinoma of the prostate treated with definitive radiotherapy: report of Radiation Therapy Oncology Group Protocol 85-31. J Clin Oncol 1997;15:1013–1021.

27. Lawton CA, Winter K, Murray K, et al. Updated results of the phase III Radiation Therapy Oncology Group (RTOG) trial 85-31 evaluating the potential benefit of androgen suppression following standard radiation therapy for unfavourable prognosis carcinoma of the prostate. Int J Radiat Oncol Biol Phys 2001;49:937–946.

28. Bolla M, Gonzalez D, Warde P, et al. Improved survival in patients with locally advanced prostate cancer treated with radiotherapy and goserelin. N Engl J Med 1997;337:295–300.

29. Bolla M, Collette L, Blank L, et al. Long-term results with immediate androgen suppression and external irradiation in patients with locally advanced prostate cancer (an EORTC study): a phase III randomised trial. Lancet 2002;360:103–108.

30. Pilepich MV, Winter K, John MJ, et al. Phase III radiation therapy oncology group (RTOG) trial 86-10 of androgen deprivation adjuvant to definitive radiotherapy in locally advanced carcinoma of the prostate. Int J Radiat Oncol Biol Phys 2001;50:1243–1252.

31. Hanks GE, Lu J, Machtay M, et al. RTOG protocol 92-02: a phase III trial of the use of long-term androgen suppression following neoadjuvant hormonal cytoreduction and radiotherapy in locally advanced carcinoma of the prostate. Proc Annu Meet Am Soc Clin Oncol 2000;19:1284.

32. Roach M III, Lu JD, Lawton C, et al. A phase III trial comparing whole-pelvic (WP) to prostate only (PO) radiotherapy and neoadjuvant to adjuvant total androgen suppression (TAS): preliminary analysis of RTOG 9413. Int J Radiat Oncol Biol Phys 2001;51(suppl 1).

33. Roach M III, Lu J, Pilepich MV, et al. Predicting long-term survival, and the need for hormonal therapy: a meta-analysis of RTOG prostate cancer trials. Int J Radiat Oncol Biol Phys 2000;47:617–627.

34. Fellows GJ, Clark PB, Beynon LL, et al. Treatment of advanced localised prostatic cancer by orchidectomy, radiotherapy or combined treatment. A Medical Research Council Study. Urological Cancer Working Party–Subgroup on Prostatic Cancer. Br J Urol 1992;70:304–309.

35. Catton C, Gospodarowicz M, Warde P, et al. Adjuvant and salvage radiation therapy after radical prostatectomy for adenocarcinoma of the prostate. Radiother Oncol 2001;59:51–60.

36. Pound CR, Partin AW, Eisenberger MA, et al. Natural history of progression after PSA elevation following radical prostatectomy. JAMA 1999;281:1591–1597.

37. Parker C, Warde P, Catton C. Salvage radiotherapy for PSA failure after radical prostatectomy. Radiother Oncol 2001;61:107–116.

6

Prostate Cancer: Immediate vs. Deferred Treatment

Mark A. Underwood and David Kirk

There continues to be controversy about the timing of treatment for localized, for locally advanced, and for metastatic prostate cancer. The decision for early radical treatments in localized disease has been based on the patient's age, general health, and preference. However, an increased understanding of the natural history of this cancer may allow us to select patients at risk for whom treatment might possibly improve survival while reducing the risk of treatment-related morbidity in those not at risk [1,2].

The survival benefits of radical treatments for localized prostate cancer still remain unclear. To date, no randomized controlled trial has demonstrated whether radical surgery or radiotherapy is more effective than watchful waiting in improving overall survival. There is evidence that radical prostatectomy may significantly reduce disease specific mortality when compared to watchful waiting, but watchful waiting may be a viable option for some men [2].

Results from hormonal treatment in early prostate cancer (EPC Trial) demonstrate that irrespective of whether patients received radical prostatectomy or radiotherapy as standard care there was a significant reduction in disease and prostate-specific antigen (PSA) progression rates [3–5].

Thus, a picture seems to be emerging that immediate treatment for certain patients with localized disease might reduce disease-specific mortality. The evidence that any benefits from

early treatment of advanced disease especially in asymptomatic men outweigh treatment related complications is still not clear.

Why Defer Treatment?

Prostate cancer is perhaps unique among soft tissue malignancies in that it is accepted that there are many patients for whom treatment is not needed, at least on first diagnosis. Indeed, it would be considered unusual not to defer treatment in a man of 85 in whom a well-differentiated tumor is identified in the chips from a transurethral resection of the prostate (TURP) done for apparently benign disease. Although a poorly differentiated tumor in a man of 50 is clearly likely to be life threatening, it is recognized that many men undergoing radical treatment for "curable" disease will not live long enough to benefit from it. Although in "advanced disease" there are clear indications for hormone treatment—metastatic prostate cancer presenting with bone pain or other symptoms, ureteric obstruction, retention of urine in an elderly man—many men with advanced disease are asymptomatic. It is here that the possibility of deferring treatment arises. Treatment at diagnosis would be expected to prolong survival, but even this has been disputed [6]. Although some response is seen in most patients, it will be temporary and relapse will occur, usually within 2 years. Although radiotherapy and other palliative measures may then be helpful in relieving symptoms, relapse after hormone therapy usually is fatal within a matter of months [7]. On the other hand, treatment delayed until symptoms occur could be followed by a further asymptomatic period and survival might be similar [8].

The balance between the benefits of treatment on the one hand and its side effects and toxicity on the other is a further consideration. This is accentuated by recent improvements in diagnostic techniques, which have created new categories of "advanced disease." Examples are lymph node involvement found at radical prostatectomy, and PSA-detected relapse after definitive treatment for localized disease [9]. In earlier days, these patients would not yet have had their disease diagnosed. These patients, as with those undergoing curative treatment for localized disease, will survive for many years, may not die from prostate cancer, and yet if treated will be exposed to any side effects for all of this time.

Immediate or Deferred Treatment: The Swinging Pendulum

The paradigm in oncology is that early diagnosis and treatment should enhance survival. This is the basis for the policy of screening for breast and cervical cancer, and similar benefits are proposed by those who advocate screening for prostate cancer. Indeed, the arguments concerning screening and those about deferred treatment are inextricably entwined.

Just as the timing of hormonal treatment for advanced disease is controversial and definitions of immediate and deferred treatments still remain unclear, so do the arguments about which patients should undergo radical treatment for localized disease. Certainly in the United Kingdom, this is a new dimension, as radical prostatectomy was rarely considered an option before the mid-1980s, partly because of failure to diagnose the disease at an early stage, and radiotherapy was largely used for locally advanced disease. As more and more men are diagnosed with confined disease, radical prostatectomy initially confined to a few specialist centers is now widely practiced. Yet its evidence base remains unsure. As disease suitable for this treatment is at an early stage and normally does not progress

rapidly, there is an argument in favor of a period of PSA monitoring to identify those with progressive disease who would be most likely to benefit [10].

The idea of deferring treatment in advanced disease was considered in the 1940s [11], and has been a recurring theme ever since. Overoptimism about the results of treatment, based on the use of historical controls, left unquestioned for several years the effectiveness of hormone treatment in prolonging survival. The Veterans Administration Cooperative Urological Research Group (VACURG) studies [9] seemed to have indicated that deferring treatment until progression occurred might not affect survival. Reanalysis of the data, however, has suggested that cancer-specific survival rates were actually lower and early benefits of immediate hormone therapy were lost secondary to the complications of estrogen treatment [10].

The development of new methods of hormone manipulation, such as luteinizing hormone-releasing hormone (LHRH) analogues, seemed to reduce the disadvantages of hormone treatment, thus favoring early treatment [12]. At the same time, these new treatments are expensive, and added an economic component to the argument in favor of deferred treatment.

There are potential advantages to deferring treatment, with any side effects resulting from treatment occurring for a shorter period of time and the possibility that many patients might not need treatment, as they would die first from an unrelated cause. However, a number of potential harmful effects could arise from delaying treatment [13] (Table 6.1), but these in turn must be balanced against the long-term toxicity of chronic androgen deprivation, which has been recognized, with particular concern about osteoporosis [14].

Thus, the decision to start treatment continues to be a balance between its advantages and its side effects and toxicity. The debate started over 50 years ago continues. Where are we in 2005?

Clinical Trials

A common finding in prostate cancer trials is for a highly significant improvement in disease-specific survival in those treated immediately, associated with less, usually insignificant,

Table 6.1. Potential hazards of delaying treatment in advanced prostate cancer

---

Deferring treatment may reduce survival

Prostate cancer may become less hormone sensitive as it progresses

Local progression in the absence of treatment increases the number of patients requiring transurethral resection of the prostate (TURP) for recurrent outflow obstruction and those who develop ureteric obstruction

Catastrophic events such as spinal cord compression and pathological fractures may occur in untreated patients

The absence of specific symptoms might mask a general malaise associated with uncontrolled cancer

Patients managed by deferred treatment may die from prostate cancer without receiving hormone therapy

---

improvement in overall survival. Interpretation of trial data often assumes erroneously that where a difference is not significant (i.e., $p \geq .05$) this is proof of no difference. In other words, the effect on prostate cancer survival does not benefit the patient, as he will live no longer. For this truly to be so, the treatment itself would have to increase mortality from other causes, something that did occur with estrogen therapy as used in the 1950s but has not been shown conclusively with other agents. The true interpretation should perhaps be somewhat different [11].

Prostate cancer occurs in an elderly population, which will experience comorbidity and have a reduced life expectation (Table 6.2). Even if their survival from prostate cancer is similar, as men get older their overall survival, the product of life expectancy and the prostate cancer survival, will decrease. Thus, an intervention that significantly extends prostate cancer survival and clearly improves the overall survival of a group of 60-year-olds will have a negligible effect on that of men in their 80s. It is this effect of age and comorbidity that reduces the statistical significance of overall survival because of the high number of coincidental deaths. Trials large enough to demonstrate differences in disease-specific survival are underpowered for overall survival, and thus are erroneously ascribed a negative interpretation. Improved survival from prostate cancer should be seen as a bonus on top of the patients' other risks of dying but one that will only be realized by a small proportion of men in their 80s.

Localized Disease

The cited natural history data show that there are subgroups of patients who are not at risk of dying from prostate cancer even within 15 years. The identification of cancers that can be treated by watchful waiting with acceptable safety, the pattern and duration of follow-up, and the trigger points for treatment are crucial elements for developing policies of delaying or completely avoiding aggressive treatments.

Table 6.2. Hypothetical relationship between disease-specific and overall survival (percent alive after 10 years) in men with prostate cancer at different ages

Age	10-year survival life expectation)	Disease-specific survival	Overall survival
60	75%	60%	45%
70	50%	60%	30%
80	25%	60%	15%
Effects of a treatment that reduces disease specific mortality from 40% to 28%			
60	75%	72% vs 60%	54% vs 45%
70	50%	72% vs 60%	36% vs 30%
80	25%	72% vs 60%	18% vs 15%

Note: Overall survival is the product of disease-specific survival and life expectation. It assumes that disease-specific survival is not affected by age, and treatment has no adverse survival effects.

The Scandinavian Prostatic Cancer Group conducted a randomized trial to assess the efficacy of radial prostatectomy for treating early prostate cancer. The investigators enrolled 695 men with newly diagnosed prostate cancer (stage T1b, T1c, or T2) from October 1989 through February 1999 and followed them through 2000 [3]. Seventy-five percent had palpable disease on digital examination of the prostate. The investigators excluded men with very high levels of PSA or poorly differentiated cancer with urinary tract obstruction. Participants were assigned to watchful waiting or to radical prostatectomy.

After a median follow-up period of 6.2 years, the all-cause mortality rate was lower in the surgery group (53 men died in the surgery group vs. 62 in the watchful waiting group). Also, of the 47 men who died of prostate cancer, 16 were in the surgery group and 31 were in the watchful waiting group. The absolute difference in prostate-specific mortality in favor of surgery was 2% (confidence interval [CI], −0.8% to 4.8%) at 5 years and 6.6% (CI, 2.1% to 11.1%) at 8 years. In terms of overall mortality, however, the difference was small and the hazard ratio was 0.83 (CI, 0.57 to 1.2; $p \geq .2$). It would be necessary to treat 17 patients with radical prostatectomy to prevent one death from prostate cancer in an 8-year period.

Of note, the trial began before PSA testing was widely available in Scandinavia, and the results apply only to a group of men with clinically detected well-differentiated or moderately differentiated adenocarcinoma of the prostate. Also, the benefits of treatment must be weighted against the known side effects of surgery. The lack of a statistically significant difference in overall survival has been addressed above and reflects the death rate from other causes. Because of this, the trial is probably not of sufficient power to demonstrate an absolute survival benefit. There is unlikely to be a significant treatment-related mortality (there was only one postoperative death among the patients undergoing radical prostatectomy). What this emphasizes is that many men with early prostate cancer die not from the disease but from other conditions, and that these men are not going to benefit from radical treatment. This study also emphasizes that this a very complicated treatment decision, and that active surveillance (watchful waiting) may be a viable option for some patients.

The use of adjuvant treatment in confined disease, as tamoxifen is used in breast cancer [15], is currently the subject of a large international study. The ongoing bicalutamide EPC program, the largest prostate cancer intervention trial in history, compared the nonsteroidal antiandrogen bicalutamide (150 mg/day), plus standard care (radical prostatectomy, radiotherapy, or watchful waiting) with placebo plus standard care in 8113 patients with localized or locally advanced prostate cancer. At the first analysis conducted after a median of 3 years' follow-up, survival data were immature, with 6% overall mortality and <2% of patients dying of prostate cancer. However, overall data show a 42% reduction in the risk of objective progression, 13.8% vs. 9%. The reduced risk of disease progression was observed in both localized and locally advanced disease. There was also a 33% reduction in the risk of bone metastasis (7.9% vs. 5.3%), and a 59% reduction in the risk of PSA progression (33% vs. 17%) with bicalutamide 150 mg compared with standard care alone. Exploratory subgroup analyses showed that a reduction in objective progression occurred irrespective of the type of standard care. The tolerability of bicalutamide is closely related to its pharmacology, with gynecomastia and breast pain being the most common adverse events. These adverse events were mild to moderate in ≥90% of cases. This study must be interpreted with caution, as the data are immature. Longer follow-up will determine whether the reduced risk of disease progression will translate into a survival benefit [3–5].

Although the EPC program has been reported enthusiastically to reduce the risk of progression, the results must be interpreted with caution. The ability of hormone therapy to delay progression is not at issue. The single snapshot of the 2-year bone scan does not prove that bone metastases are prevented, only that their appearance is delayed. The issue is whether, as with advanced disease, prevention or delay in progression, rather than treatment when progression has occurred, confers survival or other benefits, and only long-term data will tell us this. Retrospective data from a recent multicenter database analysis have demonstrated that early hormonal therapy administered for PSA recurrence after prior radical prostatectomy was an independent predictor of delayed clinical metastases only for high-risk cases at current follow-up [16]. Again longer follow-up will help resolve these issues.

Locally Advanced Disease

The results of the VACURG studies were considered inconclusive, but more recent studies have not fully answered these questions. The study sponsored by the British Medical Research Council (MRC) [17], which finished recruitment in 1993, provided evidence in favor of early treatment, as has the outcome of studies of adjuvant hormone treatment in patients receiving radiotherapy, reported from the European Organization for Research and Treatment of Cancer (EORTC) [18] and Radiation Therapy Oncology Group (RTOG) [19]. The MRC trial PR03 demonstrated not only an improvement in survival, but also a reduction in complications resulting from progression [20]. The increased risk seemed to continue even after treatment had been started in those in whom treatment was deferred, suggested as being due to disease progression during the period of deferred treatment and only being partly reversed when treatment is finally started. Further studies by the EORTC on somewhat different groups of patients are underway [21], but may be able to report results soon, and a meta-analysis of trials of immediate versus deferred treatment by the Prostate Cancer Trialists' Collaborative Group is being prepared for publication. As data are accumulated from these studies, a clearer picture may develop. It does not answer the question of immediate or deferred treatment, but has focused the issues, both in terms of advising patients of the options and in directing future research.

Of practical significance to all practitioners managing men with early prostate cancer is what to do with men with involved lymph nodes or positive margins at surgery, or when PSA-detected relapse occurs after definitive treatment. Anecdotal studies have shown that radiotherapy and/or hormonal treatment is effective in reducing the PSA. However, there is a risk in managing prostate cancer in the modern era that the patient's PSA is treated rather than his disease. Suffice it to say that currently there is a lack of trial evidence to support early treatment in these circumstances; a fall in PSA will occur, but how much impact this has on later development of the disease remains to be determined. One randomized study of early vs. deferred treatment of patients with positive lymph nodes has been presented [22]. Although showing a statistically significant advantage for early treatment, both in terms of progression and survival, the overall numbers were too small (46 early vs. 52 deferred, with six deaths in the early vs. 18 in the deferred group) for the result to be reliable. The results from the larger study from the EORTC are awaited.

Essentially, in these patients the balance between benefit and deficit is much more polarized. With adjuvant treatment, many patients will have been cured by definitive treatment, thus being unable to benefit from hormone treatment. In others, including those with detectable PSA after treatment, the prognosis is such that clinical progression and death may be years away, and possibly they will have died from another disease before clinical progression occurs. On the other hand, treatment will be taken for years and thus the risks of toxicity are exaggerated compared with those treated for advanced disease.

A number of strategies can be considered. Deferred treatment is considered on the basis that many of these patients will be incurable, but have slowly progressive disease that may not threaten life or health for some years. Although it is inappropriate to extrapolate from trials in advanced disease (such as MRC trial PR03) to earlier disease, data from MRC PR03 would favor this approach for elderly patients. Thirty percent of men with M0 disease over the age of 80 died from other causes before requiring treatment. However, the main recruitment into MRC PR03 took place prior to the full impact of PSA testing and transrectal ultrasound (TRUS) biopsy took place. Most patients were diagnosed following a TURP, and even then substantial numbers required further TURP for local progression, a risk substantially reduced in those treated immediately. Now, the diagnosis is more likely to result from a needle biopsy. Patients presenting with symptoms of outflow obstruction will require treatment, whereas others might progress to obstruction in its absence. For the symptomatic man, a TURP will palliate the symptoms, but without further treatment may only be a temporary expedient.

Although early T3 tumors can be managed by surgery [23], in most centers radiotherapy or hormone treatment, or a combination, would be considered. Radiotherapy, usually now preceded by neoadjuvant treatment [24], is logical for localized disease, for which systemic treatment is perhaps inappropriate. However, there is clear evidence that hormone treatment is effective in controlling localized disease. An earlier MRC study (PR02) demonstrated no difference between radiotherapy or hormone treatment in terms of TURP rates during follow-up, although numbers were small and radiotherapy techniques have moved on. Adjuvant hormone treatment has been shown to improve survival compared to radiotherapy alone [19]. Is this the result of the combination, or would survival have been as good if patients had received only hormone treatment? Studies exploring this possibility by comparing hormone therapy alone versus combined treatment are underway in Canada, the United States, and the U.K.

It should be noted that although hormone therapy might be as effective initially in local control, radiotherapy may be more durable. In the authors' unit, a rise in PSA is taken as a signal to reassess the patient, and if it is due to local progression, radiotherapy is considered *before* clinically significant progression occurs.

Metastatic Disease

It is probably advisable to consider treatment in the majority of men with metastatic disease. Clearly, where metastases are symptomatic, treatment is mandatory. Deferring treatment will only delay its need for a few months. In MRC trial PR03 it was in men with M1 disease at presentation that the risk of spinal cord compression and pathological fractures was greatest [20, 25]. Men with metastatic disease will not usually survive long enough to allow long-term ill effects from androgen deprivation to be experienced. In the short term, an improvement in nonspecific well-being from reduction in tumor load may well outweigh any side effects. In MRC PR03, the increased need for TURP was as common in patients with M1 as with M0 disease. A possible source of troublesome morbidity in terminal disease is with the 10% of patients needing a TURP in the last year of their life [24].

Where deferred treatment is considered, perhaps at the request of the patient, clear criteria can be identified as to suitability. The patient with a large metastasis in the spine, endangering the cord (or elsewhere with bone destruction threatening pathological fracture), the patient who is anemic or suffers from other, more subtle causes of ill health, or who has a large aggressive primary tumor, especially if the tumor is poorly differentiated, should probably be advised to start treatment immediately. When treatment is deferred, it should be with the full cooperation and understanding of the patient and his general practitioner that regular checkups, close monitoring, and initiating treatment as soon as significant progression occurs are essential. It follows that where the patient is unable (perhaps due to living in a remote place) or unwilling to comply with close follow-up, deferred treatment is unsuitable.

Is the Case for Immediate Treatment Proved?

Confirmation of definite advantages from immediate treatment is reflected in the improved survival seen in the EORTC study of adjuvant treatment with radiotherapy [18], although in the study of the RTOG, this was noted only in those with high-grade disease [19]. Hormone treatment also reduces the risk of complications from local progression. The increased risk of spinal cord compression seems to transcend the start of deferred treatment, warning that disease progression occurring during the period without treatment may not be reversed when treatment is started. There is also the risk that, for whatever reason, the appropriate time of starting treatment may be missed.

On the other hand, are there problems with immediate treatment? The immediate side effects of impotence, hot flushes, and so on have been long recognized. However, just as studies have started to show that clear benefits may result from immediate treatment, so has the possibility emerged that serious harmful effects may result from androgen treatment. Some of these are specific to particular therapies, such as cardiovascular complications of estrogens, and liver toxicity of antiandrogens. However, testosterone deficiency, including androgen deprivation from orchiectomy or LHRH analogues, long considered "safe" options, is now recognized to cause weight increase, loss of muscle mass, and loss of energy [26]. Anemia may be a particular problem in patients treated with combined androgen blockade [27]. Osteoporosis has been described as a significant problem after androgen deprivation, analogous to that in post-menopausal women [14].

The difference between disease-specific and overall survival has been noted, and discussed earlier. If the reduction or delay in prostate cancer deaths was counteracted by treatment-induced mortality, it should be apparent from an increased death rate from other causes, as was noted in the VACURG studies for patients receiving oestrogens [9]. No such excess of noncancer deaths was noted in MRC trial PR03 [20,28]. Unpublished data from the Prostate Cancer Trialists' Collaborative Group's meta-analysis confirms an excess death rate from estrogen treatment but not for patients treated with LHRH analogues or orchiectomy. To the body of evidence on hormonal treatment in advanced disease, we can now add one randomized study of radical prostatectomy versus watchful waiting.

Immediate or Deferred Treatment in 2005

Studies in rat prostate cancer models support the use of immediate hormone therapy, which is most effective in terms of survival when initiated at the time of, or early after, tumour implantation [29,30]. For patients with locally advanced prostate cancer who receive radiotherapy, several prospective randomized controlled multicenter trials have indicated that adjuvant hormone therapy (goserelin or orchiectomy) extends progression-free survival and may also improve overall survival in some patients [30,31]. Although data on the use of adjuvant hormone therapy after radical prostatectomy are currently more limited, results from two studies support this approach in patients with an unfavorable prognosis [32].

Supporting the case for early intervention in the adjuvant setting, one study showed benefits with androgen deprivation therapy in terms of reduced PSA levels, reduced tumor volume, improved margin status, pathological downstaging, and reduced risk of progression (4).

Taken together the evidence provides a rational basis for the early initiation of hormone therapy. However, the question of exactly how early to treat remains unanswered.

We still have a dilemma with hormone treatment. Not treating cancer is a difficult concept for patients and many doctors. Treatment has possible benefits, benefits that recent trial data have made firmer. Yet treatment is also a source of side effects and potential toxicity. Hormone treatment is only temporarily beneficial; hormone refractory relapse is inevitable. Future clinical research must address a number of issues: quality of life, specific monitoring of potential toxicity, osteoporosis, and treatment-related death. Meanwhile, in the laboratory, the mechanism of hormone refractory relapse and treatment-related toxicity must be addressed. Prevention of androgen insensitivity would change hormone therapy from a palliative to a curative treatment. Hormone treatments with the benefits and without the toxicity would further shift the balance; immediate treatment might then hold undisputed sway.

Meanwhile, practitioners who manage men with prostate cancer have to use the tools available at the moment. Imperfect though they are, current methods of hormone treatment are effective to an extent that is not available for many other types of cancer. We must recognize that this is a disease that varies in its impact from individual to individual. One notable aspect of participating in MRC trial PR03 was the effect of information on the patient. Having received a balanced account of the arguments for and against immediate treatment, and despite knowing that the trial was based on uncertainty, many men were clear which approach they wanted for themselves. Although this adversely affected trial recruitment, it tells us a lot about men's attitude to treatment of prostate cancer. Our patients deserve this level of information. They need to share our uncertainties, and ultimately our role is to help them make a decision as to which method of management is right for them. We then need to be aware of the risks associated with the course of action chosen, and be alert to the possible problems that might occur. In the interests of our patients, we need to show due humility about these uncertainties. Urologists or oncologists who have concluded that they know the answer to the question of immediate or deferred treatment and treat all their patients accordingly may well cause some patients to suffer from their unfounded certainty.

Conclusion

There is increasing evidence both in localized and in advanced disease that treatment has a beneficial effect on survival. But two questions remain: First, what proportion of men will benefit, and for how many men will treatment be unnecessary? Second, to what extent does the burden of treatment-related toxicity outweigh any survival benefit? Future research should be directed at identification of aggressive tumors in patients likely to benefit from treatment, and developing treatments with reduced toxicity.

References

1. McPherson CP. Quality of life in patients with prostate cancer. Semin Oncol Nurs 2001;17:138–146.
2. Wu H. Watchful waiting and factors predictive of secondary treatment for localised prostate cancer. J Urol 2004;171:1111–1116.
3. Holmberg L. A randomised trial comparing radical prostatectomy with watchful waiting in early prostate cancer. N Engl J Med 2002;347:781–789.
4. See WA. The bicalutamide early prostate cancer program: demography. Urol Oncol 2001;6:43–47.
5. Wirth M. Bicalutamide (Casodex) 150 mg as immediate therapy in patients with localised or locally advanced prostate cancer significantly reduces the risk of disease progression. Urology 2001;58:146–151.
6. See W. Immediate treatment with bicalutamide 150 mg as adjuvant therapy significantly reduces the risk of PSA progression in early prostate cancer. Eur Urol 2003;44(5):512–518.
7. Lepor H, Ross A, Walsh PC. The influence of hormonal therapy on survival of men with advanced prostatic cancer. J Urol 1982;128:335–340.
8. Beynon LL, Chisholm GD. The stable state is not an objective response in hormone-escaped carcinoma of the prostate. Br J Urol 1984;56:702–705.
9. Byar DP The Veterans Administration Cooperative Research Group's studies of cancer of the prostate. Cancer 1973;32:1126–1130.
10. Kirby RS. Avoidance and management of rising prostate-specific antigen after radical prostatectomy. In: Belldegrun A, Kirby RS, Newling DWW, eds. New Perspectives in Prostate Cancer, 2nd ed. Oxford: Isis Medical, 2000:147–155.
11. Nesbit RM, Baum WC. Endocrine control of prostatic cancer. Clinical survey of 1818 cases. JAMA 1950;143:1317–1320.
12. Kozlowski JM, Ellis WJ, Grayhack JT. Advanced prostatic carcinoma. Early versus late endocrine therapy. Urol Clin North Am 1991;15:15–24.
13. Kirk D. Deferred treatment for advanced prostatic cancer. In: Waxman J, Williams G, eds. Urological Oncology. Seven Oaks: Edward Arnold, 1991: 117–125.
14. Daniell HW. Osteoporosis after orchiectomy for prostate cancer. J Urol 1997;157:439–444.
15. Early Breast Cancer Trialists' Collaborative Group. Systemic treatment by hormonal, cytotoxic or immune therapy. Lancet 1992;339:1–15.
16. Moul JW. Early vs delayed hormonal therapy for prostate specific antigen only recurrence of prostate cancer after radical prostatectomy. J Urol 2004;171:1141–1147.
17. Kirk D. Trials and tribulations in prostatic cancer. Br J Urol 1987;59:375–379.
18. Bolla M, Gonzalez D, Ward P, et al. Improved survival in patients with locally advanced prostate cancer treated with radiotherapy and goserelin. N Engl J Med 1997;337:295–300.
19. Pilepich MV, Caplin R, Byhardt RW, et al. Phase III trial of androgen suppression using goserelin in unfavourable-prognosis carcinoma of the prostate treated with definitive radiotherapy: report of Radiation Therapy Oncology Group Protocol 85-31. J Clin Oncol 1997;15:1013–1021.
20. Kirk D. Prostate cancer: immediate vs. deferred treatment. In: Waxman J, ed. Treatment Options in Urological Cancer. Oxford: Blackwell Science, 2002:205–219.
21. Schröder FH. Endocrine treatment of prostate cancer – recent developments and the future. Part 1: maximal androgen blockade. Early vs delayed endocrine treatment and side effects. Br J Urol Int 1999;83(European Urology Update Series):161–170.
22. Messing E, Manola J, Wilding G, Sarosdy M, Crawford D, Trump D. Immediate hormonal therapy vs observation for node positive prostate cancer following radical prostatectomy and pelvic lymphadenectomy: a randomised phase III Eastern Cooperative Oncology Group Trial. J Urol 1999;161(suppl):175.
23. Zinke H, Utz DC, Benson RC, Patterson DE. Bilateral lymphadenectomy and radical retropubic prostatectomy for stage C prostate cancer. Urology 1984;24:532–539.
24. Dearnaley DP. Combined modality treatment with radiotherapy and hormonal treatment in localised prostate cancer. In: Belldegrun A, Kirby RS, Newling DWW, eds. New Perspectives in Prostate Cancer, 2nd ed. Oxford: Isis Medical, 2000:169–180.
25. Kirk D, and Medical Research Council Prostate Cancer Working Party Investigators Group. MRC immediate versus deferred treatment study: how

important is local progression in advanced prostate cancer (abstract). Br J Urol 1998;81 (suppl 4):30.

26. Morley JE, Kaiser FE, Hajjar R, Perr HM III. Testosterone and frailty. Clin Geriatr Med 1997; 13:655–695.

27. Strum SB, Mcdermed JE, Scholz MC, Johnson H, Tisman G. Anaemia associated with androgen deprivation in patients receiving combined hormone blockade. Br J Urol 1997;79:933–941.

28. Kirk D, on behalf of Medical Research Council Prostate Cancer Working Party Investigators Group. Does hormonal treatment for prostate cancer cause excess deaths: data from the MRC immediate versus deferred hormone treatment study (abstract). Br J Urol Int 1999;83(suppl 4): 9.

29. Shally AV. Combination of long acting microcapsules of the D-tryptophan-6 analog of luteinizing hormone releasing hormone with chemotherapy: investigation in the rat prostate cancer model. Proc Natl Acad Sci USA 1985;82:2498–2502.

30. Issacs JT. The timing of androgen ablation therapy and/or chemotherapy in the treatment of prostate cancer. Prostate 1984;5:1–17.

31. Bolla M. Long term results with immediate androgen suppression and external irradiation in patients with locally advanced prostate cancer (an EORTC study): a phase III randomised trial. Lancet 2002;360:103–106.

32. Prayer-Galletti T. Disease free survival in patients with pathological C stage prostate cancer at radical retropubic prostatectomy submitted to adjuvant hormonal treatment. Eur Urol 2000;38: 504a(abstract 48).

7

Surgical Treatment of Prostate Cancer

Mark R. Feneley and Roger S. Kirby

Surgery for prostate cancer has evolved, with the main purpose of curing one of the most common male malignancies at an early stage in its natural history, and preventing the morbidity otherwise associated with unchecked disease progression to more advanced, incurable stages. The operation by which this may be achieved, radical prostatectomy, advanced considerably during the 20th century through developments in anatomical knowledge and surgical experience. It is now a routine surgical procedure in urological oncology carried out through a range of surgical approaches, each with its own advantages and disadvantages.

The first radical prostatectomy operations were done through a perineal approach, adapted from contemporaneous techniques for stone surgery. Theodore Bilroth is credited with the first radical prostatectomy, carried out in 1866; however, the use of this operation was slow to develop owing to its considerable morbidity and mortality. In 1905, Hugh Hampton Young [1] at the Johns Hopkins Hospital, Baltimore, Maryland, described the surgical technique for radical perineal prostatectomy and his results. This was the only definitive treatment available for prostate cancer at that time, preceding Huggins' important work on hormone sensitivity of this disease by 40 years. His technique and its description enabled surgeons to carry out prostatectomy for cure of prostate cancer with substantially lower mortality than previously possible (17%), and a 5-year cure rate of 62% [2]. Incontinence, stricture, fistula, and erectile impotence were nevertheless common and bothersome complications.

Retropubic Prostatectomy

The retropubic approach to radical prostatectomy did not develop until Terence Millin's description of his now classical operation for benign disease, the transcapsular prostatectomy. He adapted this operation to total (radical) prostatectomy, which had not been possible with the transvesical procedures with which surgeons had hitherto become familiar [3]. During the ensuing years, the perineal and retropubic approaches for radical prostatectomy each had its advocates. Radical prostatectomy nevertheless remained a formidable procedure, particularly the retropubic approach, with the risk of uncontrolled hemorrhage from Santorini's plexus. In spite of encouraging cancer-specific outcomes in patients undergoing radical prostatectomy for organ-confined cancer, the surgical difficulties persisted, and rudimentary understanding of surgical anatomy precluded any substantial progress. Complications related, first, to the undocumented course of the periprostatic veins and bleeding consequent to unreliable control, and second, to the unrecognized functional significance of the neurovascular bundles posterolateral to the prostate. Both were described 40 years after Millin's contribution, by Patrick Walsh, at the Johns Hopkins Hospital.

The anatomy of Santorini's plexus and the surgical technique for its control were described by Reiner and Walsh [4] in 1979. This was a landmark contribution, and enabled retropubic radical prostatectomy to be undertaken with a substantially lesser risk of hemorrhage. Surgical control of the dorsal venous complex, and the prospect of a relatively bloodless operative field for the apical dissection of the prostate and urethral preservation were essential steps toward future technical refinements.

Walsh et al.'s [5–7] second pivotal contribution was the anatomical description of the neurovascular bundles and the importance of their formal surgical preservation for postoperative recovery of potency. Walsh et al. showed that the bundles could be separated from the prostate by dissection of the prostatic fascia, along an anterolateral plane, thereby avoiding their injury (by traction or disruption). Applying these two discoveries, Walsh [8] described and subsequently refined the anatomical surgical technique routinely used today. The technique for excision of the neurovascular bundle was described later, along with its indications and impact on outcomes [9].

Perineal Prostatectomy

Retropubic prostatectomy continues to be undertaken with excellent results, though some surgeons prefer the perineal approach. The perineal approach avoids the bleeding sometimes encountered from the dorsal venous complex, as the prostate is removed behind this plane. As a result, the anterior surgical margin can be compromised, and this may have some adverse therapeutic significance in some patients, particularly those with extensive or anterior tumors. Complications specific to this approach relate mostly to anal or rectal injury, with a risk of fecal incontinence, infection, and fistula, but such sequelae are uncommon.

The perineal route does not allow for assessment or removal of pelvic lymph nodes; however, when this is considered important, pelvic lymphadenectomy may need to be carried out as a prior open or laparoscopic procedure. Perineal prostatectomy, therefore, may not be ideal in patients at high risk of a non—organ-confined pathological stage.

Laparoscopic Prostatectomy

Laparoscopic radical prostatectomy has developed within the past 10 years, recognizing the many potential benefits of laparoscopic surgery. It was first described by Schuessler et al. [10] in 1992, and at that time presented significant challenges [11]. Reduction in the extent of surgical incisions, postoperative pain, and analgesic requirement, and shorter convalescence including reduced hospital stay contribute to its potential advantages. Disadvantages relate to the considerable specific skills and experience that need to be acquired and maintained. Procedure-specific advantages and disadvantages must also be considered in relation to open surgery [12].

Operative blood loss in laparoscopic prostatectomy may be minimal by comparison with the open procedure. In experienced hands blood transfusion is rarely required, though this may also apply for the open procedure. For the surgeon, laparoscopy provides an excellent magnified visual field via a monitor, although two-dimensional, and a technological approach to precise operative manipulation. Surgeons undertaking the open procedure may use magnification loupes. The risk of deep vein thrombosis and potentially fatal pulmonary embolism associated with major surgery is always a concern, even with appropriate prophylaxis, and may be increased with prolonged operative times.

Laparoscopic radical prostatectomy became an alternative standard of care to open surgery following the success published by Guillonneau and Vallancien [13] in 2000. Specific advantages, in addition to those generally offered by the laparoscopic approach, arise in the fashioning of the urethrovesical anastomosis. The anastomosis can be made with a continuous suture under direct vision. The magnified field of view allows this to be done with considerable precision, achieving accurate apposition without traction. A watertight anastomosis may minimize potential sequelae of urinary leak and promote functional recovery. Mobilization of the bladder as part of the surgical dissection may also contribute to an apparently more rapid return of urinary continence, and some surgeons have incorporated equivalent maneuvers in the "open" operation for this reason. The urethral catheter can generally be removed at 3 days, and continence appears to be quickly achieved. Overall continence rates appear as good as those achieved by the open procedure. Technical ability and experience substantially influence operative time, which may may be considerable until substantial experience is gained [14]. Throughout the evolution of today's operation, surgeons have been careful to ensure that the various technical changes introduced would not compromise cancer control. This remains a cornerstone principle in many of the more recent adaptations. The specific challenges of complex laparoscopic surgery have stimulated further advances in surgical technology with the development robotic systems such as AESOP™ (Computer Motion, CA now Intuitive Surgical Corp., Sunnyuale, CA), DaVinca™ (Intuitive Surgical Corp., Sunnyuale, CA) and Zeus™ (Computer Motion, CA, now Intuitive Surgical Corp., Sunnyuale, CA) [15,16]. These systems enable surgeons conventionally trained in open procedures to adapt their skills to use instruments via portals without some of the physical constraints of a laparoscopic environment [14,17,18]. They provide capabilities for precise and remote surgical manipulation, and three-dimensional vision.

Using the robotic approach, extremely favorable early results have been reported from the Vattikuti Institute of Prostatectomy (VIP). Hospital stay is routinely less than 24 hours [19]. Specific modifications incorporated in this form of prostatectomy aim to maximally preserve the cavernosal nerves. The nerves and neurovascular bundles are freed by an anterior dissection of the prostatic fascia, creating on each side a block of tissue referred to as a "veil of Aphrodite." The limited urethral dissection employed may contribute to rapid return of continence, achieved in 90% by 5 months.

Principles of Radical Prostatectomy

Radical prostatectomy is generally carried out with the intent of achieving long-term disease-free survival and thereby cure of early-stage prostate cancer [20]. Secondary, but nevertheless important, concerns are the maintenance of quality of life, in particular continence and erectile function. In some countries, interest is growing in a potentially palliative role in patients with more advanced and noncurable disease. Favorable long-term survival in patients with pathologically organ-confined tumors has been recognized since Young's early experience [21]. In spite of early concerns, nerve sparing does not compromise cure rate [22]. Today, alongside the shift of pathological stage toward organ-confined disease at diagnosis, neurovascular bundles are routinely preserved and bilateral excision is rarely necessary, giving optimal opportunity for maintaining quality of life and functional recovery.

Cancer Control

Cancer specific outcomes observed after radical prostatectomy have improved substantially within the past 20 years owing to the possibility of detection of earlier stage disease [23]. This is almost entirely attributable to the discovery of prostate-specific antigen (PSA), its increasing availability and clinical use, together with the increasingly prevalent proactive approach toward men's health. Though dependent on patient selection, 10 year biochemical recurrence rates less than 30% can be expected in men with clinically localised cancer, and progression to metastatic disease is rare even without secondary treatment (<10%). Radical prostatectomy is therefore generally not recommended where life expectancy is less than 10 years, particularly in populations exposed to regular PSA testing.

The natural history of prostate cancer following radical prostatectomy is predicted strongly by pathological stage [24]. Although pathological stage can be determined only following surgical treatment, preoperative variables can be combined to provide a useful prediction of pathological stage for individual patients [25]. These variables include clinical stage, serum PSA, and biopsy findings, principally Gleason grade, and each independently correlates with pathological stage. Age also contributes to outcome, and increasing age is associated with less favorable pathological features [26,27]. These pre- and postoperative factors also relate to the risk of metastatic progression following definitive treatment [28].

other than potency are inevitable, including changes in perception of orgasm, ejaculation, and libido. The effect of these consequences may vary substantially between individuals.

Outcomes

Outcomes for the retropubic, perineal, and laparoscopic approaches as carried out in the centers of greatest experience are impressive yet extremely difficult to compare. Procedure modifications must be taken into account, such as nerve sparing, which is known to influence outcome, and technical demands specific to the surgical approach, as well as preoperative baseline differences in patients' age, comorbidity, and erectile function [36]. For such reasons, published results based on a surgical series or single centers may not be truly representative of wider outcomes [42–44]. Difficulties in comparing postsurgical morbidity between centers are compounded by the lack of consistency and objectivity in the assessment and definition of continence and potency. Various outcome measures have been used, including physician-reported outcomes, patient-reported outcomes, and neutral data collectors using standardized data collection instruments, which may influence outcome perceptions [43]. Also of concern, factors that determine quality of life and sexual functioning seem to have less than precise relationships with disease and treatment-related morbidity.

Interest has centered on case volume as a factor contributing to outcome following radical prostatectomy, with particular focus on surgeon volume and institution volume. Excellent outcomes have been reported for single-institution, individual surgeon-reported series [13,19, 45–47]. Outcomes reported from high-volume centers suggest lower morbidity and greater consistency; however, favorable outcome does not always follow for high-volume surgeons [48]. Outcomes may be biased by many factors, and those established clinical and operative considerations discussed in previous sections of this chapter should be included for prospectively useful analysis. Individual training and the environment of professional practice may also be significant in influencing outcomes [49]. The importance of operating on a large number of patients to maintain skills and gain experience is widely recognized. Outcomes do vary among individual patients, and although the reliability of auditing this variability relates to case numbers, there may be nonuniformity of institution-, surgeon-, and patient-related factors influencing outcome. For such reasons, valid comparisons are difficult to make, and inevitably the very best outcomes cannot be guaranteed for all patients. Good outcomes, however, can be achieved by appropriately trained and experienced surgeons practicing in institutions of excellence.

Conclusion

Excellent cancer control and quality of life outcomes can be achieved by radical prostatectomy. The key, historical developments emphasize the importance of early diagnosis and consistency in surgical technique. Radical prostatectomy can be carried out by a variety of surgical approaches, and each has advantages and disadvantages. Technological development and application will increasingly influence future surgical practice by improving discrimination of those early-stage tumors that require definitive treatment and more consistently limiting treatment-related morbidity. The results of ongoing randomized controlled trials will add to the evidence base supporting the role of this important treatment option for the many men diagnosed with localized prostate cancer.

References

1. Young HH. The early diagnosis and radical cure of carcinoma of the prostate: being a study of 40 cases and presentation of a radical operation which was carried out in four cases. Johns Hopkins Hosp Bull 1905;16:315–321.

2. Young HH, Davis DM. Neoplasms of the urogenital tract. In: Young's Practice of Urology. Philadelphia: WB Saunders, 1926;653–654.

3. Millin T. Retropubic prostatectomy: a new extravesical technique report on 20 cases. Lancet 1945;693–696.

4. Reiner WG, Walsh PC. An anatomical approach to the surgical management of the dorsal vein and Santorini's plexus during radical retropubic surgery. J Urol 1979;121(2):198–200.

5. Walsh PC, Donker PJ. Impotence following radical prostatectomy: insight into etiology and prevention. J Urol 1982;128(3):492–497.

6. Walsh PC, Lepor H, Eggleston JC. Radical prostatectomy with preservation of sexual function: anatomical and pathological considerations. Prostate 1983;4(5):473–485.

7. Lepor H, Gregerman M, Crosby R, Mostofi FK, Walsh PC. Precise localization of the autonomic nerves from the pelvic plexus to the corpora cavernosa: a detailed anatomical study of the adult male pelvis. J Urol 1985;133:207–212.

8. Walsh PC. Anatomic radical prostatectomy: evolution of the surgical technique. J Urol 1998;160: 2418–2424.

9. Walsh PC, Epstein JI, Lowe FC. Potency following radical prostatectomy with wide unilateral excision of the neurovascular bundle. J Urol 1987; 138(4):823–827.

10. Schuessler WW, Kavoussi LR, Clayman RV, Vancaille TH. Laparoscopic radical prostatectomy: initial case report. J Urol 1992;147(4):246.

11. Schuessler WW, Schulam PG, Clayman RV, Kavoussi LR. Laparoscopic radical prostatectomy: initial short-term experience. Urology 1997;50(6): 854–857.

12. Cadeddu JA, Kavoussi LR. Laparoscopic radical prostatectomy: is it feasible and reasonable? Urol Clin North Am 2001;28(3):655–661.

13. Guillonneau B, Vallancien G. Laparoscopic radical prostatectomy: the Montsouris experience. J Urol 2000;163(2):418–422.

14. Bollens R, Roumeguere T, Vanden Bossche M, Quackels T, Zlotta AR, Schulman CC. Comparison of laparoscopic radical prostatectomy techniques. Curr Urol Rep 2002;3(2):148–151.

15. Guillonneau B, Cappele O, Martinez JB, Navarra S, Vallancien G. Robotic assisted, laparoscopic pelvic lymph node dissection in humans. J Urol 2001; 165(4):1078–1081.

16. Abbou CC, Hoznek A, Salomon L, et al. Laparoscopic radical prostatectomy with a remote controlled robot. J Urol 2001;165(6 pt 1):1964–1966.

17. Prasad SM, Maniar HS, Soper NJ, Damiano RJJ, Klingensmith ME. The effect of robotic assistance on learning curves for basic laparoscopic skills. Am J Surg 2002;183(6):702–707.

18. Stolzenburg JU, Truss MC. Technique of laparoscopic (endoscopic) radical prostatectomy. BJU Int 2003;91(8):749–757.

19. Menon M. Robotic radical retropubic prostatectomy. BJU Int 2003;91(3):175–176.

20. Han M, Partin AW, Pound CR, Epstein JI, Walsh PC. Long-term biochemical disease-free and cancer-specific survival following anatomic radical retropubic prostatectomy. The 15-year Johns Hopkins experience. Urol Clin North Am 2001;28(3):555–565.

21. Jewett HJ, Bridge RW, Gray GFJ, Shelley WM. The palpable nodule of prostatic cancer. Results 15 years after radical excision. JAMA 1968;203(6): 403–406.

22. Walsh PC. Radical prostatectomy, preservation of sexual function, cancer control. The controversy. Urol Clin North Am 1987;14(4):663–673.

23. Han M, Partin AW, Piantadosi S, Epstein JI, Walsh PC. Era specific biochemical recurrence-free survival following radical prostatectomy for clinically localized prostate cancer. J Urol 2001;166(2): 416–419.

24. Han M, Partin AW, Zahurak M, Piantadosi S, Epstein JI, Walsh PC. Biochemical (prostate specific antigen) recurrence probability following radical prostatectomy for clinically localized prostate cancer. J Urol 2003;169(2):517–523.

25. Partin AW, Mangold LA, Lamm DM, Walsh PC, Epstein JI, Pearson JD. Contemporary update of prostate cancer staging nomograms (Partin Tables) for the new millennium. Urology 2001; 58(6):843–848.

26. Khan MA, Han M, Partin AW, Epstein JI, Walsh PC. Long-term cancer control of radical prostatectomy in men younger than 50 years of age: update 2003. Urology 2003;62(1):86–91.

27. Carter HB, Epstein JI, Partin AW. Influence of age and prostate-specific antigen on the chance of curable prostate cancer among men with nonpalpable disease. Urology 1999;53(1):126–130.

28. Pound CR, Partin AW, Eisenberger MA, Chan DW, Pearson JD, Walsh PC. Natural history of progression after PSA elevation following radical prostatectomy. JAMA 1999;281(17):1591–1597.

29. Partin AW, Borland RN, Epstein JI, Brendler CB. Influence of wide excision of the neurovascular bundle(s) on prognosis in men with clinically localized prostate cancer with established capsular penetration. J Urol 1993;150(1):142–146.

30. Smith RC, Partin AW, Epstein JI, Brendler CB. Extended followup of the influence of wide excision of the neurovascular bundle(s) on prognosis in men with clinically localized prostate cancer and extensive capsular perforation. J Urol 1996; 156(2 pt 1):454–457.

31. Shah O, Robbins DA, Melamed J, Lepor H. The New York University nerve sparing algorithm decreases the rate of positive surgical margins following radical retropubic prostatectomy. J Urol 2003;169(6):2147–2152.

32. Walsh PC. Anatomic radical retropubic prostatectomy. In: Walsh PC, Retik AB, Vaughan ED, Wein AJ, eds. Campbell's Urology. Philadelphia: WB Saunders 2002;3107–3129.

33. de Koning HJ, Auvinen A, Berenguer SA, et al. Large-scale randomized prostate cancer screening trials: program performances in the European Randomized Screening for Prostate Cancer trial

and the Prostate, Lung, Colorectal and Ovary Cancer Trial. Int J Cancer 2002;97(2):237–244.

34. Donovan J, Mills N, Smith M, et al. Quality improvement report: Improving design and conduct of randomised trials by embedding them in qualitative research: Protect (prostate testing for cancer and treatment) study. Commentary: presenting unbiased information to patients can be difficult. BMJ 2002;325:766–770.

35. Holmberg L, Bill-Axelson A, Helgesen F, et al. A randomized trial comparing radical prostatectomy with watchful waiting in early prostate cancer. N Engl J Med 2002;347(11):781–789.

36. Stanford JL, Feng Z, Hamilton AS, et al. Urinary and sexual function after radical prostatectomy for clinically localized prostate cancer: the Prostate Cancer Outcomes Study. JAMA 2000; 283(3):354–360.

37. Talcott JA, Rieker P, Propert KJ, et al. Patient-reported impotence and incontinence after nerve-sparing radical prostatectomy. J Natl Cancer Inst 1997;89(15):1117–1123.

38. Holzbeierlein J, Peterson M, Smith JA Jr. Variability of results of cavernous nerve stimulation during radical prostatectomy. J Urol 2001;165(1): 108–110.

39. Walsh PC, Marschke P, Catalona WJ, et al. Efficacy of first-generation Cavermap to verify location and function of cavernous nerves during radical prostatectomy: a multi-institutional evaluation by experienced surgeons. Urology 2001;57(3):491–494.

40. Walsh PC, Marschke P, Ricker D, Burnett AL. Use of intraoperative video documentation to improve sexual function after radical retropubic prostatectomy. Urology 2000;55(1):62–67.

41. Kim ED, Nath R, Slawin KM, Kadmon D, Miles BJ, Scardino PT. Bilateral nerve grafting during radical retropubic prostatectomy: extended follow-up. Urology 2001;58(6):983–987.

42. Fowler FJ, Roman A, Barry MJ, Wasson J, Lu-Yao G, Wennberg JE. Patient-reported complications and follow-up treatment after radical prostatectomy: the national Medicare experience: 1988–1990 (updated June 1993). Urology 1993;42: 622–629.

43. Talcott JA, Rieker P, Clark JA, et al. Patient-reported symptoms after primary therapy for early prostate cancer: results of a prospective cohort study. J Clin Oncol 1998;16(1):275–283.

44. Heathcote PS, Mactaggart PN, Boston RJ, James AN, Thompson LC, Nicol DL. Health-related quality of life in Australian men remaining disease-free after radical prostatectomy. Med J Aust 1998;168(10):483–486.

45. Catalona WJ, Carvalhal GF, Mager DE, Smith DS. Potency, continence and complication rates in 1,870 consecutive radical retropubic prostatectomies. J Urol 1999;162(2):433–438.

46. Rabbani F, Stapleton AM, Kattan MW, Wheeler TM, Scardino PT. Factors predicting recovery of erections after radical prostatectomy. J Urol 2000; 164(6):1929–1934.

47. Walsh PC, Marschke P, Ricker D, Burnett AL. Patient-reported urinary continence and sexual function after anatomic radical prostatectomy. Urology 2000;55(1):58–61.

48. Begg CB, Riedel ER, Bach PB, et al. Variations in morbidity after radical prostatectomy. N Engl J Med 2002;346(15):1138–1144.

49. Eastham JA, Kattan MW, Riedel E, et al. Variations among individual surgeons in the rate of positive surgical margins in radical prostatectomy specimens. J Urol 2003;170(6 pt 1):2292–2295.

8

Hormone Therapy for Prostate Cancer

Gairin J. Dancey and Jonathan Waxman

Prostate cancer is now the most prevalent of all male malignancies and the second most common cause of male cancer deaths. Death rates have trebled over the last 30 years, and changes in mortality during this period are shown in Table 8.1 [1].

Prostate cancer is initially an androgen-dependent tumor, and treatment aims to reduce androgen supply to it. It is over a century since the first treatment for prostate cancer was introduced by an English surgeon, who castrated patients with benign and malignant prostatic conditions and observed the responses. Since that time there have been refinements of treatment so that we are now able to deal more humanely with this condition. We understand more about the toxicities of treatment and the value of second-line therapies. This has led to an improvement in survival. Our hope for the future is that new developments and therapeutic options will result from our increased understanding of the molecular basis of prostate cancer. This chapter surveys the current state of hormonal treatment for prostate cancer.

Localized Disease

The happy triumvirate of watchful waiting, radiotherapy, and surgery are offered patients with localized small-volume prostate cancer. There have been only two randomized trials comparing watchful waiting or radiotherapy with surgery, and they have involved small numbers of patients. In the most recent study, watchful waiting was compared to radical prostatectomy in 695 patients, and there was an increased risk of death in the watchful waiting group as compared with the surgical group, with a relative risk of progression to metastatic disease for watchful waiting as compared to surgery of 0.63 (95% confidence interval 0.41–0.96). The advantage to surgery was mostly apparent in those patients with poor prognosis histology [2].

The results of radiotherapy have never been subjected to any significant critical analysis that would stand scrutiny in modern times. Virtually all studies have described results of treatment in single institutions. However, the radiotherapists have managed to climb out of this critical abyss by conducting a significant number of well-organized studies that have examined the role of adjuvant antiandrogen treatment in combination with radiotherapy for localized prostate cancer. In summary, there have been 20 such studies, 14 retrospective and six prospective. Virtually all of the studies have shown an advantage to adjuvant hormonal therapy in terms of the local control of the tumor. However, the situation is distinctly different when one analyzes overall survival. Eighteen of the studies have shown no advantage, and two showed a survival advantage to treatment [3].

The two studies that describe a survival advantage merit further analysis. The first of these studies conducted by the Radiation Therapy Oncology Group (RTOG) is summa-

Table 8.1. Prostate cancer mortality

1964	3,370	1965	3,982
1966	3,915	1967	3,903
1968	3,939	1969	4,000
1970	3,906	1971	4,027
1972	4,181	1973	4,236
1974	4,313	1975	4,421
1976	4,611	1977	4,605
1978	4,730	1979	4,837
1980	5,038	1981	5,151
1982	5,291	1983	5,619
1984	6,248	1985	6,628
1986	8,434	1987	7,166
1988	7,458	1989	7,861
1990	8,098	1991	8,570
1992	8,735	1993	8,605
1994	8,689	1995	8,866
1996	8,782	1997	8,531
1998	8,573	1999	8,533
2000	8,293	2001	8,936
2002	8,973		

Source: Office for National Statistics, 2003 [1].

Table 8.2. Radiotherapy and adjuvant hormonal therapy for localised prostatic cancer: RTOG 8–31

	Goserelin adjuvant	Goserelin on progression	P
Patients	488 (477)	489 (468)	
Nodes + ve	337	345	
Gleason 8–10	139	137	
Local failure	78	135	<0.0001
Distant failure	82	136	<0.0001
Absolute survival	131	138	N.S.

Source: JCO 1997:15;1013.

lin. Kaplan-Meier predictions of 5-year survival showed an improved prospect for those patients treated with adjuvant hormonal therapy [4], and this result was confirmed when the EORTC published in 2000 an update of this trial with actual survival figures (Table 8.4) [5].

The Hormonal Treatment of Locally Advanced and Metastatic Prostate Cancer

The history of hormonal therapy for prostate cancer dates back to the 1890s, when patients with prostatic diseases, which included cancer, were treated by orchiectomy, and their condition improved. Scientific analyses of the results of treatment emerged nearly a century later, and, after enormous resistance from the urological surgical community, medical therapies for prostate cancer began to replace orchiectomy as a standard treatment for the condition. The urologists argued from the surgical viewpoint that

rized in Table 8.2. In this study there was a significant advantage to patients prescribed adjuvant treatment with goserelin as compared with those patients who received goserelin on progression of their tumor. There are echoes in these results of the 1997 randomized surgical study in this radiotherapy trial, with the significant improvement in survival confined to those patients with high Gleason grade tumors (Table 8.3). The second study published, in the same year and conducted by the European Organization for Research and Treatment of Cancer (EORTC), randomized patients to radiotherapy with or without 3 years' treatment with gosere-

Table 8.3. Radiotherapy and adjuvant hormonal therapy for localised prostatic cancer: RTOG 85–31

	Goserelin adjuvant		Goserelin on progression		
	Cancer deaths	Other causes	Cancer deaths	Other causes	P
Gleason 2–7	20	52	22	47	N.S.
Gleason 8–10	25	23	40	20	<0.0001

Source: JCO 1997:15;1013.

Table 8.4. Eortc radiotherapy and adjuvant hormonal therapy trial: the update

Patients:	415 (412)
Median FU:	5.5 yrs
5 year DFS:	40% (95% Cl 32–48%) RT 74% (95% Cl 67–81%) RT + AA
5 year OS:	62% (95% Cl 52–72%) RT 78% (95% Cl 72–84%) RT + AA
5 year disease specific survival:	79% (95% Cl 72–86%) RT 94% (95% Cl 90–98%) RT + AA

Source: Lancet 2002:360;103.

orchiectomy was a simple procedure, and that patients treated in this way could forget about their condition. Medical oncologists argued that it seemed a pretty bad stroke of luck to get cancer, but to be castrated because you had this initial piece of bad luck seemed an unfair twist of fate.

Some 20 years after the initial introduction of the concept of luteinizing hormone–releasing hormone (LHRH) agonist treatment for prostate cancer, treatment with these agents is now accepted as standard. So much so, that the sales of these drugs constituted the biggest oncology earner for big pharmaceutical companies in the late 1990s. These agents are conventionally thought of as acting to downregulate the pituitary gonadal axis. They do this by tight binding to the gonadotropin-releasing hormone (GnRH) receptors in the pituitary. The conformational change resulting from the amino acid substitution leads to greater stability of the molecule, such that the pituitary arymilidases are less able to break down the altered peptide. The result of this is prolonged binding to the receptor and its subsequent downregulation with decreased levels of luteinizing hormone (LH), follicle-stimulating hormone (FSH), and gonadal steroidal hormones. Although this is the convention, it should be noted that there is also a direct effect at the level of the tumor of the GnRH agonists. Hormone-dependent cell lines but not independent lines have higher affinity receptors for these agonists. Both hormone-dependent and -independent cell lines produce GnRH-like peptides, which provide evidence for activity of an autocrine loop in this cancer, and this is

confirmed by the presence in human tumors of the GnRH receptor [6].

Combined Antiandrogen Treatment

Labrie, a French Canadian, has made a great contribution to prostate cancer treatment, and suggested that in a disease that is androgen sensitive it is important to eliminate all sources of androgen. Labrie advocated the use of a combination of an antiandrogen with an LHRH agonist in the treatment of prostate cancer. The sources of androgen supplied to the prostate are dietary, adrenal, and testicular. The use of an antiandrogen, such as flutamide, potentially has the benefit of acting synergistically with GnRH agonist. Labrie's early work was not based on any randomized study, and so was not greeted with universal acceptance, but rather the opposite! However, his opinion has been vindicated by randomized controlled trials and meta-analyses of these studies. The randomized trials show a 7-month survival advantage to combination antiandrogen treatment. The meta-analyses, however, do not look at survival advantage, but at overall 5-year survival, and these report a 3% benefit to combination therapy as compared with monotherapy at 5 years. This would appear to be a bizarre time point to use as an assessment, in a disease with a median survival of 3 years. For the clear reason that there is a 7-month survival advantage, it would appear that the appropriate practice recommendation is for combination therapy.

Intermittent Hormonal Therapy

Among the most important quality of life issues for patients with prostate cancer is the loss of sexual function with treatment. For this reason many men delay treatment or take treatment intermittently. There is no evidence whatsoever that intermittent treatment is less successful than continuous therapy. Indeed, if one examines the effects of hormonal treatment on prostate cancer cells growing in culture, then a single exposure to antiandrogen therapy is seen to cause devastating destruction of cell cultures rather akin to the effects of chemotherapy.

There is no rational basis for continuous therapy, and so the intermittent treatment approach can be supported. This point was brought home to me by the clinical course of a patient advocate on one of the trust boards of the Prostate Cancer Charity. He presented with metastatic disease and took hormonal treatment for a period of 6 weeks. He responded well and discontinued treatment until he suddenly presented 4 years later with cord compression, a course of events that might have occurred if he had taken continuous therapy. This anecdote, though hardly hard science, if taken in context and considered in the light of the many side effects of hormonal therapy, could be used to support the case for a randomized trial of intermittent therapy. Certainly this approach is currently more widely advocated and is under investigation [7].

The Treatment of Recurrent Prostate Cancer

There is clinical evidence of prostate-specific antigen (PSA) progression after a median period of 13 months' hormonal therapy. Some 2 years after this evidence emerges, clinical symptoms develop, to be followed a median of 7 months later by death, and this course of events is not what we want for our patients. The biological basis for relapse is of more than passing interest. If patients' biopsy specimens are compared at presentation and relapse, mutations are seen within the androgen receptor in 45% to 55% of patients. It is these mutations that facilitate tumor progression. The androgen receptor is a transcription factor that binds to coactivators and co-repressors together with heat shock proteins, and by this process initiates gene transcription. It may well be that in patients who do not have obvious mutations of the androgen receptor, mutations of coactivators or co-repressors of the androgen receptor are responsible for tumor progression (Fig. 8.1).

These mutations have a practical significance. This significance is that the tumor has changed from being responsive to antiandrogen treatment to becoming dependent on it. In this situation withdrawal of the antiandrogen leads to a transient response, and this is seen in 20% to 40% of patients [8]. Upon further progression, treatment with low-dose steroids leads to a transient response in 10% to 20% of patients. It is very doubtful whether there is any benefit from other agents, such as ketoconazole, tamoxifen, or a progestogen. Platelet-derived growth factor receptor (PDGFR) positivity is reported in 10% to 70% of patients' biopsy specimens. For this reason, inhibitors of PDGFR action have been investigated in prostate cancer. Agents inhibiting PDGFR may do so through a number of routes, varying from direct blockade of the receptor itself to inhibition of downstream effector mechanisms. There is no evidence to date that these agents have activity in prostate cancer, though there has been interest recently in the combination of such agents with cytotoxic chemotherapy, and in one such study docetaxel in combination with imatinib has been shown to be of interest [9].

The Side Effects of Hormonal Therapy

In the treatment of any group of patients, there is a historical paradigm to clinical reportage. The initial publication describes an effect of a new treatment. The follow-up publications confirm this effect. A third group of publications then emerge comparing the effect of the new treatment to a standard therapy option, and then finally the side effects of the new treatment are reported. This has been the case with the hormonal treatment of prostate cancer. The initial reports of estrogen activity have been followed by overwhelming evidence of toxicity. This includes a 40% incidence of gastrointestinal toxicity, gynecomastia that is not prevented by the irradiation of breast buds, and cardiovascular toxicity that is not prevented by low-dose anticoagulation [10]. Nevertheless, estrogens are still prescribed in the United Kingdom, although their prescription is proscribed in many other countries in the European Union.

As time has progressed, the GnRH agonists have also been shown to have side effects. These include memory loss, parkinsonism, anemia, and osteoporosis, in addition to the hot flushes and impotence that were obvious from their first use. The most important of the side effects phys-

Fig. 8.1. The androgen receptor pathway in prostate cancer. (Courtesy of Dr. Charlotte Bevan, Prostate Cancer Research Group, Department of Cancer Medicine, Faculty of Medicine, Imperial College London, Hammersmith Campus, London, England.)

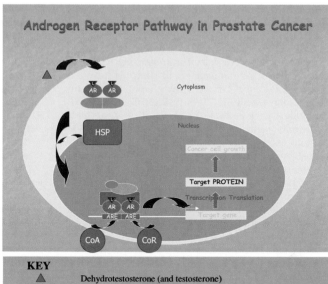

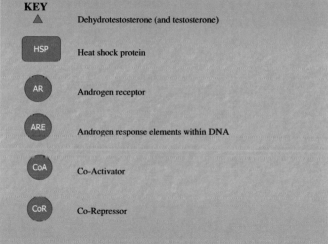

iologically is osteoporosis, with a loss of bone mass of nearly 10% per annum. Although bisphosphonates have been shown to be of little effect in prostate cancer in terms of limiting pain and tumor progression, which are the main benefits of their use in breast cancer and myeloma, this group of agents is of significant use in limiting osteoporosis in prostate cancer [11].

Conclusion

Over the years the treatment of prostate cancer has certainly become more humane. The most significant area of interest in this disease re-mains the exploration of the molecular basis for response and relapse. In understanding this, our hope is to provide more effective treatment for prostate cancer.

References

1. Office for National Statistics. Mortality Statistics: Cause (Series DH2). HMSO, 2003.
2. Holmberg L, Bill-Axelson A., Helgesen F, et al. A randomized trial comparing radical prostatectomy with watchful waiting in early prostate cancer. N Engl J Med 2002;347:781–789.
3. Pilepich MV, Caplan R, Byhardt RW, et al. Phase III trial of androgen suppression using goserelin in unfavorable-prognosis carcinoma of the prostate

treated with definitive radiotherapy: report of Radiation Therapy Oncology Group Protocol 85-31. J Clin Oncol 1997;15:1013–1021.

4. Vicini FA, Kini VR, Spencer W, Diokno A, Martinez AA. The role of androgen deprivation in the definitive management of clinically localized prostate cancer treated with radiation therapy. Int J Radiat Oncol Biol Phys 1999;43:707–713.

5. Bolla M, Collette L, Blank L, et al. Long-term results with immediate androgen suppression and external irradiation in patients with locally advanced prostate cancer (an EORTC study): a phase III randomised trial. Lancet 2002;360: 103–106.

6. Qayum A, Gullick W, Clayton RC, Sikora K, Waxman J. The effects of gonadotrophin releasing hormone analogues in prostate cancer are mediated through specific tumour receptors. Br J Cancer 1990;62:96–99.

7. Goldenberg SL, Bruchovsky N, Gleave ME, Sullivan LD, Akakura K. Intermittent androgen suppression in the treatment of prostate cancer: a preliminary report. Urology 1995;45:839–845.

8. Scher HI, Kelly WK. Flutamide withdrawal syndrome: its impact on clinical trials in hormone-refractory prostate cancer. J Clin Oncol 1993;11: 1566–1572.

9. Mathew P, Thall PF, Jones D, et al. Platelet-derived growth factor receptor inhibitor imatinib mesylate and docetaxel: a modular phase I trial in androgen-independent prostate cancer. J Clin Oncol 2004;22:3323–3329.

10. Bishop MC. Experience with low-dose oestrogen in the treatment of advanced prostate cancer: a personal view. Br J Urol 1996;78:921–927.

11. Dhillon T, Waxman J. Osteoporosis and prostate cancer. Br J Cancer 2003;89:779–780.

9

Chemotherapy in Prostate Cancer

Srikala S. Sridhar and Malcolm J. Moore

Prostate cancer is now most frequently diagnosed malignancy and the second leading cause of cancer-related death [1]. Death rates have increased over the past 20 years and mortality may approach that of lung cancer within 15 years [2]. For patients with advanced disease, the response rate to hormonal therapy is about 80%, but this is not durable, and all patients will eventually develop hormone-refractory prostate cancer (HRPC) [3]. Chemotherapy has been shown to have palliative benefit in symptomatic HRPC, but has not yet been demonstrated to prolong survival. Median life expectancy for patients with HRPC is only 12 to 18 months, underscoring the urgent need for new therapeutic approaches [4].

Historically, the role of aggressive systemic chemotherapy in HRPC had been questioned because elderly patients with poor marrow reserve, concomitant illnesses, and poor performance status tolerated it poorly. Coupled with this, chemotherapy trials before 1991 reported response rates of only 5%. In the last decade, the role of chemotherapy in prostate cancer has been revisited, with the development of less toxic regimens, which can significantly improve overall quality of life. Some recent trials in prostate cancer have used quality of life and cancer symptoms as end points. The use of prostate-specific antigen (PSA) has also provided a measure to evaluate the efficacy of newer agents in phase II studies, as most patients with HRPC have disease in bone and do not have conventionally measurable lesions. This chapter dis-

cusses the various chemotherapy regimens and recent advances in the systemic management of prostate cancer.

Hormone-Refractory Prostate Cancer

Hormone-refractory prostate cancer is defined as disease that progresses despite castrate testosterone levels, and is refractory to all hormonal manipulations including withdrawal of antiandrogen therapy. Until recently, there had been no standard chemotherapeutic approach for HRPC. Several agents had been evaluated in clinical trials, but many older studies suffered from methodological deficits such as small numbers of patients, heterogeneity of enrolled patients, and lack uniform response criteria [5]. Overall there have been very few recent phase III trials completed in HRPC (Table 9.1) making it difficult to draw firm conclusions about the efficacy of many regimens. However, it would appear that chemotherapy at a minimum does provide a palliative benefit.

Non–chemotherapy-based approaches to palliation also exist. External beam radiotherapy, for example, remains the mainstay of treatment for patients with bone pain, spinal cord compression, or painful urinary obstructive symptoms. In patients with more widespread bone disease, radioisotopes such as strontium-89, rhenium, or samarium may provide some pain

Table 9.1. Summary of recent (1996–2003) phase III trials in hormone refractory prostate cancer (HRPC)

First author, year (reference)	Regimen	No. of patients	>50% PSA decline	Palliative benefit	Time to progression (months)	Overall survival (months)	Median survival (months)
Tannock, 1996 (17)	Mitoxantrone + prednisone vs. prednisone	161	33%* 23%	38% 21%	6.0* 2.5	12.1 11.8	
Kantoff, 1999 (20)	Mitoxantrone + prednisone vs. prednisone	242	38%* 22%		3.7 2.3	12.3 12.6	
Berry, 2002 (21)	Mitoxantrone + prednisone vs. prednisone (asymptomatic)	120	48%* 24%		8.1* 4.1		23 19
Ernst, 2003 (8)	Mitoxantrone + prednisone + clodronate vs. mitoxantrone + prednisone	209	29.7% 28.6%	46% 39%			10.8 11.5
Small, 2000 (53)	Suramin + prednisone vs. prednisone	460	33% 16%	43%* 28%			10.2 10.0
Hudes, 1999 (26)	Vinblastine + estramustine vs. vinblastine	201	25.2% 3.2%		3.7* 2.2		11.9* 9.2

PSA, prostate-specific antigen.
* Statistically significant.

relief [6]. Low-dose corticosteroids both with and without chemotherapy are another option for relief of pain and constitutional symptoms [7].

Another class of agents showing palliative benefit in small phase II trials was the bisphosphonates. These are stable analogues of calcium pyrophosphate that inhibit osteoclast activity in bone, and are approved by the Food and Drug Administration (FDA) for use in the palliation of bone pain due to metastases from breast cancer and myeloma. A phase III trial by Ernst et al. [8], however, failed to demonstrate improvements in palliative response or overall quality of life when the bisphosphonate clodronate, was added to chemotherapy. Similarly, pamidronate, another bisphosphonate, did not significantly palliate bone pain or reduce skeletal-related events (SRE) when compared with placebo [9]. To date, only zoledronic acid, a newer bisphosphonate, appears to significantly reduce SRE and therefore may be a viable option in patients with HRPC [10].

In the past, HRPC patients were identified solely on the basis of symptoms occurring due to increasing tumor burden; but now with the use of the PSA test and imaging studies, patients are often diagnosed with HRPC at a time when they are asymptomatic with a PSA that is starting to rise. The increase in median survival seen in recent HRPC chemotherapy trials when compared with older studies, may thus be less reflective of more effective treatment, but rather represent lead-time bias due to the inclusion of these asymptomatic early-stage patients.

Response to Therapy

One of the more challenging aspects of treating prostate cancer is adequately assessing response to therapy. This is particularly true in the hormone-refractory setting, where disease is often limited to bone, and change in the size or intensity of bone lesions is difficult to interpret. Also, the findings on bone scans may worsen as healing occurs with the initiation of therapy, and may only subsequently slowly improve. Bone scan progression for the purpose of clinical trial entry is now being defined as the appearance of at least one new lesion. Unfortunately, restricting trials to patients with bidimensionally measurable soft tissue disease is not a feasible option either, because few patients present this way, and this would exclude otherwise eligible patients.

The PSA, a 34-kd serine protease secreted by both benign and malignant prostate epithelium, is elevated in approximately 95% of patients with advanced metastatic disease, and has been adopted as a surrogate end point in most prostate cancer trials [11]. However, in some settings PSA changes do not show good correlation with firm end points such as survival, leading to the suggestion that the PSA may require validation for the specific clinical setting and therapeutic agent under investigation [12]. There is also no consistent reporting of changes in PSA, making comparisons between trials difficult.

In an attempt to standardize PSA reporting, the PSA working group has created a guideline that defines PSA response as a decline of at least 50% or more, confirmed with a second PSA value at least 4 weeks later (in the absence of clinical or radiographic disease progression). This definition is based on previous studies that suggest a statistically significant survival advantage associated with a PSA decrease of 50% or more [13,14]. Similarly, response duration and time to PSA progression may also be important clinical end points, but have yet to be validated. The PSA is a relatively simple test to obtain, and although it may not be the ideal surrogate marker, it may help to quickly identify those treatments that warrant further investigation at the phase III level.

Measures of response such as PSA do not necessarily indicate whether a patient is benefiting from therapy. Survival and quality of life are the most important measures of patient benefit in the evaluation of treatments in HRPC. Several studies now incorporate palliative end points such as pain, analgesic use, physical activity level, fatigue, appetite, constipation, urinary difficulties, relationships, mood, and overall well-being, through the use of questionnaires such as the Present Pain Intensity (PPI) Index or the Prostate Cancer-Specific Quality of Life Instrument (PROSQOLI). In fact, on the basis of quality of life improvements alone, the chemotherapy regimen of mitoxantrone and prednisone has been approved for use in HRPC.

Mitoxantrone and Prednisone

Mitoxantrone is a synthetic anthraquinone drug that belongs to the anthracenedione class of compounds. It has a symmetrical structure comprising a tricyclic planar chromophore and two basic side chains [15]. The exact mechanism of action of this cell cycle phase nonspecific drug is unclear, but it does appear to (1) intercalate DNA, resulting in inter- and intrastrand crosslinks; (2) bind DNA phosphate backbone, inducing strand breaks; and (3) inhibit topoisomerase II activity. Clinically, mitoxantrone is well tolerated, but due to structural similarity to doxorubicin, it shares the dose-limiting side effect of cardiotoxicity. Other side effects include nausea, vomiting, and myelosuppression [16].

A Canadian study led by Tannock et al. [17] randomized 161 symptomatic patients with HRPC to receive either mitoxantrone every 3 weeks with daily prednisone or prednisone alone. The primary end point of this study was palliative response, which was defined as a significant improvement in either pain or analgesic usage or both (neither could get worse). In the mitoxantrone arm, a statistically significant improvement in pain relief (29% vs. 12%, $p = .01$) and a prolonged duration of this palliative response (43 weeks vs. 18 weeks, $p < .0001$) was demonstrated. These patients also reported improvements in physical and social functioning, global quality of life, anorexia, drowsiness, constipation, and other symptoms [18]. The use of mitoxantrone was also associated with a higher PSA response rate and time to progression. There was no survival benefit of chemotherapy, although a crossover to mitoxantrone in patients who progressed on prednisone was allowed and may have impacted on the survival analysis. An economic analysis of this study by Bloomfield et al. [19] further suggested a benefit to these patients receiving mitoxantrone and prednisone. Overall, these results were consistent with a Cancer and Leukemia Group B (CALGB) study that showed a trend toward greater pain control in the mitoxantrone arm, but no improvement in overall survival (the primary end point). The toxicities of mitoxantrone included neutropenia, thrombocytopenia, and cardiac dysfunction, but in both studies the incidence of serious toxicity was very low [20].

These two critical studies led to FDA approval of mitoxantrone and prednisone for symptomatic patients with HRPC. Its use in earlier stage asymptomatic HRPC patients was recently evaluated in a phase III study by Berry et al. [21], which again suggested no survival benefit. The PSA response in this study (48%) was higher than that seen in the Tannock or CALGB studies (33%), and median survival was also increased to 23 months, as compared to only 12 months in the Canadian and CALGB studies. This may be due to patients having lower median baseline PSA on trial entry, and the lead-time bias introduced by including these early-stage patients.

Estramustine/Taxane-Based Therapy

Estramustine phosphate, a conjugate of estradiol and nitrogen mustard, with hormonal and non-hormonal cytotoxic effects in vitro, has also been evaluated in HRPC [22]. Unlike other alkylating agents, estramustine does not directly damage DNA but depolymerizes cytoplasmic microtubules and microfilaments, binds to microtubule associated proteins, disrupts the nuclear matrix, and inhibits P-glycoprotein [23]. Based on in vitro data suggesting synergy, several phase II studies have been completed using estramustine in combination with etoposide, vinblastine, and the taxanes.

The combination of estramustine and etoposide, which showed in vitro activity, was initially attractive because both drugs target microtubules and could be administered orally. Results from several trials suggest the response rate to be approximately 50%, but this was accompanied by significant toxicity. As a result, this regimen is not in phase III trials [24,25].

Vinblastine, an agent chosen for its distinct antimicrotubule effects, lack of cross-resistance, and nonoverlapping toxicities with estramustine, has also been evaluated. Hudes et al. [26], in a phase III trial, compared estramustine plus vinblastine with vinblastine alone. Response rates in the combined arm were 25.2% versus only 3.2% in the vinblastine alone arm. There was acceptable toxicity, and no survival advantage with the combined arm, but this study was underpowered to detect slight survival improvements. A similar PSA response rate, 24.9%, was reported in a recent study by Albrect et al. [27] for the combination of estramustine and vinblastine. But this was less than the response rate for single-agent estramustine, which was 28.9%.

Furthermore, toxicity in the combined arm in this trial was felt to be unacceptable. The difference in tolerability between the trials could be explained by differences in estramustine dosing, or the inclusion of more advanced, poorer performance status patients in the latter trial. Nonetheless, it illustrates the difficulties encountered when testing new agents in HRPC where trial design, drug dosing, and patient selection can play a critical role.

The taxanes (paclitaxel and docetaxel), which also target microtubules, have shown encouraging results when combined with estramustine (Table 9.2). By binding to tubulin, the taxanes induce microtubule stabilization, G2/M phase cell cycle arrest, and apoptosis. They also induce apoptosis through activation of the proapoptotic protein bax, and inactivation of bcl-2, an antiapoptotic protein often overexpressed in HRPC. Initial studies with the combination of paclitaxel and estramustine showed activity, but excessive toxicity necessitated dose reductions prior to the phase II trial by Hudes et al. This dose reduction did not compromise antitumor activity, and PSA responses were seen in 53.1% of patients, with a 5.6-month time to progression and a median survival of 17 months [22]. This study also reported a decrease in pain and analgesic requirements, and an improvement in overall quality of life. This combination is now being evaluated in phase III trials.

Despite lowered doses, toxicities due to estramustine, primarily nausea and thromboembolism (requiring prophylactic anticoagulation) continue to be a problem. Berry et al. [28], with the U.S. Oncology Group, conducted a phase II randomized trial comparing estramustine and paclitaxel with paclitaxel alone. Though PSA response rates (48% vs. 25% $p = .01$) and the trend to median survival were higher in the combined arm, there were fewer thromboembolic complications in the paclitaxel only arm, indicating that single-agent paclitaxel may be an option for patients with a history of thromboembolic problems.

Another member of the taxane family that is more potent than paclitaxel and easier from a dosing standpoint is docetaxel. Petrylak et al. [29] treated chemonaive HRPC patients with a combination of estramustine and docetaxel. The PSA responses rates were favorable (74%), but again significant estramustine-related toxicity has led some to question whether single-agent

Table 9.2. Summary of phase II clinical trials of estramustine plus a taxane in patients with hormone-refractory prostate cancer

First author, year (reference)	Regimen	No. of patients	>50% PSA decline	Response in measurable disease	Median survival (months)	1-year survival
Petrylak, 1999 (29)	Docetaxel + estramustine	35	74%	4/7 (57%)	22	77%
Sinibaldi, 2002 (59)	Docetaxel + estramustine	40	45%	3/13 (23%)	N/A	N/A
Savarese, 2001 (60)	Docetaxel + hydrocortisone + estramustine	44	68%	12/24 (50%)	20	
Sitka, 2001 (61)	Docetaxel + estramustine	30	76%	17/30 (57%)		
Hudes, 1997 (22)	Paclitaxel + estramustine	34	53%	4/9 (44.4%)		
Hudes, 2001 (62)	Paclitaxel + estramustine	63	58.1%	6/22 (27.3%)		
Berry, 2001 (31)	Paclitaxel + estramustine	166	48%		15.1	
Athanasiadis, 2003 (63)	Paclitaxel + estramustine	41	58.5%	9/41 (22%)	17	

docetaxel is equally effective with less toxicity [29]. A phase II single-agent docetaxel trial by Picus and Schultz [30] showed PSA responses of 45%, with tolerable toxicities. Similarly, Berry et al. [31] reported that in mitoxantrone-pretreated HRPC patients, docetaxel showed a response rate of 41%, with toxicities less than those seen in the estramustine plus docetaxel regimen. Beer et al. [32], using weekly dosing of docetaxel, reported PSA response rate of 47% and pain response of 33%, and the toxicities were all less than 10%. Overall, the positive results with taxane-based therapies have led to its evaluation in several phase III trials (Table 9.3).

Two phase III studies comparing docetaxel-based regimens with mitoxantrone and prednisone have recently been reported. The TAX 327 trial, a prospective, nonblinded, three-arm study, randomized more than 1000 patients to receive docetaxel plus prednisone (a weekly regimen or every 3 weeks) or the current standard, mitoxantrone and prednisone. End points included overall survival, PSA response, and palliative response. Docetaxel every three weeks led to superior survival (18.9 mo vx. 16.5 mo) and improved rates of response in terms of pain, serum PSA, and quality of life as compared with mitoxantrone plus prednisne [32a]. The Southwest Oncology Group (SWOG) 9916 phase III study randomized 674 patients to receive estra-

mustine and docetaxel or to mitoxantrone and prednisone, with the primary end point being overall survival. The docetaxel and estramustine arm again showed an improvement in overall survival (17.5 mo vs. 15.6 mo) compared with the mitoxantrone arm [32b]. Based on these two large trials, taxane based therapy is quickly becoming the standard of care for hormone refractory prostate cancer.

By combining mitoxantrone, docetaxel, and low-dose prednisone in a phase II multicenter trial, Freeman [33] showed a PSA response rate of 69% and a trend toward improvement in quality of life end points after two cycles of chemotherapy. This is another regimen that will be investigated further.

Triplet Combinations

Triplet combinations of estramustine, paclitaxel, and carboplatin in a small study have shown a 67% PSA response rate but lacked palliative benefit. Other three-drug regimens—estramustine, etoposide, and paclitaxel; paclitaxel, estramustine, and carboplatin; and estramustine, etoposide, and vinorelbine—have shown PSA responses but yet no palliative improvements [34–37]. The value of these three-drug regimens at this time remains largely unknown.

Table 9.3. Summary of phase II trials using a single-agent taxane in patients with hormone-refractory prostate cancer

First author, year (reference)	Taxane regimen	No. of patients	>50% PSA decline	Response in measurable disease	Time to progression (months)	Survival (months)
Picus, 1999 (30)	Docetaxel 75 mg/m^2 q 3 weeks	35	46%	7/25 (28%)	9	27
Berry, 2001 (31)	Docetaxel 36 mg/m^2/ week ×6 of an 8-week cycle	59	41%	2/6 (33%)	5.1	9.4
Beer, 2001 (32)	Docetaxel 36 mg/m^2/ week ×6 of an 8-week cycle	24	46%	2/5 (40%)	NR	NR
Friedland, 1999 (64)	Docetaxel 75 mg/m^2 q 3 weeks	16	38%	6/9 (67%)	NR	NR
Trivedi, 2000 (65)	Paclitaxel 150 mg/m^2/ week	18	39%	4/8 (50%)	NR	NR

NR, no results.

Chemotherapy in Hormone-Sensitive Disease

Neoadjuvant Chemotherapy

The use of systemic chemotherapy earlier in the course of treatment, an effective strategy in some malignancies, has been explored to a small degree in prostate cancer. The objectives of neoadjuvant chemotherapy are to downstage the cancer, decrease the incidence of positive surgical margins, and eliminate micrometastases. In addition, chemotherapy may eradicate both androgen-independent clones and androgen-sensitive clones, the latter by synergizing with hormonal ablation.

Several pilot neoadjuvant chemotherapy trials have now been reported, and suggest that from a surgical standpoint this is a feasible approach (Table 9.4). Pettaway et al. [38] treated patients with high-risk localized disease with 12 weeks of ketoconazole and doxorubicin alternating with vinblastine and estramustine (KAVE) and androgen ablation followed by radical prostatectomy (RP). The primary end point, a 20% pathological complete response (pCR), was not achieved, but there were fewer positive margins. Clark et al. [39] reported similar results, but increased thromboembolic events, using a neoadjuvant regimen of etoposide and estramustine. The taxanes have also been evaluated in the neoadjuvant setting. Single-agent docetaxel

administered prior to RP was well tolerated, with final efficacy results pending at this time [40,41]. Based on encouraging phase II results of the neoadjuvant regimen of docetaxel and estramustine, the CALGB has initiated a phase III randomized study in patients with high-risk disease [42,43]. Other neoadjuvant combinations being studied are docetaxel with mitoxantrone [44], and the CALGB 99811 study of paclitaxel, estramustine, and carboplatin with an luteinizing hormone–releasing hormone (LHRH) agonist.

Administering chemotherapy prior to radical radiation therapy has been studied, but the lack of pathological specimens posttreatment makes interpretation of response somewhat difficult. Zelefsky et al [45] found that neoadjuvant and concomitant estramustine (which may act as a radiosensitizer) and vinblastine with high-dose conformal radiotherapy were well tolerated, but the authors did not draw any conclusions about efficacy. Ben-Josef et al. [46] used a regimen of estramustine and etoposide in patients with high-risk disease preradiotherapy and showed a favorable local control rate (71% vs. 54%) and 5-year disease-free survival (73% vs. 29%) compared with historical controls. In a study by Oh et al. [47], neoadjuvant liposomal doxorubicin chemotherapy prior to androgen ablation plus radiotherapy for high-risk disease showed no activity and significant toxicity.

Although preliminary data suggest that neoadjuvant chemotherapy can be safely administered, larger randomized controlled trials are necessary to determine its actual benefit. At the present time there is no indication for neoadjuvant chemotherapy outside of a well-designed clinical trial.

Adjuvant Therapy

To date, there are only a few studies published on adjuvant chemotherapy in prostate cancer (Table 9.5). The National Prostate Cancer Project has conducted two randomized trials. Patients postsurgery or post-external beam irradiation were randomized to observation or cyclophosphamide or estramustine. No overall survival benefit in the chemotherapy arm was noticed but an increased progression-free survival was found in patients receiving estramustine [48]. Three additional studies are currently underway. These include the SWOG 9921 phase II study,

randomizing post-RP patients to androgen deprivation with Casodex and Zoladex, mitoxantrone and prednisone, or to androgen deprivation alone. RTOG 9902 randomizes patients post–external beam radiotherapy to combined androgen blockade plus four cycles of paclitaxel, etoposide, and estramustine or to combined androgen blockade alone. A third nonrandomized study in high-risk post-RP patients is underway looking at the use of single-agent docetaxel (without androgen ablation).

Targeted Therapies

Our current treatment approaches rely heavily on standard cytotoxic therapies; however, greater insight at the molecular level into cell growth and proliferation has led to the development of targeted biological therapies that offer hope for improved efficacy with minimal toxicity.

Table 9.4. Summary of neoadjuvant chemotherapy trials in prostate cancer

First author, year (reference)	Regimen	Maximum treatment duration (weeks)	Local treatment	No. of patients	+ Margin (%)	Organ confined (%)	Extracapsular extension (%)
Pettaway, 2000 (38)	KAVE + androgen ablation	12	RP	33	17	33	67
Clark, 2001 (39)	Estramustine + etoposide	12	RP	18		31	69
Dreicer, 2001 (40)	Docetaxel	6	RP				
Oh, 2001 (41)	Docetaxel	24	RP				
Hussain, 2003 (42)	Docetaxel + estramustine	18	10 RP 11 RTX	21	30		
Eastham, 2003 (43)	Docetaxel + estramustine	18	RP				
Garzotto, 2002 (66)	Docetaxel + mitoxantrone	16	RP	14			
Kelly, 2001 (35)	Paclitaxel + estramustine + carboplatin	16	RTX	56			
Zelefsky, 2000 (45)	Estramustine + vinblastine	24	RTX	27			
Ben-Josef, 2001 (46)	Estramustine + etoposide	6	RTX	18			
Oh, 2003 (47)	Doxil + androgen ablation	8	RTX	7			

KAVE, ketoconazole, doxorubicin, vinblastine, estramustine, RP, radical prostatectomy; RTX, radiotherapy.

Table 9.5. Summary of adjuvant chemotherapy trials in prostate cancer

Author	Adjuvant regimen	Local therapy	Overall survival
National Prostate Cancer Project (48)	Cyclophosphamide + estramustine	Radical prostatectomy, 170 pts; prostate radiotherapy, 233 pts	No benefit
SWOG 9921	Mitoxantrone + prednisone + Casodex + Zoladex	Radical prostatectomy	
RTOG 9902	Paclitaxel + etoposide + estramustine + Casodex + Zoladex	Prostate radiotherapy	
NCI	Docetaxel	Radical prostatectomy	

NCI, National Cancer Institute; pts, patients; RTOG, Radiation Therapy Oncology Group; SWOG, Southwest Oncology Group.

Suramin

One of the first biological agents to be studied in prostate cancer was suramin, a polysulfonated aromatic compound initially synthesized as an antiparasitic agent. Suramin was later shown also to interfere with cell signaling, DNA replication, and angiogenesis, and it showed promising cytotoxic activity against prostate cancer cells in vitro [49]. In the clinical setting, patients failing antiandrogen therapy were treated with suramin, which was coadministered with a steroid to prevent adrenal suppression. The original clinical trials suggested this was an active compound; however, subsequent studies proved disappointing. Nonetheless, several key lessons were learned during this drug's development.

The importance of antiandrogen withdrawal and steroid use, for example, and the need to control for these confounding variables when designing clinical trials in HRPC, became readily apparent when each of these maneuvers independently demonstrated PSA response rates of 20% to 30%. This likely contributed to the inflated response rates of 70% seen initially in the uncontrolled suramin trials [12]. Another key realization was that PSA was not always a reliable marker of response to therapy as evidenced by trials showing a drop in PSA but no tumor regression or survival benefit, and whether this is a feature common to all biological therapies remains to be determined [12]. Suramin has significant neurological and other side effects owing to its large volume of distribution and long terminal half-life, raising the important issue of appropriate dosing of biological therapies [12]. In summary, the low response rate, lack of survival advantage, and toxicities of suramin have halted its further development, but the lessons learned from this experience can undoubtedly be applied to all future trials of novel therapies in HRPC.

Epidermal Growth Factor Receptor Inhibitors

The epidermal growth factor receptor (EGFR) superfamily of receptors, which comprises four distinct receptors known as EGFR, Human Epidermal growth Factor Receptor, HER2, HER3, and HER4, is a potential therapeutic target in prostate cancer where overexpression is seen in up to 80% of metastasis, and is generally associated with a poorer overall prognosis. Several EGFR targeting agents are now available, including tyrosine kinase inhibitors and monoclonal antibodies. To date, the tyrosine kinase inhibitor gefitinib has undergone the most investigation in prostate cancer. Three phase II trials, with gefitinib alone, and in combination with either docetaxel and estramustine, or mitoxantrone and prednisone, have completed accrual, with final results pending at this time. Two studies, reported in abstract form only, suggest that single-agent gefitinib does not have significant activity [50,51].

Angiogenesis Inhibitors

Targeting angiogenesis is another novel approach. Angiogenesis is a physiological process that is fundamental to cell growth and division. It is initiated by the release of proteases from activated endothelial cells, leading to degradation of the basement membrane, migration of endothelial cells into the interstitial space, and subsequent endothelial proliferation and differentiation into mature blood vessels [52]. Several agents targeting angiogenesis have been tested in prostate cancer, including suramin, thalidomide, matrix metalloproteinase inhibitors, endostatin, angiostatin, vascular endothelial growth factor (VEGF) inhibitors, and cell adhesion inhibitors, to name a few. These are all currently in early stages of development.

Immunotherapy

Another avenue of research in HRPC is immunotherapy, which is dependent on a suitable target antigen being presented to the immune system by an antigen-presenting cell (APC), such as the dendritic cell. The dendritic cell was chosen specifically because it is the most potent in eliciting a T-cell immune response. This approach has been evaluated in a randomized, placebo-controlled, phase III trial in HRPC patients with the drug APC8015. This is a product consisting of autologous dendritic cells loaded ex vivo with a recombinant fusion protein of prostatic acid phosphatase linked to granulocyte-macrophage colony-stimulating factor. This treatment was well tolerated and antigen-specific immunity was evident, but only in the subset of patients with a low Gleason score was there a trend toward improvement in median time to progression. A confirmatory phase III trial in these patients is now underway [53].

Vaccine-based therapies are also being evaluated. In one randomized phase II study, for example, recombinant pox viruses expressing PSA and the b7.1 co-stimulatory molecule were given to patients with nonmetastatic HRPC. Both immunologic activity and a delay in the development of metastatic disease at 6 months was seen [54]. Overall, targeting the immune system provides an exciting and novel approach to treating prostate cancer.

Combinations of Targeted and Cytotoxic Therapy

Targeted therapy in combination with chemotherapy is another area of active research. Several trials have assessed the combination of targeted therapies such as thalidomide, calcitriol, and exisulind with docetaxel. Thalidomide glutarimide is a synthetic glutamic acid derivative that was initially used for morning sickness but was taken off the market due to teratogenicity and neuropathies. Thalidomide has antiangiogenesis effects, inhibits cytokines including tumor necrosis factor-α, and can alter cell adhesion molecules. In a randomized phase II trial with 75 HRPC patients, comparing thalidomide and docetaxel with docetaxel alone, Leonard et al [55] reported a PSA response rate of 50%, and an increase in median survival by 14 months. Gastrointestinal, neurological, and thromboembolic toxicities were reported, the latter necessitating the use of prophylactic anticoagulation. Larger trials incorporating palliative end points, and more data on toxicity are needed to determine whether this combination is a viable option in HRPC.

Another interesting combination is high-dose calcitriol and docetaxel. Calcitriol, at supraphysiological concentrations, is a natural ligand for the vitamin D receptor and its analogues and has several mechanisms of action. Calcitriol causes G0/G1 arrest, changes in p21 (Waf1) and p27 (kip1) expression, dephosphorylation of retinoblastoma protein, downregulation of bcl-2, inhibition of angiogenesis, induction of apoptosis, and changes in several growth factor systems including EGF, transforming growth factor-β (TGF-β), and insulin-like growth factor (IGF). Preclinical studies suggest it enhances cytotoxic activity of docetaxel, paclitaxel, and platinum compounds, and is active in prostate cancer. In the study by Beer [56], HRPC patients treated with oral calcitriol and docetaxel had PSA responses of 81% and tolerated it well. Currently a phase II/III calcitriol study is underway.

Exisulind in an oral agent that selectively induces apoptosis via inhibition of cyclic guanosine monophosphate (cGMP) phosphodiesterase, leading to a sustained increase in cGMP, activation of protein kinase G, and jun kinase, and downstream effects culminating in cell death. Initial clinical studies with exisulind and docetaxel suggest PSA response rates of 44%, but due to toxicities dose reductions are necessary prior to further evaluation [57].

Trials are also currently underway evaluating the drug G3139 with docetaxel. G3139 is an antisense oligonucleotide to bcl-2, an antiapoptotic protein, overexpressed in prostate cancer, and a negative prognostic indicator. This combination has shown PSA responses of 48% and is well tolerated [58]. Other trials using antisense technology are also being initiated.

Taken together, targeted therapies either alone or in combination with chemotherapy are an area of active research that shows promising PSA responses and tolerability.

Summary

Chemotherapy in prostate cancer is an established treatment only for symptomatic hormone-refractory disease, where it can improve symptoms and quality of life but does not impact overall survival. Its role in earlier stage disease is currently being evaluated. Certainly, advancing chemotherapy may eliminate hormone-resistant clones early, thereby slowing the natural progression of this disease. Of the various cytotoxic agents currently under study, the taxanes show the most promise, combining encouraging PSA response rates with tolerability. Targeted therapies both alone or in combination may also prove effective, especially as we gain insight into prostate cancer at the molecular level and learn how best to use these agents. Phase III well-controlled clinical trials of the most promising regimens will then be needed to define the best regimens available.

References

1. Greenlee RT, Hill-Harmon MB, Murray T, Thun M. Cancer statistics, 2001. CA Cancer J Clin 2001; 51(1):15–36.
2. Waxman J, Roylance R. New drugs for prostate cancer? Eur J Cancer 1998;34(4):437.
3. Garnick MB. Prostate cancer: screening, diagnosis, and management. Ann Intern Med 1993; 118(10):804–818.
4. Ripple GH, Wilding G. Drug development in prostate cancer. Semin Oncol 1999;26(2):217–226.
5. Di Lorenzo G, Autorino R, De Laurentiis M, et al. Is there a standard chemotherapeutic regimen for hormone-refractory prostate cancer? Present and future approaches in the management of the disease. Tumori 2003;89(4):349–360.
6. Porter AT, McEwan AJ, Powe JE, et al. Results of a randomized phase-III trial to evaluate the efficacy of strontium-89 adjuvant to local field external beam irradiation in the management of endocrine resistant metastatic prostate cancer. Int J Radiat Oncol Biol Phys 1993;25(5):805–813.
7. Moore MJ, Tannock IF. Overview of Canadian trials in hormonally resistant prostate cancer. Semin Oncol 1996;23(6 suppl 14):15–19.
8. Ernst DS, Tannock IF, Winquist EW, et al. Randomized, double-blind, controlled trial of mitoxantrone/prednisone and clodronate versus mitoxantrone/prednisone and placebo in patients with hormone-refractory prostate cancer and pain. J Clin Oncol 2003;21(17):3335–3342.
9. Small EJ, Smith MR, Seaman JJ, et al. Combined analysis of two multicenter, randomized, placebo-controlled studies of pamidronate disodium for the palliation of bone pain in men with metastatic prostate cancer. J Clin Oncol 2003;21(23): 4277–4284.
10. Saad F, Schulman CC. Role of bisphosphonates in prostate cancer. Eur Urol 2004;45(1):26–34.
11. Kelly WK, Scher HI, Mazumdar M, Vlamis V, Schwartz M, Fossa SD. Prostate-specific antigen as a measure of disease outcome in metastatic hormone-refractory prostate cancer. J Clin Oncol 1993;11(4):607–615.
12. Kaur M, Reed E, Sartor O, et al. Suramin's development: what did we learn? Invest New Drugs 2002;20(2):209–219.
13. Bubley GJ, Carducci M, Dahut W, et al. Eligibility and response guidelines for phase II clinical trials in androgen-independent prostate cancer: recommendations from the Prostate-Specific Antigen Working Group. J Clin Oncol 1999;17(11):3461–3467.
14. Scher HI, Eisenberger M, D'Amico AV, et al. Eligibility and outcomes reporting guidelines for clinical trials for patients in the state of a rising prostate-specific antigen: recommendations from the Prostate-Specific Antigen Working Group. J Clin Oncol 2004;22(3):537–556.
15. Myers C. Anthracyclines. Cancer Chemother Biol Response Modif 1988;10:33–39.
16. Calabresi P, Chabner BA. Antineoplastic agents. In: Gilman A, Rall TW, Nies AS, eds. Goodman and Gilman's The Pharmacological Basis of Therapeutics. San Francisco: McGraw-Hill, 1993:1241–1244.
17. Tannock IF, Osoba D, Stockler MR, et al. Chemotherapy with mitoxantrone plus prednisone or prednisone alone for symptomatic hormone-resistant prostate cancer: a Canadian randomized trial with palliative end points. J Clin Oncol 1996;14(6):1756–1764.
18. Osoba D, Tannock IF, Ernst DS, et al. Health-related quality of life in men with metastatic prostate cancer treated with prednisone alone or mitoxantrone and prednisone. J Clin Oncol 1999; 17(6):1654–1663.
19. Bloomfield DJ, Krahn MD, Neogi T, et al. Economic evaluation of chemotherapy with mitoxantrone plus prednisone for symptomatic hormone-resistant prostate cancer: based on a Canadian randomized trial with palliative end points. J Clin Oncol 1998;16(6):2272–2279.
20. Kantoff PW, Halabi S, Conaway M, et al. Hydrocortisone with or without mitoxantrone in men

with hormone-refractory prostate cancer: results of the cancer and leukemia group B 9182 study. J Clin Oncol 1999;17(8):2506–2513.

21. Berry W, Dakhil S, Modiano M, et al. Phase III study of mitoxantrone plus low dose prednisone versus low dose prednisone alone in patients with asymptomatic hormone refractory prostate cancer. J Urol 2002;168(6):2439–2443.

22. Hudes GR, Nathan F, Khater C, et al. Phase II trial of 96-hour paclitaxel plus oral estramustine phosphate in metastatic hormone-refractory prostate cancer. J Clin Oncol 1997;15(9):3156–3163.

23. Perry CM, McTavish D. Estramustine phosphate sodium. A review of its pharmacodynamic and pharmacokinetic properties, and therapeutic efficacy in prostate cancer. Drugs Aging 1995; 7(1):49–74.

24. Pienta KJ, Redman BG, Bandekar R, et al. A phase II trial of oral estramustine and oral etoposide in hormone refractory prostate cancer. Urology 1997;50(3):401–406, discussion 406–407.

25. Dimopoulos MA, Panopoulos C, Bamia C, et al. Oral estramustine and oral etoposide for hormone-refractory prostate cancer. Urology 1997;50(5):754–758.

26. Hudes G, Einhorn L, Ross E, et al. Vinblastine versus vinblastine plus oral estramustine phosphate for patients with hormone-refractory prostate cancer: a Hoosier Oncology Group and Fox Chase Network phase III trial. J Clin Oncol 1999;17(10):3160–3166.

27. Albrecht W, Van Poppel H, Horenblas S, et al. Randomized Phase II trial assessing estramustine and vinblastine combination chemotherapy vs estramustine alone in patients with progressive hormone-escaped metastatic prostate cancer. Br J Cancer 2004;90(1):100–105.

28. Berry WG, Dakhil M, Hathorn S, et al. Phase II randomized trial of weekly paclitaxel (Taxol®) with or without estramustine phosphate in patients with symptomatic, hormone-refractory, metastatic carcinoma of the prostate (HRMCP). Proc Am Soc Clin Oncol 2001;20:696(abstract 175a).

29. Petrylak DP, Macarthur R, O'Connor J, et al. Phase I/II studies of docetaxel (Taxotere) combined with estramustine in men with hormone-refractory prostate cancer. Semin Oncol 1999;26(5 suppl 17):28–33.

30. Picus J, Schultz M. Docetaxel (Taxotere) as monotherapy in the treatment of hormone-refractory prostate cancer: preliminary results. Semin Oncol 1999;26(5 suppl 17):14–18.

31. Berry W, Dakhil S, Gregurich MA, et al. Phase II trial of single-agent weekly docetaxel in hormone-refractory, symptomatic, metastatic carcinoma of the prostate. Semin Oncol 2001;28(4 suppl 15):8–15.

32. Beer TM, Pierce WC, Lowe BA, et al. Phase II study of weekly docetaxel in symptomatic androgen-

independent prostate cancer. Ann Oncol 2001; 12(9):1273–1279.

32a Tannock IF, de Wit R, Berry WR, et al. Docetaxel plus prednisone or mitoxantrone plus prednisone for advanced prostate cancer. N Engl J Med 2004;351:1502–1512.

32b. Petrylak DP, Tangen CM, Hussain MHA, et al. Docetaxel and Estramustine compared with mitoxantrone and prednisone for advanced refractory prostate cancer. N Engl J Med 2004;351: 1513–1520.

33. Freeman S. A phase II study of the combination of docetaxel/mitoxantrone/low-dose prednisone in men with hormone refractory cancer (HRPC). Proc Am Soc Oncol 2003;22:432(abstract 1735).

34. Colleoni M, Graiff C, Vicario G, et al. Phase II study of estramustine, oral etoposide, and vinorelbine in hormone-refractory prostate cancer. Am J Clin Oncol 1997;20(4):383–386.

35. Kelly WK, Curley T, Slovin S, et al. Paclitaxel, estramustine phosphate, and carboplatin in patients with advanced prostate cancer. J Clin Oncol 2001;19(1):44–53.

36. Smith DC, Esper P, Strawderman M, et al. Phase II trial of oral estramustine, oral etoposide, and intravenous paclitaxel in hormone-refractory prostate cancer. J Clin Oncol 1999;17(6):1664–1671.

37. Gilligan T, Kantoff PW. Chemotherapy for prostate cancer. Urology 2002;60(3 suppl 1):94–100, discussion 100.

38. Pettaway CA, Pisters LL, Troncoso P, et al. Neoadjuvant chemotherapy and hormonal therapy followed by radical prostatectomy: feasibility and preliminary results. J Clin Oncol 2000;18(5): 1050–1057.

39. Clark PE, Peereboom DM, Dreicer R, et al. Phase II trial of neoadjuvant estramustine and etoposide plus radical prostatectomy for locally advanced prostate cancer. Urology 2001;57(2):281–285.

40. Dreicer R, Klein EA. Preliminary observations of single-agent docetaxel as neoadjuvant therapy for locally advanced prostate cancer. Semin Oncol 2001;28(4 suppl 15):45–48.

41. Oh WK, George DJ, Kaufman DS, et al. Neoadjuvant docetaxel followed by radical prostatectomy in patients with high-risk localized prostate cancer: a preliminary report. Semin Oncol 2001; 28(4 suppl 15):40–44.

42. Hussain M, Smith DC, El-Rayes BF, et al. Neoadjuvant docetaxel and estramustine chemotherapy in high-risk/locally advanced prostate cancer. Urology 2003;61(4):774–780.

43. Eastham JA, Kelly WK, Grossfeld GD, et al. Cancer and Leukemia Group B (CALGB) 90203: a randomized phase 3 study of radical prostatectomy alone versus estramustine and docetaxel before radical prostatectomy for patients with high-risk localized disease. Urology 2003;62(suppl 1):55–62.

44. Beer TM, Garzotto M, Lowe BA, et al. Phase I study of weekly mitoxantrone and docetaxel before prostatectomy in patients with high-risk localized prostate cancer. Clin Cancer Res 2004;10(4): 1306–1311.

45. Zelefsky MJ, Kelly WK, Scher HI, et al. Results of a phase II study using estramustine phosphate and vinblastine in combination with high-dose three-dimensional conformal radiotherapy for patients with locally advanced prostate cancer. J Clin Oncol 2000;18(9):1936–1941.

46. Ben-Josef E, Porter AT, Han S, et al. Neoadjuvant estramustine and etoposide followed by concurrent estramustine and definitive radiotherapy for locally advanced prostate cancer: feasibility and preliminary results. Int J Radiat Oncol Biol Phys 2001;49(3):699–703.

47. Oh WK, Kaplan ID, Febbo P, et al. Neoadjuvant doxil chemotherapy prior to androgen ablation plus radiotherapy for high-risk localized prostate cancer: feasibility and toxicity. Am J Clin Oncol 2003;26(3):312–316.

48. Schmidt JD, Gibbons RP, Murphy GP, et al. Adjuvant therapy for clinical localized prostate cancer treated with surgery or irradiation. Eur Urol 1996;29(4):425–433.

49. Takano S, Gately S, Neville ME, et al. Suramin, an anticancer and angiosuppressive agent, inhibits endothelial cell binding of basic fibroblast growth factor, migration, proliferation, and induction of urokinase-type plasminogen activator. Cancer Res 1994;54(10):2654–2660.

50. Moore MJ, Winquist E, Pollak M, et al. Randomized phase II study of two doses of gefitinib ("Iressa," ZD1839) in hormone-refractory prostate cancer: a trial of the National Cancer Institute of Canada-Clinical Trials Group. Ann Oncol 2002; 13(suppl 5):90.

51. Rosenthal MT, Gurney GC, Davis H, et al. Inhibition of the epidermal growth factor receptor (EGFR) in hormone refractory prostate cancer (HRPC): initial results of a phase II trial of gefitinib. Proc Am Soc Clin Oncol 2003;22:416 (abstract 1671).

52. Sridhar SS, Shepherd FA. Targeting angiogenesis: a review of angiogenesis inhibitors in the treatment of lung cancer. Lung Cancer 2003;42(suppl 1):S81–91.

53. Small EJ, Fratesi P, Reese DM, et al. Immunotherapy of hormone-refractory prostate cancer with antigen-loaded dendritic cells. J Clin Oncol 2000; 18(23):3894–3903.

54. Arlen PM, Gulley JL, Tsang KY, Schlom J. Strategies for the development of PSA-based vaccines for the treatment of advanced prostate cancer. Expert Rev Vaccines 2003;2(4):483–493.

55. Leonard GDD, Gulley WL, Arlen JL, Figg PM. Docetaxel and thalidomide as a treatment option for androgen-independent, nonmetastatic prostate cancer. Rev Urol 2003;5(suppl 3):S65–70.

56. Beer TM. Development of weekly high-dose calcitriol based therapy for prostate cancer. Urol Oncol 2003;21(5):399–405.

57. Pruitt-Scott DE, Ryan CW, Stadler WM, et al. Exisulind (EXI) plus docetaxel (DOC) for hormone-refractory prostate cancer (HRPC). Proc Am Soc Clin Oncol 2002;21:161b(abstract 2460).

58. Chi K, Murray RN, Gleave ME, et al. A phase II study of oblimersen sodium (G3139) and docetaxel (D) in patients (pts) with metastatic hormone-refractory prostate cancer. Proc Am Soc Clin Oncol 2003;22:393(abstract 1580).

59. Sinibaldi VJ, Carducci MA, Moore-Cooper S, Laufer M, Zahurak M, Eisenberger MA. Phase II evaluation of docetaxel plus one-day oral estramustine phosphate in the treatment of patients with androgen independent prostate carcinoma. Cancer 2002;94(5):1457–1465.

60. Savarese DM, Halabi S, Hars V, et al. Phase II study of docetaxel, estramustine, and low-dose hydrocortisone in men with hormone-refractory prostate cancer: a final report of CALGB 9780. Cancer and Leukemia Group B. J Clin Oncol 2001;19(9):2509–2516.

61. Sitka Copur M, Ledakis P, Lynch J, et al. Weekly docetaxel and estramustine in patients with hormone-refractory prostate cancer. Semin Oncol 2001;28(4 suppl 15):16–21.

62. Hudes GRM, Conroy J, Habermann J, Wilding T. Phase II study of weekly paclitaxel (P) by 1-hour infusion plus reduced-dose oral estramustine (EMP) in metastatic hormone-refractory prostate carcinoma (HRPC): a trial of the Eastern Cooperative Oncology Group. Proc Am Soc Clin Oncol 2001;20:175a(abstract 697).

63. Athanasiadis A, Tsavdaridis D, Rigatos SK, Athanasiadis I, Pergantas N, Stathopoulos GP. Hormone refractory advanced prostate cancer treated with estramustine and paclitaxel combination. Anticancer Res 2003;23(3C):3085–3088.

64. Friedland D, Cohen J, Miller R Jr, et al. A phase II trial of docetaxel (Taxotere) in hormone-refractory prostate cancer: correlation of antitumor effect to phosphorylation of Bcl-2. Semin Oncol 1999;26(5 suppl 17):19–23.

65. Trivedi C, Redman B, Flaherty LE, et al. Weekly 1-hour infusion of paclitaxel. Clinical feasibility and efficacy in patients with hormone-refractory prostate carcinoma. Cancer 2000;89(2):431–436.

66. Garzotto M, Higano C, Lowe B, et al. Neoadjuvant weekly docetaxel and mitoxantrone in patients with high risk localized prostate cancer: a phase I trial. Proc Am Soc Clin Oncol 2002;21:155b (abstract 2434).

10

Proteomic Approaches to Problem Solving in Prostate Cancer

Simon C. Gamble

Background

The term *proteomics* was coined to parallel the term *genomics;* however, proteomics encompasses more that just the study of the protein equivalent of the genome. The proteome, that is, all the proteins and their multiple isoforms and modified forms expressed in any one cell type or biological fluid, is responsible for the active work undertaken by a cell, and even reflective of the status of the entire organism, where fluids such as urine and blood serum are studied. The proteome is therefore dynamic and reflective of cell status and activity. Where RNA levels or gene mutations may give a certain amount of information, the amount and functionality of the corresponding protein is a vital part of our understanding of what makes the cell function, whether that function is normal or aberrant. Proteomic studies not only can tell us how much of a certain protein is present in a sample, but also can indicate posttranslational modifications, such as cleavage to form active or inactive isoforms, phosphorylation, acetylation, and glycosylation. None of these changes in the active status of a protein or enzyme would be detectable via genomic studies; therefore, proteomics allows us a more profound insight into the activity of cellular processes.

The majority of early proteomic studies relied on three major technologies: two-dimensional electrophoresis of proteins, mass spectrometry, and Internet database searches. Recent advances in all three areas have allowed a massive surge in proteomic studies in the past 5 years, with 62 proteomics papers being listed on Medline for 1999, compared with 1418 listed for 2003. Further advances in a variety of matrix desorption ionization-based techniques (surface-enhanced laser desorption and lonisation [SELDI] SELDI-TOFF, SEAC) and electrospray mass spectrometry have resulted in expansion of the types of data that can be obtained, including protein–protein and DNA–protein interactions. This means that proteomics now encompasses a variety of experimental techniques, each with its own particular advantages, all of which can be useful in the study of prostate cancer.

Techniques in Proteomics

Two-Dimensional Gel Electrophoresis (2DGE)

Proteins in a biological mixture, whether it be a fluid such as urine, blood serum, or cell lysates, are separated first according to their charge, by isoelectric focusing (IEF), and then second according to their molecular weight, using standard sodium dodecyl sulfate–polyacrylamide gel electrophoresis (SDS-PAGE) techniques. Isoelectric focusing relies on the charges of the various amino acids in an individual protein sequence, resulting in an overall charge for that protein. Proteins of the same molecular weight may have vastly different overall electrical charge and therefore will focus at different points on a pH gradient when a current is applied, migrating through the gradient until their charge is neutralized by the surrounding pH. This technique uses immobilized pH gradient (IPG) gel strips, where a gradient of charged amino groups is cross-linked to the acrylamide gel, making the charge gradient immobile and therefore incapable of drifting during focusing.

Once separated according to their charge, the proteins in the sample are then subjected to standard SDS-PAGE, usually on large-format gels, which give a greater area for isolating different protein spots. Many of the current protocols allow for separation over an area of 18 to 24 cm width and 20 to 25 cm depth, which allows for separation of many hundreds and even thousands of proteins, although small gels are still frequently used by some laboratories.

Protein Detection and Analysis

Detection of samples is now also much easier than before. Originally 2DGEs were silver stained or Coomassie stained; however, with the advent of fluorescent dyes such as Syproruby, reproducible and sensitive detection of proteins is possible, as these dyes do not interfere with subsequent identification of the proteins by mass spectrometry. Other methods of detection include radioisotope labeling with either phosphorous 32 or sulfur 35. Orthophosphate ^{32}P labeling is used to identify phosphorylated proteins and ^{35}S-labeled methionine and cysteine label can be incorporated into newly synthesized proteins. Silver-stained or Coomassie-stained gels are converted to digital images using a scanning densitometer, radiolabeled gels can be visualized using autoradiography and densitometry or using storage phosphorescence technology, and fluorescent dyes may be visualized using gel scanners in fluorescence mode.

Once visualized, comparison of the protein-spot patterns of the data groups is carried out to distinguish differences between the groups and highlight which proteins may be of interest for further analysis. Many software packages are available to do this.

Having used the software to detect which proteins are of interest for further study, the final task that remains is to identify them. This is now relatively straightforward, due to the recent developments in mass spectrometry technology and database searching on the Internet. Initially the protein features of interest need to be removed from the gel in order to be analyzed. This can be done manually with a scalpel, a pipette tip, or a "spot cutter," or automatically using a robot spot cutter, directly linked to the analysis software program. The goal is to remove the protein spot with minimal contamination from neighboring spots or excess gel, in order to allow easy digestion of the protein without contamination.

Mass Spectrometry to Identify Proteins

The majority of identification techniques now involve tryptic digest of the protein in the gel plug removed from the gel, followed by mass spectrometry, such as matrix-assisted laser desorption ionization (MALDI) and time of flight (TOF) mass spectrometry. Peptide samples are placed on a matrix, the surface of which is then scanned with a laser, resulting in ionization of the bound peptides. The peptides then ionize and desorb from the matrix. Often a chemical enhancer coating is used to increase the laser absorption and energy transfer to the peptides. Upon desorption, the peptides are propelled by electrical fields to a detector. The ratio of the mass of the peptide to its charge results in differing time of flight to the detector, meaning that peptides of different sequence will arrive at the detector at different times. Using known molecules for calibration, the masses of the peptides can then be calculated. These masses are then used to determine the amino acid sequences of the peptides, which are then submitted to a database search in order to find matching sequences for the peptide mass "fingerprint" obtained and give a positive identification of the protein spot removed from the gel. Spots may also be cut from membranes such as, polyvinylidene flouride, PVDF for analysis, following staining with Coomassie blue, although now that sensitive gel methods are possible, this is less common.

Once the identities of the discriminatory spots have been determined, confirmation of regulation is usually required either by Western blotting, if an antibody is available, or by reverse-transcription polymerase chain reaction (RT-PCR). If regulation is confirmed, either at the level of transcription, translation, or posttranslational modification, then the function of the identified protein can be further investigated.

Surface-Enhanced Laser Desorption

Surface-enhanced laser desorption (SELDI) involves the creation of a matrix to which molecules are fixed that will interact with proteins in a biological fluid. These molecules may be inorganic, such as metal ions, hydrophobic substances, chemical moieties, or organic, such as antibodies, fragments of antibodies, DNA sequences, and receptor proteins. Small quantities of biological fluids are added to these surfaces, allowing proteins to bind to the immobilized molecules. Several wash stages then allow removal of nonspecifically bound proteins. Then MALDI-TOF is used to ionize the bound proteins as described above, detecting a wide spectrum of whole proteins rather than peptides. If differences in the proteins are detected between cancer and noncancer samples, the sample may then be reanalyzed using trypsin digestion as part of the laser desorption process. The resultant tryptic peptides can then be compared against those in the Web-based databases, and identities assigned to the discriminatory proteins.

Early Proteomic Studies into the Prostate and Prostate Cancer

Until very recently the number of prostate-related proteomics or 2DGE-based publications was decidedly small, due to the inherent problems in carrying out such studies. In 1989 a study was carried out by Sherwood et al. [1], comparing the profiles of proteins obtained from stromal and epithelial cells from patients undergoing prostatectomy for benign prostatic hyperplasia (BPH). Differences were noted for cytokeratin levels and also vimentin, which was shown to be present in stromal cells via immunoblotting, as were three potential markers of stromal cell types named SM1, SM2, and SM3. As the existing technology did not yet allow identification of these markers, no identities were obtained for them.

In 1992 2DGE was carried out on isolated androgen receptor, revealing two isoforms of the receptor at the isoelectric point, pI 5.3 and 7.2 and molecular weight 90 to 95 kd in both prostate and foreskin [2]. A further study by Xia et al. [3] discovered three isoforms of the androgen receptor using IEF, which seemed to vary in presence between individuals, regardless of disease state.

Although the information in these studies was not very useful, due to limitations of technology, they proved that proteomic studies in prostate cancer merited further research.

Current Studies and Their Aims

Proteins Differing Between Normal and Cancerous Prostate

One of the most appealing studies that one can carry out with proteomics technology is the investigation of proteins with differing expression levels between normal and cancerous prostate. The first directly prostate-cancer related proteomics paper appeared in 1997, in which Partin et al. [4] identified a protein, PC-1, that was present in prostate cancer but not in normal or hyperplastic prostate. The protein, to which an antibody was subsequently raised, was then used in experiments to investigate its potential use in prostate cancer screening via immunohistochemistry. Despite encouraging results, this study does not appear to have been developed further.

A study of prostate cancer can be further broken down into the investigation of different stages of cancer, from prostatic intraepithelial neoplasia (PIN) to hormone therapy–resistant cancer, and all stages in between. Although the technology now exists to make this task possible, the problems that dog any other similar study on genetics or gene expression also apply to proteomics: intact and pure samples are required to enable a clear differentiation between proteins expressed or modified in the study groups.

Tissue Culture Studies

Tissue from prostate cancers is often difficult to obtain, and tissue from normal prostate even more so, meaning that only small amounts of protein are available for study. In contrast, cell-culture studies allow the production of large amounts of protein, and for this reason some studies have concentrated on the differences between prostate cancer cell lines [5,6]. Many studies have been carried out on the LNCaP cell line, due to its retaining a functional androgen receptor and therefore being androgen responsive [7–9]. Although cells in culture are always a surrogate for cells *in situ*, the advantage of proteomic studies on cell lines is homogeneity of sample. A cell line consists of only a single phenotype, therefore allowing differences between cells to be investigated fully.

However, there are major disadvantages of using cultured cells. Put simply, the act of culturing cells results in many phenotypic changes, meaning that the cultured cells no longer behave like the cells in the body. Obtaining cells from prostate cancers that will grow in culture, without further deliberate genetic alteration such as transformation with simian virus 40 (SV40), is an immensely difficult task. Human cells in culture grow for only a limited number of cell divisions, and prostate cells appear to be reluctant to do even this much. Then there are problems caused by the change in cellular environment. Cells in the body do not exist in a homogeneous monolayer, but are surrounded by a variety of other cells and cell types, all secreting molecules that give clues and instructions as to the phenotype that the cell should have. Mimicking intracellular signaling between cell types in culture is possible, but only through complicated procedures. As a result, the genes expressed and therefore the proteins detected in cell-only studies are not likely to be representative of the true state of cells in their original context. This argument applies to any tissue culture study. There is an inherent level of artifice involved, which means that results obtained may not be truly representative of the actual biological facts. For this reason many studies have painstakingly obtained biopsy and surgical specimens in order to carry out proteomic studies.

Biopsy Studies

Despite the difficulties in obtaining prostate tissue, several studies have already been published comparing either normal or BPH tissue to malignant prostate. Alaiya et al. [10] used 19 benign and malignant radical prostatectomy samples to carry out 2DGE and obtained 23 identities of differentially expressed proteins, including heat shock 70 and cytochrome P-450 7A1. Meehan et al. [11] used 2DGE of matched normal and malignant tissue from 34 radical prostatectomy specimens to identify 20 proteins lost in the process of malignant transformation. These included three proteins (NEDD8, calponin, and a follistatin-related protein) not previously detected in normal prostate, the loss of which may be significant for development of malignant phenotype and therefore worthy of further investigation for potential therapeutic or diagnostic purposes.

Laser Capture Microscopy

Tissue obtained from prostate surgery is rarely homogeneous in cell type (a fact admitted in Alaiya et al.'s [10] report) and contains not only tumor cells but also possibly multiple clonal variants of the tumor, nontumorous epithelial cells, undifferentiated epithelial cells, and stromal cells. Such a sample, therefore, is likely to give confusing results, as the protein profiles obtained would be far from representative of any particular cell type, unless the cancer cells were in the vast majority and even then subtle but important differences may be lost. To overcome this problem, laser capture microdissection of tissue samples is now being used. This technique uses lasers to remove small sections, sometimes cell by cell, from tissue slices on slides, in order to allow a homogeneous sample to be obtained. The downside to this technique is the painstaking microscopy and the length of time needed to capture enough cells to make a proteomic study worth carrying out. However, there have been encouraging results from several laboratories using this method. For example, Ahram et al. [12] used laser capture microdissection in conjunction with manual dissection to carry out a joint proteomic and genomic study of samples obtained from matched normal epithelial and high-grade prostate cancer. The results demonstrated few consistent changes at the protein level, possibly reflecting the wide variety of ways in which prostate cancer can arise. Paweletz et al. [13] used laser capture microscopy and reverse SELDI, where the samples are hybridized to the membrane and probed with antibodies for proteins of interest, to investigate prostate cancer progression. The reverse SELDI data showed increased Akt phosphorylation, decreased phosphorylation pathways, and decreased phosphorylation of ERK associated with prostate cancer progression, demonstrating that good biological data can be obtained from these studies.

Further Development of Identified Proteins

The aim of these studies is to identify proteins that have altered expression, modification, or turnover rate in neoplastic cells. There are several useful clinical applications of these data. First, any protein for which there is an antibody may be used as a marker of cancer. This may not be possible in all cases, as many will be intracellular and therefore detectable only by immunohistochemistry. Such markers may be useful in defining which cancers are likely to grow and develop rapidly or metastasize. Indeed such markers have been discovered by other methods and are reported in the literature, if not seen in the clinics. The examples cited above all have shown that such markers exist and yet they remain undeveloped for clinical use [4,10,12].

The second use of differentially detected proteins in cancer is the potential for treatment. For example, aberrant expression of cell signaling proteins can lead to the abnormal growth of cancer cells. If the protein is upregulated in cancer, the use of drugs or gene therapy to interrupt the protein's activity may cause the cells to revert to a less aggressive or noncancerous form, or result in apoptosis. The reintroduction of proteins of which expression has been lost in cancer, such as tumor-suppressor genes, may potentially be corrected by gene therapy. Hence, the further proteomic study of proteins with aberrant expression in prostate cancer may yield potential targets for these therapeutic approaches.

Second-Line Therapies

It is well known that the treatment of advanced prostate cancer with antiandrogens and other hormone therapies is successful only for a limited time. The cancer inevitably progresses to hormone independence, in which treatment by antiandrogens is no longer effective, or at worst stimulates cancer growth.

Growth-related proteins, downstream from the androgen receptor, may be targets of therapy themselves, so that when antiandrogen treatment fails, therapy aimed at these downstream targets can stop the growth of the cancer. The majority of studies to date have been at the genetic level [14,15], using standard protein expression techniques such as Western blotting to corroborate results. In one instance proteomics was used in conjunction with complementary DNA (cDNA) microarray to establish androgen-regulated proteins, detecting 351 regulated genes and 32 regulated proteins [7]. Nelson et al. [16] also used cDNA microarray in conjunction with proteomics in LNCaP cells, and M12 cells transfected with androgen receptor, to detect androgen-regulated proteins. Relatively few regulated proteins were detected, but among them was the metastasis suppressor protein nm23, which was upregulated following androgen exposure. In our own laboratory we have used proteomics alone to look at androgen responsive proteins [9], again identifying 32 regulated proteins, including one, prohibitin, that was downregulated following exposure of the cells to androgens and had a negative effect on cell cycle in LNCaP cells. Wright et al. [8] used androgen stimulation of LNCaP cells in conjunction with isotope coded affinity tags (ICATs) and mass spectrometry to detect levels of 1064 proteins, which were then grouped into 45 categories based on cellular function and process.

Further development of any of these proteins as potential target for therapy requires careful choice, based on the magnitude of the regulation observed, specificity to the prostate to avoid side effects of treatment, and careful reading of available literature. It is clear, however, that these studies have the potential to highlight new targets for therapy.

The Androgen Receptor and Proteomics

Fundamental to the treatment of prostate cancer is the action of antiandrogens on the androgen receptor. Investigation of hormone-resistant prostate cancer has demonstrated that in the majority of cases, the androgen signaling growth pathway is intact in these cells and either is responding to nonclassical ligands, such as the antiandrogens themselves, or the receptor is massively upregulated, resulting in massive oversensitivity to the ligand [17,18]. As well as these mechanisms, failure of these treatments may be due to alteration in the balance of the regulatory cofactors required by the receptor to carry out its function. Very little proteomic work has been done directly involving the androgen receptor itself. Early studies showed the presence of three isoforms of the receptor [3]. It is known that different phosphoisoforms of the receptor do exist [19] and that they have some functional significance.

It is possible that using modification-specific antibodies, for example, antiphospho- or acetyl group antibodies, the function of androgen receptor modifications may be dissected. It is also possible that certain isoforms may correlate with androgen insensitivity in prostate cancer and may therefore present possible roads to therapeutic stimulation or blocking of certain modification events.

Functional Proteomics

Functional proteomics implies an additional level of information to that of standard proteomics, in that function of related proteins is being investigated. Most commonly, this involves immunoprecipitation of protein complexes followed by 2DGE or electrospray mass spectrometry, which could be carried out with molecules such as hormone receptors or transcription and translation machinery. By immunoprecipitating the molecule of interest, say a hormone receptor, in addition to providing a catalogue of proteins normally associated with the receptor, this method allows the identification of proteins associated with the receptor in cancer cells, such as cofactors involved in gene transcription or gene repression. It is possible that such molecules themselves may also be potential targets for therapy. The technique has so far been used with other protein complexes such as the proteosome [20] and the chaperonin GroEL [21], and therefore should be capable of dissecting complexes based around molecules such as the androgen receptor, possibly giving information on other molecules known to be involved in prostate cancer formation.

New Diagnostic Markers

The holy grail of prostate cancer research is probably the discovery of new diagnostic markers. There are currently several markers available for diagnostic purposes in prostate cancer [22], although mostly these are used in immunohistochemical grading of cancer, with an aim to indicating the grade, and possible aggressiveness of the cancer. Various secreted proteins are also known, and have even proved useful in the clinic, such as prostate-specific antigen (PSA). It is likely, given these examples, that other, more accurate markers of disease presence, stage, and prognosis exist, which may be detected using proteomic techniques. An organ with a very specific function such as the prostate produces a large number of proteins, enzymes, and possibly cell surface markers that are produced only by that organ, and therefore have the potential to indicate the aberrant growth or function of that organ and the cells that form it. Proteomic investigation of the prostate could therefore yield any number of markers that may indicate various stages of neoplasia, as the specific function of that organ and the cells that form it become deregulated.

Cell Surface Markers

Cell surface markers of prostate cancer may have greater potential for therapy development than differentiated proteins found within the cells. It is possible that by linking molecules to the antibodies for cell surface markers, the antibody may be used as a delivery system for a drug or molecule that would specifically attack the prostate cancer cells expressing that cell surface marker. Experiments aimed at discovering these markers come up against one of the major drawbacks with 2DGE technology, which is the poor representation of membrane proteins in 2D gels. By definition, these proteins tend to be largely hydrophobic and therefore poorly soluble in a water-based buffer systems. As a result, it is often difficult to make cell preparations that adequately represent the membrane-bound fraction of the proteome. Technical studies have found ways to enhance their representation (see Molloy [23] for a review), so the possibility of such future experiments yielding useful data is now more likely.

The study of glycoproteins in disease is becoming more popular, due to advances in mass spectrometry capabilities. The modification of cell-surface proteins with glycans, resulting in recognizable cell–cell interaction motifs, appears to change with disease state in many cases. It is therefore possible that cell surface glycoproteins in prostate cancer may be different from those in the normal state. Currently the best way to detect such changes is by direct mass spectrometry analysis, though detection with digoxigenin conjugation or Schiff staining and 2DGE is also possible. Given that this group may include internal proteins, externally expressed cell surface markers, and excreted proteins, it is highly likely that the glycoprotein component of the proteome will reveal potential targets, either for delivery of drugs where a specific cancer marker is found or by exposing hitherto unknown biological processes involved in the formation of prostate cancer.

Serum Markers for Prostate Cancer

The discovery and development of PSA in the 1980s revolutionized the diagnosis of prostate cancer. The marker, which is simple to detect, easy to access, and relatively noninvasive for the patient, is an ideal find. It is now firmly established that PSA is one of the most reliable cancer markers currently in use. It is also true, however, that there are a very high number of false-positive and false-negative diagnoses obtained via PSA testing, and for this reason the use of PSA as a screening test in the United Kingdom has always been avoided. It is worthy of note, however, that its application in the United States has led to an increased number of diagnoses and arguably a drop in mortality. This demonstrates the value of such screening regimes in saving lives. It therefore follows that an accurate and informative blood test for prostate cancer would be invaluable in the clinics, allowing early diagnosis and possibly even informing the type of treatment required for each patient.

In attempting to discover such a marker, several groups have used proteomics to characterize the serum of men with prostate cancer. One such study concentrated on PSA itself, which, when subjected to 2DGE analysis, was seen to have several isoforms, based on differing charge and molecular weight [24]. The ratio of standard weight PSA to the smaller isoform detected was found to discriminate between prostate cancer and BPH sera, possibly due to protease activity in the BPH samples. Despite this, the study does not appear to have translated to the clinics, perhaps due to the relative difficulty in routinely carrying out 2DGE analysis, compared to standard PSA testing.

The very existence of the PSA hints at the possibility that better markers remain to be discovered. Several limitations affect this type of study, however. The vast majority of the protein "space" in the serum of a patient is taken up by very few, highly abundant proteins such as albumen and immunoglobulins. The presence of such highly abundant species has two effects on the results of 2DGE experiments. First, it means that out of any sample loaded, if, say, >80% of the sample is taken up with a few proteins there is very little loading space on a gel for less abundant and possibly more significant proteins. Second, the presence of a highly abundant protein will cause problems with the separation of the other proteins, in that the proteins will not focus on an IPG strip and will run aberrantly on the 2D gel. It is therefore necessary to remove such proteins before running the 2D gels, or to avoid this technology altogether. In either method, employing a technique for the removal of high-abundance proteins will enrich the presence of less abundant proteins, although there is some danger of accidentally also removing less abundant proteins that may be of interest. Incubation of samples with antibodies attached to a column or Sepharose beads in solution can allow the removal of several species of proteins in one step. Once cleared of these proteins, the resultant serum may be subjected to 2DGE or some other technique such as SELDI.

Several serum-based studies have already been carried out and have yielded encouraging results. For example, there has been the recent discovery of a protein NMP48 [25], with sequence similarity to vitamin D–binding protein, which was present in the serum of patients with prostate cancer or PIN, but not in patients with BPH or no prostate disease. It was found that the marker could accurately diagnose between 70% and 96% of samples. Meanwhile Lehrer et al. [26] used SELDI to isolate three low molecular weight (15.2 to 17.5 kd) proteins that were present in BPH and cancer sera, but not in normal patients, with a protein at 15.9 kd being present in nine of 11 cancer sera but none of the BPH sera. Interestingly, a protein of 17.5 kd was present in higher amounts in stage T1 cancer than in stage T2 cancer, indicating that markers may exist for a range of cancer stages, and that a panel of these markers may allow diagnosis of cancer stage.

Even with the detection of a small tumor, the treatment required is not always apparent, and given that many men die *with* prostate cancer but not *of* it, it would be of clinical benefit to be able to distinguish which cancers are likely to be aggressive from those that will remain latent. Out of those that have already spread, to be able to determine which are likely to relapse rapidly following hormone treatment could be of clinical value. Whether some of the markers discovered for detection of cancer will also allow diagnosis to be made regarding aggressiveness or invasiveness of that cancer is not clear. It is more likely that another set of markers would be required to make those distinctions. Furthermore, it may not be a single marker that denotes any of these factors, but combined alterations, a "signature," which could perhaps be detected by mass spectrometry. Yasui et al. [27] used SELDI to generate signature profiles for prostate cancer, BPH, and normal sera, which worked well in differentiating between normal and diseased prostate, but did not clearly distinguish between cancer and BPH when the profiles were used to diagnose test samples. Other studies have obtained similar or better results [28,29], though some have been criticized for not identifying the proteins responsible for the signature [30], the suggestion being that some of the proteins in the fingerprint may be produced by the invaded tissues surrounding the cancer and that tests developed from the study may be confounded by other similar responses such as the immune response. It can still be argued that in such studies, the identities of the distinguishing proteins become irrelevant to the test, as it is the combined variables that make up the fingerprint. If this pattern can be easily distinguished in an inexpensive and rapid clinical test, then the aim of the research has been achieved. Subsequent identification is recommended, however, as the proteins involved in producing the fingerprint signature for cancer may themselves be potential targets for therapy. Some proteins may be purely of diagnostic value, such as PSA, but others may be related to cell–cell signaling and therefore growth and metastasis.

Summary

If the major areas of prostate cancer research needing further development are discovering new targets for therapy, a better understanding of prostate cancer development, and discovery of new markers for more accurate diagnosis of prostate disease, then proteomic studies can contribute hugely to these areas. The relevance of protein rather than DNA and RNA information to such studies is that protein activity is the machinery of cell action; therefore, changes in protein profiles in cancer can be used on many levels, to detect, to understand, and finally to treat the cancer.

References

1. Sherwood ER, et al. Two-dimensional protein profiles of cultured stromal and epithelial cells from hyperplastic human prostate. J Cell Biochem 1989;40(2):201–214.
2. Stamatiadis D, et al. Isoelectric focusing and 2D electrophoresis of the human androgen receptor. J Steroid Biochem Mol Biol 1992;41(1):43–51.
3. Xia SJ, Hao GY, Tang XD. Androgen receptor isoforms in human and rat prostate. Asian J Androl 2000;2(4):307-310.
4. Partin AW, et al. Preliminary immunohistochemical characterization of a monoclonal antibody (PRO:4-216) prepared from human prostate cancer nuclear matrix proteins. Urology 1997; 50(5):800–808.
5. Liu X, et al. Proteomic analysis of the tumorigenic human prostate cell line M12 after microcell-mediated transfer of chromosome 19 demonstrates reduction of vimentin. Electrophoresis 2003;24(19–20):3445–3453.
6. Nagano K, et al. Differential protein synthesis and expression levels in normal and neoplastic human prostate cells and their regulation by type I and II interferons. Oncogene 2004;23(9):1693–1703.
7. Waghray A, et al. Identification of androgen-regulated genes in the prostate cancer cell line LNCaP by serial analysis of gene expression and proteomic analysis. Proteomics 2001;1(10):1327–1338.
8. Wright ME, et al. Identification of androgen-coregulated protein networks from the microsomes of human prostate cancer cells. Genome Biol 2003;5(1):R4.
9. Gamble SC, et al. Androgens target prohibitin to regulate proliferation of prostate cancer cells. Oncogene 2004;23(17):2996–3004.
10. Alaiya AA, et al. Identification of proteins in human prostate tumor material by two-dimensional gel electrophoresis and mass spectrometry. Cell Mol Life Sci 2001;58(2):307–311.
11. Meehan KL, Holland JW, Dawkins HJ. Proteomic analysis of normal and malignant prostate tissue

to identify novel proteins lost in cancer. Prostate 2002;50(1):54–63.

12. Ahram M, et al. Proteomic analysis of human prostate cancer. Mol Carcinog 2002;33(1):9–15.

13. Paweletz CP, et al. Reverse phase protein microarrays which capture disease progression show activation of pro-survival pathways at the cancer invasion front. Oncogene 2001;20(16):1981–1989.

14. Nelson PS, et al. The program of androgen-responsive genes in neoplastic prostate epithelium. Proc Natl Acad Sci USA 2002;99(18): 11890–11895.

15. Eder IE, et al. Gene expression changes following androgen receptor elimination in LNCaP prostate cancer cells. Mol Carcinog 2003;37(4):181–191.

16. Nelson PS, et al. Comprehensive analyses of prostate gene expression: convergence of expressed sequence tag databases, transcript profiling and proteomics. Electrophoresis 2000; 21(9):1823–1831.

17. Koivisto P, et al. Androgen receptor gene and hormonal therapy failure of prostate cancer. Am J Pathol 1998;152(1):1–9.

18. Visakorpi T, et al. In vivo amplification of the androgen receptor gene and progression of human prostate cancer. Nat Genet 1995;9(4):401–406.

19. Wang LG, Liu XM, Kreis W, Budman DR. Phosphorylation/dephosphorylation of androgen receptor as a determinant of androgen agonistic or antagonistic activity. Biochem Biophys Res Commun 1999;259(1):21–28.

20. Mason GG, et al. Phosphorylation of ATPase subunits of the 26S proteasome. FEBS Lett 1998; 430(3):269–274.

21. Houry WA, et al. Identification of in vivo substrates of the chaperonin GroEL. Nature 1999; 402(6758):147–154.

22. Ross JS, et al. Morphologic and molecular prognostic markers in prostate cancer. Adv Anat Pathol 2002;9(2):115–128.

23. Molloy MP. Two-dimensional electrophoresis of membrane proteins using immobilized pH gradients. Anal Biochem 2000;280(1):1–10.

24. Charrier JP, et al. Differential diagnosis of prostate cancer and benign prostate hyperplasia using two-dimensional electrophoresis. Electrophoresis 2001; 22(9):1861–1866.

25. Hlavaty JJ, et al. Identification and preliminary clinical evaluation of a 50.8-kDa serum marker for prostate cancer. Urology 2003;61(6):1261–1265.

26. Lehrer S, et al. Putative protein markers in the sera of men with prostatic neoplasms. BJU Int 2003;92(3):223–225.

27. Yasui Y, et al. A data-analytic strategy for protein biomarker discovery: profiling of high-dimensional proteomic data for cancer detection. Biostatistics 2003;4(3):449–463.

28. Petricoin EF 3rd, et al. Serum proteomic patterns for detection of prostate cancer. J Natl Cancer Inst 2002;94(20):1576–1578.

29. Adam BL, et al. Proteomic approaches to biomarker discovery in prostate and bladder cancers. Proteomics 2001;1(10):1264–1270.

30. Diamandis EP. Re: serum proteomic patterns for detection of prostate cancer. J Natl Cancer Inst 2003;95(6):489–490; author reply 490–491.

11

Gene Therapy for Prostate Cancer

Danish Mazhar and Roopinder Gillmore

Prostate cancer has recently become the most commonly diagnosed male malignancy in industrialized countries and the second leading cause of cancer-related mortality in men. Over the last 30 years death rates from prostate cancer have more than doubled in England and Wales [1]. It is argued that disease confined to the prostate can be successfully treated by radiation or surgery, with adjuvant hormonal therapy. However, up to half of men with clinically localized disease are not cured by these approaches [2]. In the United Kingdom over 60% of men with prostate cancer have either locally advanced or metastatic disease at presentation and are incurable. These patients are treated by androgen ablation, but the efficacy of this approach is limited by the development of hormone-refractory disease. Although chemotherapy can have a role to play in patients with advanced prostate cancer, response rates are modest and the survival benefit marginal. There is thus clearly a need for novel therapies to improve current prospects for survival.

Significant advances have been made in gene therapy over recent years as a result of developments in molecular and cell biology. These include the improvement of both viral and nonviral gene delivery systems, the discovery of new therapeutic genes, better understanding of mechanisms of disease progression, and the emergence of better prodrug systems.

Prostate cancer displays several features that make it a good candidate for gene therapy. First, the primary tumor site is easy to access and image. Thus, treatments can be readily and accurately injected into the tumor, assisted for example by transrectal ultrasonography. Second, although many prostate cancer–associated target molecules are also expressed on normal prostate tissue, because the prostate is not a vital organ, any damage to adjacent normal prostate tissue would not be a contraindication to initiating treatment.

Delivery Systems for Gene Therapy

Gene therapy for cancer currently necessitates the transfer of recombinant DNA into human cells in order to achieve an antitumor effect, and efficient gene transfer requires the use of a vector. All vectors contain at a minimum the transgene of interest linked to a promoter to drive its expression. The ideal vector should be specific to the target cell and deliver DNA efficiently into cells. It should be nontoxic to the patient and environment, nonimmunogenic, nonmutagenic, and ideally produced cheaply at high concentrations. There are an increasing number of vectors and delivery methods available for gene transfer. Factors that may determine which vector is most ideal for a particular study include maximal transgene size permissible, tendency to provoke inflammatory/immune responses, persistence of gene transfer, the ability to deliver the transgene to nondividing cells, target cell specificity, and transduction efficiency.

Viral Delivery Systems

Viral vectors are used in the vast majority of gene therapy trials owing to their relatively high gene transfer efficiency. They may be either RNA or DNA virus based. The DNA viruses include adenovirus, vaccinia, and herpes simplex viruses. The RNA viruses include retroviruses and lentiviruses. To improve their safety, viral vectors may be designed to be replication-deficient, with no further virus particles generated following infection of the target cells. Alternatively, they may be replication-competent or replication-attenuated, in which case viral replication can occur in permissive cells.

Retroviruses

Because of their stable integration into the target cell genome and transmission to the progeny of the transduced parent cell, retroviral vectors can potentially lead to sustained transgene expression. However, retroviral entry into the cell nucleus is cell-division–dependent, which may be a significant problem when considering the treatment of cancers with low mitotic rates, such as prostate cancer. Other limitations include relatively low transduction rates in vivo, the rapid inactivation of retroviruses by human complement, as well as the potential to induce insertional mutagenesis and secondary malignancies.

Lentiviruses

Lentiviruses, such as the human immunodeficiency virus, are a subfamily of retroviruses that are able to integrate into nondividing cells. Lentivirus vectors are also able to sustain prolonged transgene expression. Safety concerns, however, including the risk of insertional mutagenesis, have limited the use of these vectors.

Adenoviruses and Adeno-Associated Vectors

Adenovirus vectors are the most common viral vehicles used for prostate cancer gene therapy in human clinical trials. This is because of the advantages of efficient transduction and easy manipulation in vitro. It is also relatively straightforward to produce high titers of purified virus. Moreover, adenoviruses infect both dividing and nondividing cells, and their DNA is not incorporated into the host genome, minimizing concerns about insertional mutagenesis. The major disadvantages are the transient expression of its DNA insert and the immune responses generated in response to the vector. A major consequence of the antiadenovirus immune response is a marked reduction of transgene expression following multiple dosing, which appears to result mainly from stimulation of neutralizing antibody responses, although adenovirus-specific cytotoxic T lymphocytes (CTLs) have been detected. In addition to specific antiadenovirus transgene–directed immune responses, nonspecific inflammation can also significantly reduce transgene expression. It has been possible to increase the duration of adenovirus gene expression through the use of CTL blocking agents [3] or immunosuppressive drugs [4].

Safety, however, is still an issue with systemic use of adenovirus vectors because this has been associated with acute liver injury, resulting from the release of cytokines, in several mouse models. However, low doses of modified E1-deleted viruses can be used with minimal toxicity even in animals with damaged livers, although in some cases a lower level of transgene expression was seen [5]. It is still to be determined exactly how much these mouse models truly reflect the possible toxicities in humans.

New adenoviral vectors have been developed that have no adenoviral genes within their genome but retain sequences essential for replication and packaging of the genome. These "gutless" vectors can carry very large DNA inserts of up to 35 kilobase (kb), compared with 8 kb in the former adenoviral vectors, and do not express viral proteins, which has the additional advantage of limiting the host immune response.

The adeno-associated virus vector is replication-deficient and is unique in that it requires co-infection with another adenovirus for productive infection in cell cultures. Though adeno-associated viruses may infect nondividing cells and elicit little immune response, they have lost their ability to integrate specifically into the target cell genome, raising concerns of potential insertional mutagenesis.

Vaccinia and Herpes Viruses

The vaccinia virus, a member of the pox virus family, is naturally cytopathic but can be engineered to a noncytopathic form that retains its infectious activity. It has several characteristics that offer a potential advantage for gene therapy. Vaccinia has a large genome of 186 kb, allowing the incorporation of a large transgene insert, and it replicates DNA and transcribes RNA in the cytoplasm without being transported to the cell nucleus, thus avoiding any potential insertional mutagenesis. Disadvantages include systemic toxicity, high immunogenicity, and only transient transgene expression. Vaccinia virus–based vectors have been used mainly for the delivery of antigens to tumors to elicit host cell immune responses as a means of targeting the cancer cells for immune-based destruction.

The main advantages of herpes viruses are their large insert size of 35 kb and their ability to infect dividing and nondividing cells. However, they are limited by their potential pathogenicity, poor transduction efficiency, and transient gene expression.

Nonviral Delivery Systems

Nonviral gene transfer systems include chemical methods, such as the use of liposomes, and physical methods, such as microinjection electroporation. Liposomes are relatively cheap, nontoxic, nonimmunogenic lipids, and can be used for DNA coating to protect DNA from degradation until it reaches the target cell. The lipid envelope fuses with the target cell membrane, and the gene is delivered directly to the cytoplasm. However, the low efficiency of transgene delivery is the main limiting step. On the other hand, the safety of this technique has been verified in a phase I study in which liposomes containing the interleukin-2 (IL-2) gene were injected into the prostates of patients with advanced prostate cancer [6].

Hybrid vectors, combining viral and synthetic approaches, have been devised to overcome their respective limitations. Adenovirus-liposome complexes have resulted in a 1000-fold increase in gene transfer efficiency relative to naked plasmid. Transgenes of up to 48 kb

have been successfully transferred using this technique [7].

The most basic form of delivery strategy is to deliver the plasmid directly to the desired site, i.e., the tumor. Although this method is cheap and can be simple to perform, the cellular uptake of the plasmid DNA/RNA and expression of the transgene occur with low efficiency. Furthermore, DNA that is internalized into the cell is susceptible to endonuclease activity, thus limiting the duration of transgene expression. However, because no immune responses are generated with this system, research is ongoing to try and bypass the present limitations.

Gene Therapy Strategies in Prostate Cancer

There are currently four main approaches to prostate cancer gene therapy: the replacement of deficient tumor-suppressor genes with genes that enhance apoptosis, the introduction of an effector gene that can stimulate the host's immune response by activating tumor-specific CTLs, suicide gene therapies involving transfection of tumor cells with a gene that produces an enzyme that converts a prodrug into a toxic agent, and the use of oncolytic viruses.

Enhancing Apoptosis

Mutations in the tumor-suppressor gene $p53$ are observed in 25 to 75% of prostate cancers, more commonly in advanced tumors [8]. The ability of overexpressed $p53$ to inhibit the growth of primary cultures derived from radical prostatectomy specimens has been demonstrated, even when the $p53$ status is normal [9]. The further potential therapeutic efficacy of II $p53$ gene delivery has been suggested by the observation that prostate cancer cell lines infected with wild-type $p53$ adenovirus were not tumorigenic [10]. Furthermore, when recombinant adenoviruses encoding $p53$ were injected intratumorally (IT) into established PC-3 tumors in vivo, a delay in tumor growth was seen [11]. Similar results were seen when the gene for p21, a critical downstream mediator of $p53$-induced growth suppression, was introduced using a recombinant adenoviral vector. In vivo studies in mice with established subcutaneous prostate tumors revealed a decreased rate of growth and final tumor volume. In addition, the survival of tumor-bearing animals was extended [12]. The therapeutic effects of *p53* gene delivery are likely to be due to enhancement of apoptosis as well as other "bystander" mechanisms such as antiangiogenesis. Clinical trials using replication-deficient adenoviral vectors encoding *p53* directly injected into the prostate gland under ultrasonic or magnetic resonance imaging are underway.

A study has also demonstrated growth inhibition of prostate cancer by an adenovirus expressing a "novel" tumor-suppressor gene, *pHyde* [13]. *In vitro* introduction of this recombinant vector led to a decrease in growth of the human prostate cancer cell lines DU145 and LNCaP in culture. In vivo injection of the virus reduced DU145 tumors in nude mice compared with untreated control or viral control–treated DU145 tumors. Introduction of the *pHyde* gene resulted in apoptosis and stimulated *p53* expression.

Oncogenes that may be activated in prostate cancer include c-*myc*, *bcl-2*, c-*met*, and *ras*. Disruption of c-*myc* overexpression using antisense c-*myc* transduced by a replication-deficient retrovirus led to a 95% reduction in the tumor volume of DU145 prostate cancer cell xenografts [14]. The *bcl-2* gene is overexpressed in androgen-independent prostate cancer [15]. A hammerhead ribozyme designed to disrupt *bcl-2* expression in LNCaP prostate cancer cells has been shown to have proapoptotic activity [16].

It has been shown that proteolytic activation of caspase-7 is a common event in LNCaP cells undergoing apoptosis [17]. The overexpression of caspase-7 induced by transfection of LNCaP cells with an adenoviral vector expressing the gene resulted in apoptosis of these cells after 72 hours. It was possible to induce apoptosis despite the overexpression of the apoptosis suppressor gene *bcl-2*.

Godbey and Atala [18] were also able to induce apoptosis in targeted prostate cancer cells. In this study the polycation poly(ethylenimine) was used to nonvirally introduce the genes into the target cells. The plasmid introduced was under the control of the cyclooxygenase-2 (COX-2) promoter because constitutive COX-2 overexpression has been implicated in tumorigenesis. Thus, coculture of normal cells and COX-2 overexpressing prostate cancer cells (PC3) revealed a higher reporter expression in the cancer cells. This targeting method was then used to direct the expression of inducible forms of caspases 3 and 9 following which the cells underwent apoptosis. Thus, in this particular study, the heightened COX-2 expression levels of the cancer cells were used for guidance of gene expression in transfected cells.

Enhancing Immunological Responses

Prostate cancer has several factors that make it a good candidate for adoptive immunotherapy. Although prostate cancer is a visceral tumor, the primary tumor site is relatively easy to access and image. Effector immune cells can be readily and accurately injected directly into the tumor assisted by transrectal ultrasonography. In addition, prostate cancer expresses a number of unique tumor and tissue markers including prostate-specific antigen (PSA), prostate-specific membrane antigen (PSMA), and members of the *ErbB* gene family. These markers not only can serve for screening and monitoring of prostate cancer, but also those markers expressed on the cell surface may provide useful targets for active and passive immunotherapy. Finally, although many of these prostate cancer–associated antigens are also expressed on normal prostate tissue, the prostate is not a vital organ and thus any damage to neighboring cells can be accepted as a consequence of treatment.

However, active immunization against prostate cancer may be of limited efficacy because in many cases the tumor cells are of low immunogenicity. Defects in major histocompatibility complex (MHC) class I expression are observed in 85% of primary and 100% of metastatic tumors [19], suggesting that evasion of MHC class I tumor-associated antigens is important in tumor development.

One method of generating an immune response despite downregulation of MHC class I is the use of lymphocytes possessing chimeric receptors. Pinthus et al. [20] have used "chimeric-immune receptors" that possess antibody-like specificity linked to T cell triggering domains in order to redirect immune effector cells toward tumors. This approach combines the effector functions of T cells with the ability of antibodies to recognize a presented antigen with high specificity and without MHC restriction. Using this approach, anti-*erbB2* chimeric receptors were introduced into human lymphocytes and tested against human prostate cancer xenografts in a severe combined immunodeficiency disease (SCID) mouse model. Local delivery of *erbB2*-specific chimeric receptor-bearing lymphocytes, together with systemic IL-2 administration, resulted in retardation of both tumor growth and PSA secretion, prolongation of survival, and complete tumor elimination in a significant number of mice.

Antitumor responses can also be enhanced by presenting tumor antigens in the context of high levels of transduced cytokines. Granulocyte-macrophage colony-stimulating factor (GM-CSF) has emerged as a cytokine with significant efficacy in the induction of an antitumor immune response [21]. GM-CSF may be transduced into autologous or allogeneic tumor cells ex vivo using a viral vector. The transduced tumor cells are then irradiated both to minimize malignant potential and to improve immunogenicity. The cells are then reintroduced by vaccination into the patient. Tumor cell vaccine-expressed GM-CSF may activate quiescent antigen-presenting cells, which then present processed antigen to both CD4 (helper) and CD8 (cytotoxic) T cells, activating a systemic antitumor immune response. A phase I trial of eight immunocompetent patients treated with autologous GM-CSF vaccine prepared from ex vivo retroviral transduction of surgically harvested cells showed that the technique was safe and that antitumor immune responses were inducible [22]. Phase II studies have commenced with GM-CSF generated allogeneic vaccines. Preliminary analysis of the initial trial approved to use direct transrectal prostatic gene therapy injection has suggested that this approach is safe [23].

Studies employing other cytokine genes such as *IL-2* are also underway. In a phase II trial intratumoral injection of a plasmid coding for *IL-2* formulated in a liposomal, cationic lipid mixture vehicle led to decreases in serum PSA levels at 2 weeks postinjection in 80% of the patients, with no grade 3 or 4 toxicity reported [24].

Another vaccine strategy is the DNA vaccine. In this approach, an expression cassette containing the transgene against which an immune response is desired, is injected directly into host cells. The expression of the transfected gene in vivo then promotes immune responses. DNA vaccines are easier to prepare than peptide- or viral-based vaccines and are safe, as they are nonreplicating. Efficacy can be improved by fusion of the desired transgene with the sequence for a pathogen-derived gene to elicit a stronger immune response. The preclinical testing of a PSA-based DNA vaccine in mice resulted in a strong humoral immune response against PSA-positive tumors [25].

The major drawback with the strategy of cytoreductive immunotherapy is the limited tumor burden the immune system can eliminate, and thus applicability may be limited to low bulk disease. Also, the harvesting and culture of autologous or allogeneic tumor or immune cells for ex vivo gene therapy is costly and challenging technically.

Suicide Gene Therapy

Suicide gene therapy involves the conversion of an inactive prodrug into toxic metabolites that can lead to cell cycle arrest and death. Active drug is limited spatially to the transduced cells and adjacent surrounding cells, facilitating higher drug concentrations without increased normal tissue toxicity. Bystander mechanisms markedly enhance efficacy of tumor destruction such that tumors can be eradicated following transduction of only 10% of neoplastic cells with suicide genes. Activation of ganciclovir by herpes simplex virus thymidine kinase (HSV-tk) has been the most widely investigated system. Other enzyme-prodrug systems that generate antimetabolites as the cytotoxic agent include cytosine deaminase/5-fluorocytosine and deoxycytidine kinase/cytosine arabinoside. Enzyme-prodrug systems that generate alkylating agents have also been described including *Escherichia coli* (*E. coli*) nitroreductase/CB1954, carboxypeptidase/CMDA, and cytochrome P-450/cyclophosphamide. In addition, there are examples of enzyme-prodrug systems that generate toxic agents that kill by mechanisms not involving DNA damage such as cytochrome P-450/paracetamol. As stated earlier, importantly, all of these systems can kill bystander cells, eliminating the need for 100% gene delivery.

The HSV-tk system is characterized by the highly effective phosphorylation of ganciclovir. The toxic product of this process cannot cross cell membranes, allowing it to accumulate within the cell. Incorporation into newly synthesized DNA causes termination of synthesis and cell death. Marked tumor growth inhibition and suppression of spontaneous and induced metastases have been demonstrated after injection of the vector containing the HSV-tk gene directly into prostate tumors with subsequent treatment with ganciclovir in the orthotopic mouse model [26]. A phase I clinical trial has now been carried out in patients with recurrent prostate cancer using a replication-deficient adenovirus vector containing the thymidine kinase gene injected directly into the prostate followed by intravenous ganciclovir [27]. A statistically significant prolongation of the PSA doubling time from a mean of 9.8 months to 13.3 months was achieved after the first cycle of gene therapy. Grade 4 toxicity was encountered after the vector injection in only one of 18 patients. Even after repeated injections, side effects were generally mild and self-limiting. An additive response was observed in patients receiving a second cycle of gene therapy with further prolongation of the mean PSA doubling time.

The cytosine deaminase (CD) gene isolated from E. coli encodes for an enzyme that is not normally present in mammalian cells that transforms cytosine to uracil. This enzyme converts 5-fluorocytosine to 5-fluorouracil, which inhibits RNA and DNA synthesis. Preclinical studies have shown greater efficacy in killing tumor cells compared with the herpes simplex thymidine kinase/ganciclovir system [28]. Clinical studies are now being initiated.

The E. coli nitroreductase/CB1954 combination is also an attractive candidate for clinical evaluation because it generates a potent DNA cross-linking agent that can kill both dividing and nondividing cells by induction of apoptosis via a p53-independent mechanism. Furthermore, the efficacy that has been demonstrated in xenograft models required only three cycles of prodrug administration. Djeha et al. [29] injected a replication-deficient adenovirus expressing high levels of nitroreductase intratumorally and combined this with systemic CB1954 treatment. They found that a single injection of the virus (7.5×10^9 to 2×10^{10} particles) followed by CB1954 resulted in a decrease in tumor growth of human prostate cancer xenografts (PC3 cell line) in nude mice.

Several trials are currently taking place looking at the potential of combining radiotherapy with gene therapy treatments. Chhikara et al. [30] treated subcutaneous murine prostate tumors with an intratumoral injection of an adenovirus expressing the HSV-tk gene followed by systemic ganciclovir or local radiation therapy or the combination of gene and radiotherapy. Both single-therapy modalities resulted in a 38% decrease in tumor growth compared to untreated controls, but the combined treatment resulted in a decrease of 61%. Preliminary data suggest that this approach is also safe in humans. Teh et al. [31] have treated men with newly diagnosed prostate cancer with a combination of radiotherapy, in situ gene therapy consisting of an adenovirus expressing the thymidine kinase gene, together with valacyclovir, and in high-risk patients hormonal therapy. At a median follow up of 5 months, the acute toxicities were limited, with no patient experiencing a grade 3 or greater acute toxicity. More recently at a median follow-up of 22.3 months, no grade 3 or greater late toxicity was seen [32]. Further trials assessing the efficacy of this treatment are taking place.

To further increase the effectiveness of suicide gene therapy, several groups have developed approaches to deliver both the cytosine deaminase and HSV-tk genes and treat with both 5-fluorocystine and ganciclovir. Freytag et al. [33] have developed a lytic replication-competent adenoviral vector encoding an HSV-tk–CD fusion protein and used it for the treatment of patients with a local recurrence of prostate cancer at least 1 year after the completion of definitive radiotherapy treatment. The virus was injected intratumorally into 16 patients, followed by systemic treatment with ganciclovir and 5-fluorocystine. The treatment was well tolerated with a reduction in PSA in nearly 50% of patients. Furthermore, two patients showed a lack of detectable carcinoma at their 1 year follow-up biopsies. Freytag et al. [34] have also used the same gene therapy in combination with radiotherapy for the treatment of patients with newly diagnosed intermediate- to high-risk prostate cancer. The authors reported no significant side effects, and acute urinary and gastrointestinal toxicities were similar to those expected with the radiotherapy treatment. Also as expected, because all the patients received radiotherapy, all patients experienced a decline in their PSA levels. However, the mean PSA half-life in patients given more than 1 week of prodrug therapy was significantly shorter than that of patients receiving prodrugs for only 1 week and markedly shorter than that reported previously for patients treated with radiotherapy alone.

Oncolytic Viruses

Viruses alone can infect and kill tumor cells without the insertion of a cytotoxic transgene. Certain viruses, including adenoviruses and HSV, have as part of their normal life cycle a lytic phase that is lethal to the host cell.

The use of oncolytic HSV for the treatment of cancer has progressed to phase I clinical trials, although this is for the treatment of gliomas. G207 is a replication-competent HSV that is mutated so that viral propagation is confined to tumor cells and to limit neurovirulence. Although G207 is mainly being assessed clinically for the treatment of gliomas, with regard to prostate cancer G207 was capable of conferring cytotoxicity to several prostate tumor cell lines and either growth retardation or tumor eradication of mouse xenografts [35].

The cytotoxic application of adenoviruses has also been investigated. Several prostate-specific constructs have been developed and tested *in vitro* as well as in humans. CG7060 (previously known as CN706 and CV706) expresses the *E1A* gene (a viral gene product that promotes viral replication and induces cell death) under the control of a PSA minimal promoter enhancer. This construct showed potent PSA-selective cytotoxic activity in preclinical testing [36], and a phase I trial has been carried out [37]. A total of 20 patients with locally recurrent prostate cancer following radiotherapy were treated. The study revealed that intratumoral injection of the construct was safe, and it led to a decrease in PSA in a dose-responsive manner. Additional studies have demonstrated that combination treatment of CG7060 and radiation leads to synergistic prostate tumor cytotoxicity [38].

Conclusion

The main limiting factors for the development of an effective gene therapy are efficiency of gene transfer, selectivity of tumor targeting, and the immunogenic properties of the vectors as well as general safety considerations. The findings of the early clinical trials of gene therapy have been promising, and results of several ongoing clinical trials are awaited. More recent trials have focused on combining gene therapy with conventional hormonal, chemotherapeutic, and radiation strategies in an attempt to overcome such problems as cellular heterogeneity and tumor resistance.

The expanding field of genomics provides an exciting new resource for the design of prostate-specific gene therapy strategies. The obstacles to the development of gene-based human therapeutics are significant but the rewards are great. Recent developments in molecular biology and virus delivery together with the ability to individualize molecular profiles point to a promising future for gene therapy for prostate cancer.

References

1. Department of Health. London: HMSO, 1996.
2. Brawley OW, Giovannucci E, Kramer BS. Epidemiology of Prostate Cancer. Philadelphia: Lippincott Williams & Wilkins, 2000.
3. Kay MA, Holterman AX, Meuse L, et al. Long-term hepatic adenovirus-mediated gene expression in mice following CTLA4Ig administration. Nat Genet 1995;11(2):191–197.
4. Dai Y, Schwarz EM, Gu D, et al. Cellular and humoral immune responses to adenoviral vectors containing factor IX gene: tolerization of factor IX and vector antigens allows for long-term expression. Proc Natl Acad Sci USA 1995;92(5):1401–1405.
5. Nakatani T, Kuriyama S, Tominaga K, et al. Assessment of efficiency and safety of adenovirus mediated gene transfer into normal and damaged murine livers. Gut 2000;47(4):563–570.
6. Belldegrun A, Tso CL, Zisman A, et al. Interleukin 2 gene therapy for prostate cancer: phase I clinical trial and basic biology. Hum Gene Ther 2001;12(8):883–892.
7. Cotten M, Wagner E, Zatloukal K, et al. High-efficiency receptor-mediated delivery of small and large 48 kilobase gene constructs using the endosome-disruption activity of defective or chemically inactivated adenovirus particles. Proc Natl Acad Sci USA 1992;89(13):6094–6098.
8. Heidenberg HB, Sesterhenn IA, Gaddipati JP, et al. Alteration of the tumor suppressor gene p53 in a high fraction of hormone refractory prostate cancer. J Urol 1995;154(2 pt 1):414–421.
9. Asgari K, Sesterhenn IA, McLeod DG, et al. Inhibition of the growth of pre-established subcutaneous tumor nodules of human prostate cancer

cells by single injection of the recombinant adenovirus p53 expression vector. Int J Cancer 1997; 71(3):377–382.

10. Ko SC, Gotoh A, Thalmann GN, et al. Molecular therapy with recombinant p53 adenovirus in an androgen-independent, metastatic human prostate cancer model. Hum Gene Ther 1996;7(14): 1683–1691.

11. Gotoh A, Kao C, Ko SC, et al. Cytotoxic effects of recombinant adenovirus p53 and cell cycle regulator genes (p21 WAF1/CIP1 and p16CDKN4) in human prostate cancers. J Urol 1997;158(2): 636–641.

12. Eastham JA, Hall SJ, Sehgal I, et al. In vivo gene therapy with p53 or p21 adenovirus for prostate cancer. Cancer Res 1995;55(22):5151–5155.

13. Steiner MS, Zhang X, Wang Y, Lu Y. Growth inhibition of prostate cancer by an adenovirus expressing a novel tumor suppressor gene, pHyde. Cancer Res 2000;60(16):4419–4425.

14. Steiner MS, Anthony CT, Lu Y, Holt JT. Antisense c-myc retroviral vector suppresses established human prostate cancer. Hum Gene Ther 1998; 9(5):747–755.

15. McDonnell TJ, Troncoso P, Brisbay SM, et al. Expression of the protooncogene bcl-2 in the prostate and its association with emergence of androgen-independent prostate cancer. Cancer Res 1992;52(24):6940–6944.

16. Dorai T, Olsson CA, Katz AE, Buttyan R. Development of a hammerhead ribozyme against bcl-2. I. Preliminary evaluation of a potential gene therapeutic agent for hormone-refractory human prostate cancer. Prostate 1997;32(4):246–258.

17. Marcelli M, Cunningham GR, Walkup M, et al. Signaling pathway activated during apoptosis of the prostate cancer cell line LNCaP: overexpression of caspase-7 as a new gene therapy strategy for prostate cancer. Cancer Res 1999;59(2):382–390.

18. Godbey WT, Atala A. Directed apoptosis in Cox-2-overexpressing cancer cells through expression-targeted gene delivery. Gene Ther 2003;10(17):1519–27.

19. Blades RA, Keating PJ, McWilliam LJ, George NJ, Stern PL. Loss of HLA class I expression in prostate cancer: implications for immunotherapy. Urology 1995;46(5):681–686; discussion 686–687.

20. Pinthus JH, Waks T, Kaufman-Francis K, et al. Immuno-gene therapy of established prostate tumors using chimeric receptor-redirected human lymphocytes. Cancer Res 2003;63(10):2470–2476.

21. Dranoff G, Jaffee E, Lazenby A, et al. Vaccination with irradiated tumor cells engineered to secrete murine granulocyte-macrophage colony-stimulating factor stimulates potent, specific, and long-lasting anti-tumor immunity. Proc Natl Acad Sci USA 1993;90(8):3539–3543.

22. Simons JW, Mikhak B, Chang JF, et al. Induction of immunity to prostate cancer antigens: results of a clinical trial of vaccination with irradiated autologous prostate tumor cells engineered to secrete granulocyte-macrophage colony-stimulating factor using ex vivo gene transfer. Cancer Res 1999;59(20):5160–5168.

23. Steiner MS, Gingrich JR. Gene therapy for prostate cancer: where are we now? J Urol 2000;164(4): 1121–1136.

24. Pantuck AJ, Zisman A, Belldegrun AS. Gene therapy for prostate cancer at the University of California, Los Angeles: preliminary results and future directions. World J Urol 2000;18(2):143–147.

25. Kim JJ, Trivedi NN, Wilson DM, et al. Molecular and immunological analysis of genetic prostate specific antigen (PSA) vaccine. Oncogene 1998; 17(24):3125–3135.

26. Thompson TC. In situ gene therapy for prostate cancer. Oncol Res 1999;11(1):1–8.

27. Herman JR, Adler HL, Aguilar-Cordova E, et al. In situ gene therapy for adenocarcinoma of the prostate: a phase I clinical trial. Hum Gene Ther 1999;10(7):1239–1249.

28. Singhal S, Kaiser LR. Cancer chemotherapy using suicide genes. Surg Oncol Clin North Am 1998; 7(3):505–536.

29. Djeha AH, Thomson TA, Leung H, et al. Combined adenovirus-mediated nitroreductase gene delivery and CB1954 treatment: a well-tolerated therapy for established solid tumors. Mol Ther 2001;3(2):233–240.

30. Chhikara M, Huang H, Vlachaki MT, et al. Enhanced therapeutic effect of HSV-tk+GCV gene therapy and ionizing radiation for prostate cancer. Mol Ther 2001;3(4):536–542.

31. Teh BS, Aguilar-Cordova E, Kernen K, et al. Phase I/II trial evaluating combined radiotherapy and in situ gene therapy with or without hormonal therapy in the treatment of prostate cancer—a preliminary report. Int J Radiat Oncol Biol Phys 2001;51(3):605–613.

32. Teh BS, Aguilar-Cordova E, Aguilar L, et al. Late toxicity of a phase I/II trial evaluating combined radiotherapy and in-situ gene-therapy with or without hormonal therapy in the treatment of prostate cancer. Int J Radiat Oncol Biol Phys 2003;57(2 suppl):S275.

33. Freytag SO, Khil M, Stricker H, et al. Phase I study of replication-competent adenovirus-mediated double suicide gene therapy for the treatment of locally recurrent prostate cancer. Cancer Res 2002;62(17):4968–4976.

34. Freytag SO, Stricker H, Pegg J, et al. Phase I study of replication-competent adenovirus-mediated double-suicide gene therapy in combination with conventional-dose three-dimensional conformal radiation therapy for the treatment of newly diag-

nosed, intermediate- to high-risk prostate cancer. Cancer Res 2003;63(21):7497–7506.

35. Oyama M, Ohigashi T, Hoshi M, et al. Oncolytic viral therapy for human prostate cancer by conditionally replicating herpes simplex virus 1 vector G207. Jpn J Cancer Res 2000;91(12):1339–1344.

36. Rodriguez R, Schuur ER, Lim HY, et al. Prostate attenuated replication competent adenovirus (ARCA) CN706: a selective cytotoxic for prostate-specific antigen-positive prostate cancer cells. Cancer Res 1997;57(13):2559–2563.

37. DeWeese TL, van der Poel H, Li S, et al. A phase I trial of CV706, a replication-competent, PSA selective oncolytic adenovirus, for the treatment of locally recurrent prostate cancer following radiation therapy. Cancer Res 2001;61(20):7464–7472.

38. Chen Y, DeWeese T, Dilley J, et al. CV706, a prostate cancer-specific adenovirus variant, in combination with radiotherapy produces synergistic antitumor efficacy without increasing toxicity. Cancer Res 2001;61(14):5453–5460.

Part II

Bladder Cancer

12

Molecular Biology of Bladder Cancer

Margaret A. Knowles

Knowledge of the molecular biology of bladder cancer has advanced dramatically in recent years. Much information concerns common genetic alterations, but there is also information on global changes in gene expression. Almost all comes from studies of transitional cell carcinoma (TCC), the major histopathological type of bladder cancer in Western countries, and only these tumors are discussed here.

There is now a well-defined model for the molecular pathogenesis of TCC that is compatible with clinical observations. There is also an extensive repertoire of genes and genomic regions that are altered in TCC and ongoing studies are analyzing the functional consequences of the alterations seen. Impetus for such studies is generated by the hypothesis that tumor phenotype is determined largely by genotype. The predicted rewards of these efforts are the identification of markers for diagnosis, disease monitoring prediction of prognosis and response to therapy, and of targets for rational drug design. This chapter summarizes our current knowledge of the molecular biology of transitional cell carcinoma and gives some examples of the potential clinical utility of this information.

Pathogenesis of Bladder Cancer

Bladder tumors comprise two major groups. The majority of tumors at presentation (70% to 80%) are low grade, non muscle-invasive (pTa/T1),

papillary tumors [1]. Carcinoma in situ (CIS) is by definition noninvasive, but it is considered a high-risk lesion, more appropriately grouped with the invasive tumors. Low-grade superficial TCC frequently recurs (~70%) but often with no increase in grade or progression to muscle invasion. Patients may have multiple recurrences over many years but only 10% to 20% progress to invade muscle. In contrast, the 20% of tumors that are invasive at diagnosis have a much poorer prognosis with a 50% 5-year survival for pT2 tumors [2]. Like the muscle invasive tumors, CIS has a poor prognosis [3].

Multifocality and frequent recurrence is characteristic of urothelial tumors. The macroscopically "normal" urothelium in many cases shows areas of microscopic dysplasia [4], so that it is easy to envisage how new lesions develop after resection of the primary tumor. There has been much discussion over the clonality of bladder tumors. One possibility is that the entire urothelium is unstable and many different clones of altered cells are present that give rise to polyclonal tumors, the so-called field effect. In fact, there is little evidence for this, and most studies have found only monoclonal tumors. The presence of shared genetic changes in all tumors resected from individual patients suggests that these are related lesions that have evolved from a single altered cell clone. Divergence between the genetic changes found in such related tumors has been used to determine the likely timing of events. Nevertheless, there are some examples of more than one unrelated monoclonal tumor in the same bladder, and this is not surprising, given the association of TCC risk with smoking and the pan-urothelial carcinogenic insult associated with it [reviewed in ref. 5].

Molecular Alterations in Superficial Transitional Cell Carcinoma

Bladder cancer is commonly categorized as superficial or invasive, depending on the degree of invasion of the submucosa and the muscle wall of the bladder. In light of current genetic data, this subdivision appears inappropriate, and the current thinking is that low-grade superficial papillary tumors (pTa G1/2) should be considered as distinct from those tumors that have penetrated the basement membrane and invade the submucosa (pT1) and from the high-grade

lesion CIS, all of which have been grouped together in the past. These latter are high-risk lesions that commonly progress to invade muscle [6]. High-grade Ta tumors (pTaG3) are also at increased risk of progression to invasion, and this is reflected in a spectrum of molecular changes and genetic instability similar to that seen in T2 tumors. A grouping into genetically stable (low-grade pTa) and genetically unstable superficial tumors is therefore recommended.

Low-grade (G1-2) pTa tumors show few molecular alterations. Despite efforts from many laboratories that have examined hundreds of such tumors, only two common alterations are found: deletions involving chromosome 9 and mutations of the FGF receptor 3 (*FGFR3*) (Table 12.1). Three major approaches have been used to search for genomic alterations: karyotypic analysis, loss of heterozygosity (LOH) analysis, and comparative genomic hybridization (CGH).

Karyotypic analysis has revealed that such tumors are often near diploid, and loss of chro-

Table 12.1. Genetic alterations of known genes in transitional cell carcinoma

Gene (cytogenetic location)	Alteration	Frequency/clinical association
	Oncogenes	
HRAS (11p15)	Activating mutation	10–15% overall (high grade) [127–129]
FGFR3 (4p16)	Activating mutation	30–80% [42, 47]
ERBB2 (17q)	Amplification/overexpression	Amplified 10–14% high grade/stage [73,74,130]
CCND1(11q13)	Amplification/overexpression	10–20% all grades and stages [131,132]
MDM2 (12q13)	Amplification/overexpression	4% amplification, high grade
		~30% overexpression, low grade [76,133]
	Tumor-suppressor genes	
CDKN2A (Ha1) (9p21)	Homozygous deletion/ methylation/mutation	20–30% high grade/stage [24,25,134]
		LOH 60% all grades/stages, immortalization in vitro [135]
RB1 (13q14)	Deletion/mutation	10–15% overall [95–97]
		37% muscle invasive
TP53 (17p13)	Deletion/mutation	70% muscle invasive [83,86,87] high grade and stage
PTEN (10q23)	Homozygous deletion/mutation	10q LOH in 35% muscle invasive [106,108]
		6.6% superficial
PTCH (9q22)	Deletion/mutation	LOH 60% all grades/stages [18,27]
		Mutation frequency low
TSC1 (9q34)	Deletion/mutation	LOH 60% all grades/stages [30–32]
		Mutation frequency 13%
DBC1 (9q32–33)	Deletion/methylation	LOH 60% all grades/stages [38,136]
DCC/SMAD (18q)	Deletion	LOH 30% high grade/stage [137]

LOH, loss of heterozygosity.

Table 12.2. Common regions of deletion detected by loss of heterozygosity (LOH) analysis in transitional cell carcinoma

Cytogenetic location	Frequency (%)	Association with clinical parameters
3p	48	Stage [138]
4p	22	None [46,139]
4q	24	High grade/stage [139]
8p	23	High grade/stage [140–142]
9q	60	None [14,143]
11p	40	Grade [9,144]
11q	15	None [9]
14q	10–40	Stage [145]

mosome 9 is by far the most common cytogenetic finding [7]. Apart from chromosome 9 loss, only loss of the Y chromosome has been found at significant frequency. Loss of heterozygosity analysis has revealed little apart from that for chromosome 9 (Table 12.2). 11p LOH is found in ~40% of bladder tumors, including some pTa tumors, though there appears to be a higher frequency in tumors of higher grade and stage [8,9]. Comparative genomic hybridization analysis has identified a few other copy number changes, such as gain of 1q and 17 and some amplifications of 11q, but none is frequent (Table 12.3). Amplifications of 11q include the cyclin D1 gene *(CCND1)*, which is involved in regulation of cell cycle progression from G1 to S phase via the Rb pathway. In contrast, high-grade pTa tumors (pTaG3) resemble invasive tumors in the alterations they contain (see below).

As bladder cancer is a disease of the middle to late decades of life, it is predicted that multiple heritable changes are required for tumor development. Thus it is surprising that so few changes have been identified in low-grade pTa tumors, which represent the major group at diagnosis. Efforts are in progress using expression and genomic microarray technology to identify other genetic or epigenetic events that may contribute to the development of these tumors, but as yet no other common changes have been described.

Low-grade pTa tumors are genetically very stable. There have been several studies of synchronous or metachronous tumors from the same patient, and in general these show a striking identity in the genetic alterations found [10,11]. Chromosome 9 LOH is the least divergent event, and other genetic events differ in different tumors from the same patient. This indicates that LOH of chromosome 9 is likely to be an early change, whereas other events occur during independent evolution of different tumor sub-clones [11].

Chromosome 9

Chromosome 9 LOH is found in more than 50% of all bladder tumors regardless of grade and stage [8,12,13]. The finding that many TCCs have loss of the entire chromosome, commonly with reduplication of the other homologue, implies that loss of function of tumor-suppressor genes on both chromosome arms contributes to tumor development. Identification of these target genes is considered pivotal to understanding the pathogenesis of the disease and to providing useful clinical markers and targets. Some tumors have regions of LOH affecting only part of the chromosome, and this has allowed mapping of "common" or "critical" regions of LOH on both

Table 12.3. Common comparative genomic hybridization (CGH) findings in transitional cell carcinoma[1]

Tumor stage	Losses	Gains	Amplification
Ta	9p, 9q, Y	1q, 17	11q
T1	2q, 4p, 4q, 5q, 6q, 8p, 9p, 9q, 10q, 11p, 11q, 13q, 17p, 18q, Y	1q, 3p, 3q, 5p. 6p, 8q, 10p, 17q, 20q	1q22–24, 3p24–25, 6p22, 8p12, 8q22, 10p12–14, 10q22–23, 11q13, 12q12–21, 17q21, 20q13
T2–4	As for T1 + 15q	As for pT1 + 7p, Xq	As for pT1

[1] Data from refs, 10,70,113,146–148.

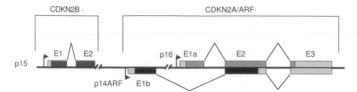

Fig. 12.1. Genomic organization of the 9p21 loci *CDKN2B* and *CDKN2A/ARF* encoding p15, p16, and p14ARF. p16 and p14ARF share exons 2 and 3 but have distinct exons 1. Transcripts read in different reading frames generate two different protein products. Coding regions are shown in black (p15 and p14 ARF) or grey (p16).

9p and 9q. Where small primary tumors have been studied, the frequency of smaller deletions appears higher, suggesting that initially small regions of LOH may develop and coalesce during tumor development [14–16]. Loss of a copy of chromosome 9 has also been visualized by fluorescence in situ hybridization (FISH) in urothelial dysplasia and in morphologically normal urothelium in patients with bladder cancer [17], providing additional evidence that chromosome 9 loss is an early event in TCC development.

Currently, one region of loss is mapped on 9p (9p21), and at least three regions on 9q (at 9q22, 9q32–q33 and 9q34) [14,18–21]. Candidate genes within these regions are *CDKN2A/ARF* (p16/p14ARF) and *CDKN2B* (p15) at 9p21 [22–26], *PTCH* (Gorlin syndrome gene) at 9q22 [18,27], *DBC1* (a novel gene) at 9q32–q33 [19,28,29], and *TSC1* (tuberous sclerosis syndrome gene 1) at 9q34 [30–32].

The *CDKN2A/ARF* locus on 9p21 encodes two proteins, p16 and p14ARF, both of which are key cell cycle regulators (Fig. 12.1). These genes share coding region in exons 2 and 3 but have distinct exons 1. The protein products are translated in different reading frames to generate two entirely different proteins, one of which, p16, plays a key role in the Rb pathway and the other, p14ARF, in the p53 pathway (Fig. 12.2). Both genes are commonly inactivated in TCC via homozygous co-deletion. In the same region of 9p21 is the related gene *CDKN2B* encoding the cell cycle regulator p15, and in many cases, though not all, this gene is also homozygously deleted. Point mutations of p16 are infrequent, but hypermethylation of the promoter is found as a mechanism of inactivation of the second allele, though there is controversy over the exact frequency [33,34]. There is no consensus on whether 9p21 homozygous deletion is related to TCC grade and stage. Loss of heterozygosity of 9p21 is as common in low-grade pTa as in invasive (≥pT2) TCC, though homozygous deletion is reported to be associated with larger tumor size and reduced recurrence free interval [35]. This may indicate that, as suggested by knockout mouse studies [reviewed in ref. 36] and *in vitro* experiments on mouse cells [37], haploinsufficiency of p16 and/or p14ARF is significant.

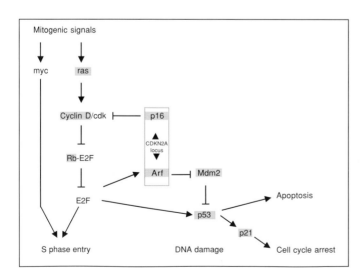

Fig. 12.2. Relationship of the p53 and Rb pathways in controlling cell cycle progression and response to stress (DNA damage). The CDKN2A locus (boxed) encodes both p16 and p14ARF and links the two pathways. Genes commonly altered either genetically or at the expression level in transitional cell carcinoma (TCC) are shaded in gray. Arrowheads indicate stimulatory effects and barred lines indicate inhibitory effects.

Three genes on 9q are implicated. *PTCH*, the Gorlin syndrome gene, maps within a small region of deletion at 9q22. Mutations of the gene are infrequent in TCC [27] but reduction in messenger RNA (mRNA) expression is common, and it has been suggested that this gene may be haploinsufficient in the urothelium [18]. At 9q33, a novel gene, *DBC1*, is the only gene within the common region of deletion. Homozygous deletion has been found in a few tumors [28,29], and although there is no evidence of mutational inactivation, there is common transcriptional silencing by hypermethylation of the promoter [19,38]. The function of *DBC1* is not yet clear, but it has been shown that ectopic expression can induce a nonapoptotic form of cell death [39], and in cells that survive, there is a delay in the G1 phase of the cell cycle [40].

The third gene at 9q34 is the tuberous sclerosis gene *TSC1*. Germline mutation of *TSC1* is associated with the familial hamartoma syndrome tuberous sclerosis complex (TSC). In bladder tumors, mutations of *TSC1* are found in ~13% of cases [30,31]. Interestingly, some of these are in tumors without 9q34 LOH, indicating the possible role of haploinsufficiency [30]. The *TSC1* gene product hamartin acts in complex with the *TSC2* gene tuberin in the phosphatidylinositol (PI)3-kinase pathway to negatively regulate mTOR, a central molecule in the control of protein synthesis and cell growth [41].

FGFR3

Recently, mutations in the fibroblast growth factor (FGF) receptor gene *(FGFR3)* have been identified in many bladder tumors [42–45]. *FGFR3* maps to 4p16.3 within a common region of LOH in TCC [46], but mutations do not appear to be related to LOH status [47]. Rather, *FGFR3* appears to be an oncogene activated by mutation in TCC. The frequency of *FGFR3* mutation detected varies (Table 12.1). Mutation is strongly associated with low tumor grade and stage, with up to 80% of low-grade pTa tumors showing mutation [43], and this appears to indicate lower risk of tumor recurrence in noninvasive TCC [45]. Mutations have also been found in urothelial papilloma [48]. The mutations detected are the same as germline mutations found in inherited dwarfism syndromes [reviewed in ref. 49]. The most common mutation found in TCC to date is S249C, which when present in the

germline causes thanatophoric dysplasia type I, a lethal form of achondroplasia. All of the mutations found are confined to a few hot spots in exons 7, 10 and 15, where the effect of mutation is predicted to cause constitutive activation of the kinase activity of the receptor [50] (Fig. 12.3).

Interestingly, despite quite extensive studies of other major adult tumor types, *FGFR3* mutation is only found at significant frequency in bladder cancer. A small number of mutations have been described in multiple myeloma, where they occur in association with the translocation t(4;14) and also in cervical carcinoma [42], but none in a wide range of the common adult solid tumors [44,51]. This dramatic bladder tumor specificity may represent a significant opportunity for the development of tumor-specific therapy. The predominance of mutation in superficial bladder tumors lends itself well to the development of novel forms of intravesical therapy.

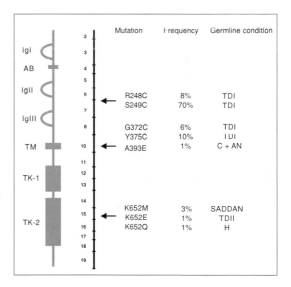

Fig. 12.3. Structure of the FGFR3 protein, showing positions of exons and positions and frequency of mutations identified in TCC. Igl, II, III, immunoglobin domains; AB, acid box; TM, transmembrane domain; TK-1, TK-2, tyrosine kinase domains; TDI, thanatophoric dysplasia type I; TDII, thanatophoric dysplasia type II; C+AN, Crouzon syndrome with acanthoma nigricans; SADDAN, severe achondroplasia with developmental delay and acanthosis nigricans. H, hypochondroplasia.

Risk of Recurrence and Progression in Superficial Transitional Cell Carcinoma

Key issues in the clinical management of superficial bladder cancer are the provision of adequate disease monitoring after resection of a primary tumor and prediction of the risk of recurrence and progression to invasive disease. Accurate assessment of risk of recurrence could allow less frequent monitoring by cystoscopy and if urine-based analyses could be used, this would reduce costs and the cystoscopy-associated morbidity and anxiety suffered by patients. A wide range of molecular alterations has been assessed, but to date there is no marker that has sufficient predictive power to be used routinely in the clinic.

Several studies have reported that markers associated with cell proliferation (e.g., Ki-67 labeling) are predictive [e.g., 52,53]) though not all studies agree [54]. An altered cytokeratin 20 (CK20) staining pattern has also been reported to predict recurrence. Normal urothelium shows staining confined to the superficial and upper intermediate cell layers of the urothelium. In some superficial tumors, this pattern is disrupted, with staining throughout all layers, and this is associated with higher risk of recurrence [55]. Monosomy 9 and 4 regions of LOH (9pter-p22, 9q22.3, 9q33, and 9q34) have been reported to be associated with increased risk of recurrence [56]. In a second study, monosomy 9 or LOH in the region of TSC1 but not p16 or DBC1 was associated with increased risk of recurrence [57]. This may indicate that loss of TSC1 is critical, and this should now be tested in a larger tumor panel.

FGFR3 mutation may be a useful marker, as the recurrence rate for tumors with mutation appears lower than for tumors without mutation [45]. In a recent study, a combination of FGFR3 mutation status and immunohistochemistry for MIB-1 was found to be superior to pathological grading for prediction of outcome (recurrence, progression, and disease-free survival) [58]. FGFR3 mutation screening has also been applied to urine sediments. Mutations were detected in 67% of patients undergoing transurethral resection TCC and in 28% of patients who subsequently underwent cystectomy [59]. FGFR3 mutation screening outperformed cytology in both groups, but in the low-grade superficial tumors it was markedly better than cytology (68% vs. 32%). In another prospective study, paired tumor and urine samples were analyzed for FGFR3 mutation and for microsatellite alterations. The same alterations were detected in tumor and urine from the same patients, and combined sensitivity was 89% for all types of tumor [60]. These studies clearly indicate that molecular detection and grading of tissues and urine samples can add significant information.

Other molecular changes reported to be predictive of increased risk of recurrence include low matrix metalloproteinase-9 (MMP-9), tissue inhibitor of metalloproteinase-1 (TIMP-1) ratio [61], CDKN2A/p14^{ARF} promoter methylation [62], DAPK (death associated protein kinase) promoter methylation [63], reduced expression of E-cadherin [64], expression of the imprinted H19 gene [65], and expression of the antiapoptotic protein survivin [66].

Although many molecular alterations are associated with high tumor grade and stage and with adverse clinical outcome (see below), these do not necessarily represent risk factors for progression from pTa. Risk of progression is difficult to assess, as few of the low-grade pTa tumors progress to muscle invasion, and hence large tumor banks are required to ensure an adequate sample size. TP53 alteration has been suggested as a risk factor [67]. However, most studies that have assessed TP53 and other molecular alterations have grouped pTa and pT1 tumors together, and it is likely that in most cases it is the pT1 tumors that show TP53 and other alterations. Molecular changes that have been proposed as potential markers for high risk of progression from pTa include loss of expression of E-cadherin [68], loss of p63 expression [69], and in pT1 tumors various cytogenetic alterations [70].

Molecular Alterations in Invasive Transitional Cell Carcinoma

Muscle invasive bladder tumors commonly have many genetic alterations in addition to chromosome 9 deletions (Tables 12.1 to 12.3). There are both alterations to known genes and many genomic alterations for which the target genes are currently unknown. Karyotype studies have identified losses of 1p, 6q, 9p, 9q, and 13q, and gains of 5p in more than 15% of cases; CGH and LOH analyses have confirmed and extended these findings (Tables 12.2 and 12.3).

Oncogenes

ERBB2 (17q23) encodes a receptor tyrosine kinase of the *EGFR* gene family. It is amplified in 10% to 20% and overexpressed in 10% to 50% of invasive TCC [71–74]. Thus, in contrast to the situation in breast carcinoma, there are many cases of TCC where gene amplification is not the mechanism whereby expression is increased. The underlying mechanism has not been elucidated. A similar situation exists in the case of the EGF receptor; 30% to 50% of invasive tumors overexpress EGFR, and this is associated with poor prognosis [75], but only a small percentage show gene amplification.

MDM2 (12q14) is amplified in a few cases of TCC (4% to 6%) [76]. MDM2 acts in an autoregulatory loop with p53 and its overexpression represents an alternative mechanism by which p53 function may be inactivated in some TCCs. Several immunohistochemical studies have shown upregulation of expression of MDM2 in TCC samples, but there is no consensus on the relation of this to tumor grade, stage, or prognosis [e.g.,54,77,78].

HRAS is mutated in some TCCs, but there are conflicting estimates of the frequency of mutation (Table 12.1). *In vitro* experiments on human tumor cells indicate that HRAS can upregulate EGFR expression (commonly found in invasive TCC) and induce an invasive phenotype [79,80]. However, in transgenic mice engineered to express mutant HRAS in the urothelium, this leads to the development of papillary tumors rather than muscle invasive tumors [81]. Further studies in animal models may help to clarify whether HRAS can participate in the development of both major forms of TCC. No clear association of *HRAS* mutation with tumor phenotype has been described. Other members of the *RaS* gene family have not been comprehensively studied.

Tumor Suppressor Genes

Tumor suppressor genes are defined as genes whose functional inactivation contributes to tumor development. These have a wide range of negative regulatory functions in the cell, ranging from control of cell cycle progression to influences on cellular adhesion. Several of the tumor suppressor genes implicated in invasive TCC, including *TP53*, *RB*, *CDKN2A/ARF* (also altered in many superficial tumors), and *PTEN*, are major players in other human cancers.

p53 and Rb and Their Pathways

The interconnecting pathways controlled by p53 and Rb regulate cell cycle progression and responses to stress, processes that are almost universally deregulated in malignant cells [reviewed in ref. 82] (Fig. 12.2). p53 plays a key role in determining cellular response to various stress signals. In the absence of stress stimuli, p53 protein levels are low, but when activated protein levels rise and transcription of a wide range of genes is activated. p53 activation induces apoptosis in some circumstances and cell cycle arrest in others, depending on the cell type and the nature of the stimulus. Mutation of *TP53* is found in many muscle invasive bladder cancers [83–87]. As many mutations increase the half-life of the protein, detection of high levels of protein by immunohistochemistry provides a useful surrogate marker for mutation [88] and has been used extensively to measure *TP53* alteration. p53 accumulation has been associated with adverse prognosis in all types of TCC [67,89–91], and it has been suggested that this might be used as a prognostic marker in the clinic. Similarly, expression of the cyclin-dependent kinase p21, which acts downstream of p53, has a reported association with better prognosis [92]. It has also been reported that patients with tumors that retain p21 expression even with *TP53* mutation have outcomes similar to those with wild-type *TP53* [92,93]. Not all studies have confirmed these findings, though a meta analysis of more than 3000 tumors indicated a small but significant association between p53 positivity by immunohistochemistry and poor prognosis [94].

Rb acts in a pathway that regulates progression from G1 to S phase of the cell cycle (Fig. 12.2). It binds to members of the E2F transcription factor family, and this complex recruits histone deacetylases (HDACs) to E2F responsive promoters. Cdk-mediated phosphorylation of Rb prevents association with E2F and enables

E2F-mediated gene expression and progression into S phase. The *RB* gene is large and has not been screened for small mutations, but some homozygous deletions, LOH of 13q14, and loss of Rb protein expression have been detected in TCC. The frequency of loss of Rb, as for inactivation of *TP53*, is higher in tumors of high grade and stage [95–98].

As indicated above, *CDKN2A* (encoding p16 and p14^{ARF}) is commonly deleted in TCC of all grades and stages. These proteins interact with and link the Rb and p53 pathways (Fig. 12.2), and inactivation of both of these together is likely to provide further freedom from the G1 checkpoint than conferred by either p53 of Rb inactivation alone. There are therefore several ways in which tumors may evade the checkpoint and it would be predicted that those with p53 and Rb or p16 loss would be more aggressive than those with either p53 or Rb loss alone. Rb and p53 have been assessed together in several studies, and this prediction is borne out with double mutant tumors showing worse prognosis [99–101]. To date, an assessment of all genes known to be involved in this G1 checkpoint has not been carried out on a single patient series, but such an analysis may achieve much greater predictive power than single or two-marker analyses.

Cyclin D1 is overexpressed in some bladder tumors, including some superficial tumors by virtue of DNA amplification. However, the frequency of amplification is insufficient to explain all cases with overexpression. Interestingly, cyclin D1 is a possible target of the Wnt/β-catenin pathway, and recently it was reported that some high-grade bladder tumors (3/59 studied) had mutations in β-catenin [102]. This represents an alternative mechanism for cyclin D1 activation in these tumors that is accompanied by *myc* overexpression and appears to be associated with a more aggressive phenotype than the overexpression associated with gene amplification, found in low-grade tumors with papillary architecture [103].

PTEN

PTEN (phosphatase and tensin homologue deleted on chromosome 10) maps to 10q23, a region of common LOH in TCC of high grade and stage [104–106]. PTEN has a phosphatase domain that acts on both lipid and protein sub-strates. The major substrate appears to be the signaling lipid PtIns(3,4,5)P$_3$, a major product of PI3-kinase, which is activated by various tyrosine kinase receptors. Thus PTEN is a negative regulator of this major signaling pathway, which affects cell phenotype in various ways including effects on proliferation, apoptosis and cell migration [107]. Heterozygous knockout mice (Pten +/−) show widespread proliferative changes, suggesting that loss of one allele in tumors may provide a advantage at the cellular level. Mutation screening in TCC has revealed some mutations of the second allele in tumors with LOH and in bladder cell lines [108–110]. Some homozygous deletions have also been found. Gene replacement studies have been carried out in two bladder tumor cell lines that lack functional PTEN. In both cases this suppressed proliferation and induced G1 arrest [111].

Other Genetic Changes in Invasive Transitional Cell Carcinoma

Large numbers of changes have been detected by karyotyping, CGH, and LOH analyses in muscle invasive TCC. Numerically most common are losses of 2q, 5q, 8p, 9p, 9q, 10q, 11p, 18q, and Y. These are summarized in Tables 12.2 and 12.3. Gains of 1q, 5p, 8q, and 17q are frequent, and several high-level amplifications have been found. [More detailed information, including frequencies of involvement of all chromosome arms, is given is ref. 6.]

This group of tumors displays genetic instability. This can be detected as rapid and major divergence in the genetic changes identified in related tumors from the same patient and is commonly chromosomal instability (CIN) rather than microsatellite instability (MIN) [112]. The genetic differences between minimally invasive (pT1) and more deeply invasive tumors (≥pT2) are not significant, suggesting that tumors with the ability to break through the epithelial basement membrane are aggressive lesions. Some studies have suggested that certain genetic changes are associated with tumor progression in this group [70]. In one CGH study, muscle-invasive tumor samples were compared with paired metastatic samples. In general, alterations were shared, and no significant metastasis-associated markers were identified [113].

Carcinoma in Situ

Carcinoma in situ is a fragile lesion that is difficult to sample as unfixed tissue. By definition, CIS has normal urothelial thickness, and commonly the cells, which are highly anaplastic, are only weakly adherent and tend to fragment during cystoscopy. Thus most specimens are only recognized retrospectively in paraffin-embedded samples. For this reason, only a few studies have attempted to assess genetic changes in such lesions. In general, the findings are similar to those for invasive tumors [114].

Prognostic Markers in Invasive Transitional Cell Carcinoma

Prediction of risk of recurrence and metastasis would be beneficial in localized muscle-invasive disease, and for all patients prediction of response to available therapies is desirable. As discussed above, alterations in genes affecting the G1 checkpoint have prognostic significance, and to date the potential clinical utility of *TP53* alteration has received most attention. Some other single-marker studies have also reported an association with overall patient survival, though none are adequately confirmed and there are conflicting reports for some. These include overexpression of ERBB2 [115], overexpression of EGFR [116], and reduced expression of thrombospondin [117].

Studies on molecular changes associated with specific responses to therapy are in their infancy. There is controversy over the relationship of

TP53 status to response, and no other genetic markers have yet been assessed. However, other molecules such as glutathione and metallothionein may affect resistance to cisplatin [reviewed in ref. 118]. Undoubtedly this area will receive much attention in the future.

Genetic Model for Bladder Tumor Development

Based on molecular and histopathological observations, a model for molecular pathogenesis of TCC has been developed (Fig. 12.4). Almost certainly it is too simple, but it does provide a useful anchor for genetic studies. Mutation of *FGFR3* appears to define the large group of superficial tumors, and two recent studies confirm that *FGFR3* and *TP53* mutation are virtually mutually exclusive, each confined to one of the two major groups of TCC [119,120].

There are several gaps in our current understanding. First, there may be more alterations in low-grade papillary superficial TCC that remain to be discovered. Another outstanding question is what the significance of pT1 tumors is. Are these merely muscle invasive tumors caught in their journey toward the muscle, or do they represent a distinct group? Genetic findings tend to support the former conclusion, but perhaps differences remain to be identified using novel approaches that will define these as a clear entity. No significant differences have yet been found among CIS, muscle invasive TCC, and the metastases that develop from them. Possibly this reflects the early migration of cells to

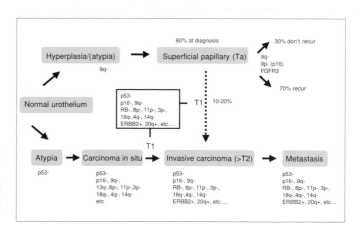

Fig. 12.4. A model for TCC progression based on molecular data and histopathological observations. Copy number losses or loss of heterozygosity (LOH) are denoted by "−" and gains or amplifications by "+." FGFR3 has activating point mutations.

distant sites without the requirement for additional changes, or possibly there are determinants of progression and metastasis yet to be identified.

Gaps in Knowledge: Application of Microarray Technology

The availability of microarray-based technologies now provides a means to interrogate the entire genome and transcriptome in tumor samples. There have been several reports of the application of these techniques to studies of TCC samples, and many alterations have been identified. As yet, most of these findings have not been fully validated, and a detailed listing of the changes recorded would be premature.

Array-based CGH uses spotted arrays of products (commonly degenerate oligonucleotide-primed polymerase chain reaction [PCR] products) from large insert human genomic DNA clones. Labeled test and reference DNAs are hybridized to the arrays rather than to metaphase chromosome preparations, and the ratio of intensity of the two signals is used to measure relative copy number of each clone. Plots of fluorescence ratio versus distance along each chromosome allow accurate visualization of the position and nature of copy number changes. This technique has been used in two studies to date, on 41 primary tumors and 22 tumor derived cell lines [121,122]. The high-resolution compared with conventional CGH has identified many new alterations and has confirmed and refined the localization of many known changes. The use on the arrays of clones from the tiling path (the overlapping array of genomic clones) used to sequence the human genome, allows direct access to information on the genmes, they contain (http://www.ensembl.org/Homo_sapiens/cytoview) [122]. Among the most interesting findings are high-level amplifications that may identify the location of as yet unknown oncogenes. Amplicons have been identified in several regions, including 6p22, 8p12, 8q22, 11q13, and 19q13 within which candidate oncogenes can be identified.

There are several reports of the use of expression microarrays to examine global gene expression profiles of bladder tumors [123–126].

It is already clear that bladder tumor-derived cell lines can be subdivided into groups that reflect known genetic alterations and the tumor type of origin [124], and similarly that tumors can be subdivided into superficial and muscle-invasive groups according to expression patterns [126].

Potential Applications of Molecular Information

The wealth of information on molecular alterations that has been acquired in recent years has yet to be applied on a large scale in the clinic. Although many potential markers have been identified, clinical associations have not been confirmed in large patient cohorts. In the case of *TP53* and *RB*, both genes whose mutation is clearly associated with high tumor grade and stage, it has been difficult to use these in a meaningful way in the clinic. It can be suggested that this is due to an incomplete picture resulting from failure to identify all tumors with similar phenotype. Larger panels of markers that cover all possible molecular mechanisms that generate the same clinical phenotype may be needed before sufficient predictive power can be achieved. In the next few years it is anticipated that basic science will be applied to real clinical benefit in the management of bladder cancer.

References

1. Raghavan D, Shipley W, Garnick M, Russell P, Richie J. Biology and management of bladder cancer. N Engl J Med 1990;322:1129–1138.
2. Cutler SJ, Heney NM, Friedell GH. Longitudinal study of patients with bladder cancer: factors associated with disease recurrence and progression. In: Bonney WW, Prout GR Jr, eds. Bladder Cancer. Baltimore: Williams and Wilkins, 1982: 35–46.
3. Farrow GM, Utz DC, Rife CC, Greene LF. Clinical observations on sixty-nine cases of in situ carcinoma of the urinary bladder. Cancer Res 1977; 37(8 pt 2):2794–2798.
4. Schade ROK, Swinney J. Pre-cancerous changes in bladder epithelium. Lancet 1968;2:943–946.
5. Hafner C, Knuechel R, Stoehr R, Hartmann A. Clonality of multifocal urothelial carcinomas: 10

years of molecular genetic studies. Int J Cancer 2002;101(1):1–6.

6. WHO. WHO Classification Tumours of the Urinary System and Male Genital Organs. Lyon: IARC Press, 2004.

7. Fadl-Elmula I, Gorunova L, Mandahl N, et al. Karyotypic characterization of urinary bladder transitional cell carcinomas. Genes Chromosomes Cancer 2000;29(3):256–265.

8. Tsai YC, Nichols PW, Hiti AL, Williams Z, Skinner DG, Jones PA. Allelic losses of chromosomes 9, 11, and 17 in human bladder cancer. Cancer Res 1990;50:44–47.

9. Shaw ME, Knowles MA. Deletion mapping of chromosome 11 in carcinoma of the bladder. Genes Chromosomes Cancer 1995;13:1–8.

10. Zhao J, Richter J, Wagner U, et al. Chromosomal imbalances in noninvasive papillary bladder neoplasms (pTa). Cancer Res 1999;59(18):4658–4661.

11. Takahashi T, Habuchi T, Kakehi Y, et al. Clonal and chronological genetic analysis of multifocal cancers of the bladder and upper urinary tract. Cancer Res 1998;58(24):5835–5841.

12. Cairns P, Shaw ME, Knowles MA. Initiation of bladder cancer may involve deletion of a tumour-suppressor gene on chromosome 9. Oncogene 1993;8:1083–1085.

13. Linnenbach AJ, Pressler LB, Seng BA, Simmel BS, Tomaszewski JE, Malkowicz SB. Characterization of chromosome 9 deletions in transitional cell carcinoma by microsatellite assay. Human Mol Gen 1993;2(9):1407–1411.

14. Simoneau M, Aboulkassim TO, LaRue H, Rousseau F, Fradet Y. Four tumor suppressor loci on chromosome 9q in bladder cancer: evidence for two novel candidate regions at 9q22.3 and 9q31. Oncogene 1999;18(1):157–163.

15. van Tilborg AA, de Vries A, de Bont M, Groenfeld LE, van der Kwast TH, Zwarthoff EC. Molecular evolution of multiple recurrent cancers of the bladder. Hum Mol Genet 2000; 9(20):2973–2980.

16. Louhelainen J, Wijkstrom H, Hemminki K. Initiation-development modelling of allelic losses on chromosome 9 in multifocal bladder cancer. Eur J Cancer 2000;36(11):1441–1451.

17. Hartmann A, Moser K, Kriegmair M, Hofstetter A, Hofstaedter F, Knuechel R. Frequent genetic alterations in simple urothelial hyperplasias of the bladder in patients with papillary urothelial carcinoma. Am J Pathol 1999;154(3):721–727.

18. Aboulkassim TO, LaRue H, Lemieux P, Rousseau F, Fradet Y. Alteration of the PATCHED locus in superficial bladder cancer. Oncogene 2003; 22(19):2967–2971.

19. Habuchi T, Luscombe M, Elder PA, Knowles MA. Structure and methylation-based silencing of a gene (DBCCR1) within a candidate bladder cancer tumor suppressor region at 9q32–q33. Genomics 1998;48(3):277–2788.

20. Czerniak B, Chaturvedi V, Li L, et al. Superimposed histologic and genetic mapping of chromosome 9 in progression of human urinary bladder neoplasia: implications for a genetic model of multistep urothelial carcinogenesis and early detection of urinary bladder cancer. Oncogene 1999;18(5):1185–1196.

21. Wada T, Berggren P, Steineck G, et al. Bladder neoplasms—regions at chromosome 9 with putative tumour suppressor genes. Scand J Urol Nephrol 2003;37(2):106–111.

22. Cairns P, Mao L, Merlo A, et al. Rates of p16 (MTS1) mutations in primary tumors with 9p loss. Science 1994;265(5170):415–417.

23. Devlin J, Keen AJ, Knowles MA. Homozygous deletion mapping at 9p21 in bladder carcinoma defines a critical region within 2cM of IFNA. Oncogene 1994;9:2757–2760.

24. Orlow I, Lacombe L, Hannon GJ, et al. Deletion of the p16 and p15 genes in human bladder tumors. J Natl Cancer Inst 1995;87:1524–1529.

25. Williamson MP, Elder PA, Shaw ME, Devlin J, Knowles MA. p16 (CDKN2) is a major deletion target at 9p21 in bladder cancer. Hum Mol Genet 1995;4:1569–1577.

26. Berggren P, Kumar R, Sakano S, et al. Detecting homozygous deletions in the CDKN2A (p16(INK4a))/ARF(p14(ARF)) gene in urinary bladder cancer using real-time quantitative PCR. Clin Cancer Res 2003;9(1):235–242.

27. McGarvey TW, Maruta Y, Tomaszewski JE, Linnenbach AJ, Malkowicz SB. PTCH gene mutations in invasive transitional cell carcinoma of the bladder. Oncogene 1998;17(9):1167–1172.

28. Nishiyama H, Takahashi T, Kakehi Y, Habuchi T, Knowles MA. Homozygous deletion at the 9q32–33 candidate tumor suppressor locus in primary bladder cancer. Genes Chromosomes Cancer 1999;26:171–175.

29. Stadler WM, Steinberg G, Yang X, Hagos F, Turner C, Olopade OI. Alterations of the 9p21 and 9q33 chromosomal bands in clinical bladder cancer specimens by fluorescence in situ hybridization. Clin Cancer Res 2001;7(6):1676–1682.

30. Knowles MA, Habuchi T, Kennedy W, Cuthbert-Heavens D. Mutation spectrum of the 9q34 tuberous sclerosis gene TSC1 in transitional cell carcinoma of the bladder. Cancer Res 2003; 63:7652–7656.

31. Hornigold N, Devlin J, Davies AM, Aveyard JS, Habuchi T, Knowles MA. Mutation of the 9q34 gene TSC1 in sporadic bladder cancer. Oncogene 1999;18:2657–2661.

32. Adachi H, Igawa M, Shiina H, Urakami S, Shigeno K, Hino O. Human bladder tumors with 2-hit

mutations of tumor suppressor gene TSC1 and decreased expression of p27. J Urol 2003;170(2 Pt 1):601–604.

33. Chang LL, Yeh WT, Yang SY, Wu WJ, Huang CH. Genetic alterations of p16INK4a and p14ARF genes in human bladder cancer. J Urol 2003;170(2 Pt 1):595–600.

34. Florl AR, Franke KH, Niederacher D, Gerharz CD, Seifert HH, Schulz WA. DNA methylation and the mechanisms of CDKN2A inactivation in transitional cell carcinoma of the urinary bladder. Lab Invest 2000;80(10):1513–1522.

35. Orlow I, LaRue H, Osman I, et al. Deletions of the INK4A gene in superficial bladder tumors. Association with recurrence. Am J Pathol 1999; 155(1):105–113.

36. Serrano M. The INK4a/ARF locus in murine tumorigenesis. Carcinogenesis 2000;21(5):865–869.

37. Carnero A, Hudson JD, Price CM, Beach DH. p16INK4A and p19ARF act in overlapping pathways in cellular immortalization. Nat Cell Biol 2000;2(3):148–155.

38. Habuchi T, Takahashi T, Kakinuma H, et al. Hypermethylation at 9q32–33 tumour suppressor region is age-related in normal urothelium and an early and frequent alteration in bladder cancer. Oncogene 2001;20:531–537.

39. Wright KO, Messing EM, Reeder JE. DBCCR1 mediates death in cultured bladder tumor cells. Oncogene 2004;23(1):82–90.

40. Nishiyama H, Gill JH, Pitt E, Kennedy W, Knowles MA. Negative regulation of G1/S transition by the candidate bladder tumour suppressor gene DBCCR1. Oncogene 2001;20:2956–2964.

41. Manning BD, Cantley LC. United at last: the tuberous sclerosis complex gene products connect the phosphoinositide 3–kinase/Akt pathway to mammalian target of rapamycin (mTOR) signalling. Biochem Soc Trans 2003;31(pt 3): 573–578.

42. Cappellen D, De Oliveira C, Ricol D, et al. Frequent activating mutations of FGFR3 in human bladder and cervix carcinomas. Nat Genet 1999; 23(1):18–20.

43. Billerey C, Chopin D, Aubriot-Lorton MH, et al. Frequent FGFR3 mutations in papillary non-invasive bladder (pTa) tumors. Am J Pathol 2001; 158(6):1955–1959.

44. Sibley K, Stern P, Knowles MA. Frequency of fibroblast growth factor receptor 3 mutations in sporadic tumours. Oncogene 2001;20(32):4416–4418.

45. van Rhijn BW, Lurkin I, Radvanyi F, Kirkels WJ, van der Kwast TH, Zwarthoff EC. The fibroblast growth factor receptor 3 (FGFR3) mutation is a strong indicator of superficial bladder cancer with low recurrence rate. Cancer Res 2001;61(4): 1265–1268.

46. Elder PA, Bell SM, Knowles MA. Deletion of two regions on chromosome 4 in bladder carcinoma: definition of a critical 750 kB region at 4p16.3. Oncogene 1994;9(12):3433–3436.

47. Sibley K, Cuthbert-Heavens D, Knowles MA. Loss of heterozygosity at 4p16.3 and mutation of FGFR3 in transitional cell carcinoma. Oncogene 2001;20:686–691.

48. van Rhijn BW, Montironi R, Zwarthoff EC, Jobsis AC, van der Kwast TH. Frequent FGFR3 mutations in urothelial papilloma. J Pathol 2002; 198(2):245–251.

49. Passos-Bueno MR, Wilcox WR, Jabs EW, Sertie AL, Alonso LG, Kitoh H. Clinical spectrum of fibroblast growth factor receptor mutations. Hum Mutat 1999;14(2):115–125.

50. Ornitz DM, Itoh N. Fibroblast growth factors. Genome Biol 2001;2(3):3005.1–3005.12.

51. Karoui M, Hofmann-Radvanyi H, Zimmermann U, et al. No evidence of somatic FGFR3 mutation in various types of carcinoma. Oncogene 2001;20(36):5059–5061.

52. Zlotta AR, Noel JC, Fayt I, et al. Correlation and prognostic significance of p53, p21WAF1/CIP1 and Ki-67 expression in patients with superficial bladder tumors treated with bacillus Calmette-Guerin intravesical therapy. J Urol 1999;161(3): 792–798.

53. Liukkonen T, Rajala P, Raitanen M, Rintala E, Kaasinen E, Lipponen P. Prognostic value of MIB-1 score, p53, EGFr, mitotic index and papillary status in primary superficial (Stage pTa/T1) bladder cancer: a prospective comparative study. The Finnbladder Group. Eur Urol 1999;36(5):393–400.

54. Pfister C, Moore L, Allard P, et al. Predictive value of cell cycle markers p53, MDM2, p21, and Ki-67 in superficial bladder tumor recurrence. Clin Cancer Res 1999;5(12):4079–4084.

55. Harnden P, Mahmood J, Southgate J. Cytokeratin 20 expression redefines uroepithelial papillomas of the bladder. Lancet 1999;353:974–977.

56. Simoneau M, LaRue H, Aboulkassim TO, Meyer F, Moore L, Fradet Y. Chromosome 9 deletions and recurrence of superficial bladder cancer: identification of four regions of prognostic interest. Oncogene 2000;19(54):6317–6323.

57. Edwards J, Duncan P, Going JJ, Watters AD, Grigor KM, Bartlett JM. Identification of loci associated with putative recurrence genes in transitional cell carcinoma of the urinary bladder. J Pathol 2002;196(4):380–385.

58. van Rhijn BW, Vis AN, van der Kwast TH, et al. Molecular grading of urothelial cell carcinoma with fibroblast growth factor receptor 3 and MIB-1 is superior to pathologic grade for the prediction of clinical outcome. J Clin Oncol 2003; 21(10):1912–1921.

59. Rieger-Christ KM, Mourtzinos A, Lee PJ, et al. Identification of fibroblast growth factor receptor 3 mutations in urine sediment DNA samples complements cytology in bladder tumor detection. Cancer 2003;98(4):737–744.

60. van Rhijn BW, Lurkin I, Chopin DK, et al. Combined microsatellite and FGFR3 mutation analysis enables a highly sensitive detection of urothelial cell carcinoma in voided urine. Clin Cancer Res 2003;9(1):257–263.

61. Durkan GC, Nutt JE, Marsh C, et al. Alteration in urinary matrix metalloproteinase-9 to tissue inhibitor of metalloproteinase-1 ratio predicts recurrence in nonmuscle-invasive bladder cancer. Clin Cancer Res 2003;9(7):2576–2582.

62. Dominguez G, Carballido J, Silva J, et al. p14ARF Promoter hypermethylation in plasma DNA as an indicator of disease recurrence in bladder cancer patients. Clin Cancer Res 2002;8(4):980–985.

63. Tada Y, Wada M, Taguchi K, et al. The association of death-associated protein kinase hypermethylation with early recurrence in superficial bladder cancers. Cancer Res 2002;62(14):4048–4053.

64. Lipponen PK, Eskelinen MJ. Reduced expression of E-cadherin is related to invasive disease and frequent recurrence in bladder cancer. J Cancer Res Clin Oncol 1995;121(5):303–308.

65. Ariel I, Sughayer M, Fellig Y, et al. The imprinted H19 gene is a marker of early recurrence in human bladder carcinoma. Mol Pathol 2000;53(6):320–323.

66. Swana HS, Grossman D, Anthony JN, Weiss RM, Altieri DC. Tumor content of the antiapoptosis molecule survivin and recurrence of bladder cancer. N Engl J Med 1999;341(6):452–453.

67. Sarkis AS, Zhang Z-F, Cordon-Cardo C, et al. p53 nuclear overexpression and disease progression in Ta bladder carcinoma. Int J Oncol 1993;3:355–360.

68. Bringuier PP, Umbas R, Schaafsma E, Karthaus HFM, Debruyne FMJ, Schalken JA. Decreased E-cadherin immunoreactivity correlates with poor survival in patients with bladder tumors. Cancer Res 1993;53:3241–3245.

69. Urist MJ, Di Como CJ, Lu ML, et al. Loss of p63 expression is associated with tumor progression in bladder cancer. Am J Pathol 2002;161(4):1199–1206.

70. Richter J, Wagner U, Schraml P, et al. Chromosomal imbalances are associated with a high risk of progression in early invasive (pT1) urinary bladder cancer. Cancer Res 1999;59(22):5687–5691.

71. Lipponen P. Expression of c-erbB-2 oncoprotein in transitional cell bladder cancer. Eur J Cancer 1993;29A(5):749–753.

72. Gardiner RA, Samaratunga ML, Walsh MD, Seymour GJ, Lavin MF. An immunohistological demonstration of c-erbB-2 oncoprotein expression in primary urothelial bladder cancer. Urol Res 1992;20(2):117–120.

73. Coombs LM, Pigott DA, Sweeney E, et al. Amplification and over-expression of c-erbB-2 in transitional cell carcinoma of the urinary bladder. Br J Cancer 1991;63(4):601–608.

74. Sauter G, Moch H, Moore D, et al. Heterogeneity of erbB-2 gene amplification in bladder cancer. Cancer Res 1993;53:2199–2203.

75. Neal DE, Sharples L, Smith K, Fennelly J, Hall RR, Harris AL. The epidermal growth factor receptor and the prognosis of bladder cancer. Cancer 1990;65(7):1619–1625.

76. Habuchi T, Kinoshita H, Yamada H, et al. Oncogene amplification in urothelial cancers with p53 gene mutation or MDM2 amplification. J Natl Cancer Inst 1994;86:1331–1335.

77. Tuna B, Yorukoglu K, Tuzel E, Guray M, Mungan U, Kirkali Z. Expression of p53 and mdm2 and their significance in recurrence of superficial bladder cancer. Pathol Res Pract 2003;199(5):323–328.

78. Schmitz-Drager BJ, Kushima M, Goebell P, et al. p53 and MDM2 in the development and progression of bladder cancer. Eur Urol 1997;32(4):487–493.

79. Theodorescu D, Cornil I, Fernandez BJ, Kerbel RS. Overexpression of normal and mutated forms of HRAS induces orthotopic bladder invasion in a human transitional cell carcinoma. Proc Natl Acad Sci USA 1990;87(22):9047–9051.

80. Theodorescu D, Cornil I, Sheehan C, Man MS, Kerbel RS. Ha-ras induction of the invasive phenotype results in up-regulation of epidermal growth factor receptors and altered responsiveness to epidermal growth factor in human papillary transitional cell carcinoma cells. Cancer Res 1991;51:4486–4491.

81. Zhang ZT, Pak J, Huang HY, et al. Role of Ha-ras activation in superficial papillary pathway of urothelial tumor formation. Oncogene 2001;20(16):1973–1980.

82. Sherr CJ, McCormick F. The RB and p53 pathways in cancer. Cancer Cell 2002;2(2):103–112.

83. Sidransky D, von Eschenbach A, Tsai YC, et al. Identification of p53 gene mutations in bladder cancers and urine samples. Science 1991;252:706–709.

84. Fujimoto K, Yamada Y, Okajima E, et al. Frequent association of p53 gene mutation in invasive bladder cancer. Cancer Research 1992;52:1393–1398.

85. Williamson MP, Elder PA, Knowles MA. The spectrum of TP53 mutations in bladder carci-

noma. Genes Chromosomes Cancer 1994;9:108–118.

86. Habuchi T, Takahashi R, Yamada H, et al. Influence of cigarette smoking and schistosomiasis on p53 gene mutation in urothelial cancer. Cancer Res 1993;53:3795–3799.

87. Spruck CH III, Rideout WM III, Olumi AF, et al. Distinct pattern of p53 mutations in bladder cancer: relationship to tobacco usage. Cancer Res 1993;53:1162–1166.

88. Esrig D, Spruck CHd, Nichols PW, et al. p53 nuclear protein accumulation correlates with mutations in the p53 gene, tumor grade, and stage in bladder cancer. Am J Pathol 1993; 143(5):1389–1397.

89. Esrig D, Elmajian D, Groshen S, et al. Accumulation of nuclear p53 and tumor progression in bladder cancer. N Engl J Med 1994;331:1259–1264.

90. Sarkis AS, Dalbagni G, Cordon-Cardo C, et al. Association of p53 nuclear overexpression and tumor progression in carcinoma in situ of the bladder. J Urol 1994;152:388–392.

91. Sarkis AS, Dalbagni G, Cordon-Cardo C, et al. Nuclear overexpression of p53 protein in transitional cell bladder carcinoma: a marker for disease progression. J Natl Cancer Inst 1993;85: 53–59.

92. Stein JP, Ginsberg DA, Grossfeld GD, et al. Effect of p21WAF1/CIP1 expression on tumor progression in bladder cancer. J Natl Cancer Inst 1998; 90(14):1072–1079.

93. Qureshi KN, Griffiths TR, Robinson MC, et al. Combined p21WAF1/CIP1 and p53 overexpression predict improved survival in muscle-invasive bladder cancer treated by radical radiotherapy. Int J Radiat Oncol Biol Phys 2001; 51(5):1234–1240.

94. Schmitz-Drager BJ, Goebell PJ, Ebert T, Fradet Y. p53 immunohistochemistry as a prognostic marker in bladder cancer. Playground for urology scientists? Eur Urol 2000;38(6):691–699; discussion 700.

95. Cairns P, Proctor AJ, Knowles MA. Loss of heterozygosity at the RB locus is frequent and correlates with muscle invasion in bladder carcinoma. Oncogene 1991;6:2305–2309.

96. Logothetis CJ, Xu H-J, Ro JY, et al. Altered expression of retinoblastoma protein and known prognostic variables in locally advanced bladder cancer. J Natl Cancer Inst 1992;84:1256–1261.

97. Cordon-Cardo C, Wartinger D, Petrylak D, et al. Altered expression of the retinoblastoma gene product: prognostic indicator in bladder cancer. J Natl Cancer Inst 1992;84:1251–1256.

98. Xu H-J, Cairns P, Hu S-X, Knowles MA, Benedict WF. Loss of RB protein expression in primary bladder cancer correlates with loss of heterozygosity at the RB locus and tumor progression. Int J Cancer 1993;53:781–784.

99. Cordon-Cardo C, Zhang Z-F, Dalbagni G, et al. Cooperative effects of p53 and pRB alterations in primary superficial bladder tumors. Cancer Res 1997;57:1217–1221.

100. Cote RJ, Dunn MD, Chatterjee SJ, et al. Elevated and absent pRb expression is associated with bladder cancer progression and has cooperative effects with p53. Cancer Res 1998;58(6):1090–1094.

101. Grossman HB, Liebert M, Antelo M, et al. p53 and RB expression predict progression in T1 bladder cancer. Clin Cancer Res 1998;4(4):829–834.

102. Shiina H, Igawa M, Shigeno K, et al. Beta-catenin mutations correlate with over expression of C-myc and cyclin D1 Genes in bladder cancer. J Urol 2002;168(5):2220–2226.

103. Wagner U, Suess K, Luginbuhl T, et al. Cyclin D1 overexpression lacks prognostic significance in superficial urinary bladder cancer. J Pathol 1999; 188(1):44–50.

104. Kagan J, Liu J, Stein JD, et al. Cluster of allele losses within a 2.5 cM region of chromosome 10 in high-grade invasive bladder cancer. Oncogene 1998;16(7):909–913.

105. Cappellen D, Gil Diez de Medina S, Chopin D, Thiery JP, Radvanyi F. Frequent loss of heterozygosity on chromosome 10q in muscle-invasive. Oncogene 1997;14(25):3059–3066.

106. Aveyard JS, Skilleter A, Habuchi T, Knowles MA. Somatic mutation of PTEN in bladder carcinoma. Br J Cancer 1999;80:904–908.

107. Yamada KM, Araki M. Tumor suppressor PTEN: modulator of cell signaling, growth, migration and apoptosis. J Cell Sci 2001;114(pt 13):2375–2382.

108. Cairns P, Evron E, Okami K, et al. Point mutation and homozygous deletion of PTEN/MMAC1 in primary bladder cancers. Oncogene 1998;16(24): 3215–3218.

109. Liu J, Babaian DC, Liebert M, Steck PA, Kagan J. Inactivation of MMAC1 in bladder transitional-cell carcinoma cell lines and specimens. Mol Carcinog 2000;29(3):143–150.

110. Wang DS, Rieger-Christ K, Latini JM, et al. Molecular analysis of PTEN and MXI1 in primary bladder carcinoma. Int J Cancer 2000;88(4):620–625.

111. Tanaka M, Koul D, Davies MA, Liebert M, Steck PA, Grossman HB. MMAC1/PTEN inhibits cell growth and induces chemosensitivity to doxorubicin in human bladder cancer cells. Oncogene 2000;19(47):5406–5412.

112. Gonzalez-Zulueta M, Ruppert JM, et al. Microsatellite instability in bladder cancer. Cancer Res 1993;53:5620–5623.

113. Hovey RM, Chu L, Balazs M, et al. Genetic alterations in primary bladder cancers and their metastases. Cancer Res 1998;58(16):3555–3560.

114. Rosin MP, Cairns P, Epstein JI, Schoenberg MP, Sidransky D. Partial allelotype of carcinoma *in situ* of the human bladder. Cancer Res 1995;55:5213–5216.

115. Lonn U, Lonn S, Friberg S, Nilsson B, Silfversward C, Stenkvist B. Prognostic value of amplification of c-erb-B2 in bladder carcinoma. Clin Cancer Res 1995;1(10):1189–1194.

116. Mellon K, Wright C, Kelly P, Horne CH, Neal DE. Long-term outcome related to epidermal growth factor receptor status in bladder cancer. J Urol 1995;153(3 pt 2):919–925.

117. Grossfeld GD, Ginsberg DA, Stein JP, et al. Thrombospondin-1 expression in bladder cancer: association with p53 alterations, tumor angiogenesis, and tumor progression. J Natl Cancer Inst 1997;89(3):219–227.

118. Raghavan D. Molecular targeting and pharmacogenomics in the management of advanced bladder cancer. Cancer 2003;97(8 suppl):2083–2089.

119. Bakkar AA, Wallerand H, Radvanyi F, et al. FGFR3 and TP53 gene mutations define two distinct pathways in urothelial cell carcinoma of the bladder. Cancer Res 2003;63(23):8108–8112.

120. van Rhijn BW, van der Kwast TH, Vis AN, et al. FGFR3 and P53 characterize alternative genetic pathways in the pathogenesis of urothelial cell carcinoma. Cancer Res 2004;64(6):1911–1914.

121. Veltman JA, Fridlyand J, Pejavar S, et al. Array-based comparative genomic hybridization for genome-wide screening of DNA copy number in bladder tumors. Cancer Res 2003;63(11):2872–2880.

122. Hurst CD, Fiegler H, Carr P, Williams S, Carter NP, Knowles MA. High-resolution analysis of genomic copy number alterations in bladder cancer by microarray-based comparative genomic hybridization. Oncogene 2004;23:2250–2263.

123. Sanchez-Carbayo M, Socci ND, Lozano JJ, et al. Gene discovery in bladder cancer progression using cDNA microarrays. Am J Pathol 2003;163(2):505–516.

124. Sanchez-Carbayo M, Socci ND, Charytonowicz E, et al. Molecular profiling of bladder cancer using cDNA microarrays: defining histogenesis and biological phenotypes. Cancer Res 2002;62(23):6973–6980.

125. Dyrskjot L, Thykjaer T, Kruhoffer M, et al. Identifying distinct classes of bladder carcinoma using microarrays. Nat Genet 2003;33(1):90–96.

126. Thykjaer T, Workman C, Kruhoffer M, et al. Identification of gene expression patterns in superficial and invasive human bladder cancer. Cancer Res 2001;61(6):2492–2499.

127. Knowles MA, Williamson M. Mutation of H-ras is infrequent in bladder cancer: confirmation by single-strand conformation polymorphism analysis, designed restriction fragment length polymorphisms, and direct sequencing. Cancer Res 1993;53(1):133–139.

128. Ooi A, Herz F, Ii S, et al. Ha-*ras* codon 12 mutation in papillary tumors of the urinary bladder: a retrospective study. Int J Oncol 1994;4:85–90.

129. Fitzgerald JM, Ramchurren N, Rieger K, et al. Identification of H-ras mutations in urine sediments complements cytology in the detection of bladder tumors. J Natl Cancer Inst 1995;87:129–133.

130. Sato K, Moriyama M, Mori S, et al. An immunohistologic evaluation of c-*erb*B-2 gene product in patients with urinary bladder carcinoma. Cancer 1992;70:2493–2498.

131. Proctor AJ, Coombs LM, Cairns JP, Knowles MA. Amplification at chromosome 11q13 in transitional cell tumours of the bladder. Oncogene 1991;6:789–795.

132. Bringuier PP, Tamimi J, Schuuring F, Amplification of the chromosome 11q13 region in bladder tumours. Urol Res 1994;21:451.

133. Lianes P, Orlow I, Zhang Z-F, et al. Altered patterns of MDM2 and TP53 expression in human bladder cancer. J Natl Cancer Inst 1994;86:1325–1330.

134. Cairns P, Tokino K, Eby Y, Sidransky D. Homozygous deletions of 9p21 in primary human bladder tumors detected by comparative multiplex polymerase chain reaction. Cancer Res 1994;54:1422–1424.

135. Yeager TR, DeVries S, Jarrard DF, et al. Overcoming cellular senescence in human cancer pathogenesis. Genes Dev 1998;12(2):163–174.

136. Habuchi T, Yoshida O, Knowles MA. A novel candidate tumour suppressor locus at 9q32–33 in bladder cancer: localisation of the candidate region within a single 840 kb YAC. Hum Mol Genet 1997;6:913–919.

137. Brewster SF, Gingell JC, Browne S, Brown KW. Loss of heterozygosity on chromosome 18q is associated with muscle-invasive transitional cell carcinoma of the bladder. Br J Cancer 1994;70:697–700.

138. Presti JC, Jr., Reuter VE, Galan T, Fair WR, Cordon-Cardo C. Molecular genetic alterations in superficial and locally advanced human bladder cancer. Cancer Res 1991;51(19):5405–5409.

139. Polascik TJ, Cairns P, Chang WYH, Schoenberg MP, Sidransky D. Distinct regions of allelic loss on chromosome 4 in human primary bladder carcinoma. Cancer Res 1995;55:5396–5399.

140. Takle LA, Knowles MA. Deletion mapping implicates two tumor suppressor genes on chromosome 8p in the development of bladder cancer. Oncogene 1996;12(5):1083–1087.

141. Ohgaki K, Iida A, Ogawa O, Kubota Y, Akimoto M, Emi M. Localization of tumor suppressor gene associated with distant metastasis of urinary bladder cancer to a 1–Mb interval on 8p22. Genes Chromosomes Cancer 1999;25(1):1–5.

142. Choi C, Kim MH, Juhng SW, Oh BR. Loss of heterozygosity at chromosome segments 8p22 and 8p11.2–21.1 in transitional-cell carcinoma of the urinary bladder. Int J Cancer 2000;86(4):501–505.

143. Habuchi T, Devlin J, Elder PA, Knowles MA. Detailed deletion mapping of chromosome 9q in bladder cancer: evidence for two tumour suppressor loci. Oncogene 1995;11:1671–1674.

144. Fearon ER, Feinberg AP, Hamilton SH, Vogelstein B. Loss of genes on the short arm of chromosome 11 in bladder cancer. Nature 1985;318:377–380.

145. Chang WY-H, Cairns P, Schoenberg MP, Polascik TJ, Sidransky D. Novel suppressor loci on chromosome 14q in primary bladder cancer. Cancer Res 1995;55:3246–3249.

146. Simon R, Burger H, Brinkschmidt C, Bocker W, Hertle L, Terpe HJ. Chromosomal aberrations associated with invasion in papillary superficial bladder cancer. J Pathol 1998;185(4):345–351.

147. Richter J, Beffa L, Wagner U, Schraml P, Gasser TC, Moch H, et al. Patterns of chromosomal imbalances in advanced urinary bladder cancer detected by comparative genomic hybridization. Am J Pathol 1998;153(5):1615–1621.

148. Kallioniemi A, Kallioniemi O-P, Citro G, et al. Identification of gains and losses of DNA sequences in primary bladder cancer by comparative genomic hybridisation. Genes Chromosomes and Cancer 1995;12:213–219.

13

Treatment Options in Superficial (pTA/pT1/CIS) Bladder Cancer

Jeremy L. Ockrim and Paul D. Abel

Bladder cancer is the fourth most common cancer in men and the eighth most common cancer in women worldwide, and the incidence continues to rise. In the United Kingdom, 13,600 new cases per annum contribute 5% to the national cancer burden [1]. Over 100,000 diagnostic, check, and interventional cystoscopies each year are performed in surveillance protocols in attempting to monitor for disease progression. In the United States, there were approximately 57,500 new cases and 12,500 deaths in 2003, resulting in an annual expenditure ($2.2 billion/year) almost twice that for prostate cancer [2]. These figures reflect the lifelong commitment to surveillance and intervention for recurrent and progressive disease. The difficulties involved in this complex process were emphasized in McFarlane et al.'s [3] seminar in 1996, where considerable divergence of opinion was noted among clinicians presented with a variety of clinical scenarios. This chapter provides an overview of the current rationale behind the therapeutic options available for superficial bladder cancer treatment. In this way, it is hoped to empower clinicians with a broad sweep of the evidence on which therapy is based.

Current Issues in Superficial Bladder Cancer Classification

The current system of bladder tumor classification is based on the International Union Against Cancer (UICC) revision of 1997 [4].

Superficial bladder cancer is the term used to describe transitional cell carcinomas with histopathological categories pTa and pT1 as well as carcinoma in situ (CIS); pTa tumors are confined to the urothelium bordered by the basement membrane, whereas pT1 tumors have penetrated into the lamina propria. Much debate has been concerned with the inclusion of pT1 tumors as "superficial," with an implication of indolent natural history. In fact, the depth of penetration into and beyond the lamina propria may be the single most important prognostic factor for "superficial" bladder cancers [5,6] (both vascular and lymphatic invasion have also been suggested as important prognostic factors [7,8]). As such, subcategorization of pT1 tumors has been proposed, dividing pT1 tumors into "up to muscularis mucosae" (pT1a), "into muscularis mucosae" (pT1b), and "beyond muscularis mucosae" (pT1c) [8,9]. The dependence of the urologist on the uropathologist is fundamental to this classification. Concern persists that even experienced uropathologists may vary in their interpretation of tissue, not only among themselves, but also with themselves over time [10]. One study has demonstrated that pathologists often overstage but undergrade bladder specimens [11]. The importance of good-quality resection specimens, including the underlying detrusor muscle (see Role of Transurethral Resection and Tumor Surveillance, below) and of good liaison between urologist and uropathologist (which ideally should be centralized within a multidisciplinary setting) is clear.

Natural History of Superficial Bladder Cancer and Prognostic Factors

Because the type and timing of adjuvant therapy for superficial bladder cancer depends on the prediction of biological change from an indolent to an aggressive phenotype, a good understanding of the natural history of the disease is essential for the working practice of urologists and oncologists. Because even patients with low-grade, low-stage superficial bladder cancers are now subjected to adjuvant therapy, contemporary data of untreated tumors are sparse. This is of particular relevance to high-risk tumor groups, where it is now unacceptable for modern trials to contain an "untreated" arm. As a result, outcomes have to be compared to historical data. All analyses and any conclusions from data must be assessed with this limitation in mind.

Grade

Many series have shown the importance of tumor grade in rates of recurrence and progression. The National Bladder Cancer Collaborative Group (NBCCG) trial [12] reported progression rates for World Health Organization tumor grades I, II, and III of 2%, 11%, and 45%, respectively, figures reflected in many similar studies [5,13].

Stage

Between 70% and 80% of new bladder tumors are superficial on presentation: 70% pTa and 30% pT1 [14]. Despite the presumption that bladder cancer develops through a logical sequence of biological events from superficial to invasive disease, pTa and pT1 tumors show substantial differences in their potential to progress to muscle invasion. Several series have shown that progression is nearly always associated with pT1 disease. The NBCCG demonstrated that progression occurs in only 3% of pTa tumors, compared with 30% of pT1 tumors [12]. The risk of progression is closely correlated with mortality. The 5-year mortality rate for pTa tumors is less than 1%, whereas the 5-year mortality for pT1 tumors is as high as 24% [5,15]. As such, separate protocols for pTa and pT1 cysto-

scopic surveillance have been proposed [15] (Fig. 13.1).

Frequency of Recurrence

The intervals between tumor recurrences are of central importance. Recurrence rates steadily decrease with the length of disease-free interval, such that the risk of further disease is less than 10% after 5 years of negative cystoscopic examination [16,17]. Fitzpatrick et al. [18] demonstrated that the first check cystoscopy also pointed to future tumor activity; 80% of those with a clear 3-month cystoscopy remained disease free, whereas those with recurrent disease at 3 months had only a 10% chance of remaining disease free in the 2 years thereafter. The European Organization for the Research and Treatment of Cancer–Genitourinary Group (EORTC-GU) also reviewed the importance of initial treatment failure as a prognostic factor for long-term outcome [16]. The overall recurrence rate following transurethral tumor ablation was approximately 50% to 70%. This rate was substantially affected by the early clinical response; over 75% of those with rapidly recurrent lesions developed subsequent recurrences. It is important to recognize that early tumor recurrence may also be related to surgical technique (see Role of Transurethral Resection and Tumor Surveillance, below).

Multifocality and Tumor Size

Multicentric presentation and tumor volume are also important prognostic factors. At diagnosis, 30% of lesions are multiple [17], and these carry a poorer prognosis than solitary tumors, with shorter disease-free intervals and higher progression rates [19,20]. Tumor sizes greater than 3 cm and 5 cm have also been correlated with poorer outcome [12,20].

Carcinoma in Situ (CIS)

Carcinoma in situ is defined as a flat (nonpapillary) high-grade transitional cell carcinoma that has not penetrated the basement membrane of the epithelium. Such lesions are considered distinct entities from papillary (pTa/pT1) tumors, with profound implications for prognosis. Clinically, CIS can be divided into diffuse (velvety erythematous elevations) or focal (thickened

Fig. 13.1. Suggested surveillance protocols for newly diagnosed superficial bladder cancers. (From Abel PD. Follow-up of patients wih a "superficial" transitional cell carcinoma of the bladder: the case for a change in policy. Br J Urol 1993;72(2):135–142, Blackwell Publishing Ltd.)

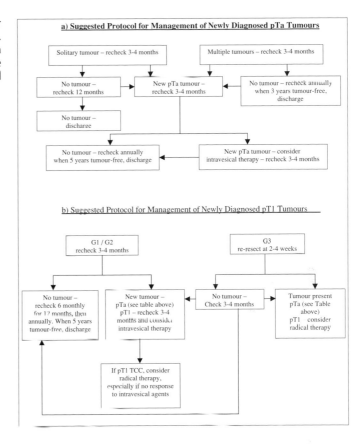

white metaplasia) lesions. Diffuse CIS is nearly always reflected in filling (storage) bladder symptoms and positive urine cytology, whereas focal CIS is frequently a marker for subsequent papillary tumor development. These two subsets of CIS have marked differences in invasive potential. In Lamm's [21] review, an overall progression rate of 54% was reported for untreated CIS. Riddle et al. [22] showed muscle invasion occurring in 58% of those with diffuse disease, compared with only 8% of those with focal urothelial (CIS) abnormalities. Association with papillary tumors increases the risk. The series reported by Althausen et al. [23] and Herr et al. [24] showed progression rates of 83% and 71% when CIS and papillary tumor were noted together. Moreover, with diffuse CIS, occult disease of the distal ureters and prostatic urethra may be present in as many as 60% [25]. In cases of suspected (diffuse) CIS, sampling of the prostatic urethra is essential, especially as positive biopsies would preclude orthotopic bladder reconstruction.

Relative Risk of Clinical Prognostic Factors

The factors that predict the biological potential of superficial lesions must be correctly weighted before deciding on cystoscopic surveillance protocols and adjuvant therapy. The relative importance of the prognostic factors was measured by multivariate analyses of two Medical Research Council (MRC) trials [26] and two EORTC-GU trials [20]. In the MRC analyses, tumor number at presentation and tumor recurrence at the first follow-up cystoscopy at 3 months were statistically better at predicting recurrence than all other prognostic factors. The confidence of these observations compared with the (subjective) interpretation of other histopathological data led Hall et al. [27] to propose a cystoscopic and adjuvant chemotherapy protocol based on these two factors alone. In the EORTC-GU analyses, the relative risk of disease progression was assessed [20]. The

Table 13.1. Risk index for patients in various subgroups

Recurrence rate (per year)	<1			1 to 3			>3		
Tumor size (cm)	<1.5	1.5–3	>3	<1.5	1.5–3	>3	<1.5	1.5–3	>3
G1	1	1	1	1	2	2	2	2	3
G2	1	2	2	2	2	3	3	3	3
G3	2	2	2	2	3	3	3	3	3

Note: Each cell gives the risk index pertaining to progression and disease-specific mortality. Risk index estimated from the Cox model including only three factors: tumor size, G grade, and recurrence rate. The estimated Cox models for progression is 0.51 recurrence rate + 0.84 G grade + 0.48 tumor size, and for death is 0.89 recurrence rate + 0.73 G grade + 0.44 tumor size. Adapted from Kurth et al. [20].

greatest risk was in those with frequent disease recurrence, followed by tumor grade and size. Surprisingly, the T stage at presentation (pTa/pT1) did not add to the prognostic calculation. The authors proposed stratification of superficial bladder tumors into three different prognostic (risk) groups on which clinicians may decide the necessity of adjuvant therapy (Table 13.1). Although these tables are interesting research tools, most clinicians assess risk according to all the available clinical and histological information (Table 13.2), applied on an individual basis, and according to the needs of the patient.

Molecular Markers

The search to find alternate prognostic factors on which to base treatment decisions (conservative versus radical intervention for high-risk tumors) has shifted to the molecular level. Many markers have been proposed, including altered expression of *p53, p21, Ki-67, bcl-2, EGFR, c-erb B2,* cyclooxygenase-2 (COX-2), and E-cadherin [28]. Of these, the most studied is the *p53* tumor-suppressor gene. Overexpression of *p53* is correlated with stage and grade, and in some studies has been linked to an increased risk of disease progression [29]. Unfortunately, a recent meta-analysis [30] of 138 publications on the predictive value of *p53*, including nearly 4000 patients, failed to find to any significant correlation that could be applied in daily clinical practice. Moreover, *p53* expression has not been useful in predicting response to adjuvant (bacille Calmette-Guerin [BCG]) therapy [29]. As yet, the potential of molecular makers remains unfulfilled.

Table 13.2. Suggested prognostic factors influencing management of superficial bladder tumors

Low risk (conservative management)	High risk (surgical management*)
No involvement of muscularis mucosae (<pT1b)	Involvement into or beyond the muscularis mucosae (pT1b and pT1c)
Small (less than 1.5 cm)	Large (greater than 1.5 cm) tumor
Solitary tumor	Multifocal tumors
Absence of associated carcinoma in situ	Presence of carcinoma in situ (especially if distant to papillary tumor site)
Second endoscopic resection showing no residual tumor (at 3 months)	Second endoscopic resection showing residual tumor (at 3 months)
Good response to intravesical chemotherapy/immunotherapy	Poor response to intravesical chemotherapy/immunotherapy
No tumor recurrence during the first year of surveillance cystoscopy	Early recurrence less than 6 months after initial resection

* Surgical management (cystectomy/cystoprostatectomy) for high-grade, high-stage (G3pT1) disease.

Role of Transurethral Resection (TUR) and Tumor Surveillance (Recurrence and New Occurrence)

Cystoscopic visualization of the bladder remains the primary modality of diagnosis, surveillance, and treatment of superficial bladder tumors. Attention to and accurate documentation of the relevant clinical prognostic factors are essential components for future therapeutic decisions. This should include estimation of tumor number, size, position, and configuration as well as the intervals between recurrences. Tissue sampling by TUR is advocated from all the affected areas to document the worst stage and tumor grade, and the presence of muscle in the biopsy specimen is essential to allow the uropathologist to accurately stage the tumor (see Natural History of Superficial Bladder Cancer and Prognostic Factors, above). Routine (random) biopsies of macroscopically normal urothelium to identify dysplasia are not useful, as less than 10% of normal-appearing urothelium in either pTa or pT1 disease will show an abnormality [31]. Moreover, significant variations in the interpretation of histological samples may in fact hinder rather than benefit therapeutic decisions [32].

It was previously assumed that the incidence of recurrence is low following cystoscopic extirpation of tumor, and that most treatment failure is a result of new occurrences in remote areas of de novo urothelial dysplasia. It is now apparent that as many as 50% of recurrences are due to tumor reimplantation at the time of original resection, as evidenced by molecular studies that demonstrate that many synchronous and metachronous lesions are of similar clonal origin [33,34]. Early tumor recurrences, which are multifocal and orientated toward the bladder dome (which occur in less than 5% of first presentations), are more likely to be as a result of the mechanical dispersion of "freed" tumor cells during resection (which gravitate upward) rather than genuine new occurrences. Later recurrences are more likely to be of disparate clonal derivation and represent genuine new occurrences. It is interesting to note that it is only the incidence of early tumor recurrence that is reduced by intravesical chemotherapy; the rate of later recurrences is unchanged (see Intravesical Therapy and Dose Scheduling, below) [35].

It is accepted that conventional light cystoscopy is an insensitive method of visualizing all superficial tumors and areas of subtle urothelial abnormality. Up to one third of tumors may be missed using conventional light sources, and inadequate resection is commonplace [36]. In one series of pT1 disease [37], recurrent tumor was detected in 43% of those subjected to repeat resection of the original resection site, emphasizing the importance of second look cystoscopy, re-resection, and early (3-month) surveillance. This is particularly relevant for high-risk tumors. Several series have demonstrated that up to 30% of these tumors are upstaged to muscle-invasive disease with a second resection [38]. Recent attempts to overcome the limitations of conventional white light cystoscopy, using the protoporphyrin 5-aminolevulinic acid (ALA) and blue light, have been reported to enhance visualization and direct tumor ablation [39]. Rates of local recurrence may also be reduced using laser ablation, which may be exploited to more precisely ablate lesions (and less likely to disperse cells) than the standard TUR diathermy loop [40]. These techniques have been successful in reducing recurrence rates by up to 15% in small, uncontrolled series [39,40]. Although these methods have considerable development ahead, they highlight the importance of scrupulous TUR technique to all operating clinicians.

Role of Intravesical Therapy in Tumor Prophylaxis

The purpose of intravesical adjuvant therapy is threefold: to eradicate residual tumor, to reduce the rate of recurrence, and to reduce the risk of tumor progression. Many different topical instillation agents have been proposed and tried over three decades. However, only two classes of cytotoxic agent and one immunotherapeutic modulator have been established with (limited) clinical efficacy, and are in common use. These are the anthracycline antibiotics Adriamycin and epirubicin, the alkylating agents thiotepa and mitomycin C (MMC), and the mycobacterium bacille Calmette-Guerin (BCG).

Intravesical Chemotherapy and Recurrence/Progression Rates

Intravesical chemotherapy agents were traditionally administered as delayed bladder instillations initiated at least 1 week following transurethral resection of the tumor and continued for up to 6 weeks. Such regimes were originally intended as prophylaxis against new occurrences, and had been demonstrated in many series to effect significant reductions in the short-term tumor recurrence rates. Early recurrence rates (within 1 year) for low-grade (G1 or G2), low-stage (pTa) superficial tumors can be reduced by up to 33% using anthracyclines [41] and 33% to 50% using MMC [42], although these rates are adversely affected by increasing tumor stage and grade [43]. Unfortunately, good initial responses have proven less durable with prolonged tumor surveillance. In a review of 2861 patients enrolled in controlled studies up to 1992 [42], the long-term reduction in tumor recurrence averaged only 17%. Indeed, in those followed 5 years or more, the recurrence rate increased to that achieved using transurethral extirpation alone [44]. Neither has this figure improved significantly by protracted maintenance therapy [45,46]. The cumulative data from such studies suggests that the overall reduction in recurrence rates using intravesical chemotherapy is approximately 12% to 15% [47]. Even more disappointing is the failure of chemotherapy to affect overall progression rates. The EORTC-GU/MRC meta-analysis demonstrated that intravesical chemotherapy has no impact on either stage progression or overall survival [48]. No study to date has demonstrated a significant improvement in these parameters using chemotherapy agents.

Intravesical Immunotherapy and Recurrence/Progression Rates

Intravesical immunotherapy using BCG was first proposed by Morales et al. [49] in 1976. Conventional prophylactic regimes of 6 weekly instillations, similar to those used for chemotherapy, resulted in complete response rates of 60% to 100% at 1 year, 55% to 75% after 2 years, and mean recurrence-free intervals of 10 to 22.5 months [50]. Although the long-term response rates with BCG are less enduring, the reduction in recurrence appears to be better than the rates achieved using most chemotherapy agents. This superiority is supported by comparative studies of BCG and anthracycline agents, which suggest that BCG has a roughly twofold advantage over Adriamycin and epirubicin (with an overall BCG tumor recurrence rate reduction of approximately 30%) [51]. In contrast, trials comparing MMC directly with BCG have been less consistent in outcome, and passionately debated. Of the published comparative MMC-BCG studies, three have suggested that MMC may have therapeutic equivalence to BCG for patients with low risk stage pTa and lower grade 1 and 2 tumors [52–54]. The inter- and cross-trial inconsistencies (inclusion criteria) and the interpretation of clinical and pathological factors have compounded the problems of analyses. However, in each of these three studies, the BCG schedules used were suboptimal. The balance of evidence still suggests an (small) advantage for BCG immunotherapy. Series reported by the Finnbladder Group [55] and Lundholm et al. [56] showed short-term response rates between 49% and 65% for BCG, compared with 34% and 38% for MMC. The Southwest Oncology Group (SWOG) trial 8795 was terminated early when a significant advantage for high-risk patients was demonstrated for those in the BCG arm [57]. In a recent meta-analysis of published and unpublished MMC-BCG comparative studies, seven of the 11 trials demonstrated superiority for BCG with mean 2-year recurrence rates of 46.4% and 38.6%, respectively [58]. It must be recognized that it has not yet been established whether this advantage is durable. The current American Urological Association (AUA) guidelines (published in 1999) still recommend the use of either MMC or BCG for the prophylaxis of pT1 and high-grade pTa disease [59].

Despite many studies, definitive evidence that BCG immunotherapy improves the overall survival for those with superficial bladder cancer has not been established. However, BCG may affect the rate of disease progression. Some of the largest studies that have attempted to assess the risk of progression are shown in Table 13.3. These studies can be criticized for their inclusion criteria, power (most having an insufficient number of patients to detect small differences in outcome) and ill-defined end points. Accepting these limitations, there now exists a body of evi-

Table 13.3. Selected studies of disease progression following bacille Calmette-Guérin (BCG) immunotherapy

Study (year)	Study design	No. of patients	Follow-up (months)	Progression*
Herr (86) (1988)	TUR alone vs. BCG induction	86	72	37% TUR vs. 28% BCG ($p = .01$)
Martinez-Pineiro (87) (1990)	BCG induction vs. thiotepa induction and maintenance monthly (year) vs. Adriamycin induction and maintenance monthly (year)	176	36	1.5% BCG vs. 3.6% thiotepa vs. 7.5% Adriamycin
Lamm (88) (1991)	BCG induction and maintenance 6 monthly (2 years) vs. Adriamycin induction and monthly maintenance (year)	131	65	6% BCG vs. 16% Adriamycin (not significant)
Pagano (89) (1991)	TUR alone vs. BCG induction and maintenance monthly (year) and quarterly (second year)	126	21	17% TUR vs. 4% BCG ($p < .05$)
Lamm (69) (2000)	BCG induction vs. BCG induction and six monthly maintenance (3 years)	384	60	30% induction vs. 24% maintenance ($p = .04$)
Millan-Rodriguez (90) (2000)	Retrospective analysis of TUR alone vs. BCG vs. chemotherapy	1529	50	Relative risk of progression decreased 0.3 for BCG
Sylvester (60) (2002)	Meta-analysis of 24 trials	4863	30	9.8% BCG vs. 13.8% controls ($p = .001$)

TUR, transurethral resection.
* The wide variation in progression rates reflects the widely different inclusion criteria and definitions of disease progression used in different studies.

dence that suggests that BCG therapy may delay stage progression or delay the necessity for radical (cystectomy or radiotherapy) intervention for those with high-risk disease. This view is supported by Sylvester et al.'s [60] meta-analysis of 4863 patients enrolled in 24 trials (see Treatment Options in G3pT1 Disease, below) [60].

Intravesical Therapy and Dose Scheduling

The traditional induction regimen of six weekly instillations of chemotherapy, initiated a week after resection, was based on original work using BCG immunotherapy. Delayed bladder instillation was intended as a *prophylactic* therapy for a secondary new occurrence, presuming that all previous tumors have been eradicated. It is now increasingly apparent that intravesical chemotherapy is best intended as an *ablative* therapy to "mop up" loose cells released at the time of extirpation and to prevent tumor reimplantation. Longitudinal studies have shown that tumor recurrences occur in two time-dependent peaks. The groups with early recurrence peaks are sensitive to chemotherapy, whereas those with delayed recurrences are generally resistant [35]. It is not surprising, therefore, that the influential study of the MRC demonstrated that immediate instillation of MMC within 24 hours of transurethral resection was as effective as conventional 6-week courses [61]. Indeed, more recent studies have suggested that intravesical chemotherapy should be administered as soon after resection as possible, with most of the advantage being lost within the first 24 hours [62]. Immediate bladder instillation appears to be safe as long as there is no risk of perforation and the bleeding has been adequately controlled. For those with extensive resection, the risk of systemic absorption and side effects should be considered. Cutaneous reactions often involving the genitalia and palms have been noted in up to 9% of patients receiving MMC [63]. BCG immunotherapy should never be given in the perioperative setting, as this increases the risk of systemic absorption and infection.

The optimal BCG treatment schedule remains a matter of some debate. A second 6-week cycle of BCG therapy improves the overall response rate from 50% to 70% [64], and 30% to 50% of those who fail an initial course of BCG respond to a second 6-week induction course [64,65]. As a result, many trials have attempted to improve BCG efficacy using "maintenance" regimens of continued weekly, biweekly, or monthly instillations [66], as well as longer induction courses [67]. Although one review of 14 such trials [68] suggested that response rates were maximized with additional BCG courses and led to a more durable long-term advantage over single-induction regimens, only one randomized study has proven any (statistically significant) advantage for progression. The SWOG 8507 study [69] showed a disease-free improvement from 40% to 61% and a 6% reduction in the rate of surgical intervention in patients receiving 3-week maintenance instillations at 3 and 6 months and every 6 months thereafter over 3 years. However, only 16% of the 243 patients were able to tolerate the complete 3-year regimen due to the local side effects. Overall, only a third to one half of the patients in these studies were able to tolerate regular BCG instillations due to the cumulative BCG-induced cystitis [68,69]. The toxicity of maintenance regimes (consisting of up to 27 instillations over a 3-year period) has also been addressed by the EORTC-GU group. The analysis of their own and other studies [19,70,71] suggests that the toxicity is mostly incurred during the induction phase, and lowering the dose of the maintenance (one-third dose) could reduce the limiting toxicity to 20%. It remains to be seen if the EORTC results can be translated into the common experience of most urology practices. For most, the therapeutic advantages of maintenance regimes are compromised by significant increases in local toxicity.

Role of Bacille Calmette-Guérin in the Treatment of Carcinoma in Situ

To date, BCG remains the treatment of choice for CIS disease. Although cytotoxic chemotherapy agents have shown initial response rates as good as 48% using anthracyclines and 53% for MMC, most series have demonstrated that this response is time limited, with fewer than 20% remaining disease free at 5 years [72]. This apparent chemoresistance may well reflect the high grade of CIS disease, whereas higher grade may imply greater antigenicity and therefore susceptibility to BCG immunotherapy. Bacille Calmette-Guerin therapy gives complete response rates of 60% to 70% with a median duration beyond 3 years and projected 5-year responses of 45%. Nevertheless, 30% to 40% of patients with CIS disease do not respond to a single induction course of BCG [72]. The response rates and the durability of response may be improved with maintenance therapy. Advocates of long-term maintenance refer to the SWOG 8507 study (see above) [69], although this was not specific for CIS. Further credence to maintenance BCG therapy has been offered by the more recent meta-analysis of Sylvester et al. [60]. Of the 403 patients with CIS disease treated with maintenance regimens, the relative advantage over no therapy was 35% and the overall risk of progression was 13.9% after 2.5 years. If patients are committed to repeated BCG courses, judicious monitoring for disease recurrence and progression (including extravesical sites) is paramount. Each consecutive induction course following CIS recurrence has a diminishing therapeutic value and an increased risk of disease progression. Current European Association of Urologists (EAU) guidelines recommend a second course for patients who fail primary therapy, and consideration of radical intervention (cystectomy) thereafter [73].

Treatment Options in G3pT1 Disease

G3pT1 forms the watershed of therapeutic intervention, with advocates of conservative and radical intervention equally persuaded in their differing interpretation of the available data. The historical series suggest that untreated G3pT1 has a recurrence rate between 70% and 80%, and progression rates ranging from 29% to as high as 50% [74]. In Birch and Harland's [75] review, 40% of G3pT1 cases followed beyond 24 months developed muscle-invasive disease. Although it is now accepted that treatment with transurethral resection for G3pT1 disease alone is inadequate, it is also apparent that a significant proportion of G3pT1 patients do not experience disease progression, and for these patients (early) cystectomy would represent an overtreatment. The challenge remains to find a way of identifying and reducing the risk of progression while safely conserving the bladder.

The decision to opt for conservative (bladder-sparing) treatment obligates the use of adjuvant BCG immunotherapy, despite an acceptance that the impact of BCG therapy on G3pT1 tumors has been difficult to assess. This is due in part to the limited number of patients with G3pT1 disease available for study (who will accept enrollment in a study arm with no adjuvant therapy), but also to the interdependence of other factors such as concomitant CIS, tumor multifocality, tumor size, and previous recurrence rates. The non-standardization of BCG treatment protocols has also limited direct comparisons of data. Historical reports of response rates following BCG therapy have varied from 25% to 75% for recurrence and 7% to 54% for progression [76–78]. Important differences would account for the large variation in responses. For example, in Herr's [76] 1991 series, where progression rates were high (54%) all the selected patients had

multiple tumor recurrences. In contrast, in Cookson and Sarosdy's [77] study, in which post-BCG progression rates were significantly lower (19%), only 30% of the patients had had a prior recurrence. In Serretta et al.'s [78] series, patients were treated with various chemotherapy and combination regimens; all the patients with poor (clinical) prognostic indicators of response were excluded, resulting in progression rates of only 12%. The lack of a randomized control throws open the question of whether this apparent success was due to the chemotherapy or the patient selection process. Some of the more recent series using BCG therapies alone are summarized on Table 13.4.

Although the numbers of patients enrolled in studies with "unpolluted" G3pT1 disease are limited, clinicians are obliged to take guidance from the evidence base as a whole. The recent meta-analysis of Sylvester et al. [60] of all superficial bladder cancers enrolled in randomized studies of BCG therapy suggests a 27% reduction in the odds of progression, but only for those receiving maintenance protocols over a period of 3 years. There was no statistically significant benefit for either overall or disease-specific survival, raising the question of the durability of the benefit beyond 3 years. For those who received only single or a duplicate course of BCG the progression rate was similar to that of resection alone. From the accumulation of such data has emerged a "rule of threes," in which a third of those with G3pT1 disease treated by BCG survive with their bladder in situ, a third survive after cystectomy, and a third die from their disease despite all interventions [10].

Table 13.4. Recent studies of BCG immunotherapy for G3pT1 disease

Study (year)	Study design	No. of patients	Follow-up (years)	Result
Cookson (91) (1997)	BCG (one or more induction)	48	15	Progression 35% within 5 years, 16% 5–10 years, 10% 10–15 years
Pansadoro (92) (2002)	BCG (induction and maintenance)	81	6.3	Recurrence 33%; progression 15%
Patard (93) (2002)	TUR alone or delayed BCG and BCG primary induction	80	5	Progression TUR alone or delayed BCG 53% vs. BCG primary induction 36%
Shahin (10) (2003)	TUR alone and BCG (one or more induction)	153	5.3	Recurrence TUR alone 75% vs. BCG 70%; progression TUR alone 36% vs. BCG 33%

Although cystectomy can result in recurrence free rates as good as 78% at 10 years [79], those who advocate a conservative policy argue that such results simply reflect the natural history of the disease. Nevertheless, the preservation of the bladder in situ, even as a temporized objective, could be considered a worthwhile benefit to some patients.

Other Immunomodulators

The relative success of BCG has stimulated interest in other immunomodulators for use as adjuvant intravesical agents. Interferons (IFNs) are key components of the cytokine response, causing increased expression of major histocompatibility complex antigens on transitional cells, activating T cells, lymphokine activated killer cells, and natural killer cells. Intravesical IFN-α2b has demonstrated the most activity against bladder cancer. Several small studies have now been reported [80–82]. These early data have shown moderate tumor responses (recurrence rates reduced by approximately 15%), although the responses and the relapse rates are inferior to those for BCG and MMC [81,82]. Although it is likely that BCG (as well as MMC) as monotherapy is superior, in vitro studies have suggested that the combination of IFN-α and standard intravesical agents may have a synergistic effect [82]. Pilot studies have already shown a synergistic action of IFN-α with epirubicin [83], MMC [84], and BCG [85], whereas the combination of BCG and IFN-α effected a 55% secondary response in 40 patients who were prior BCG failures [51]. The numbers in these preliminary studies have all been small and the follow-up limited. Further large-scale trials are awaited before interferon therapy is more widely adopted.

Conclusion

Many patients with bladder cancer are elderly, with extended comorbidity, and a careful approach to their treatment is necessary. Attention to and accurate documentation of relevant clinical and histopathological prognostic factors allows stratification into low-, intermediate-, and high-risk groups. Diffuse carcinoma in situ is considered a separate and aggressive disease category. The timing of future surveillance cystoscopy and interventional adjuvant therapy are dependent on these criteria. A change in risk classification should prompt a reevaluation of patient status.

In all patients, the initial approach is to attempt cystoscopic tumor ablation. Adjuvant intravesical therapy is decided by the prognostic status and the dynamic of stage change. For those with low- or intermediate-risk lesions, ablative chemotherapy immediately following resection is the first choice. High-risk lesions including G3pT1 disease and CIS should be treated with intravesical BCG immunotherapy. Maintenance regimens may confer a reduction in progressive potential but at a cost of increased risk of toxicity. Concomitant poor prognostic factors or failure of BCG therapy (reappearance of tumor or positive urine cytology) is an indication for more aggressive therapy. In these patients radical cystectomy is indicated.

The role of alternative immunomodulators, combination and dose-modulated instillation protocols, and molecular prognosticators is promising, although their potential is dependent on further large-scale study.

References

1. Office of National Statistics. Cancer trends Table 3.1: Bladder cancer, key statistics. www.statistics.gov.uk/StatBase/xsdataset.asp.
2. Jemal A, Tiwari RC, Murray T, et al. Cancer statistics, 2004. CA Cancer J Clin 2004;54(1):8–29.
3. McFarlane JP, Ellis BW, Harland SJ. The management of superficial bladder cancer: an interactive seminar. Br J Urol 1996;78(3):372–378.
4. International Union Against Cancer. Urinary Bladder. In: Sobin LH, Wittekind Ch, eds. TNM Classification of Malignant Tumours. New York: Wiley-Liss, 1997:187–190.
5. Anderstrom C, Johansson S, Nilsson S. The significance of lamina propria invasion on the prognosis of patients with bladder tumors. J Urol 1980;124(1):23–26.
6. Abel PD, Hall RR, Williams G. Should pT1 transitional cell cancers of the bladder still be classified as superficial? Br J Urol 1988;62(3):235–239.
7. Lopez JI, Angulo JC. The prognostic significance of vascular invasion in stage T1 bladder cancer. Histopathology 1995;27(1):27–33.
8. Smits G, Schaafsma E, Kiemeney L, Caris C, Debruyne F, Witjes JA. Microstaging of pT1 tran-

sitional cell carcinoma of the bladder: identification of subgroups with distinct risks of progression. Urology 1998;52(6):1009–1013.

9. Angulo JC, Lopez JI, Grignon DJ, Sanchez-Chapado M. Muscularis mucosa differentiates two populations with different prognosis in stage T1 bladder cancer. Urology 1995;45(1):47–53.

10. Shahin O, Thalmann GN, Rentsch C, Mazzucchelli L, Studer UE. A retrospective analysis of 153 patients treated with or without intravesical bacillus Calmette-Guerin for primary stage T1 grade 3 bladder cancer: recurrence, progression and survival. J Urol 2003;169(1):96–100.

11. Witjes JA, Kiemeney LA, Schaafsma HE, Debruyne FM. The influence of review pathology on study outcome of a randomized multicentre superficial bladder cancer trial. Members of the Dutch South East Cooperative Urological Group. Br J Urol 1994; 73(2):172–176.

12. Heney NM, Ahmed S, Flanagan MJ, et al. Superficial bladder cancer: progression and recurrence. J Urol 1983;130(6):1083–1086.

13. Malmstrom PU, Busch C, Norlen BJ. Recurrence, progression and survival in bladder cancer. A retrospective analysis of 232 patients with greater than or equal to 5-year follow-up. Scand J Urol Nephrol 1987;21(3):185–195.

14. Donat SM. Evaluation and follow-up strategies for superficial bladder cancer. Urol Clin North Am 2003;30(4):765–776.

15. Abel PD. Follow-up of patients with "superficial" transitional cell carcinoma of the bladder: the case for a change in policy. Br J Urol 1993;72(2): 135–142.

16. Brausi M, Collette L, Kurth KH, et al. Variablity in the recurrence rate at first follow-up cystoscopy after TUR in stage TaT1 transitional cell carcinoma of the bladder: a combined analysis of seven EORTC studies. Eur Urol 2002;41(5):523–531.

17. Heney NM, Proppe K, Prout GR Jr, Griffin PP, Shipley WU. Invasive bladder cancer: tumor configuration, lymphatic invasion and survival. J Urol 1983;130(5):895–897.

18. Fitzpatrick JM, West AB, Butler MR, Lane V, O'Flynn JD. Superficial bladder tumors (stage pTa, grades 1 and 2): the importance of recurrence pattern following initial resection. J Urol 1986; 135(5):920–922.

19. Dalesio O, Schulman CC, Sylvester R, et al. Prognostic factors in superficial bladder tumors. A study of the European Organization for Research on Treatment of Cancer: Genitourinary Tract Cancer Cooperative Group. J Urol 1983;129(4): 730–733.

20. Kurth KH, Denis L, Bouffioux C, et al. Factors affecting recurrence and progression in superficial bladder tumours. Eur J Cancer 1995; 31A(11):1840–1846.

21. Lamm DL. Carcinoma in situ. Urol Clin North Am 1992;19(3):499–508.

22. Riddle PR, Chisholm GD, Trott PA, Pugh RC. Flat carcinoma in Situ of bladder. Br J Urol 1975; 47(7):829–833.

23. Althausen AF, Prout GR Jr, Daly JJ. Non-invasive papillary carcinoma of the bladder associated with carcinoma in situ. J Urol 1976;116(5):575–580.

24. Herr HW, Wartinger DD, Fair WR, Oettgen HF. Bacillus Calmette-Guerin therapy for superficial bladder cancer: a 10-year followup. J Urol 1992; 147(4):1020–1023.

25. Utz DC, Farrow GM. Carcinoma in situ of the urinary tract. Urol Clin North Am 1984;11(4): 735–740.

26. Parmar MK, Freedman LS, Hargreave TB, Tolley DA. Prognostic factors for recurrence and followup policies in the treatment of superficial bladder cancer: report from the British Medical Research Council Subgroup on Superficial Bladder Cancer (Urological Cancer Working Party). J Urol 1989;142(2 pt 1):284–288.

27. Hall RR, Parmar MK, Richards AB, Smith PH. Proposal for changes in cystoscopic follow up of patients with bladder cancer and adjuvant intravesical chemotherapy. BMJ 1994;308(6923): 257–260.

28. Soloway MS, Sofer M, Vaidya A. Contemporary management of stage T1 transitional cell carcinoma of the bladder. J Urol 2002;167(4):1573–1583.

29. Smith ND, Rubenstein JN, Eggener SE, Kozlowski JM. The p53 tumor suppressor gene and nuclear protein: basic science review and relevance in the management of bladder cancer. J Urol 2003; 169(4):1219–1228.

30. Schmitz-Drager BJ, Goebell PJ, Ebert T, Fradet Y. p53 immunohistochemistry as a prognostic marker in bladder cancer. Playground for urology scientists? Eur Urol 2000;38(6):691–699.

31. van der Meijden AP, Oosterlinck W, Brausi M, Kurth KH, Sylvester R, de Balincourt C. Significance of bladder biopsies in Ta,T1 bladder tumors: a report from the EORTC Genito-Urinary Tract Cancer Cooperative Group. EORTC-GU Group Superficial Bladder Committee. Eur Urol 1999;35(4):267–271.

32. Richards B, Parmar MK, Anderson CK, et al. Interpretation of biopsies of "normal" urothelium in patients with superficial bladder cancer. MRC Superficial Bladder Cancer Sub Group. Br J Urol 1991;67(4):369–375.

33. Sidransky D, Frost P, Von Eschenbach A, Oyasu R, Preisinger AC, Vogelstein B. Clonal origin bladder cancer. N Engl J Med 1992;326(11):737–740.

34. Takahashi T, Habuchi T, Kakehi Y, et al. Clonal and chronological genetic analysis of multifocal

cancers of the bladder and upper urinary tract. Cancer Res 1998;58(24):5835–5841.

35. Hinotsu S, Akaza H, Ohashi Y, Kotake T. Intravesical chemotherapy for maximum prophylaxis of new early phase superficial bladder carcinoma treated by transurethral resection: a combined analysis of trials by the Japanese Urological Cancer Research Group using smoothed hazard function. Cancer 1999;86(9):1818–1826.

36. Zaak D, Kriegmair M, Stepp H, et al. Endoscopic detection of transitional cell carcinoma with 5-aminolevulinic acid: results of 1012 fluorescence endoscopies. Urology 2001;57(4):690–694.

37. Klan R, Loy V, Huland H. Residual tumor discovered in routine second transurethral resection in patients with stage T1 transitional cell carcinoma of the bladder. J Urol 1991;146(2):316–318.

38. Herr HW. The value of a second transurethral resection in evaluating patients with bladder tumors. J Urol 1999;162(1):74–76.

39. Filbeck T, Pichlmeier U, Knuechel R, Wieland WF, Roessler W. Clinically relevant improvement of recurrence-free survival with 5-aminolevulinic acid induced fluorescence diagnosis in patients with superficial bladder tumors. J Urol 2002; 168(1):67–71.

40. Beisland HO, Seland P. A prospective randomized study on neodymium-YAG laser irradiation versus TUR in the treatment of urinary bladder cancer. Scand J Urol Nephrol 1986;20(3):209–212.

41. Richie JP. Intravesical chemotherapy. Treatment selection, techniques, and results. Urol Clin North Am 1992;19(3):521–527.

42. Lamm DL. Long-term results of intravesical therapy for superficial bladder cancer. Urol Clin North Am 1992;19(3):573–580.

43. Mishina T, Oda K, Murata S, Ooe H, Mori Y. Mitomycin C bladder instillation therapy for bladder tumors. J Urol 1975;114(2):217–219.

44. Lamm DL, Torti FM. Bladder cancer, 1996. CA Cancer J Clin 1996;46(2):93–112.

45. Flamm J. Long-term versus short-term doxorubicin hydrochloride instillation after transurethral resection of superficial bladder cancer. Eur Urol 1990;17(2):119–124.

46. Huland H, Kloppel G, Feddersen I, et al. Comparison of different schedules of cytostatic intravesical instillations in patients with superficial bladder carcinoma: final evaluation of a prospective multicenter study with 419 patients. J Urol 1990;144(1):68–71.

47. Traynelis CL, Lamm DL. Current status of intravesical therapy for bladder cancer. In: Rous SN, ed. Urology Annual. New York: Norton, 1994:113–143.

48. Pawinski A, Sylvester R, Kurth KH, et al. A combined analysis of European Organization for Research and Treatment of Cancer, and Medical Research Council randomized clinical trials for the prophylactic treatment of stage TaT1 bladder cancer. European Organization for Research and Treatment of Cancer Genitourinary Tract Cancer Cooperative Group and the Medical Research Council Working Party on Superficial Bladder Cancer. J Urol 1996;156(6):1934–1940.

49. Morales A, Eidinger D, Bruce AW. Intracavitary Bacillus Calmette-Guerin in the treatment of superficial bladder tumors. 1976. J Urol 2002;167(2 pt 2):891–893.

50. Mungan NA, Witjes JA. Bacille Calmette-Guerin in superficial transitional cell carcinoma. Br J Urol 1998;82(2):213–223.

51. O'Donnell MA, Krohn J, DeWolf WC. Salvage intravesical therapy with interferon-alpha 2b plus low dose bacillus Calmette-Guerin is effective in patients with superficial bladder cancer in whom bacillus Calmette-Guerin alone previously failed. J Urol 2001;166(4):1300–1304.

52. Debruyne FM, van der Meijden AP, Schreinemachers LM, et al. BCG-RIVM intravesical immunoprophylaxis for superficial bladder cancer. Prog Clin Biol Res 1988;269:511–524.

53. Vegt PD, Witjes JA, Witjes WP, Doesburg WH, Debruyne FM, van der Meijden AP. A randomized study of intravesical mitomycin C, bacillus Calmette-Guerin Tice and bacillus Calmette-Guerin RIVM treatment in pTa-pT1 papillary carcinoma and carcinoma in situ of the bladder. J Urol 1995;153(3 pt 2):929–933.

54. Krege S, Giani G, Meyer R, Otto T, Rubben H. A randomized multicenter trial of adjuvant therapy in superficial bladder cancer: transurethral resection only versus transurethral resection plus mitomycin C versus transurethral resection plus bacillus Calmette-Guerin. Participating Clinics. J Urol 1996;156(3):962–966.

55. Alfthan O, Jauhiainen K, Kaasinen E, Liukkonen T. Current concepts in the role of intravesical instillations in the therapy and prophylaxis of superficial transitional-cell cancer of the bladder. The Finnbladder Research Group. World J Urol 1997;15(2):89–95.

56. Lundholm C, Norlen BJ, Ekman P, et al. A randomized prospective study comparing long-term intravesical instillations of mitomycin C and bacillus Calmette-Guerin in patients with superficial bladder carcinoma. J Urol 1996;156(2 pt 1):372–376.

57. Lamm DL, Blumenstein BA, Crawford ED, et al. Randomised intergroup comparison of bacillus Calmette-Guerin immunotherapy and mitomycin C chemotherapy in superficial transitional cell carcinoma of the bladder. A Southwest Oncology Group study. Urol Oncol 1995;1:119–126.

58. Bohle A, Jocham D, Bock PR. Intravesical bacillus Calmette-Guerin versus mitomycin C for

superficial bladder cancer: a formal meta-analysis of comparative studies on recurrence and toxicity. J Urol 2003;169(1):90–95.

59. Smith JA, Labsky RF, Cockett AT, Fracchia JA, Montie JE, Rowland RG. Bladder cancer clinical guidelines panel summary report on the management of nonmuscle invasive bladder cancer (stages Ta, T1 and TIS). The American Urological Association. J Urol 1999;162(5):1697–1701.

60. Sylvester RJ, van der Meijden AP, Lamm DL. Intravesical bacillus Calmette-Guerin reduces the risk of progression in patients with superficial bladder cancer: a meta-analysis of the published results of randomized clinical trials. J Urol 2002; 168(5):1964–1970.

61. Tolley DA, Parmar MK, Grigor KM, et al. The effect of intravesical mitomycin C on recurrence of newly diagnosed superficial bladder cancer: a further report with 7 years of follow up. J Urol 1996;155(4):1233–1238.

62. Okamura K, Ono Y, Kinukawa T, et al. Randomized study of single early instillation of (2″R)-4′-O-tetrahydropyranyl-doxorubicin for a single superficial bladder carcinoma. Cancer 2002; 94(9):2363–2368.

63. Thrasher JB, Crawford ED. Complications of intravesical chemotherapy. Urol Clin North Am 1992;19(3):529–539.

64. Catalona WJ, Hudson MA, Gillen DP, Andriole GL, Ratliff TL. Risks and benefits of repeated courses of intravesical bacillus Calmette-Guerin therapy for superficial bladder cancer. J Urol 1987; 137(2):220–224.

65. Haaff EO, Dresner SM, Ratliff TL, Catalona WJ. Two courses of intravesical bacillus Calmette-Guerin for transitional cell carcinoma of the bladder. J Urol 1986;136(4):820–824.

66. Brosman SA. Experience with bacillus Calmette-Guerin in patients with superficial bladder carcinoma. J Urol 1982;128(1):27–30.

67. Gruenwald IE, Stein A, Rashcovitsky R, Shifroni G, Lurie A. A 12- versus 6-week course of bacillus Calmette-Guerin prophylaxis for the treatment of high risk superficial bladder cancer. J Urol 1997; 157(2):487–491.

68. Khanna OP, Son DL, Mazer H, et al. Multicentre study of superficial bladder cancer treated with intravesical bacillus Calmette-Guerin or Adriamycin. J Urol 1990;35(2):101–108.

69. Lamm DL, Blumenstein BA, Crissman JD, et al. Maintenance bacillus Calmette-Guerin immunotherapy for recurrent TA, T1 and carcinoma in situ transitional cell carcinoma of the bladder: a randomized Southwest Oncology Group Study. J Urol 2000;163(4):1124–1129.

70. Martinez-Pineiro JA, Flores N, Isorna S, et al. Long-term follow-up of a randomized prospective trial comparing a standard 81 mg dose of intrav-esical bacille Calmette-Guerin with a reduced dose of 27 mg in superficial bladder cancer. BJU Int 2002;89(7):671–680.

71. van der Meijden AP, Sylvester RJ, Oosterlinck W, Hoeltl W, Bono AV, EORTC Genito-urinary Tract Cancer Collaborative Group. Maintenance Bacillus Calmette-Guerin for TaT1 bladder tumors is not associated with increased toxicity: results from a European Organisation for Research and Treatment of Cancer Genito-Urinary Group Phase III Trial. Eur Urol 2003; 44(4):429–434.

72. Lamm DL. BCG immunotherapy for transitional-cell carcinoma in situ of the bladder. Oncology (Huntington) 1995;9(10):947–952, discussion 955.

73. Oosterlinck W, Lobel B, Jackse G, et al. EAU Recommendations 2001. Guidelines on bladder cancer. Eur Urol 2002;41(2):105–112.

74. Pham HT, Soloway MS. High-risk superficial bladder cancer: intravesical therapy for T1 G3 transitional cell carcinoma of the urinary bladder. Semin Urol Oncol 1997;15(3):147–153.

75. Birch BR, Harland SJ. The pT1 G3 bladder tumour. Br J Urol 1989;64(2):109–116.

76. Herr HW. Progression of stage T1 bladder tumors after intravesical bacillus Calmette-Guerin. J Urol 1991;145(1):40–43.

77. Cookson MS, Sarosdy MF. Management of stage T1 superficial bladder cancer with intravesical bacillus Calmette-Guerin therapy. J Urol 1992; 148(3):797–801.

78. Serretta V, Piazza S, Pavone C, Piazza B, Pavone-Macaluso M. Results of conservative treatment (transurethral resection plus adjuvant intravesical chemotherapy) in patients with primary T1, G3 transitional cell carcinoma of the bladder. Urology 1996;47(5):647–651.

79. Stein JP, Lieskovsky G, Cote R, et al. Radical cystectomy in the treatment of invasive bladder cancer: long-term results in 1,054 patients. J Clin Oncol 2001;19(3):666–675.

80. Glashan RW. A randomized controlled study of intravesical alpha-2b-interferon in carcinoma in situ of the bladder. J Urol 1990;144(3):658–661.

81. Boccardo F, Cannata D, Rubagotti A, et al. Prophylaxis of superficial bladder cancer with mitomycin or interferon alfa-2b: results of a multicentric Italian study. J Clin Oncol 1994; 12(1):7–13.

82. Belldegrun AS, Franklin JR, O'Donnell MA, et al. Superficial bladder cancer: the role of interferon-alpha. J Urol 1998;159(6):1793–1801.

83. Ferrari P, Castagnetti G, Pollastri CA, Ferrari G, Tavoni F, Grassi D. Chemoimmunotherapy for prophylaxis of recurrence in superficial bladder cancer: interferon-alpha 2b versus interferon-alpha 2b with epirubicin. Anticancer Drugs 1992; 3(suppl 1):25–27.

84. Engelmann U, Knopf HJ, Graff J. Interferon-alpha 2b instillation prophylaxis in superficial bladder cancer—a prospective, controlled three-armed trial. Project Group Bochum-interferon and superficial bladder cancer. Anticancer Drugs 1992;suppl 1:33–37.

85. Stricker P, Pryor K, Nicholson T, et al. Bacillus Calmette-Guerin plus intravesical interferon alpha-2b in patients with superficial bladder cancer. Urology 1996;48(6):957–961.

86. Herr HW, Laudone VP, Badalament RA, et al. Bacillus Calmette-Guerin therapy alters the progression of superficial bladder cancer. J Clin Oncol 1988;6(9):1450–1455.

87. Martinez-Pineiro JA, Jimenez LJ, Martinez-Pineiro L Jr, et al. Bacillus Calmette-Guerin versus doxorubicin versus thiotepa: a randomized prospective study in 202 patients with superficial bladder cancer. J Urol 1990;143(3):502–506.

88. Lamm DL, Blumenstein BA, Crawford ED, et al. A randomized trial of intravesical doxorubicin and immunotherapy with bacille Calmette-Guerin for transitional-cell carcinoma of the bladder. N Engl J Med 1991;325(17):1205–1209.

89. Pagano F, Bassi P, Milani C, Meneghini A, Maruzzi D, Garbeglio A. A low dose bacillus Calmette-Guerin regimen in superficial bladder cancer therapy: is it effective? J Urol 1991;146(1):32–35.

90. Millan-Rodriguez F, Chechile-Toniolo G, Salvador-Bayarri J, Palou J, Vicente-Rodriguez J. Multivariate analysis of the prognostic factors of primary superficial bladder cancer. J Urol 2000;163(1):73–78.

91. Cookson MS, Herr HW, Zhang ZF, Soloway S, Sogani PC, Fair WR. The treated natural history of high risk superficial bladder cancer: 15-year outcome. J Urol 1997;158(1):62–67.

92. Pansadoro V, Emiliozzi P, de Paula F, Scarpone P, Pansadoro A, Sternberg CN. Long-term follow-up of G3T1 transitional cell carcinoma of the bladder treated with intravesical bacille Calmette-Guerin: 18-year experience. Urology 2002;59(2):227–231.

93. Patard JJ, Rodriguez A, Leray E, Rioux-Leclercq N, Guille F, Lobel B. Intravesical Bacillus Calmette-Guerin treatment improves patient survival in T1G3 bladder tumours. Eur Urol 2002;41(6):635–641.

14

Chemotherapy for Bladder Cancer

Matthew D. Galsky and Dean F. Bajorin

Transitional cell carcinoma (TCC) of the urinary bladder is the second most common genitourinary malignancy. Each year, over 73,000 new cases are reported in Europe and over 56,000 new cases in the United States. A substantial percentage of these patients develop metastases despite initial management for presumed localized disease, whereas others have metastases at the time of presentation. Once metastasis occurs, the median survival for patients with TCC is approximately 1 year. To improve this poor survival rate, intense efforts over the past two decades have focused on the development of active chemotherapeutic regimens for use in this disease, both in the perioperative setting and in the setting of advanced disease. Chemotherapy for advanced disease is discussed here first because of its impact on the management of early-stage disease.

Older Chemotherapeutic Regimens in Metastatic Transitional Cell Carcinoma

Older Single Agents

Cisplatin is the most active single agent in urothelial TCC. During the late 1970s, trials evaluating single-agent cisplatin were initiated in patients with advanced TCC, yielding overall response (OR) rates ranging from 26% to 65%. Although uncommon, complete response (CR) rates were also observed (5% to 16%). Subsequently, additional single agents demonstrated activity in urothelial TCC. The most active of these included methotrexate (OR 30%), doxorubicin (OR 17%), and vinblastine (OR 22%) [1,2].

Combination Chemotherapy and the Development of MVAC

Multiagent chemotherapeutic regimens were developed during the 1980s in an attempt to improve upon the results with single-agent therapy. A landmark trial reported in 1985 used the combination of methotrexate, vinblastine, Adriamycin (doxorubicin), and cisplatin (MVAC). In this trial, 24 patients with advanced or unresectable urothelial TCC were treated with MVAC [3]. Remarkably, responses were observed in 71% of those treated (95% confidence interval [CI], 53–89%), with complete clinical responses in 50% (95% CI, 30–70%). A follow-up report from the same investigators confirmed these initial results with MVAC in a larger patient population [4]. Subsequent randomized trials showed improved survival with MVAC compared to single-agent cisplatin [5] and CISCA (cisplatin, cyclophosphamide, and Adriamycin) [6].

Limitations of MVAC

Despite the superiority of MVAC in phase III trials, the limitations of this regimen were readily apparent. Although many patients responded to MVAC, median survivals were consistently reported as less than 13 months. In addition, the durability of responses with MVAC was poor, with less than 4% of patients alive and continuously disease-free at 6 years or more [7]. The most limiting factor associated with MVAC was associated toxicity. Treatment-related deaths occurred in 2% to 4% of patients. Severe toxicities such as febrile neutropenia (20% to 30%) and mucositis (10% to 20%) were also common in patients treated with this regimen. Other toxicities included decreased renal function, hearing loss, and peripheral neuropathy.

Attempts to Improve MVAC

In an attempt to decrease the toxicity and enhance the efficacy of MVAC, several investigators evaluated the use of altered doses and schedules with granulocyte colony-stimulating factor (GCSF) support. Based on the potential for enhanced survival conferred by greater drug delivery, the European Organization for Research and Treatment of Cancer (EORTC) conducted a randomized trial comparing MVAC administered every 2 weeks (with GCSF) with MVAC administered every 4 weeks [8]. Although this prospective trial showed a significantly greater CR rate (21% compared to 9%, $p = .009$) and progression-free survival (hazard ratio 0.75; 95% CI, 0.58–0.98, $p = .037$) in patients receiving the every-2-week schedule there was no significant difference in the overall survival distributions. This trial, designed to detect a 50% difference in median survival with a total of 263 patients, showed a trend toward greater survival in patients receiving more intense therapy. It is possible that a survival benefit with the dose-dense regimen may have been missed due to the small sample size. However, given the modest differences in outcome, the conventional regimen given at 4-week intervals remains the standard of care.

The Impact of Prognostic Factors

Pretreatment prognostic factors play a key role in predicting the outcome of patients with advanced TCC treated with MVAC and other cisplatin-based regimens. In a retrospective analysis, a database of 203 patients with unresectable/metastatic TCC was subjected to multivariate analysis to determine which patient characteristics predicted survival [9]. Two factors had independent prognostic significance: Karnofsky performance status (KPS) ≤80% and visceral (lung, liver, or bone) metastases. The median survival for patients with 0, 1, or 2 risk factors was 33, 13.4, and 9.3 months, respectively ($p = .0001$). Clearly, the proportion of patients in these various risk categories must be considered when comparing median survivals among different phase II studies. In addition, these baseline prognostic factors can be used to stratify patients in phase III trials comparing new regimens to standard therapy. Similar differences in survival have been observed in patients treated with cisplatin, gemcitabine, and paclitaxel [10].

Newer Agents/Combinations in Metastatic Transitional Cell Carcinoma

New Active Single Agents

Given the limitations with MVAC therapy, new agents had to be developed to improve long-term outcome and reduce toxicity. Recently, several agents with activity in TCC have been identified. These new agents differ from the older drugs in that they demonstrate moderate activity as both first-line and second-line therapy, more favorable toxicity profiles, and a drug metabolism that is independent of renal excretion. Of these newer agents, the most extensively studied have been gemcitabine, the taxanes, and ifosfamide.

Gemcitabine and Cisplatin: A New Standard of Care

Based on the promising activity and favorable side-effect profile of gemcitabine, trials exploring the combination of gemcitabine and cisplatin in metastatic TCC were initiated. Several phase II studies reported OR rates of 42% to 57% and CR rates of 18 to 22% [11–13]. Subsequently, a multicenter, randomized phase III trial was performed to compare gemcitabine and cisplatin (GC) with MVAC (Table 14.1) [14], in which 405 chemotherapy-naive patients were randomized

Table 14.1. Randomized trials of cisplatin-based chemotherapy in advanced transitional cell carcinoma

Regimens	Reference	No. of patients	OR (%)	CR (%)	Survival (months)	p
MVAC	5	120	36	13	12.5	<.0002
Cisplatin		126	11	3	8.2	
MVAC	6	55	65	35	12.6	<.05
CISCA		55	46	25	10	
MVAC	64	86	59	24	12.5	.17
FAP		83	42	10	12.5	
MVAC	8	129	58	9	14.1	.122
HD-MVAC		134	72	21	15.5	
MVAC	14	205	46	12	14.8	.746
Gemcitabine + cisplatin		203	50	12	13.8	
MVAC	18	109	54	23	14.2	.025
Docetaxel + cisplatin		111	37	13	9.3	
*MVAC	28	44	40	13%	14.2	.41
Paclitaxel + carboplatin		41	28	3%	13.8	

MVAC, methotrexate, vinblastine, doxorubicin, cisplatin; CISCA, cyclophosphamide, cisplatin, doxorubicin, CMV, cisplatin, methotrexate, vinblastine; MV, methotrexate, vinblastine; FAP, 5-fluorouracil, interferon-alpha-2b, cisplatin; HD-MVAC, high-dose MVAC; OR, overall response; CR, complete response.
* Trial terminated early with only 85 patients, underpowered, preliminary results.

to GC or standard MVAC. The CR, OR, and median survival rates were similar in both arms. Although GC was associated with more grade ≥3 anemia and thrombocytopenia, MVAC was associated with a greater incidence of neutropenic fever (14% compared to 2%), neutropenic sepsis (12% compared to 1%), grade ≥3 mucositis (22% compared to 1%), and treatment-related deaths (3% compared to 1%).

Notably, this randomized trial was not designed as an equivalence trial. However, the data can be interpreted as showing that, in terms of survival, GC is comparable to MVAC. In addition, GC appears to be associated with a more favorable risk-benefit ratio. Given the trial results and this regimen's ease of administration, GC has become widely used as a standard treatment regimen for patients with metastatic TCC.

New Cisplatin Doublets

The combinations of paclitaxel or docetaxel plus cisplatin have been explored in multiple phase II studies. In an Eastern Cooperative Oncology Group (ECOG) study, 52 patients were treated with paclitaxel $175 \, mg/m^2$ and cisplatin $75 \, mg/m^2$ every 21 days [15]. Twenty-six patients

achieved an objective response (50%; 95% CI, 36–61%) with four (8%) complete responses. The toxicity of this regimen was considered moderate, with neutropenia (without fever) and neurotoxicity being most common.

Trials evaluating the combination of docetaxel and cisplatin (DC) report OR rates of 58% to 60%, with CR rates ranging from 19% to 26% [16,17]. Results of a phase III randomized trial comparing DC with MVAC plus GCSF conducted by the Hellenic Cooperative Oncology Group have recently been reported (Table 14.1) [18]. Although DC was associated with less hematologic toxicity and febrile neutropenia, response rates and survival favored the MVAC arm. The reported toxicity of the MVAC arm, administered with GCSF, was less than in previous phase III trials employing MVAC without GCSF.

New Cisplatin Triplets

The combination of ifosfamide, paclitaxel, and cisplatin (ITP) has been studied in a phase II trial [19]. Myelosuppression was the predominant toxicity (45% grade 3 to 4 neutropenia), although the risk of febrile neutropenia was low (3.3% of all cycles). Grade 3 neuropathy and renal insufficiency occurred in 9% and 11%, respectively. Thirty of 44 assessable patients (68%; 95% CI, 52–81%) achieved a major response, with 10 complete responses (23%) and 20 partial responses (45%). The reported median survival of 20 months is among the best reported results for patients with metastatic, advanced TCC, and greater than the previously observed results with MVAC (12–13 months). This regimen has not been taken to phase III evaluation.

Other cisplatin-based triplets have been explored, the most notable of which is cisplatin, gemcitabine, and paclitaxel. In a phase I/II trial of 58 patients, this regimen resulted in 16 complete responses (28%) and 29 partial responses (50%) for an overall response proportion of 77.6% (95% CI, 60–98%) [20]. The median survival time had not been reached at the time of the report. This regimen is currently being compared with gemcitabine plus cisplatin in an international randomized phase III trial conducted by the EORTC.

New Carboplatin Doublets

Given the renal, neurologic, and auditory toxicity associated with cisplatin, it was hoped that carboplatin would prove to be equivalent to cisplatin in this disease. In a review of 327 patients with advanced, metastatic TCC treated on 13 trials with single-agent carboplatin, 14% achieved an objective response [21].

The best-studied carboplatin doublet in TCC is the combination of paclitaxel and carboplatin. Phase II trials have been performed with wide variations in the doses of paclitaxel (150 to 225 mg/m^2) and carboplatin (area under the curve [AUC] 5 to 6); not unexpectedly, the OR rates vary from 14% to 65%, and the CR rates range from 0% to 40% [22–27].

Given the promising phase II results, ECOG launched a phase III trial comparing MVAC with paclitaxel plus carboplatin; results were reported in preliminary form (Table 14.1). Because the study was terminated after $2^1/_2$ years of slow accrual [28], only 85 of the planned 330 patients were enrolled. Patients treated with MVAC had more severe myelosuppression, mucositis, and renal toxicity. Interestingly, a quality of life instrument revealed no significant differences between the two arms. At a median follow-up of 32.5 months, there was no significant difference

in response rate or median survival between the two arms. However, this trial was underpowered, and definitive conclusions cannot be made due to its early termination.

The combination of gemcitabine and carboplatin has also been explored. Trials have reported OR rates ranging from 44% to 68% and CR rates ranging from 6% to 23% [29–31]. An Italian randomized phase II study comparing gemcitabine plus cisplatin versus gemcitabine plus carboplatin has been reported in preliminary form. Overall and complete response rates favored the cisplatin-containing regimen (Table 14.1) [32]. A phase III trial comparing the gemcitabine plus carboplatin regimen to the three-drug regimen of carboplatin plus methotrexate plus vinblastine has been initiated by the EORTC in patients who cannot tolerate cisplatin therapy.

New Carboplatin Triplets

Several carboplatin triplets have been studied including: paclitaxel plus carboplatin plus methotrexate [33], paclitaxel plus carboplatin plus gemcitabine [34], and methotrexate plus carboplatin plus vinblastine (M-CAV) [35]. In general, these regimens have been associated with slightly higher response proportions and slightly increased toxicity compared with historical trials of carboplatin doublets. No phase III trials have explored the activity of these triplets relative to standard therapy.

Carboplatin Compared to Cisplatin

Despite the similar response proportions of single-agent carboplatin compared to single-agent cisplatin, controversy still exists regarding the relative value of carboplatin in TCC, particularly in combination regimens. The randomized phase II trials exploring combination regimens with cisplatin compared to carboplatin consistently report higher overall and complete response rates for the cisplatin-containing regimens [32,35,36]. Consequently, in patients with advanced TCC without absolute contraindications (e.g., poor creatinine clearance, solitary kidney, poor performance status), cisplatin-based therapy should be considered the treatment of choice.

Nonplatinum Combinations

In an alternate attempt to improve the efficacy and tolerability of combination chemotherapy in advanced TCC, regimens devoid of platinum analogues have been developed. These regimens include paclitaxel plus ifosfamide [37], paclitaxel plus gemcitabine [38,39], and docetaxel plus gemcitabine [40]. Several of these trials were performed in patients who had previously received cisplatin-based therapy. Overall, these regimens were well tolerated. However, hematologic toxicity was prominent, particularly in the pretreated population. Noteworthy activity was seen with these regimens, including varying rates of complete responses, but the role of these regimens in the treatment of patients with metastatic TCC has not been defined.

Novel Therapeutic Strategies in Metastatic Transitional Cell Carcinoma

Despite the promising activity of the newer combination regimens in TCC, the majority of patients still succumb to their disease, necessitating further exploration in approaches to treatment. One novel approach is the administration of sequential dose-dense chemotherapy based on the Norton-Simon hypothesis, a mathematical prediction model of chemotherapy sensitivity derived from the Gompertzian growth rates of tumors [41]. Other studies are exploring novel targeted therapies.

Given the promising results with the Ifosfamide, pacliTaxel, and cisPlatin (ITP) regimen, a pilot study of sequenced therapy with Adriamycin (doxorubicin) and gemcitabine (AG) followed by ITP was initiated [42]. A preliminary analysis of 21 patients treated with this regimen showed a major response in 18 patients (87%; 95% CI, 71–100%) and a complete response in 43% of patients (95% CI, 22–64%) [43]. Importantly, the sequential use of ITP increased complete and partial response rates after the initial AG doublet.

Chemotherapy regimens that include new agents targeting the epidermal growth factor receptor (EGFR) pathway are also under study. The Southwest Oncology Group is evaluating trastuzumab given in combination with paclitaxel, carboplatin, and gemcitabine [44]. The selective EGFR tyrosine kinase inhibitor ZD1839, in combination with either gemcitabine/cisplatin or gemcitabine/carboplatin, is being explored as first-line therapy in two Cancer and Leukemia Group B (CALGB) trials.

Postchemotherapy Surgery in Metastatic Transitional Cell Carcinoma

The importance of postchemotherapy surgery in the setting of minimal residual disease after achieving a "near" complete response to chemotherapy has been highlighted in several analyses [45–47]. In a series of 203 patients treated on five trials with MVAC, 50 patients underwent postchemotherapy surgery for suspected or known residual disease [45]. Seventeen patients had no viable tumor found at postchemotherapy surgery. In three patients, the residual disease was unresectable. In the remaining 30, residual TCC was completely resected, resulting in a complete response to chemotherapy plus surgery. Of these 30 patients, 10 (33%) remained alive at 5 years, similar to results attained for patients achieving a complete response to chemotherapy alone. Optimal candidates for postchemotherapy resection of residual disease had prechemotherapy disease limited to the primary site or lymph nodes.

Recommendations for Treatment of Metastatic Transitional Cell Carcinoma

Over the past two decades, multiple chemotherapeutic regimens with activity in TCC have been introduced. Additionally, the importance of baseline prognostic factors, comorbidities, and postchemotherapy surgery has been recognized. Integrating this information allows the development of a rational approach to the treatment of individual patients (Fig. 14.1). Based on phase III data, GC or MVAC is recommended for patients with metastatic TCC who can tolerate cisplatin-based therapy and who have potential for long-term benefit.

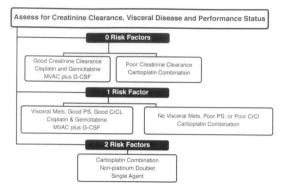

Fig. 14.1. Memorial Sloan-Kettering Cancer Center's algorithm for the management of patients with advanced/metastatic transitional cell carcinoma based on baseline prognostic factors and renal function. CrCl, creatinine clearance; Mets, metastases; PS, performance status.

Perioperative Chemotherapy for Transitional Cell Carcinoma

Despite potentially curative surgery, approximately 50% of patients with muscle-invasive TCC develop metastases and die of disease. Given the chemosensitivity of TCC, attempts to improve survival have focused on administering chemotherapy in the perioperative setting.

Neoadjuvant Chemotherapy

Administering chemotherapy prior to surgery offers several potential advantages. Systemic therapy is initiated sooner, and patients may be able to tolerate treatment better in the preoperative state. Furthermore, the response of the primary tumor to chemotherapy can be assessed, which is of prognostic significance. In a study of patients treated with neoadjuvant cisplatin-based therapy followed by definitive surgery, 91% of patients who responded to chemotherapy (defined as pathologic stage ≤T1) were alive at a median follow-up of 25 months compared to 37% of nonresponders [48].

Several randomized trials have explored neoadjuvant chemotherapy in TCC (Table 14.2). Although many of these trials failed to show a benefit for chemotherapy, the studies suffered from small sample size [49], suboptimal chemotherapy [50,51], premature closure [52], or inadequate follow-up time [53]. Recently,

well-designed trials utilizing effective chemotherapeutic regimens have shifted the treatment paradigm in muscle-invasive disease toward the use of perioperative chemotherapy [54–56].

Intergroup trial 0080 randomized patients with T2 to T4a TCC of the bladder to radical cystectomy alone (154 patients) compared to three cycles of MVAC followed by radical cystectomy (153 patients) [55]. The use of neoadjuvant chemotherapy was associated with a higher rate of complete pathologic response (38% compared to 15%, $p < .001$). At a median follow-up of 8.7 years, improvements in median survival (77 compared to 46 months, $p = .06$) and 5-year survival (57% compared to 43%, $p = .06$) favored the neoadjuvant MVAC arm. Although approximately one third of patients treated with MVAC developed grade ≥3 hematologic or gastrointestinal toxicity, there were no treatment-related deaths, and neoadjuvant chemotherapy did not adversely impact the ability to proceed with radical cystectomy or increase adverse events related to surgery.

The Medical Research Council (MRC)/EORTC performed a large trial in which 976 patients were enrolled and randomized to neoadjuvant cisplatin, methotrexate, and vinblastine (CMV) (491 patients) or no neoadjuvant chemotherapy (485 patients) [57]. Management of the primary tumor involved cystectomy, radiation therapy, or both. An 8% improvement in time to progression and a 5.5% difference in absolute 3-year survival (Hazard ratio (HR) = 0.85; 95% CI, 0.71–1.02) favoring the neoadjuvant chemotherapy arm were reported. The results of this trial were recently updated, and, at a median follow-up of approximately 7 years, a statistically significant improvement in survival was observed for patients who received neoadjuvant chemotherapy (HR = 0.85; 95% CI, 0.72–1.0; $p = .048$) [54]. This trial, well powered and with adequate follow-up, demonstrated both a survival benefit and improved locoregional control with neoadjuvant chemotherapy.

A recent meta-analysis reviewed data from 2688 patients treated on 10 randomized trials evaluating neoadjuvant chemotherapy for invasive TCC [58]. Of note, this analysis did not include data from Intergroup 0080. Compared to local treatment alone, neoadjuvant platinum-based combination chemotherapy was associated with a significant benefit in overall survival

Table 14.2. Randomized trials of adjuvant chemotherapy

Trial organization/country	No. of patients	Treatment arms	Chemotherapy survival benefit
University of Southern California, Norris Comprehensive Cancer Center (61)	91	Cyst → CAP Cyst	Yes
University of Mainz (60)	49	Cyst → M-VAC/M-VEC Cyst	Yes
Swiss Group for Clinical Cancer Research (62)	77	Cyst → C Cyst	No
Italian Uro-Oncologic Cooperative Group (59)	83	Cyst → CM Cyst	No
Stanford University (63)	50	Cyst → CMV Cyst	No
MD Anderson Cancer Center (68)	140	MVAC → Cyst → MVAC Cyst → MVAC	*

M, methotrexate; C, cisplatin; V, vinblastine; A, (Adriamycin (doxorubicin); E, epirubicin; Cyst, cystectomy.
* In this trial, both arms received perioperative chemotherapy. Patients were randomized to receive chemotherapy both pre- and postoperatively or only postoperatively. There were no significant differences in outcome between the two arms.

(HR = 0.87; 95% CI, 0.78–0.98; p = .016), a 13% decrease in the risk of death, and a 5% absolute survival benefit at 5 years (overall survival increased from 45% to 50%). When trials utilizing single-agent cisplatin were included, the survival benefit did not achieve statistical significance (HR = 0.91; 95% CI, 0.83–1.01; p = .084).

Adjuvant Chemotherapy

As with neoadjuvant chemotherapy, administration of chemotherapy after surgery is associated with potential advantages and disadvantages. Foremost, an adjuvant approach allows the administration of chemotherapy to be based on pathologic stage. Given the inaccuracies in clinical staging, this avoids overtreatment of patients who are estimated to have a reasonable outcome from surgery alone. Administration of chemotherapy after surgery also prevents delays in carrying out potentially curative surgery. The major disadvantages associated with adjuvant chemotherapy are the potential difficulties of tolerating treatment postoperatively and the lack of an objective means to assess response after the primary tumor is removed.

At least six randomized trials have evaluated the use of adjuvant chemotherapy following cys-

tectomy for muscle-invasive TCC (Table 14.3) [59–63]. Although all of these trials used cisplatin-based chemotherapy and had surgery as a control arm, two trials primarily evaluated patients with bladder-confined disease [59,62]. These latter studies did not detect a survival benefit, but patients in these studies would be expected to have a better prognosis. Of the remaining trials, two demonstrated a survival benefit with adjuvant chemotherapy [61,62].

As a consequence of small sample size, inclusion of "good-prognosis" patients, and potentially inadequate chemotherapy, the data supporting adjuvant chemotherapy are less compelling than the data supporting neoadjuvant chemotherapy. In an effort to definitively address this issue, two large cooperative group trials are under way. The EORTC is randomizing patients with pT3-T4 or node-positive disease to immediate cisplatin-based chemotherapy (MVAC or GC) or similar chemotherapy at the time of relapse. In a trial conducted by the CALGB/Clinical Trial Support Unit (CTSU), patients meeting the same pathological criteria are randomized to either the sequential doublet of AG-TP (doxorubicin plus gemcitabine followed by paclitaxel plus cisplatin) or a conventional GC regimen.

Table 14.3. Randomized trials of neoadjuvant chemotherapy

Trial organization/country	No. of patients	Treatment arms	Chemotherapy survival benefit
MRC/EORTC (54)	975	CMV → RT/Cyst/both RT/Cyst/both	Yes
INT-0080 (55)	317	MVAC → Cyst Cyst	Yes
Nordic-1 (56)	325	C+A → RT/Cyst RT/Cyst	*Yes
Nordic-2 (65)	317	M+C → Cyst Cyst	No
Italy (GUONE) (49)	206	MVAC → Cyst Cyst	No
Italy (Genoa) (66)	104	C+5-FU → Cyst Cyst	No
Spain (CUETO) (51)	122	C → Cyst Cyst	No
Australia/UK (50)	255	C → RT RT	No
MGH/RTOG (52)	123	MCV → Cyst/RT Cyst/RT	No
GISTV (53)	171	MVEC → Cyst Cyst	No
Egypt (67)	194	Carboplatin MV→ Cyst Cyst	No

MRC, Medical Research Council; EORTC, European Organization for Research and Treatment; INT, United States Intergroup; GUONE, Gruppo Uro-Oncologico del Nord Est; CUETO, Club Urologico Espagnol de Tratiemneto Oncologico; MGH, Massachussetts General Hospital; RTOG, Radiation Therapy Oncology Group; GITSV, Gruppo Italiano per lo Studio dei Tumori de la Vesicula; M, methotrexate; C, cisplatin; V, vinblastine; A, Adriamycin (doxorubicin); 5-FU, 5-fluorouracil; E, epirubicin; Cyst, cystectomy; RT, radiation therapy.
* Benefit for subset with T3–T4.

Recommendations for Treatment of Locally Advanced Transitional Cell Carcinoma

Two large randomized trials and a meta-analysis support the concept that neoadjuvant chemotherapy for patients with muscle-invasive bladder cancer imparts a survival benefit over surgery alone. This approach should be considered for patients who are candidates for cisplatin-based combination chemotherapy and radical cystectomy. For patients who have not received neoadjuvant chemotherapy and who have extravesicular or node-positive disease following cystectomy, enrollment in a clinical trial should be encouraged. If a patient is not protocol-eligible, adjuvant cisplatin-based combination chemotherapy is a reasonable consideration.

References

1. Herr H, Shipley W, Bajorin D. Cancer of the bladder. In: DeVita V Jr, Hellman S, Rosenberg S, eds. Cancer: Principles and Practice of Oncology, 6th ed. Philadelphia: Lippincott Williams & Wilkins, 2001:1396–1418.
2. Raghavan D, Shipley WU, Garnick MB, et al. Biology and management of bladder cancer. N Engl J Med 1990;322:1129–1138.
3. Sternberg CN, Yagoda A, Scher HI, et al. Preliminary results of M-VAC (methotrexate, vinblastine, doxorubicin and cisplatin) for transitional cell carcinoma of the urothelium. J Urol 1985;133: 403–407.
4. Sternberg CN, Yagoda A, Scher HI, et al. Methotrexate, vinblastine, doxorubicin, and cisplatin for advanced transitional cell carcinoma of the urothelium. Efficacy and patterns of response and relapse. Cancer 1989;64:2448–2458.
5. Loehrer PJ Sr, Einhorn LH, Elson PJ, et al. A randomized comparison of cisplatin alone or in com-

bination with methotrexate, vinblastine, and doxorubicin in patients with metastatic urothelial carcinoma: a cooperative group study. J Clin Oncol 1992;10:1066–1073.

6. Logothetis CJ, Dexeus F, Sella A, et al. A prospective randomized trial comparing CISCA to MVAC chemotherapy in advanced metastatic urothelial tumors. J Clin Oncol 1990;8:1050–1055.

7. Saxman SB, Propert KJ, Einhorn LH, et al. Long-term follow-up of a phase III intergroup study of cisplatin alone or in combination with methotrexate, vinblastine, and doxorubicin in patients with metastatic urothelial carcinoma: a cooperative group study. J Clin Oncol 1997;15:2564–2569.

8. Sternberg CN, de Mulder PH, Schornagel JH, et al. Randomized phase III trial of high-dose-intensity methotrexate, vinblastine, doxorubicin, and cisplatin (MVAC) chemotherapy and recombinant human granulocyte colony-stimulating factor versus classic MVAC in advanced urothelial tract tumors: European Organization for Research and Treatment of Cancer Protocol no. 30924. J Clin Oncol 2001;19:2638–2646.

9. Bajorin DF, Dodd PM, Mazumdar M, et al. Long-term survival in metastatic transitional-cell carcinoma and prognostic factors predicting outcome of therapy. J Clin Oncol 1999;17:3173–3181.

10. Bellmunt J, Albanell J, Paz-Ares L, et al. Pretreatment prognostic factors for survival in patients with advanced urothelial tumors treated in a phase I/II trial with paclitaxel, cisplatin, and gemcitabine. Cancer 2002;95:751–757.

11. von der Maase H, Andersen L, Crino L, et al. Weekly gemcitabine and cisplatin combination therapy in patients with transitional cell carcinoma of the urothelium: a phase II clinical trial. Ann Oncol 1999;10:1461–1465.

12. Kaufman D, Raghavan D, Carducci M, et al. Phase II trial of gemcitabine plus cisplatin in patients with metastatic urothelial cancer. J Clin Oncol 2000;18:1921–1927.

13. Moore MJ, Winquist EW, Murray N, et al. Gemcitabine plus cisplatin, an active regimen in advanced urothelial cancer: a phase II trial of the National Cancer Institute of Canada Clinical Trials Group. J Clin Oncol 1999;17:2876–2881.

14. von der Maase H, Hansen SW, Roberts JT, et al. Gemcitabine and cisplatin versus methotrexate, vinblastine, doxorubicin, and cisplatin in advanced or metastatic bladder cancer: results of a large, randomized, multinational, multicenter, phase III study. J Clin Oncol 2000;18:3068–3077.

15. Dreicer R, Manola J, Roth BJ, et al. Phase II study of cisplatin and paclitaxel in advanced carcinoma of the urothelium: an Eastern Cooperative Oncology Group Study. J Clin Oncol 2000;18:1058–1061.

16. Garcia del Muro X, Marcuello E, Guma J, et al. Phase II multicentre study of docetaxel plus cisplatin in patients with advanced urothelial cancer. Br J Cancer 2002;86:326–330.

17. Sengelov L, Kamby C, Lund B, et al. Docetaxel and cisplatin in metastatic urothelial cancer: a phase II study. J Clin Oncol 1998;16:3392–3397.

18. Bamias A, Aravantinos G, Deliveliotis C, et al. Docetaxel and cisplatin with granulocyte colony-stimulating factor (G-CSF) versus MVAC with G-CSF in advanced urothelial carcinoma: a multicenter, randomized, phase III study from the Hellenic Cooperative Oncology Group. J Clin Oncol 2004;22:1–9.

19. Bajorin DF, McCaffrey JA, Dodd PM, et al. Ifosfamide, paclitaxel, and cisplatin for patients with advanced transitional cell carcinoma of the urothelial tract: final report of a phase II trial evaluating two dosing schedules. Cancer 2000;88:1671–1678.

20. Bellmunt J, Guillem V, Paz-Ares L, et al. Phase I-II study of paclitaxel, cisplatin, and gemcitabine in advanced transitional-cell carcinoma of the urothelium. Spanish Oncology Genitourinary Group. J Clin Oncol 2000;18:3247–3255.

21. Mottet-Auselo N, Bons-Rosset F, Costa P, et al. Carboplatin and urothelial tumors. Oncology 1993;50(suppl 2):28–36.

22. Vaughn DJ, Malkowicz SB, Zoltick B, et al. Paclitaxel plus carboplatin in advanced carcinoma of the urothelium: an active and tolerable outpatient regimen. J Clin Oncol 1998;16:255–260.

23. Vaughn DJ, Manola J, Dreicer R, et al. Phase II study of paclitaxel plus carboplatin in patients with advanced carcinoma of the urothelium and renal dysfunction (E2896): a trial of the Eastern Cooperative Oncology Group. Cancer 2002;95:1022–1027.

24. Redman BG, Smith DC, Flaherty L, et al. Phase II trial of paclitaxel and carboplatin in the treatment of advanced urothelial carcinoma. J Clin Oncol 1998;16:1844–1848.

25. Pycha A, Grbovic M, Posch B, et al. Paclitaxel and carboplatin in patients with metastatic transitional cell cancer of the urinary tract. Urology 1999;53:510–515.

26. Zielinski CC, Schnack B, Grbovic M, et al. Paclitaxel and carboplatin in patients with metastatic urothelial cancer: results of a phase II trial. Br J Cancer 1998;78:370–374.

27. Small EJ, Lew D, Redman BG, et al. Southwest Oncology Group Study of paclitaxel and carboplatin for advanced transitional-cell carcinoma: the importance of survival as a clinical trial end point. J Clin Oncol 2000;18:2537–2544.

28. Dreicer R, Manola J, Roth BJ, et al. ECOG 4897: Phase III trial of methotrexate, vinblastine, doxorubicin, and cisplatin (M-VAC) versus carbo-

platin and paclitaxel in patients with advanced carcinoma of the urothelium [abstract]. Proc Am Soc Clin Oncol 2003;22:384(abstract 1542).

29. Carles J, Nogue M. Gemcitabine/carboplatin in advanced urothelial cancer. Semin Oncol 2001;28: 19–24.

30. Bellmunt J, de Wit R, Albanell J, et al. A feasibility study of carboplatin with fixed dose of gemcitabine in "unfit" patients with advanced bladder cancer. Eur J Cancer 2001;37:2212–2215.

31. Santoro A, Santoro M, Maiorino L, et al. Phase II trial of gemcitabine plus carboplatin for urothelial transitional cell carcinoma in advanced or metastatic stage. Ann Oncol 1998;9(suppl 2):647.

32. Carteni G, Dogliotti L, Crucitta A, et al. Phase II randomised trial of gemcitabine plus cisplatin (GP) and gemcitabine plus carboplatin (GC) in patients (pts) with advanced or metastatic transitional cell carcinoma of the urothelium (TCCU) [abstract]. Proc Am Soc Clin Oncol 2003;22: 384(abstract 1543).

33. Edelman MJ, Meyers FJ, Miller TR, et al. Phase I/II study of paclitaxel, carboplatin, and methotrexate in advanced transitional cell carcinoma: a well-tolerated regimen with activity independent of p53 mutation. Urology 2000;55:521–525.

34. Hussain M, Vaishampayan U, Du W, et al. Combination paclitaxel, carboplatin, and gemcitabine is an active treatment for advanced urothelial cancer. J Clin Oncol 2001;19:2527–2533.

35. Bellmunt J, Ribas A, Eres N, et al. Carboplatin-based versus cisplatin-based chemotherapy in the treatment of surgically incurable advanced bladder carcinoma. Cancer 1997;80:1966–1972.

36. Petrioli R, Frediani B, Manganelli A, et al. Comparison between a cisplatin-containing regimen and a carboplatin-containing regimen for recurrent or metastatic bladder cancer patients. A randomized phase II study. Cancer 1996;77:344–351.

37. Sweeney CJ, Williams SD, Finch DE, et al. A Phase II study of paclitaxel and ifosfamide for patients with advanced refractory carcinoma of the urothelium. Cancer 1999;86:514–518.

38. Meluch AA, Greco FA, Burris HA 3rd, et al. Paclitaxel and gemcitabine chemotherapy for advanced transitional-cell carcinoma of the urothelial tract: a phase II trial of the Minnie pearl cancer research network. J Clin Oncol 2001;19: 3018–3024.

39. Sternberg CN, Calabro F, Pizzocaro G, et al. Chemotherapy with an every-2–week regimen of gemcitabine and paclitaxel in patients with transitional cell carcinoma who have received prior cisplatin-based therapy. Cancer 2001;92:2993–2998.

40. Dreicer R, Manola J, Schneider DJ, et al. Phase II trial of gemcitabine and docetaxel in patients with advanced carcinoma of the urothelium: a trial of the Eastern Cooperative Oncology Group. Cancer 2003;97:2743–2747.

41. Norton L, Simon R. The Norton-Simon hypothesis revisited. Cancer Treat Rep 1986;70:163–169.

42. Dodd PM, McCaffrey JA, Hilton S, et al. Phase I evaluation of sequential doxorubicin gemcitabine then ifosfamide paclitaxel cisplatin for patients with unresectable or metastatic transitional-cell carcinoma of the urothelial tract. J Clin Oncol 2000;18:840–846.

43. Maluf F, Hilton S, Nanus D, et al. Sequential doxorubicin/gemcitabine (AG) and ifosfamide, paclitaxel, and cisplatin (ITP) chemotherapy (AG-ITP) in patients with metastatic or locally advanced transitional cell carcinoma of the urothelium [abstract]. Proc Am Soc Clin Oncol 2000;19: 342a(abstract 1344).

44. Hussain M, Smith DC, Vaishampayan U, et al. Trastuzumab (T), paclitaxel (P), carboplatin (C) and gemcitabine (G) in patients with advanced urothelial cancer and overexpression of HER-2. (NCI study #198) [abstract]. Proc Am Soc Clin Oncol 2003;22:391(abstract 1569).

45. Dodd PM, McCaffrey JA, Herr H, et al. Outcome of postchemotherapy surgery after treatment with methotrexate, vinblastine, doxorubicin, and cisplatin in patients with unresectable or metastatic transitional cell carcinoma. J Clin Oncol 1999;17: 2546–2552.

46. Donat SM, Herr HW, Bajorin DF, et al. Methotrexate, vinblastine, doxorubicin and cisplatin chemotherapy and cystectomy for unresectable bladder cancer. J Urol 1996;156:368–371.

47. Miller R, Freiha F, Reese J, et al. Surgical restaging of patients with advanced transitional cell carcinoma of the urothelium treated with cisplatin, methotrexate, and vinblastine: update of the Stanford University experience [abstract]. Proc Am Soc Clin Oncol 1992;10:167.

48. Splinter TA, Scher HI, Denis L, et al. The prognostic value of the pathological response to combination chemotherapy before cystectomy in patients with invasive bladder cancer. European Organization for Research on Treatment of Cancer—Genitourinary Group. J Urol 1992;147:606–608.

49. Bassi P, Pagano F, Pappagallo G, et al. Neoadjuvant M-VAC of invasive bladder cancer: G.U.O.N.E. multicenter phase III trial (abstract 567). Eur Urol 1998;33:142.

50. Wallace DM, Raghavan D, Kelly KA, et al. Neoadjuvant (pre-emptive) cisplatin therapy in invasive transitional cell carcinoma of the bladder. Br J Urol 1991;67:608–615.

51. Martinez-Pineiro JA, Gonzalez Martin M, Arocena F, et al. Neoadjuvant cisplatin chemotherapy before radical cystectomy in invasive transitional cell carcinoma of the bladder: a prospective randomized phase III study. J Urol 1995;153:964–973.

52. Shipley WU, Winter KA, Kaufman DS, et al. Phase III trial of neoadjuvant chemotherapy in patients with invasive bladder cancer treated with selective bladder preservation by combined radiation therapy and chemotherapy: initial results of Radiation Therapy Oncology Group 89-03. J Clin Oncol 1998;16:3576–3583.

53. Cortesi E. Neoadjuvant treatment for locally advanced bladder cancer: a prospective randomized clinical trial [abstract]. Proc Am Soc Clin Oncol 1995;14:237(abstract 623).

54. Hall R. Updated results of a randomised controlled trial of neoadjuvant cisplatin (C), methotrexate (M) and vinblastine (V) chemotherapy for muscle-invasive bladder cancer [abstract]. Proc Am Soc Clin Oncol 2002;21:178a(abstract 710).

55. Grossman HB, Natale RB, Tangen CM, et al. Neoadjuvant chemotherapy plus cystectomy compared with cystectomy alone for locally advanced bladder cancer. N Engl J Med 2003;349:859–866.

56. Malmstrom PU, Rintala E, Wahlqvist R, et al. Five-year followup of a prospective trial of radical cystectomy and neoadjuvant chemotherapy. Nordic Cystectomy Trial I. The Nordic Cooperative Bladder Cancer Study Group. J Urol 1996;155: 1903–1906.

57. Neoadjuvant cisplatin, methotrexate, and vinblastine chemotherapy for muscle-invasive bladder cancer: a randomised controlled trial. International collaboration of trialists. Lancet 1999;354: 533–540.

58. Neoadjuvant chemotherapy in invasive bladder cancer: a systematic review and meta-analysis. Lancet 2003;361:1927–1934.

59. Bono AV, Benvenuti C, Reali L, et al. Adjuvant chemotherapy in advanced bladder cancer. Italian Uro-Oncologic Cooperative Group. Prog Clin Biol Res 1989;303:533–540.

60. Stockle M, Meyenburg W, Wellek S, et al. Advanced bladder cancer (stages pT3b, pT4a, pN1 and pN2): improved survival after radical cystectomy and 3 adjuvant cycles of chemotherapy. Results of a controlled prospective study. J Urol 1992;148:302–306.

61. Skinner DG, Daniels JR, Russell CA, et al. The role of adjuvant chemotherapy following cystectomy for invasive bladder cancer: a prospective comparative trial. J Urol 1991;145:459–464.

62. Studer UE, Bacchi M, Biedermann C, et al. Adjuvant cisplatin chemotherapy following cystectomy for bladder cancer: results of a prospective randomized trial. J Urol 1994;152:81–84.

63. Freiha F, Reese J, Torti FM. A randomized trial of radical cystectomy versus radical cystectomy plus cisplatin, vinblastine and methotrexate chemotherapy for muscle invasive bladder cancer. J Urol 1996;155:495–499.

64. Siefker-Radtke AO, Millikan RE, Tu SM, et al. Phase III trial of fluorouracil, interferon alpha-2b, and cisplatin versus methotrexate, vinblastine, doxorubicin, and cisplatin in metastatic or unresectable urothelial cancer. J Clin Oncol 2002;20: 1361–1367.

65. Malmstrom PU, Rintala E, Wahlqvist R, et al. Neoadjuvant cisplatin-methotrexate chemotherapy of invasive bladder cancer: Nordic cystectomy trial 2: XIVth Congress of the European Association of Urology [abstract]. Eur Urol 1999;35(suppl 2):60(abstract 238).

66. Curotto A, Martorana G, Venturini M, et al. Multicenter randomized study on the comparison between radical cystectomy alone and neoadjuvant alternate chemoradiotherapy before radical cystectomy: Assessment over 104 patients. In: Giuliani L, Puppo P, eds. Urology. Genova: Monduzzi, 1992:489–493.

67. Abol-Enein H, El-Mekresh M, El-Baz M, et al. Neoadjuvant chemotherapy in treatment of invasive transitional bladder cancer: a controlled prospective randomized study [abstract]. Br J Urol 1997;80(suppl 2):49(abstract 191).

68. Millikan R, Dinney C, Swanson D, et al. Integrated therapy for locally advanced bladder cancer: final report of a randomized trial of cystectomy plus adjuvant M-VAC versus cystectomy with both preoperative and postoperative M-VAC. J Clin Oncol 2001;19:4005–4013.

Gene Therapy of Urothelial Malignancy

Sunjay Jain and J. Kilian Mellon

The basic principle of gene therapy centers on the use or manipulation of genetic material to achieve a therapeutic effect. The term, therefore, encompasses a huge number of treatment strategies. Clinically gene therapy for cancer is still in its infancy but there are many experimental studies that suggest it will have a useful role. This chapter summarizes the current status of gene therapy for bladder cancer; there is very little data on its use in upper tract urothelial tumors.

When considering patients with bladder cancer it is important to appreciate the wide range of clinical presentations with very different standard treatment strategies. Four main groups can be identified:

1. Low- to medium-risk superficial disease, currently managed with cystoscopic surveillance and intravesical chemotherapy
2. High-risk superficial disease (carcinoma in situ [CIS] and G3pT1 tumors), which, although mostly managed by endoscopic measures and intravesical bacille Calmette-Guérin (BCG), are at high risk of progression and may require radical treatment
3. Invasive, nonmetastatic disease suitable for attempted curative treatment by radical cystectomy or radiotherapy; overall cure rates are unsatisfactory at approximately 50%; adjuvant chemotherapy may improve outcome
4. Metastatic disease, where any treatment is palliative and prognosis is poor

There is certainly scope for improvement in groups 2 to 4. Intravesical administration of gene therapy is the most commonly utilized method of delivery, and it is hoped that this will improve upon BCG in reducing progression of high-risk superficial disease. Adjuvant gene therapy prior to attempted curative treatment of muscle invasive disease is likely to be used in conjunction with chemotherapy. Intratumoral injection, intravesical therapy, and systemic administration could be used. It is in patients with metastatic disease that initial clinical trials are likely to take place, and there is already phase I data from other cancer types. Clearly in this situation balancing the safety and efficacy of systemic gene therapy is paramount.

This chapter describes the technical aspects of gene therapy in relation to transitional cell cancers, and methods in which gene therapy has been applied in bladder malignancy. A discussion of the ethical aspects of gene therapy is beyond the scope of this chapter.

Vectors for Transfer of Genetic Information

Effective and safe gene delivery to the target cells is the cornerstone of successful gene therapy. Methods remain far from perfect.

The gene delivery system (vector) is most conveniently divided into nonviral and viral.

Nonviral Methods

Nonviral gene delivery systems have to overcome the physical barrier of the cell membrane, and in vivo this is most often achieved by surrounding the DNA in a cationic lipid liposome. This is then endocytosed by cells. Although liposomes have minimal toxicity, they are a poorly efficient method of gene delivery. In bladder tumors this method of gene delivery has been described in a murine orthotopic bladder cancer model [1]. Other methods described include bombardment with high-speed micropellets and electrotransfection using a pulsed direct current after direct injection of the vector [2]. In these experiments reasonable gene transfer was achieved; however, it was performed directly into surgically exposed bladder and therefore not really comparable with clinical situations. Overall the present data suggest that nonviral methods are likely to be poor in vivo and most suitable to those diseases in which cells can be manipulated outside the body and then returned (e.g., bone marrow for the treatment of hematological disease).

Viral Methods

Viruses have evolved to be efficient in introducing their DNA into host cells, where it is converted into protein product and hence are obvious methods of gene delivery for therapy. There are clearly drawbacks in terms of toxicity, both from the viruses themselves and due to the immunogenicity of viral antigens.

The vector in most bladder cancer gene therapy experiments has been the adenovirus, and this will be discussed in some detail. There are many other DNA virus types that have been used in individual experiments, but the differences are subtle. The poxvirus vaccinia is the only one used in a human study. Retroviruses are not commonly used in bladder cancer but will be described because of their fundamental differences from DNA viruses.

Adenovirus

This virus attaches to cells via a specific receptor the Coxsackie and adenovirus receptor (CAR). Transfection can be very efficient, but the adenovirus can carry only relatively small genes and expression is transient (4 to 8 weeks). Thus

repeated dosing is required. The virus can be highly immunogenic, and patients report systemic upset with flu-like symptoms. In vivo work has suggested possible liver toxicity [3], although this has not been borne out during short-term administration in initial phase I studies [4].

One issue with adenoviral gene transfer concerns reports that bladder cancer cell lines express variable levels of CAR, and this may affect the efficiency of transduction [5]. Indeed it has recently been demonstrated immunohistochemically that CAR expression is decreased in more aggressive human bladder cancers [6]. This may be because the CAR functions as an adhesion molecule. Despite this potential difficulty, adenoviral gene transfer seems the most promising method for urothelial cancers at present. Methods to overcome the CAR receptor problem include the use of drugs to increase CAR expression in bladder cells such as sodium butyrate [7] and sodium valproate [8]. It has also been shown that coadministration of CAR DNA along with the therapeutic gene results in increased viral transduction [9].

Bypassing the CAR receptor has been attempted by engineering viruses that can enter the cell via other adhesion sites. In one study both the epidermal growth factor receptor (EGFR) and epithelial cell adhesion molecule (Ep-CAM) have been targeted [10]. The EGFR seemed most promising, increasing transgene expression by up to 12.5 times. As EGFR is overexpressed in many bladder cancers, this form of targeting may increase the specificity of gene therapy for tumor cells compared to normal urothelium. Chimeric viruses that utilize parts of other viruses that do not enter bladder cells via CAR have also been recently described [11].

Although improving the transfer of adenovirus to superficial cells is clearly important and likely to be improved by the above techniques, penetration deeper into the tissue remains a problem. Experiments on intact urothelium (from normal ureters) have demonstrated this [12]. The deeper layers do possess CAR, and so there are likely to be other factors responsible probably related to the natural barrier function of the urothelium. A major component of this innate immunity is the glycosaminoglycans (GAG) layer. Disruption of this layer using ethanol [13] and hydrochloric acid

[14] has been shown to improve adenoviral transduction in rat models. These methods, however, are likely to be toxic in clinical practice. More subtle methods have used specific polyamides that are capable of increasing viral transgene expression in the bladder without damaging the umbrella cell layer of urothelium [15]. For example, the polyamide Syn3, when injected intravesically into mouse bladder, increases gene transfer [16]. Kuball et al. [17] have investigated intravesical gene transfer in the clinical setting using adenovirus. They used the polyamide, *N,N-615-(3-D-glucoamidropgl) chloramide*, Big CHAP to enhance viral transduction. Histological assessment revealed that virus had penetrated all layers of the urothelium and was also in the submucosal tissue. Interestingly, when tissue cultures of normal urothelium and transitional cell carcinoma are compared, the latter is susceptible to viral transduction at much lower doses [12]. This is likely to be due to loss of barrier function in the tumor tissue.

Pox Viruses

Pox viruses are used extensively in gene therapy, but there are only a few reports of use in the bladder. A phase I trial to assess the feasibility of using vaccinia for intravesical gene transfer showed some promise [18]. In this study patients scheduled to undergo cystectomy for muscle-invasive bladder cancer received intravesical vaccinia three times in the 2 weeks prior to surgery. Mild dysuria was the only reported side effect. There was marked immune response in the bladder and histological evidence of viral infection. Recent in vivo work has suggested that pox viruses are more efficient at gene transfer than adenoviral vectors when the intravesical route is used [19].

Retroviruses

Retroviral gene transfer is unique in allowing integration of the therapeutic gene into the target cells nuclear DNA. This leads to more prolonged gene expression and allows the gene to be passed to daughter cells. However, there are risks of insertional mutagenesis at the points where the retrovirus integrates into the host genome. Although retrovirus-mediated gene transfer is probably the commonest method used in cancer gene therapy, there are far fewer examples of retrovirus mediated gene transfer in bladder cancer compared to adenovirus. No clinical trials have yet taken place.

The advantages and disadvantages of the various methods of gene transfer described are summarized in Table 15.1.

Gene Therapy Strategies in Bladder Cancer

There are three main approaches to gene therapy of cancer (Table 15.2):

Table 15.1. Various vectors for gene therapy

Type of vector	Advantages	Disadvantages
Nonviral	1. Noninfectious 2. Can often carry large amounts of DNA	1. Poor transduction in vivo
Adenoviral	1. High infectivity 2. Efficient transfer 3. Infects resting cells	1. Highly immunogenic 2. Limits on size of gene 3. Possible liver toxicity
Pox virus	1. High infectivity 2. Can carry large amount of DNA	1. Possible pathogenesis
Retrovirus	1. Prolonged expression 2. Good transduction in replicating cells	1. Potential for insertional mutagenesis 2. Low infectivity 3. Immunogenic

Table 15.2. Gene therapy approaches in bladder cancer

Corrective	1. Restoration/overexpression of tumor-suppressor genes
	2. Inhibition/destruction of oncogenes and other genes associated with tumor growth
Cytotoxic	1. Suicide gene therapy
	2. Selective tumor cell killing
Immunological	1. Tumor vaccines
	2. In vivo transfection of cytokines

1. In the corrective approach, genetic defects thought to have a major role in the development of malignancy are targeted. These can be genes favoring cancer development (e.g., oncogenes) where an attempt is made to inactivate them, or tumor-suppressor genes that need replacing. As information about the genetics of cancer increases, so do the potential targets for corrective gene therapy.

2. Cytotoxic strategies usually employ the "suicide gene" approach. Here an enzyme is introduced into tumor cells that converts a normally harmless prodrug into a toxic one. Toxicity is usually confined to the transfected cells and those close by (bystander effect)

3. Immunological gene therapy involves introducing a gene that will enhance the local immune response against the tumor. Most commonly the gene transfected is a cytokine (e.g., interleukin-2 [IL-2]).

Corrective Strategies in Gene Therapy of Bladder Cancer

The development of bladder cancer is known to involve activation of a variety of oncogenes combined with loss of vital tumor-suppressor genes. These genes have crucial roles in control of cell proliferation, adhesion, and apoptosis, and are responsible for changes in the cancer cell phenotype from benign to malignant. The rationale of gene therapy in this situation is to restore gene expression in the cell to normal either by replacing lost genes or by inhibiting/destroying those that are overexpressed.

Restoration/Overexpression of Tumor-Suppressor Genes

Reintroducing a missing tumor-suppressor gene into cancer cells has been a popular method of gene therapy in various malignancies. Interestingly even cells that are not deficient in the suppressor gene may be affected by overexpression, extending the potential number of tumors suitable for treatment.

p53

Mutations of *p53* are common in many human cancers, and therapeutic strategies involving its replacement by gene therapy have been the subject of much research. It is highly suitable for bladder cancer, as approximately 50% of human transitional cell carcinomas (TCC) have mutations of *p53*, and these are associated with a poorer prognosis [20]. Efficacy of adenoviral *p53* gene therapy for bladder cancer was demonstrated both in vitro and with direct injection into subcutaneous mouse xenografts [21,22]. Intravesical administration was also shown to be effective in a mouse model and seemed to have minimal systemic effects [3], paving the way for clinical studies, of which two so far have been published.

The first studied the effectiveness of gene transfer in 11 patients who subsequently underwent cystectomy for locally advanced or high-grade superficial disease [17]. It was initially planned as a comparison of intratumoral and intravesical administration of an adenoviral vector containing the complete wild-type human *p53* gene, with dose escalation in both groups. However, early analysis showed a lack of *p53* transgene expression in the three patients where the vector was injected into the tumor, and this arm of the study was discontinued. In contrast, the *p53* transgene was detected in seven of the eight patients who had intravesical administration. Importantly functional activity was assessed by reverse-transcription polymerase chain reaction (RT-PCR) and immunohistochemistry of the *p53* target gene *p21/WAF1*, and this was seen in tissue from patients exposed to the highest dose of vector (7.5×10^{13} particles per instillation). There were only minor local side effects, and although dwell times had to be reduced in some patients, all completed the study.

A subsequent trial carried out at the M.D. Anderson Cancer Center involved administration of intravesical adenoviral *p53* to patients not considered suitable for cystectomy [4]. Three different doses and three regimens of repeated dosing were used and again very little toxicity was seen. Biopsies were taken at 4 to 16 days posttreatment, and unfortunately only 7 of 13 were suitable for RT-PCR to detect the *p53* transgene. Two patients were found to express the transgene, and both had received the highest dose (10^{12} viral particles). One of the reasons for the apparently lower level of successful transfection in this study may be that less tissue was available for analysis. Also while the previous study used a polyamide in an effort to increase penetration of the GAG layer, this was not the case in this trial. Although only a phase I trial, one patient was described who seemed to have significant tumor regression after *p53* therapy. Histology revealed a potent cell-mediated immune response, and the patient had not had previous BCG, so it was felt that the response may have been a nonspecific immune response to the adenoviral vector.

Phase II and III trials, when they occur, are likely to assess the effects of *p53* gene transfer in conjunction with chemotherapy regimens. There has been experimental work that suggests this is a promising strategy. When mice with subcutaneous tumors were injected intratumorally with adenoviral *p53* and also administered intravenous cisplatin, the reduction in tumor growth was greater than with either agent alone [23] (Fig. 15.1). Subsequent work in vitro has shown statistically, using the combination index, that this additional effect is synergistic rather than just additive, implying that gene therapy such as this may target chemoresistant cells [24]. This idea is further supported by work on bladder cancer cell lines known to be cisplatin-resistant, which are more susceptible to *p53* gene therapy than those that are cisplatin-sensitive [25].

p21

p21 is a key downstream mediator of *p53*, responsible for inhibition of cyclin-dependent kinase activity. This may be the mechanism for *p53*-mediated cell cycle arrest, and therefore introduction of *p21* to cancer cells might be expected to have therapeutic potential. Initial

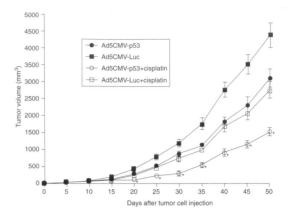

Fig. 15.1. Effect of combined treatment with Ad5CMV-p53 transfer and cisplatin on KoTCC-1 tumor growth in nude mice. Mice were treated with Ad5CMV-p53 alone, Ad5CMV-Luc alone, Ad5CMV-p53 plus cisplatin, or Ad5CMV-Luc plus cisplatin. Seven days after subcutaneous injection of 1×10^6 cells into nude mice, 200 L of Ad5CMV-p53 or Ad5CMV-Luc (1×10^7 PFU/mL) was injected intratumorally and 100 L of cisplatin (1 mg/kg) was injected intravenously twice per week for 2 weeks. Tumor volume was measured twice weekly and calculated by the following formula: length × width × depth × 0.5236. Each data point represents the mean tumor volume and standard deviation in each experimental group containing seven mice. *Significantly different from treatment with Ad5CMV-p53 alone, Ad5CMV-Luc alone, and Ad5CMV-Luc plus cisplatin ($p < .01$, Student's t-test) Ad5CMV-Luc = luciferase labelled control Ad5CMV-p53 = active agent. (From Miyake et al. [23].)

in vitro studies, however, have failed to show a consistent growth inhibitory effect for *p21* gene transfection to bladder tumor cell lines [26].

Retinoblastoma

Loss of *retinoblastoma (RB)* gene function is linked to the initiation and progression of many cancers including bladder cancer. When an adenovirus containing the *RB* gene was injected into established (> 28 days) subcutaneous *RB*-defective mouse bladder tumors, growth rate was reduced significantly [27]. Interestingly, a modified form of the *RB* gene that codes for a truncated protein missing the N-terminal 26 amino acids appeared to be more potent and actually caused tumor regression. This truncated form has previously been shown to be more stable [28]. A phase I clinical study is currently underway using a vector expressing the wild-type *RB* gene at University of California in San Francisco (E.J. Small, lead investigator).

Gelsolin

The expression of the protein gelsolin, a cell cycle regulator, is reduced or absent in many human cancers, suggesting a tumor-suppressor role. After initial in vitro experiments, the utility of introducing gelsolin into established bladder tumors via an adenovirus vector has now been assessed [29]. Tumors were produced orthotopically in mice by transvesical administration of the human cell line KU-7, and subsequently the gelsolin gene was introduced on days 2, 3, and 4, also by transvesical administration. When the mice were sacrificed after 10 days, bladder tumors in treated mice had 10% of the mass of those in the control group ($p < .05$). This experiment suggests effectiveness of this approach at the early stage of cell implantation, and further work will be needed to assess its effect on established tumors.

Inhibition/Destruction of Oncogenes and Other Genes Associated with Tumor Growth

The H-ras oncogene is associated with tumor initiation and progression in bladder cancer, and was the first gene to be targeted for studies of the effectiveness of ribozymes in bladder cancer. Ribozymes are small catalytically active RNA strands with a specific activity that hybridize with their specific messenger RNA (mRNA) targets and interfere with protein translation [30]. The H-ras ribozyme targets the mutated sequence of the oncogene and hence the normal proto-oncogene is not affected. Intratumoral injection using an adenoviral vector was studied in subcutaneous tumors in mice and was associated with significant tumor regression and even complete disappearance in some cases [31]. Another approach to inhibit the action of the H-ras oncogene has been the use of a dominant negative mutant of this gene, N116Y. This has a substitution of tyrosine for asparagine at position 116 and inhibits the function of the ras protein. Using two cell lines (KU-7 and UMUC-2), orthotopic bladder tumors were created in mice and subsequently exposed to adenovirus-carried N116Y [32]. In both models the treated group showed significantly less tumors and less overall tumor burden than in controls. The authors did point out that as N116Y originates

from a viral oncogene, there may be concerns about reversion or reactivation, but these are extremely small.

Antisense oligonucleotides are small pieces of genetic material that are complementary to their target and therefore interfere with transmission of genetic information and have shown potential for bladder cancer treatment in vitro. In a multidrug-resistant T24 cell line, anti-c-myc was associated with increased sensitivity to cisplatin [33]. Similarly anti-bcl-2 was associated with an enhanced response to Adriamycin [34]. As yet there are no in vivo studies.

Angiogenesis is crucial in tumor development, and several factors are important in stimulating it. Two of these have been studied by the same group as potential targets for antisense gene therapy. Intralesional injection of antisense basic fibroblast growth factor (bFGF) reduced growth of subcutaneous bladder tumors 10-fold in mice [35]. A further experiment using antisense IL-8 on the same model gave similar results [36]. The next stage is to try these methods in orthotopic models, as the likely benefits are in preventing invasion and metastasis.

Cytotoxic Approaches to Bladder Cancer Gene Therapy
Suicide Gene Therapy

The commonest type of cytotoxic gene therapy used in bladder cancer is based on the herpes simplex virus thymidine kinase (HSV-tk) gene. This enzyme converts a prodrug ganciclovir into the active metabolite ganciclovir monophosphate, which is then further phosphorylated by cellular kinases and inhibits DNA polymerase leading to cell death (Fig. 15.2). As the prodrug is nontoxic, the aim is to target cell killing to the tumor. Both viral and nonviral methods have been used to deliver the HSV-tk gene to orthotopic bladder tumors in animal models. Intratumoral injection of an adenovirus containing the HSV-tk gene together with intraperitoneal ganciclovir administration led to a threefold reduction in tumor growth over 21 days of treatment in one study, which was associated with improved survival [37]. Another group had similar results, with twofold reduction in tumor

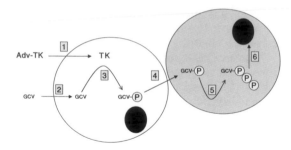

1) The adenoviral vector (AdV) delivers the Herpes simplex thymidine kinase (TK) gene to its target tumour cell.
2) Ganciclovir (GCV) enters the cell by diffusion.
3) The expressed TK phosphorylates GCV to GCV monophosphate (GCV-P), a biochemical reaction that human kinases cannot achieve.
4) GCV-P can be transported to adjacent cells through gap junctions
5) Human kinases can add two additional phosphates to GCV-P producing GCV-triphosphate (GCV-P-P-P)
6) GCV-P-P-P is incorporated into DNA; however, DNA polymerases cannot replicate DNA containing GCV-P-P-P. Mitosis is interrupted and the cell dies.

Because GCV-P can be transported to adjacent cells, not every cell needs to be transduced by the viral vector in order to be killed—the bystander effect

Fig. 15.2. Herpes simplex virus thymidine kinase (HSV-tk) suicide gene therapy.

growth [38]. This group (Baylor College of Medicine, Houston, Texas) is currently performing a phase I trial that involves intratumoral injection of HSV-tk in patients with locally advanced or refractory superficial bladder cancer. The patients undergo transurethral resection or cystectomy 2 weeks after a 14-day course of intravenous ganciclovir. Although this study is mainly looking at safety, tumor tissue will also be assessed to gauge the efficiency of transduction and histological changes.

The use of intravesical administration would probably be of more practical use clinically. Although this was not as effective as intratumoral injection in one study [38], another group demonstrated effective tumor cell killing in vivo with this approach [39].

A significant part of cell killing in cytotoxic gene therapy is from a process called the bystander effect. It has been shown that transduction of just 10% of tumor cells with HSV-tk can result in 50% cell killing within a tumor [40]. Enhancing the bystander effect by cotransfecting the gene for connexin 26 (Cx 26) with HSV-

tk shows promise. Cx 26 increases the expression of gap junctions in cells and therefore allows increased intracellular communication. Cotransfection increases the toxicity of HSV-tk/ganciclovir in vitro [41], and it will be interesting to see if this is reproduced in vivo.

Recently, nonviral transfection of HSV-tk has been described in vivo using the process of electroporation [42].

Cytotoxic gene therapy with HSV-tk/ganciclovir has been combined with several established chemotherapeutic agents in vitro [43]. Interestingly, very little additional benefit was seen, with some combinations even interfering with each other. Clearly, further work is required, and as the authors point out, the timing of the different treatments is probably crucial. The same group has looked at combining suicide gene therapy with immunological gene therapy [44]. Coadministration of HSV-tk and IL-2 did not lead to increased benefits.

Another prodrug-based cytotoxic gene therapy utilizes the enzyme horseradish peroxidase (HRP), which activates the harmless prodrug indole-3-acetic acid (IAA) [45]. This therapy was noted to be effective in anoxic conditions, and subsequent experiments combining it with radiotherapy suggested significant radiosensitization [46]. The proposed explanation was that the gene therapy worked on cells that were relatively hypoxic and therefore less prone to radiation damage.

Selective Tumor Cell Killing

Cancer cells usually have gene expression profiles that are different from those of normal cells, and this characteristic has been targeted in the use of replication competent viruses for direct cell killing. Clearly, in administering replication competent viruses, albeit attenuated, there are safety concerns with regard to systemic infection and to transmission to other individuals by the patient.

As has already been mentioned, bladder cancer has a high rate of *p53* mutations. It has been shown that adenovirus produces a protein (E1B-55) that binds wild-type *p53*, and viruses that are engineered to lack expression of this protein selectively target cells lacking functional *p53* [47]. There have already been phase I clinical trials utilizing this virus in head and neck cancers, and these crucially showed that virus was not detected in normal tissues [48]. In vitro studies have shown in bladder cancer that this virus lyses cells with mutant *p53* selectively [49], and there is therefore scope for clinical studies. Further specificity for bladder cancer cells using this virus has been demonstrated by targeting EGFR-positive cells [10].

Uroplakins, a group of integral membrane proteins, have been shown to be specifically overexpressed in transitional cell carcinomas [50]. Zhang et al. [51] engineered an adenovirus (CG8840) in which the uroplakin II promoter gene controlled expression of essential early genes and demonstrated that replication of this virus was limited to bladder cancer cells. When this virus was administered to mice with tumor xenografts, there was significant reduction of tumor growth. This effect was observed both with intratumoral and intravenous administration, and was enhanced in combination with docetaxel. This approach shows promise for patients with metastatic disease.

Other viruses have been studied in bladder cancer that are not bladder specific but cancer cell specific. PV701 is an attenuated strain of Newcastle disease virus that has been shown in a phase I trial to have tolerable toxicity levels [52]. It has several favorable characteristics, such as lack of antigenic drift, absence of human-to-human transmission, and minimal toxicity. The virus infects cancer cells at doses 1000 times lower than normal cells. Currently investigators at University of Chicago Cancer Research Center are undertaking a phase I trial of intravesical administration of PV701 prior to cystectomy (W.M. Stadler, lead investigator). The herpes simplex virus G207 also shows potential and has been demonstrated to be effective in an orthotopic bladder cancer model [53]. Histological studies showed no viral infection of normal urothelium or distant organs.

Immunological Gene Therapy

The purpose of immunological gene therapy is to enhance the host immune response against the tumor.

Tumor Vaccines

Initial studies transfected tumor cell lines with cytokines in vitro and demonstrated that tumor formation was prevented when these cells were administered to experimental animals. This led to the development of so-called tumor vaccines. In this approach cancer cells transfected with a cytokine-producing gene are administered to animals with established tumors of the same cell line. By inducing specific immunity, an antitumor effect is seen.

Connor et al. [54] studied the cytokines IL-2 and interferon-γ (IFN-γ). Retroviral vectors were used to transfect the bladder cancer cell line MBT-2 with these cytokines and they were then inactivated by X-irradiation. Mice with orthotopic bladder tumors derived from MBT-2 cells were then vaccinated intraperitoneally with these cell lines (individually or combined), once weekly for 3 weeks. IL-2 vaccination had a significant inhibitory effect on tumor growth, and three of five mice tumors regressed completely. Interferon-γ had a less marked effect but still showed antitumor activity. There was no benefit for combined treatment. The same group showed in a subsequent study that granulocyte-macrophage colony-stimulating factor (GM-CSF) could similarly be used as a tumor vaccine and was almost as effective as IL-2 [55].

In an effort to increase further the immunogenicity of tumor vaccines, the use of cotransfection with co-stimulatory molecules has been studied. For example, the adhesion molecule B7 is usually present on antigen-presenting cells and reacts with CD28 to activate T cells. When mice with MBT-2 bladder tumors received a combination of IL-2 transfected cells followed by B7 transfected cells, tumor regression was significantly enhanced [1]. This was not the case if B7 was administered before IL-2, and the implication is that B7 has a role in the induction of a cytotoxic T lymphocyte (CTL) response after it has been activated by IL-2. A human study of tumor cell vaccination using this model is proposed. Another co-stimulatory molecule is CD40 ligand, which interacts with CD40 on antigen-presenting cells. Although vaccination with tumor cells expressing CD40 ligand was successful in preventing subsequent tumor development, unfortunately a significant response was not seen in preexisting tumors [56].

In Vivo Cytokine Transfection

An alternative method of immune-mediated gene therapy is to transfect tumor cells directly in vivo with cytokines. This would obviate the need to perform the technically demanding process of culturing tumor cells obtained from patients. For example intravesical administration of the IL-2 gene contained within a liposomal vector has been performed in a mouse model [57]. Results were promising, with 40% of mice alive and tumor free at 60 days, compared to 100% mortality in the control group. This treatment strategy may have potential in high-risk superficial bladder cancer as an alternative to or perhaps in combination with BCG. Indeed, a recent study has suggested a synergistic effect [58].

Interleukin-12 is a cytokine important in activation of the CTL response. It is also a potent upregulator of IFN-γ. When an adenoviral vector containing the IL-12 gene was injected directly into subcutaneously inoculated mouse bladder tumors, it led to a significant reduction in tumor growth [59]. Indeed, all six animals in the group receiving the highest dose experienced complete remission of the tumor. In a separate experiment, injection into the primary tumor was associated with reduced growth of lung metastases, thus demonstrating that this form of therapy had a systemic effect.

A similar experiment has been performed using adenoviral vectors containing the gene for interferon-β (IFN-β) [60]. This important cytokine has a multitude of actions including immune modulation and the inhibition of angiogenesis. Tumor weight in those tumors injected with the IFN-β gene was significantly less than in controls. These tumors also showed reduced angiogenesis as measured by microvessel density.

Conclusion

This chapter has summarized the large amount of experimental work exploring the potential for gene therapy in bladder cancer. Several phase I trials have now been reported, and the next decade holds out the hope of successful transfer of these therapies to the clinical situation. The future must lie with multimodality treatment, and the studies that have described synergy between chemotherapy and gene therapy are extremely encouraging. However, there is a long way to go, and, unfortunately, achieving efficacious therapy is not the only challenge, because gene therapy continues to court ethical controversy, and its success is most likely to depend on its acceptance by the general public.

References

1. Larchian WA, Horiguchi Y, Nair SK, Fair WR, Heston WD, Gilboa E. Effectiveness of combined interleukin 2 and B7.1 vaccination strategy is dependent on the sequence and order: a liposome mediated gene therapy treatment for bladder cancer. Clin Cancer Res 2000;6:2913–2920.
2. Harimoto K, Sugimura K, Lee CR, Kuratsukuri K, Kishimoto T. In vivo gene transfer methods in the bladder without viral vectors. Br J Urol 1998;81: 870–874.
3. Perrotte P, Wood M, Slaton JW, et al. Biosafety of in vivo adenovirus-p53 intravesical administration in mice. Urology 2000;56:155–159.
4. Pagliaro LC, Keyhani A, Williams D, et al. Repeated intravesical instillations of an adenoviral vector in patients with locally advanced bladder cancer: a phase I study of p53 gene therapy. J Clin Oncol 2003;21:2247–2253.
5. Li Y, Pong RC, Bergelson JM, et al. Loss of adenoviral receptor expression in human bladder cancer cells: a potential impact on the efficacy of gene therapy. Cancer Res 1999;59:325–330.
6. Sachs MD, Rauen KA, Ramamurthy M, et al. Integrin α_v and coxsackie adenovirus receptor expression in clinical bladder cancer. Urology 2002;60: 531–536.
7. Lee CT, Seol JY, Park KH, et al. Differential effects of adenovirus-p16 on bladder cancer cell lines can be overcome by the addition of butyrate. Clin Cancer Res 2001;7:210–214.
8. Sachs MD, Cohen M, Chowdhury W, Lacey D, Loening SA, Rodriguez R. Rendering bladder cancer suitable for adenoviral gene therapy. J Urol 2003;169:185(abstract 716).
9. Okegawa T, Pong RC, Li Y, Bergelson JM, Sagalowsky AI, Hsieh JT. The mechanism of the growth-inhibitory effect of coxsackie and adenovirus receptor (CAR) on human bladder cancer: a functional analysis of car protein structure. Cancer Res 2001;61:6592–6600.
10. van der Poel HG, Molenaar B, van Beusechem VW, et al. Epidermal growth factor receptor targeting of replication competent adenovirus enhances cytotoxicity in bladder cancer. J Urol 2002;168: 266–272l.
11. Matsumoto K, Freund CT, Jian W, et al. Effective suicide gene transfer strategy by a chimeric adenovirus vector to bladder cancer. J Urol 2003;169:184(abstract 713).

12. Chester JD, Kennedy W, Hall JD, Selby PJ, Knowles MA. Adenovirus-mediated gene therapy for bladder cancer: efficient gene delivery to normal and malignant human urothelial cells in vitro and ex vivo. Gene Therapy 2003;10:172–179.

13. Engler H, Anderson SC, Machemer TR, et al. Ethanol improves adenovirus-mediated gene transfer and expression to the bladder epithelium of rodents. Urology 1999;53:1049–1053.

14. Lin LF, Zhu G, Yoo JJ, Soker S, Sukhatme VP, Atala A. A system for the enhancement of adenovirus mediated gene transfer to uro-epithelium. J Urol 2002;168:813–818.

15. Connor RJ, Engler H, Machemer T, et al. Identification of polyamides that enhance adenovirus mediated gene expression in the urothelium. Gene Ther 2001;8:41–48.

16. Yamashita M, Rosser CJ, Zhou JH, et al. Syn3 provides high levels of intravesical adenoviral-mediated gene transfer for gene therapy of genetically altered urothelium and superficial bladder cancer. Cancer Gene Ther 2002;9:687–691.

17. Kuball J, Wen SF, Leissner J, et al. Successful adenovirus-mediated wild-type p53 gene transfer in patients with bladder cancer by intravesical vector instillation. J Clin Oncol 2002;20:957–965.

18. Gomella LG, Mastrangelo MJ, McCue PA, Maguire HC Jr, Mulholland SG, Lattime EC. Phase I study of intravesical vaccinia virus as a vector for gene therapy of bladder cancer. J Urol 2001;166:1291–1295.

19. Siemens DR, Crist S, Austin JC, Tartaglia J, Ratliff TL. Comparison of viral vectors: gene transfer efficiency and tissue specificity in a bladder cancer model. J Urol 2003;170:979–984.

20. Esrig D, Elmajian D, Groshen S, et al. Accumulation of nuclear p53 and tumour progression in bladder cancer. N Engl J Med 1994;331:1259–1264.

21. Harris MP, Sutjipoto S, Wills KN, et al. Adenovirus-mediated p53 gene transfer inhibits growth of human tumor cells expressing mutant p53 protein. Cancer Gene Ther 1996;3:121–130.

22. Wada Y, Gotoh A, Shirakawa T, Hamada K, Kamidono S. Gene therapy for bladder cancer using adenoviral vector. Mol Urol 2001;5:47–52.

23. Miyake H, Hara I, Hara S, Arakawa S, Kamidono S. Synergistic chemosensitization and inhibition of tumor growth and metastasis by adenovirus mediated p53 gene transfer in human bladder cancer model. Urology 2000;56:332–336.

24. Pagliaro LC, Keyhani A, Liu B, Perrotte P, Wilson D, Dinney CP. Adenoviral p53 gene transfer in human bladder cancer cell lines: cytotoxicity and synergy with cisplatin. Urol Oncol 2003;21:456–462.

25. Shirakawa T, Sasaki R, Gardner TA, et al. Drug resistant human bladder cancer cells are more sensitive to adenovirus mediated wild-type p53 gene therapy compared to drug-sensitive cells. Int J Cancer 2001;94:282–289.

26. Hall MC, Li Y, Pong RC, et al. The growth inhibitory effect of p21 adenovirus on human bladder cancer cells. J Urol 2000;163:1033–1038.

27. Xu HJ, Zhou Y, Seigne J, et al. Enhanced tumor suppressor gene therapy via replication deficient adenovirus vectors expressing an N-terminal truncated retinoblastoma protein. Cancer Res 1996;56:2245–2249.

28. Xu HJ, Xu K, Zhou Y, Benedict WF, Hu SX. Enhanced tumor cell growth suppression by an N-terminal truncated retinoblastoma protein. Proc Natl Acad Sci USA 1994;91:9837–9841.

29. Sazawa A, Watanabe T, Tanaka M, et al. Adenovirus mediated Gelsolin gene therapy for orthotopic human bladder cancer in nude mice. J Urol 2002;168:1182–1187.

30. Irie A, Kashani-Sabet M, Scanlon K, Uchida T, Baba S. Hammerhead ribozymes as therapeutic targets for bladder cancer. Mol Urol 2000;4:61–65.

31. Irie A, Anderegg B, Kashani-Sabet M, et al. Therapeutic efficacy of an adenovirus-mediated anti-H-ras ribozyme in experimental bladder cancer. Antisense Nucleic Acid Drug Dev 1999;9:341–349.

32. Watanabe T, Shinohara N, Sazawa A, et al. Adenovirus mediated gene therapy for bladder cancer in an orthotopic model using a dominant negative H-ras mutant. Int J Cancer 2001;92:712–717.

33. Mizutani Y, Fukumoto M, Bonavida B, Yoshida O. Enhancement of sensitivity of urinary bladder tumor cells to cisplatin by c-myc antisense oligonucleotide. Cancer 1994;74:2546–2554.

34. Bilim V, Kasahara T, Noboru H, Takahashi K, Tomita Y. Caspase involved synergistic toxicity of bcl-2 antisense oligonucleotides and Adriamycin on transitional cell cancer cells. Cancer Lett 2000;155:191–198.

35. Inoue K, Perrotte P, Wood CG, Slaton JW, Sweeney P, Dinney CP. Gene therapy of human bladder cancer with adenovirus-mediated antisense basic fibroblast growth factor. Clin Cancer Res 2000;6:4422–4431.

36. Inoue K, Wood CG, Slaton JW, Karashima T, Sweeney P, Dinney CP. Adenoviral-mediated gene therapy of human bladder cancer with antisense interleukin-8. Oncol Rep 2001;8:955–964.

37. Cheon J, Moon DG, Cho HY, et al. Adenovirus mediated suicide gene therapy in an orthotopic murine bladder tumor model. Int J Urol 2002;9:261–267.

38. Sutton MA, Freund CT, Berkman SA, et al. In vivo adenovirus-mediated suicide gene therapy of orthotopic bladder cancer. Mol Ther 2000;2:211–217.

39. Akasaka S, Suzuki S, Shimizu H, Igarishi T, Akimoto M, Shimada T. Suicide gene therapy for chemically induced rat bladder tumor entailing

instillation of adenoviral vectors. Jpn J Can Res 2001;92:568–575.

40. Freeman SM, Abboud CN, Whartenby KA, et al. The "bystander effect": tumor regression when a fraction of the tumor mass is genetically modified. Cancer Res 1993;53:5274–5283.

41. Tanaka M, Fraizer GC, De La Cerda J, Cristiano RJ, Liebert M, Grossman HB. Connexin 26 enhances the bystander effect in HSVtk/GCV gene therapy for human bladder cancer by adenovirus/PLL/DNA gene delivery. Gene Ther 2001;8:139–148.

42. Shibata MA, Horiguchi T, Morimoto J, Otsuki Y. Massive apoptotic cell death in chemically induced rat urinary bladder carcinomas following in situ HSV*tk* electrogene transfer. J Gene Med 2003;5:219–231.

43. Freund CT, Tong XW, Rowley D, et al. Combination of adenovirus-mediated thymidine kinase gene therapy with cytotoxic chemotherapy in bladder cancer in vitro. Urol Oncol 2003;21:197–205.

44. Freund CT, Sutton MA, Dang T, Contant CF, Rowley D, Lerner SP. Adenovirus-mediated combination suicide and cytokine gene therapy for bladder cancer. Anticancer Res 2000;20:1359–1365.

45. Greco O, Folkes LK, Wardman P, Tozer GM, Dachs GU. Development of a novel enzyme/prodrug combination for gene therapy of cancer: horseradish peroxidase/indole-3–acetic acid. Cancer Gene Ther 2000;7:1414–1420.

46. Greco O, Tozer GM, Dachs GU. Oxic and anoxic enhancement of radiation mediated toxicity by horseradish peroxidase/indole-3–acetic acid gene therapy. Int J Radiat Biol 2002;78:173–181.

47. Bischoff JR, Kirn DH, Williams A, et al. An adenovirus mutant that replicates selectively in p53 deficient human tumor cells. Science 1996;274:373–376.

48. Khuri FR, Nemunaitis J, Ganly I, et al. A controlled trial of intratumoural ONYX-015, a selectively replicating adenovirus, in combination with cisplatin and 5–fluorouracil in patients with recurrent head and neck cancer. Nat Med 2000;6:879–885.

49. Hsieh JL, Wu CL, Lai MD, Lee CH, Tsai CS, Shiau AL. Gene therapy for bladder cancer using E1B-55 deleted adenovirus in combination with adenoviral vector encoding plasminogen kringles 1–5. Br J Cancer 2003;88:1492–1499.

50. Moll R, Wu XR, Lin JH, Sun TT. Uroplakins, specific membrane proteins of urothelial umbrella cells, as histological markers of metastatic transitional cell carcinomas. Am J Pathol 1995;147:1383–1397.

51. Zhang J, Ramesh N, Chen Y, et al. Identification of human uroplakin II promoter and its use in the construction of CG8840, a urothelium-specific adenovirus variant that eliminates established bladder tumors in combination with docetaxel. Cancer Res 2002;62:3743–3750.

52. Pecora AL, Rizvi N, Cohen GI, et al. Phase I trial of intravenous administration of PV701, an oncolytic virus, in patients with advanced solid cancers. J Clin Oncol 2002;20:2251–2266.

53. Cozzi PJ, Malhotra S, McCauliffe P, et al. Intravesical oncolytic viral therapy using attenuated, replication competent herpes simplex viruses G207 and Nv1020 is effective in the treatment of bladder cancer in an orthotopic syngeneic model. FASEB J 2001;15:1306–1308.

54. Connor J, Bannerji R, Saito S, Heston W, Fair W, Gilboa E. Regression of bladder tumours in mice treated with interleukin 2 gene modified tumor cells. J Exp Med 1993;177:1127–1134.

55. Saito S, Bannerji R, Gansbacher B, et al. Immunotherapy of bladder cancer with cytokine gene-modified tumor vaccines. Cancer Res 1994;54:3516–3520.

56. Kimura T, Ohashi T, Kikucji T, Kiyota H, Eto Y, Ohishi Y. Antitumor immunity against bladder cancer induced by ex vivo expression of CD40 ligand gene using retrovirus vector. Cancer Gene Ther 2003;10:833–839.

57. Horiguchi Y, Larchian WA, Kaplinsky R, et al. Intravesical liposome mediated interleukin 2 gene therapy in orthotopic murine bladder cancer model. Gene Ther 2000;7:844–851.

58. Oyama M, Heston WD, Horiguchi Y, et al. Synergistic antitumor effect of intravesical liposome mediated interleukin 2 gene therapy plus BCG in orthotopic murine bladder cancer. J Urol 2003;169:128(abstract 497).

59. Chen L, Chen D, Block E, O'Donnel M, Kufe DW, Clinton SK. Eradication of murine bladder carcinoma by intratumor injection of a bicistronic adenoviral vector carrying cDNAs for the IL-12 heterodimer and its inhibition by the IL-12 p40 subunit homodimer. J Immunol 1997;159:351–359.

60. Izawa JI, Sweeney P, Perrotte P, et al. Inhibition of tumorigenicity and metastasis of human bladder cancer growing in athymic mice by interferon-β gene therapy results partially from various antiangiogenic effects including endothelial cell apoptosis. Clin Cancer Res 2002;8:1258–1270.

Part III

Kidney Cancer

16

Molecular Biology of Kidney Cancer

Jeffrey M. Holzbeierlein and J. Brantley Thrasher

Kidney cancer, more commonly known as renal cell carcinoma, is the sixth leading cause of cancer death in the United States [1]. It currently accounts for approximately 3% of all adult malignancies [1]. In 2001, 32,000 cases of renal cell carcinoma in the United States were documented. Of these 32,000 cases, approximately 40% will die of the disease [1]. Renal cell carcinoma is more common in males than in females, with approximately a 2:1 ratio. It typically affects patients between the ages of 50 and 70 but may occur in younger individuals, especially those who suffer from familial syndromes [2–5]. The number one risk factor for the disease is cigarette smoking. Other risk factors include obesity and hypertension, which are thought to be particular risk factors for females who develop renal cell carcinoma [3–5]. Occupational exposures such as leather finishing products and asbestos have also been associated with the development of renal cell carcinoma [6,7]. Also an increased incidence has been found in patients with end-stage renal disease and acquired renal cystic disease, especially in those who are undergoing dialysis, with the risk of renal cell carcinoma being approximately 20 times that of a normal individual [8,9]. Renal cell carcinoma is thought to be made up by four histopathological types: clear cell carcinoma, which accounts for approximately 80% to 85%; papillary renal cell carcinoma, which accounts for approximately 5% to 10%; chromophobe; and oncocytoma.

It is estimated that approximately 4% of renal cancers are familial, and that this percentage is likely to increase with the discovery of more inherited forms of the disease [10]. Currently there are four hereditary syndromes that are associated with the development of renal cell carcinoma, the most common being von Hippel–Lindau disease. Other hereditary forms of renal cell carcinoma include tuberous sclerosis, hereditary papillary renal cell carcinoma, Birt Hogg-Dube syndrome, hereditary leiomyoma renal cell carcinoma, familial renal oncocytoma, and hereditary nonpolyposis colon cancer [10]. With the identification of the familial association of some renal cell carcinomas, intense investigations into the genetic alterations leading to these tumors has been undertaken. This effort, led by researchers at the National Cancer Institute, has been successful in identifying and characterizing many genetic loci associated with familial forms of renal cell carcinoma. This chapter discusses the molecular genetics of renal cell carcinoma, some of the molecular markers associated with these types of tumors, and the familial syndromes associated with development of renal cell carcinoma, which may play an important role in the diagnosis and management of these tumors in the future.

Clear Cell Carcinoma

Clear cell carcinoma is the histopathological subtype that accounts for the majority of renal cell carcinomas. It is characterized by cells that typically have clear cytoplasm, although there is

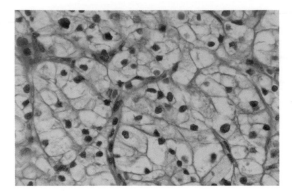

Fig. 16.1. Clear cell carcinoma.

a "granular" pattern that may occur in some tumors (Fig. 16.1) [11]. Clear cell carcinoma is thought to be the most aggressive of the histopathological subtypes with the greatest chance of metastases, and may be associated with the sarcomatoid variant in up to 5% of cases [11]. This subtype tends to be one of the better responders to immunotherapy. Clear cell carcinoma occurs in both sporadic and familial forms, and in both forms it is characterized by the loss of a tumor-suppressor gene, namely the *VHL* gene.

Von Hippel–Lindau Disease

Von Hippel–Lindau (VHL) disease is a hereditary syndrome characterized by the development of multiple tumors, both benign and malignant, affecting several different organ systems [3], including the eyes, spine, inner ear, pancreas, adrenal gland, and kidneys. Retinal angiomas, cerebellar and spinal hemangioblastomas, and renal cell carcinomas are the hallmark lesions of this disease. Renal cysts, pancreatic cysts, pancreatic carcinomas, pheochromocytomas, epididymal or broad ligament cyst adenomas, and endolymphatic sac tumors may also occur in patients who suffer from this disease. Von Hippel–Lindau disease is estimated to affect approximately 1 in 36,000 individuals and is inherited in an autosomal-dominant fashion, with estimated penetrance of 80% to 90% by the age of 65 [12,13]. Renal cell carcinoma eventually develops in approximately 28% to 45% of those individuals affected with VHL disease [3]. The tumors associated with

VHL disease are typically multicentric and are often bilateral. These tumors are predominantly of the clear cell variety.

The *VHL* gene has been localized to the short arm of chromosome 3, sub-band 25 (3p25) [14–16]. This mapping was first accomplished by Seizinger et al. [15], who used genetic linkage analysis to study nine families affected with VHL disease. The germline mutation is transmitted in an autosomal-dominant fashion, with each of the offspring having a 50% risk of inheriting the mutant allele [12]. According to Knudson's [17] "two-hit" hypothesis, the carriers of mutations in a tumor-suppressor gene have a germline mutation in one allele of the gene, and a second "hit" or somatic mutation occurs in the homologous normal allele, thus leading to tumor formation. The purpose of tumor-suppressor genes, such as the *VHL* gene, is to inhibit tumor development through regulation of self-proliferation and differentiation, and their inactivation predisposes an individual to cancer through loss of these regulatory processes.

Tory et al. [18] used restriction fragment length polymorphism (RFLP) analysis to confirm that in the VHL patients the wild-type chromosome 3p25 allele inherited from the unaffected parent had been lost. With the other allele being the abnormal germline copy of the *VHL* gene inherited from the affected parent, Tory et al. were able to demonstrate this association with the development of renal cell carcinoma. Lubensky et al. [19] subsequently demonstrated loss of the wild-type 3p allele with evidence of the inherited mutated allele in 25 of 26 renal lesions from patients affected with VHL disease. Also, the loss of heterozygosity (LOH) at 3p25 was detectable in atypical renal cysts and cysts with renal cell carcinoma in situ. These provided strong evidence that the *VHL* gene was indeed a tumor-suppressor gene, and loss of function of both gene copies appeared to be an important early step toward tumor formation.

In 1988 Seizinger et al. [15] confirmed that the *VHL* gene was linked to the locus encoding the human homologue of the *RAF1* oncogene mapping to the 3p25 chromosome. In this important report, the authors hypothesized that the defect responsible for the *VHL* phenotype was not a mutation in the *RFA1* gene itself but rather the inactivation of a putative tumor-suppressor gene, namely the *VHL* gene, and that this led to the development of renal cell carcinoma. This linkage to *RFA1* was confirmed by Hosoe et al. [20], who also reported linkage of the *VHL* gene to D3S18, a polymorphic DNA marker located at 3p26. Richards et al. [21] then demonstrated tight linkage of the *VHL* gene to the DNA probe D3S601, which was located in the region between *RAF1* and D3S18. The *VHL* gene was subsequently identified by Latif et al. [16] in 1993 through the use of yeast artificial chromosomes and cosmid phase contigs. Latif et al. demonstrated that the *VHL* gene was a single-copy gene with evolutionary conservation across several species, pointing to its essential role in cellular processes.

The *VHL* gene contains three exons with an open reading frame of 852 nucleotides that encode a protein of 213 amino acids [2,3]. Several hundred germline mutations have now been recognized in VHL kindreds [2,3]. These include microdeletions, insertions, large deletions, and missense and nonsense mutations. Chen et al. [22] studied 114 VHL families and identified mutations throughout the coding region, but clustering occurred at the 3′ end of exon 1 and the 5′ end of exon 3 with a paucity of mutations in exon 2. The importance of this is that specific mutations have now been correlated with certain phenotypic characteristics in VHL patients. For example, VHL type 1 families most frequently have large deletions, microdeletions/insertions, or nonsense mutations [12,22,23]. The specific phenotypic characteristic of these families is that they typically do not develop pheochromocytomas. However, in VHL type 2 families that do suffer from pheochromocytomas, 96% of the mutations are missense mutations [12,22,23]. Gnarra et al. [24] evaluated sporadic clear cell carcinomas and found *VHL* gene mutations in 57% of the cancers, with LOH of the gene in 98%. In these patients, they found that the mutations clustered to the 3′ end of exon 1 and at the 5′ end of exon 3; however, exon 2 also had a high frequency of mutations (approximately 45%). This high number of mutations, as well as splice-site mutations that would eliminate its translation, suggested that exon 2 may have a role in the function of the protein product. The functions of the VHL protein product have been difficult to predict as there is no important homology to other proteins [12,16]. Further characterization has been performed through cellular localization studies. Immunofluorescence microscopy demonstrated

that the protein product is located primarily in the cytoplasm but can also been found in the nucleus [3,12,25–28]. Subsequently, two biologically active VHL protein isoforms, pPVHL$_{30}$ and pVHL$_{19}$, have been demonstrated [29]. Furthermore, there is evidence to suggest that the expression of the VHL proteins in either the cytoplasm or the nucleus may be associated with clinical outcome [29]. Coimmunoprecipitation of the VHL protein revealed two proteins of 9 and 16 kilodaltons (kd), which were subsequently identified as elongin C and elongin B, respectively [3,30–32]. However, when certain missense mutations of the *VHL* gene occurred, this protein interreaction was found to be very weak or nonexistent [3,28]. This relationship of the normal VHL protein and loss of its association with other proteins due to certain mutations has led several investigators to study the protein–protein interactions in VHL much more closely.

Normally the VHL protein product binds tightly to elongin B and C, which are regulatory subunits of elongin SIII [3,30,33–35]. The VHL protein product has not been shown to bind to elongin A. Elongin SIII is known to hasten DNA transcriptional elongation by RNA polymerase II by inhibiting temporary pausing of the polymerase at certain DNA sites and by controlling its release from DNA [3,12,36,37]. With binding of elongin B and C, the VHL protein is able to abort the formation of the active heterotrimeric protein elongin SIII [3,30]. The transcription of certain genes may be downregulated as a result of these binding sequences [12,34]. As mentioned previously, a number of VHL proteins with missense gene mutations have been found to complex minimally or not at all with the elongin regulatory subunits [3,28]. This inability to inhibit the formation of elongin may lead to the loss of regulation of transcription rates of genes important in tumor suppression [12,28,35].

The association of the VHL protein with elongin B and C may function to promote a complex that is responsible for ubiquitination and proteasome degradation. Cullin-2 (CUL-2), a member of the CDC53 family of proteins, has been found to bind to VHL elongin B and C and form a stable tetrameric complex [3,38]. This complex has been noted to be crucial in the degradation of specific proteins such as hypoxia-induced factor 1α (HIF1α) [33,39]. Studies have

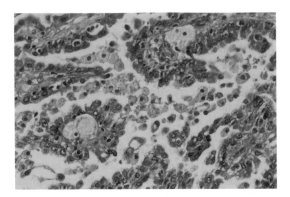

Fig. 16.3. Papillary renal cell carcinoma.

also appears to be more common in patients on chronic dialysis for end-stage renal disease [9]. The tumors associated with papillary renal cell carcinoma tend to be multifocal and arise independently of one another [2,14,74]. There are two broad classifications of the tumor: sporadic and hereditary. Papillary renal cell carcinoma has not been associated with 3p mutations as is found in clear cell carcinoma. Instead it is associated with the proto-oncogene *met*, found on chromosome 7 [2]. Unlike the *VHL* gene, studies have demonstrated that the *met* allele and c-*met* receptor are proto-oncogenes having tumorigenic properties consisting of increased proliferation, motility, extracellular invasion, and tubule formation [14,75].

Sporadic papillary carcinoma of the kidney is associated with more than one chromosomal abnormality. Roughly 80% of sporadic papillary tumors possess polysomies [74]. Some of the more common trisomies that have been observed include trisomy of chromosomes 7, 17, and 16 [2,14,74,76]. In addition, in male patients with papillary renal cell carcinoma, loss of they Y chromosome has been associated in approximately 80% to 90% of cases [77–80]. Other chromosomal abnormalities reported include LOH and somatic translocations. Thrash-Bingham et al. [81] detected LOH on chromosomes 9q, 11q, 14q, 21q, and 6p. Somatic translocations of chromosomes 1 and X have been reported as well [82–84].

Hereditary papillary renal cell carcinoma (HPRC), first established by Burton Zbar [85] in 1994, is associated with abnormalities of chromosome 7. Specifically the *met* proto-oncogene

has been strongly associated with the hereditary form of this neoplasm [86]. The *met* proto-oncogene has now been localized to the 7q 31.3 region, which codes for a transmembrane receptor tyrosine kinase [10,85,86]. Zbar et al. [85–88] performed multigenerational studies of families affected with HPRC and found germline missense mutations of the tyrosine kinase portion of the *met* gene. The *met* gene is found in a high percentage of HPRC family members as well as in a subset of sporadic papillary renal cell carcinomas. Hereditary papillary renal cell carcinoma is characterized by an autosomal-dominant inheritance pattern and is associated with bilateral and multifocal tumors.

Oncogenic properties of the *met* gene come from studies of its amplification and mutations that result in the activation of its encoded protein [89,90]. Function of the c-*met* receptor is also of special interest. It is a tyrosine kinase receptor involved in motility, proliferation, and morphogenic signals [14]. Hepatocyte growth factor/scatter factor (HGF/SF) is its ligand [91]. Normal organogenesis is dependent on the *met* receptor–HGF/SF pathway. Activation of cells possessing HGF/SF causes increased proliferation, increased motility, extracellular invasion, polarization, and tubule formation [75]. Studies of mice with increased levels of tyrosine phosphorylation and enhanced kinase activity have revealed a correlation between tumorigenesis and biological activity of this pathway [92]. The C-terminal is the docking site of this receptor. Once activated by ligand binding, the receptor is upregulated by autocatalytic pathways, ultimately increasing enzymatic and biological activity of the receptor [93,94]. It is this upregulation of the c-*met* receptor that is suspected to result in the development of papillary renal cell carcinoma in both the sporadic and hereditary forms. However, the exact function of the c-*met* receptor has not currently been fully delineated.

A second type of hereditary papillary renal cell carcinoma, known as hereditary leiomyoma renal cell carcinoma, is an autosomal-dominant condition due to a mutation in the fumarate hydratase gene [10]. This is often referred to as type 2 hereditary papillary renal cell carcinoma and is associated with a more aggressive form of the disease [10]. The fumarate hydratase gene maps to the 1q42.3-43 chromosome [10]. It is believed that fumarate hydratase is an enzyme of the Krebs cycle and is a "housekeeping" gene.

The exact function of the gene, however, is unknown. Patients afflicted with this hereditary disorder get skin leiomyomas and papillary renal cell carcinomas, which are usually single at presentation. Females afflicted with the disease may also develop uterine fibroids. This hereditary form of papillary renal cell carcinoma tends to affect patients at younger ages, usually between the ages of 20 to 35 [10].

Chromophobe Tumors

The chromophobe histological classification of renal cell carcinomas accounts for approximately 5% of renal cell carcinomas [95]. Chromophobe tumors classically contain three elements: (1) small cells with granular cytoplasm called type 1 cells, (2) cells with larger eosinophilic granular cytoplasm and characteristic clear perinuclear halos called type 2 cells, and (3) polygonal cells with clear cytoplasm called type 3 cells (Fig. 16.4). Chromophobes typically have a less aggressive clinical course than its clear cell and papillary counterparts [96]. However, one discouraging feature of chromophobe renal cell carcinomas is that they are typically unresponsive to immunotherapy. Genetically, chromophobe tumors have been associated with chromosome losses that have multiple genetic loci including chromosomes 1, 2, 6, 10, 13, 17, and 21 [95]. Recently, a new syndrome known as Birt-Hogg-Dube was associated with the development of renal tumors. This syndrome, first described by a pathologist, a dermatologist, and an internist in 1977, is a triad

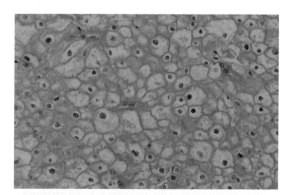

Fig. 16.4. Type 3 cells: polygonal cells with clear cytoplasm.

of skin lesions including fibrofolliculomas, trichodiscomas, and acrochordomas [97]. It was noted to develop in an autosomal-dominant fashion, usually after the age of 30. In 2002 Zbar et al. [98] described the association of Birt-Hogg-Dube with the development of renal and colonic neoplasms as well as the development of spontaneous pneumothoraces. Those patients who suffer from Birt-Hogg-Dube have approximately a 9.3 times increased incidence of developing a renal tumor, with the most common histology being chromophobe. The tumors are often multiple and are bilateral in approximately 60% of patients. In 2002 Pavlovich et al. [95] reviewed 130 solid renal tumors resected from 30 patients with Birt-Hogg-Dube. The patients had a mean of 5.3 tumors and an average age at discovery of the tumors of 50.7 years. In this series, 34% were pure chromophobes. Another 50% of the patients had a hybrid of chromophobe and oncocytoma, whereas 9% were of the clear cell variety. In this series classic papillary tumors or pure oncocytomas were rarely found. The Birt-Hogg-Dube gene has now been mapped to the 17p11.2 locus and is thought to be a tumor-suppressor gene [99]. The presence of the Birt-Hogg-Dube gene mutation is rare in sporadic renal tumors.

Renal Oncocytoma

Renal oncocytoma is a neoplasm that occurs in approximately 3% to 5% of renal cell carcinomas [74,100]. It typically has a more benign course, although metastases have been reported [101]. In a large number of tumors there are no chromosomal losses associated with oncocytomas. However, in some tumors genetic changes, including losses at chromosomes 1p, 14q, X, and Y or translocations involving 5q35 and 11q13, have been reported [1,74,102–108]. There is a familial syndrome known as familial renal oncocytoma (FRO) that was described by Weirich et al. [109] in 1998 in five families. There was no putative chromosomal loss identified in these families, and it was felt that perhaps there might be some overlap with the Birt-Hogg-Dube syndrome. The pattern of inheritance appeared to be autosomal dominant. No evidence of *VHL* germline mutations has been demonstrated in oncocytomas, and the tumors are typically viewed as nonlethal.

Collecting Duct and Medullary Carcinoma of the Kidney

Collecting duct carcinoma, also known as Bellini's tumor, is a rare form of kidney cancer accounting for approximately 0.4% to 2% of renal cancers [110]. Typically these tumors are very aggressive, with many patients presenting with metastases. Median survival has been reported to be around 11.5 months across all stages [111]. Structurally and histologically these tumors resemble papillary renal cell carcinoma (Fig. 16.5) [110]. Collecting ducts carcinomas are typically characterized by hypodiploid stem lines with chromosomes 1, X, and Y most commonly affected [112]. Additional abnormalities have been found on chromosomes 22 and 23 but are less common than those at 1, X, and Y. Kuoda et al. [110] have demonstrated LOH at 1q32.1-32.2; however, the rarity of these tumors has made it difficult to completely characterize them.

Renal medullary carcinoma is another rare renal cancer found almost exclusively in African Americans. In a study by Suartz et al. [113], 82% of the patients with medullary carcinoma were African Americans, and all had either sickle cell disease or trait. These tumors are also characterized by a very aggressive phenotype, with many presenting with metastases at diagnosis, and extremely poor survival rates. Genetically the tumors typically show no chromosomal losses or gains. Medullary carcinoma tumors have been shown to stain strongly for HIF1α and VEGF [113], the hypothesis for this being that there is chronic medullary hypoxia secondary to the sickle cell hemoglobinopathy leading to accumulation of HIF1α and VEGF with neoangiogenesis and tumor growth.

Molecular Markers

Within the last decade there has been intense research into the development of molecular markers as potential prognosticators in various malignancies. Others have evaluated the use of various prognostic factors in renal cell carcinoma such as tumor size, histologic pattern, nuclear morphometry, and DNA content; however, none of these has proved to supply information more predictive than stage and grade [114–117]. The prognostic value of cellular proliferation markers such as Ki-67, p53 mutations, growth factor expression, PTEN status, and intratumoral microvessel density have been investigated [118–122]. Also, as discussed earlier, the pattern of VHL protein (pVHL$_{19}$, pVHL$_{30}$) staining in renal cell carcinomas has been correlated with tumor aggressiveness [29]. Despite these newer markers, stage and grade remain the greatest predictive prognostic factors.

Wilms' Tumor

Wilms' tumor is the most common malignant neoplasm of the urinary tract in children and one of the most common solid tumors of children [123]. First described in 1814 by Rance and subsequently characterized by Max Wilms in 1899, Wilms' tumor has become an excellent model for the link between cancer and development. The tumor occurs with a frequency of about 1 in 10,000 live births, and approximately 350 new cases occur per year in the United States [123,124]. The peak incidence is between the third and fourth years of life, with 90% of patients presenting before the age of 7. There does not appear to be a sex predominance. Several other congenital abnormalities have been found in patients with Wilms' tumour, including aniridia, hemihypertrophy, musculoskeletal abnormalities, neurofibromatosis, and secondary malignant neoplasms (sarcomas, adenocarcinomas, and leukemias). Wilms' tumor has also been associated with other congenital

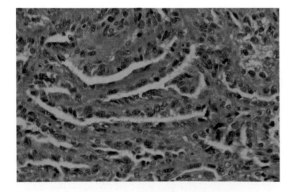

Fig. 16.5. Collecting duct carcinoma, also known as Bellini's tumor.

syndromes including Beckwith-Wiedemann, Denys-Drash, WAGR (Wilms' tumor, aniridia, genitourinary abnormalities, and mental retardation), Perlman, and Bloom syndromes [123–125]. The biology of this tumor has been studied extensively, and it is thought that its formation is due to aberrant expression of the normal developmental program. Abnormal proliferation of metanephric blastemal tissue that lacks maturation and normal differentiation is felt to be the source of this tumor [123]. Normal nephrogenesis is the product of controlled proliferation, differentiation, and apoptosis. Wilms' tumor is likely to be due to the interruption of normal signaling, proliferation, and controlled apoptosis during development [125]. Multiple chromosomal regions have been identified as playing a role in the development of Wilms' tumors; however, only the Wilms' tumor gene, WT1, has been clearly proven to play a significant role. Studies of the normal gene function of WT1 suggest that its role as a tumor suppressor and developmental regulator are crucial to normal nephrogenic development [124]. Furthermore, the presence of nephrogenic rests in Wilms' tumors supports the association of this tumor with immature blastemal tissue [125].

The WT1 gene maps to 11p13 and is expressed in normal-developing nephrogenic tissue [126–128]. Point mutations and LOH for alleles on 11p have been found in Wilms' tumors [129]. Approximately 40% of cases of Wilms' tumor have been found to have LOH at the 11p allele. The two-hit model by Knudson and Strong was based on studies of Wilms' tumor [130,131]. This model was also applied to retinoblastoma. Although the clinical observations associated with retinoblastoma fit the two-hit model appropriately, the development of Wilms' tumor appears to be more complex. The rarity of familial Wilms' tumor suggests that multiple gene abnormalities are involved.

The WT1 locus encodes four different proteins. It contains 10 exons and spans nearly 50 kilobase (kb) [124,126,127,129,130]. The gene has a zinc finger in which mutations are found. Alternative RNA splicing results in the inclusion or exclusion of different exons. This may result in as many as 16 WT1 isoforms [124]. It is the complex functions of these multiple splice variants that are involved in cellular development. Expression of the WT1 gene and function of its encoded proteins have been studied in the attempt to determine how WT1 regulates cellular maturation.

The exact function of WT1 is unknown, but it is felt that its expression results in coordinated apoptosis, differentiation, and proliferation. Haber et al. [132] have shown that wild-type WT1 can induce apoptosis in embryonal tumor cell lines. Englert et al. [133] created cell lines with WT1 expression that resulted in EGF receptor downregulation and cell apoptosis. Studies such as these support the role of WT1 as a tumor suppressor. In addition, the development by Kreidberg et al. [127] of knockout mice with a WT1 null mutation resulted in the failure of normal kidney development, suggesting WT1's role as a regulator of cell proliferation and differentiation. In vitro studies by Menke et al. [123] looked at the function of WT1 transcriptional regulators, with each having different functions and likely to be cell dependent. The specific role of WT1 as a transcriptional regulator is not clear, as the physiological rationale of splice variants and the necessary cellular environment are all unknown. One can conclude that the WT1 locus encodes data required by nephrogenic tissue to achieve normal developmental maturation.

Nephrogenic rests in kidneys removed for Wilms' tumor have been found to have mutations at WT1 [125]. Nephrogenic rests are microscopic residues of renal blastemal tissue, found in about 1 in 200 to 300 infant autopsies [125]. This immature blastemal tissue is rarely found after infancy except in kidneys removed for Wilms' tumor. It is felt that these rests are precursors for Wilms' tumor development. Nephrogenic rests also occur in other syndromes associated with an increased incidence of Wilms' tumor. There are two broad classifications of rests: perilobar and intralobar. Both may be multifocal and occasionally diffuse within the renal cortex. Grundy et al. [128] studied the association of LOH at WT1 and its association with nephrogenic rests. In the 286 Wilms' tumors analyzed, 40% of the nephrogenic rests had LOH for the alleles at 11p [129]. Intralobar rests were found to have LOH at both 11p13 and 11p15. In contrast, perilobar rests had LOH only at 11p13. The alleles at 11p15 have been implicated in other types of childhood cancer, such as Beckwith-Wiedemann syndrome, and are also felt to play a pathogenic role in the development of Wilms' tumor [125]. Consequently, this locus has been named *WT2*. Other genes found at this locus include insulin-like growth factor-2 (*IGF-2*), which may be involved in the pathogenesis of childhood cancers [125].

In summary, studies of Wilms' tumor have provided some insight into the links between cancer and development. It is known that normal renal development is dependent on controlled proliferation, differentiation, and apoptosis. Although several models have been suggested for the genetic predisposition for Wilms' tumor, it is clear that it is more complex than the two-hit model that can be applied to retinoblastoma. The association with immature blastemal tissue is still being clarified. Many chromosomal abnormalities are likely involved in its formation. The *WT1* locus is certainly a very important regulator of cell formation and apoptosis in nephrogenesis. Although *WT1* has been shown to act as a transcriptional factor regulating kidney development, its exact role has yet to be determined. The role of *WT2* and proteins encoded in or near this locus has also been an area of significant interest. Mutations at *WT1* and *WT2* have clearly been implicated in the formation of Wilms' tumor as well as in childhood syndromes associated with this tumor.

Conclusion

Great advances have been made with regard to understanding the molecular mechanisms behind the development of renal cancers (Table 16.1). Many of the renal cancers have well characterized tumor-suppressor genes or proto-oncogenes that may be good targets for future gene therapy. The discovery of new syndromes that cause renal cancer, such as Birt-Hogg-Dube, continues to provide further characterization of different forms of renal cancer and enables the clinician to offer better genetic counseling to affected families. With the great advances in the last decade, it is certain that more effective treatments for renal carcinoma will be available in the near future.

Table 16.1. Kidney Turners and Their Associated Mutations

Tumor Type	Chromsomal Alterations
Clear Cell Carcinoma	
VHL Disease	3p25.5
Sporadic Clear Cell	3p(3p13–14, 3p21–26), 17p, PTEN, p53
Hereditary Clear Cell	3p to 8q
Tuberous Sclerosis	TSC1(9q34), TSC2(11p13)
Papillary Renal Cell Carcinoma	
Sporadic Papillary	7(MET), trisomy 7, 17, 16 and X, 9q, 11q, 14q, 21q, 6p
Hereditary Papillary	7q(7q31.1–34), 7(MET)
Chromophobe	
birt-Hogg-Dube	17p11.2
Sporadic	1,2,6,10,13,17,21
Oncocytoma	1p, 14q, X, Y, 5q35 to 11q13
Collecting Duct Carcinoma	1, X, Y, 22, 23
Wilm's Tumor	WT1(11p13), WT2(11p15)

References

1. Khoo SK, Kahnoski K, Sugimura J, et al. Inactivation of BHD in sporadic renal tumors. Cancer Res 2003;63:4583–4587.
2. Walther MM, Enquist EG, Jennings SB, Gnarra JR, Zbar B, Linehan WM. Molecular genetics of renal cell carcinoma. In: Vogelzang NJ, Scardino PT, Shipley WU, Coffey DS, eds. Comprehensive Textbook of Genitourinary Oncology. Baltimore: Williams & Wilkins, 1999:116–128.
3. Linehan WM, Zbar B, Klausner RD. Renal carcinoma. In: Scriver CR, Beaudet AL, Sly WS, Valle D, Vogelstein B, eds. Metabolic and Molecular Basis of Inherited Disease. 2000.
4. Yu MC, Mack TM, Hannish R, Cicioni C, Henderson BE. Cigarette smoking and obesity, diuretic use, and coffee consumption as risk factors for renal cell carcinoma. J Natl Cancer Inst 1986;77:351–356.
5. McCredie M, Stewart JH. Risk factors for kidney cancer in New South Wales. Eur J Cancer 1992; 28A:2050–2054.
6. Malker HR, Malker BK, McLaughlin JK, Blot WJ. Kidney cancer among leather workers. Lancet 1984;1:56–57.
7. Maclure M. Asbestos and renal adenocarcinoma: a case-control study. Environ Res 1987;42:353–361.

8. Chung-Park M, Parveen T, Lam M. Acquired cystic disease of the kidneys and renal cell carcinoma in chronic renal insufficiency without dialysis treatment. Nephron 1989;53:157–161.

9. Kovacs G, Ishikawa I. High incidence of papillary renal cell tumours in patients on chronic haemodialysis. Histopathology 1993;22:135–139.

10. Choyke PL, Glenn GM, Walther MM, et al. Hereditary renal cancers. Radiology 2003;226: 33–46.

11. Farrow GM. Diseases of the kidney. In: Murphy WM, ed. Urological Pathology, 2nd ed. Philadelphia: WB Saunders, 1997:464–470.

12. Couch V, Lindor NM, Karnes PS, Michels VV. Von Hippel-Lindau disease. Mayo Clin Proc 2000;75: 265–272.

13. Maher ER, Iselius L, Yater JR, et al. Von Hippel-Lindau disease: a genetic study. J Med Genet 1991;28:443–447.

14. Iliopoulos O, Eng C. Genetic and clinical aspects of familial renal neoplasms. Semin Oncol 2000; 27:138–149.

15. Seizinger BR, Rouleau GA, Ozelius LJ, et al. von Hippel-Lindau disease maps to the region of chromosome 3 associated with renal cell carcinoma. Nature 1988;332:268–269.

16. Latif F, Tory K, Gnarra J, et al. Identification of the von Hippel-Lindau disease tumor suppressor gene. Science 1993;260:1317–1320.

17. Knudson AG Jr. Mutation and cancer: statistical study of retinoblastoma. Proc Natl Acad Sci USA 1971;68:820–823.

18. Tory K, Brauch H, Linehan WM, et al. Specific genetic change in tumors associated with von Hippel-Lindau disease. J Natl Cancer Inst 1989; 81:1097–1101.

19. Lubensky IA, Gnarra JR, Bertheau P, Walther MM, Linehan WM, Zhuang Z. Allelic deletions of the VHL gene detected in multiple microscopic clear cell renal lesions in von Hippel-Lindau disease patients. Am J Pathol 1996;149:2089–2094.

20. Hosoe S, Brauch H, Latif F, et al. Localization of the von Hippel-Lindau disease gene to a small region of chromosome 3. Genomics 1990;8: 634–640.

21. Richards FM, Maher Er, Latif F, et al. Detailed genetic mapping of the von Hippel-Lindau disease tumor suppressor gene. J Med Gent 1993; 30:104–107.

22. Chen F, Kishida T, Yao M, et al. Ge mutations in the von Hippel-Lindau disease tumor suppressor gene: correlations with phenotype. Hum Mutat 1995;5:66–75.

23. Abar B, Kishida T, Chen F, et al. Germline mutations in the von Hippel-Lindau disease (VHL) gene in families from North America, Europe, and Japan. Hum Mutat 1996;8:348–357.

24. Gnarra J, Tory K, Weng Y, et al. Mutation of the VHL tumour suppressor gene in renal carcinoma. Nature Genet 1994;7:85–90.

25. Corless Cl, Kiebel A, Iliopoulos O, Kaelin WG Jr. Immunostaining of the von Hippel-Lindau gene product (pVHL) in normal and neoplastic human tissues. Hum Pathol 1997;26:459–464.

26. Lee S, Neumann M, Stearman R, et al. Transcription-dependent nuclear-cytoplasmic trafficking is required for the function of the von Hippel-Lindau tumor suppressor protein. Mol Cell Biol 1999;19:1486–1497.

27. Lee S, Chen DY, Humphrey JS, Gnarra JR, Linehan WM, Klausner RD. Nuclear/cytoplasmic localization of the von Hippel-Lindau tumor suppressor gene product is determined by cell density. Proc Natl Acad Sci USA 1996;93:1770–1775.

28. Duan Dr. Humphrey JS, Chen DY, et al. Characterization of the VHL tumor suppressor gene product: localization, complex formation, and the effect of natural inactivating mutations. Proc Natl Acad Sci USA 1995;92:6459–6463.

29. Schraml P, Hergovitz A, Hatz F, et al. Relevance of nuclear and cytoplasmic von Hippel Lindau protein expression of renal carcinoma progression. Am J Pathol 2003;163:1013–1020.

30. Duan DR, Puase A, Burgess WH, et al. Inhibition of transcription elongation by the VHL tumor suppressor protein. Science 1995;269: 1402–1406.

31. Garrett KP, Tan S, Brasher JN, Lane WS, Conaway JW, Conaway RC. Molecular cloning of an essential subunit of RNA polymerase II elongation factor SIII. Proc Natl Acad Sci USA 1994;91: 5237–5241.

32. Garrett KP, Aso T, Brasher JN, et al. Positive regulation of general transcription factor SIII by a tailed ubiquitin homolog. Proc Natl Acad Sci USA 1995;92:7172–7176.

33. Turner KJ. Inherited renal cancer. BJU Int 2000; 86:155–164.

34. Kible A, Iliopoulos O, De Caprio JD, Kaelin WG. Binding of the von Hippel-Lindau tumour suppressor protein to elongin B and C. Science 1995; 269:1444–1446.

35. Kishida T, Stackhouse Tm, Chen F, Lerman MI, Zbar B. Cellular proteins that bind the von Hippel-Lindau gene product: mapping of binding domains and the effect of missense mutations. Cancer Res 1995;55:4544–4548.

36. Decekr JH, Weidt EJ, Brieger J. The von Hippel-Lindau tumor suppressor gene: a rare and intriguing disease opening new insight into basic mechanisms of carcinogenesis. Cancer Genet Cytogenet 1997;93:74–83.

37. Aso T, Lane WS, Conaway JW, Convawy RC. Elongin (SIII): a multisubunit regulator of elon-

gation by RNA polymerase II. Science 1995;269: 1439–1443.

38. Pause A, Lee S, Worrell RA, et al. The von Hippel-Lindau tumor-suppressor gene product forms a stable complex with human CUL-2, a member of the Cdc53 family of proteins. Proc Natl Acad Sci USA 1997;94:2156–2161.

39. Salceda S, Caro J. Hypoxia-inducible factor 1α (HIF1α) protein is rapidly degraded by the ubiquitin-proteasome system under normoxic conditions: its stabilization by hypoxia depends upon redox-induced changes. J Biol Chem 1997;272: 22642–22647.

40. Na X, Wu G, Ryan CK, et al. Overproduction of vascular endothelial growth factor related to von Hippel-Lindau tumor suppressor gene mutations and hypoxia inducible factor-1 alpha expression in renal cell carcinomas. J Urol 2003;170:588–592.

41. Siemeister G, Weindel K, Mohrs K, Barleon B, Martiny-Baron G, Marme D. Reversion of deregulated expression of vascular endothelial growth factor in human renal carcinoma cells by von Hippel-Lindau tumor suppressor protein. Cancer Res 1996;56:2299–2301.

42. Berger DP, Herstritt L, Dengler WA, Marme D, mertelsmann R, Fiebig HH. Vascular endothelial growth factor (VEGF) mRNA expression in human tumor models of different histologies. Ann Oncol 1995;6:817–825.

43. Takahashi A, Sasaki H, Kim SJ, et al. Markedly increased amounts of messenger RNAs for vascular endothelial growth factor and placenta growth factor in renal cell carcinoma associated with angiogenesis. Cancer Res 194;54:4233–4237.

44. Sato K, Terada K, Sugiama T, et al. Frequent overexpression of vascular endothelial growth factor gene in human renal cell carcinoma. Tohoku J Exp Med 1994;173:355–360.

45. Mukhopadhyay D, Kneblemann B, Cohen HT, Anath S, Sukhatme VP. The von Hippel-Lindau tumor suppressor gene product interacts with SP1 to repress vascular endothelial growth factor promoter activity. Mol Cell Biol 1997;17:5629–5639.

46. Pal S, Claffey KP, Dvorac HF, Mukhopadhyay D. The von Hippel-Lindau gene product inhibits vascular permeability factor/vascular endothelial growth factor expression in renal cell carcinoma by blocking protein kinase C pathways. J Biol Chem 1997;272:27509–27512.

47. Wizigmann-Voos S, Breier G, Risau W, Plate KH. Up-regulation of vascular endothelial growth factor and its receptors in von Hippel-Lindau disease-associated and sporadic hemangioblastomas. Cancer Res 1995;55:1358–1364.

48. Ananth S, Knebelmann B, Gruning W, et al. Transforming growth factor beta 1 is a target for the von Hippel-Lindau tumor suppressor and a critical growth factor for clear cell renal carcinoma. Cancer Res 1999;59:2210–2216.

49. Gomella LG, Sargent ER, Wade TP, Anglard P, Linehan WM, Kasid A. Expression of transforming growth factor alpha in normal human adult kidney and enhanced expression of transforming growth factors alpha and beta 1 in renal cell carcinoma. Cancer Res 1989;49:6972–6975.

50. Ohh M, Yauch RL, Lonergan KM, et al. The von Hippel-Lindau tumor suppressor protein is required for proper assembly of an extracellular fibronectin matrix. Mol Cell 1998;1:959–968.

51. Ruoslahti E. Integrins. J Clin Invest 1991;87:1–5.

52. Hynes R. Integrins: versatility, modulation, and signaling in cell adhesion. Cell 1992;69:11–25.

53. Rouslathi E. Fibronectin and its integrin receptors in cancer. Adv Cancer Res 1999;76:1–20.

54. Yoshida MA, Ohyashiki K, Ochi H, et al. Cytogenetic studies of tumor tissue from patients with nonfamilial renal cell carcinoma. Cancer Res 1986;46:2139–2147.

55. Oshida MA, Ohyashiki K, Ochi H, et al. Rearrangement of chromosome 3 in renal cell carcinoma. Cancer Genet Cytogenet 1986;19: 351–354.

56. Nordenson I, Ljungberg B, Roos G. Chromosomes in renal carcinoma with reference to intratumor heterogeneity. Cancer Genet Cytogenet 1988;32:35–41.

57. Kovacs G, Erlandsson R, Boldog F, et al. Consistent chromosome 3p deletion and loss of heterozygosity in renal cell carcinoma. Proc Natl Acad Sci USA 1988;85:1571–1575.

58. Kovacs G, Frisch S. Clonal chromosome abnormalities in tumor cells from patients with sporadic renal cell carcinomas. Cancer Res 1989;49: 651–659.

59. Anglard P, Brauch TH, Weiss GH, et al. Molecular analysis of genetic changes in the origin and development of renal cell carcinoma. Cancer Res 1991;51:1071–1077.

60. Shuin T, Kondo K, Torigoe S, et al. Frequent somatic mutations and loss of heterozygosity of the von Hippel-Lindau tumor suppressor gene in primary human renal cell carcinomas. Cancer Res 1994;54:2852–2855.

61. Reiter RE, Anglard P, Liu S, Gnarra JR, Linehan WM. Chromosome 17p deletions and p53 mutations in renal cell carcinoma. Cancer Res 1993; 53:3092–3097.

62. Foster K, Crossey PA, Cairns P, et al. Molecular genetic investigation of sporadic renal cell carcinoma: analysis of allele loss on chromosomes 3p, 5q, 11p, 17 and 22. Br J Cancer 1994;69:230–234.

63. Presti JC Jr, Reuter VE, Cordon-Cardo C, Mazumdar N, Fair WR, Jhanwir SC. Allelic

deletions in renal tumors: histopathological correlations. Cancer Res 1993;53:5780–5783.

64. Brenner W, Farber G, Herget T, et al. Loss of tumor suppressor protein PTEN during renal carcinogenesis. Int J Cancer 2002;99:53–57.

65. Cohen AJ, Li FP, Berg S, et al. Hereditary renal-cell carcinoma associated with chromosomal translocation. N Engl J Med 1979;301;592–595.

66. Melendez B, Rodriguez-Perales S, Martinez-Delgado B, et al. Molecular study of a new family with hereditary renal cell carcinoma and a translocation t(3,8)(p13,q24.1)Hum Genet 2003; 112:178–185.

67. Glassberg KI. Renal dysplasia and cystic disease of the kidney. In: Walsh P, Retik AB, Vaughan ED Jr, Wein AJ, eds. Campbell's Urology. Philadelphia: WB Saunders, 1996:1778–1781.

68. Osborne JP, Fryer A, Webb D. Epidemiology of tuberous sclerosis. Ann NY Acad Sci 1991;615: 125–127.

69. European Consortium on Tuberous Sclerosis. Identification and characterization for the tuberous sclerosis gene on chromosome 16. Cell 1993; 75:1305–1315.

70. Kandt RS, Haines JL, Smith M, et al. Linkage of an important gene locus for tuberous sclerosis to a chromosome 16 marker for polycystic kidney disease. Nat Genet 1992;2:37–41.

71. Kovacs G. Papillary renal cell carcinoma: a morphologic and cytogenetic study of 11 cases. Am J Pathol 1989;134:27–34.

72. Mancilla-Jimenez R, Stanley RJ, Blath RA. Papillary renal cell carcinoma: a clinical, radiologic and pathologic study of 34 cases. Cancer 1996; 38:2469.

73. Robson CJ, Churchill BM, Anderson W. The results of radical nephrectomy for renal cell tumours. World J Urol 1969;101:297–301.

74. Zambrano NR, Lubensky IA, Merino MJ, Linehan WM, Walther MM. Histopathology and molecular genetics of renal tumors: toward unification of a classification system. J Urol 1999;162: 1246–1258.

75. Bardelli A, Pugliese L, Comoglio PM. 'Invasive growth' signaling by the Met/HGF receptor: the hereditary renal carcinoma connection. Biochem Biophys Acta 1997;1333:M41–M51.

76. Kovacs G, Szucs S, Deriese W, Baumgartel H. Specific chromosomal aberration in human renal cell carcinoma. Int J Cancer 1978;40:171–178.

77. Kovacs G, Fuzesi L, Emanuel A, Kung HF. Cytogenetics of papillary renal cell tumors. Genes Chromosomes Cancer 1991;3:249–255.

78. Hughson MD, Johnson LD, Silva FG, Kovacs G. Nonpapillary and papillary renal cell carcinoma: a cytogenetic and phenotypic study. Mod Pathol 1993;6:449–456.

79. Henn W, Zwergel T, Wullich B, Thonnes M, Zang KD, Seitz G. Bilateral multicentric papillary renal tumors with heteroclonal origin based on tissue-specific karyotype instability. Cancer 1993;72: 1315–1318.

80. Kovacs G, Tory K, Kovacs A. Development of papillary renal cell tumours is associated with a loss of Y-chromosome-specific DNA sequences. J Pathol 1994;173:39–44.

81. Thrash-Bingham CA, Salazar H, Freed JJ, Greenberg RE, Tartof KD. Genomic alterations and instabilities in renal cell carcinomas and their relationship to tumor pathology. Cancer Res 1995; 55:6189–6195.

82. Tonk V, Wilson KS, Timmons CF, Schneider NR, Tomlison GE. Renal cell carcinoma with translocation (X;1): further evidence for cytogenetically defined subtype. Cancer Genet Cytogenet 1995; 81:72–75.

83. Kardas I, Denis A, Babinska M, et al. Translocation (X;1)(p11.2;q21) in a papillary renal cell carcinoma in a 14–year-old girl. Cancer Genet Cytogenet 1998;101:159–161.

84. Sidhar SK, Clark J, Gill S, et al. The t(X;1) (p11.2;q21.2) translocation in papillary renal cell carcinoma fuses a novel gene PRCC to the TFE3 transcription factor gene. Hum Mol Genet 1996; 5:1333–1338.

85. Zbar B, Glenn G, Lubensky I, et al. Hereditary papillary renal cell carcinoma: clinical studies in 10 families. J Urol 1995;153:907–912.

86. Duh FM, Scherer SW, Tsui LC, Lerman MI, Zbar B, Schmidt L. Gene structure of the human MET proto-oncogene. Oncogene 1997;15:1583–1586.

87. Zbar B, Tory K, Merino M, et al. Hereditary papillary renal cell carcinoma. J Urol 1994;151: 151–156.

88. Zbar B, Lerman M. Inherited carcinomas of the kidney. In: Advances in Cancer Research. 1998: 163–201.

89. Huang Z, Park WS, Pack S, et al. Trisomy 7–harboring nonrandom duplication of the mutant MET allele in hereditary papillary renal carcinomas. Nat Genet 1998;20:66–69.

90. Fischer J, Palmedo G, von Knobloch R, et al. Duplication and overexpression of the mutant allele of the MET proto-oncogene in multiple hereditary papillary renal cell tumours. Oncogene 1998;17:733–739.

91. Bottaro DP, Rubin JS, Faletto DL, et al. Identification of the hepatocyte growth factor receptor as the c-met proto-oncogene product. Science 1991;251:802–804.

92. Giordano S, Zhen Z, Medico E, Gaudino G, Galimi F, Comoglio PM. Transfer of mitogenic and invasive response to scatter factor/hepatocyte growth factor by transfection of human

MET protooncogene. Proc Natl Acad Sci USA 1993;90:649–653.

93. Naldini L, Vigna E, Ferracini R, et al. The tyrosine kinase encoded by the MET protooncogene is activated by autophosphorylation. Mol Cell Biol 1991;4:1793–1803.

94. Ponzetto C, Bardelli A, Zen Z, et al. A multifunctional docking site mediated signaling and transformation by the hepatocyte growth factor-scatter factor receptor family. Cell 1994;77:261–271.

95. Pavlovich CP, Walther MM, Eyler RA, et al. Renal tumors in the Birt-Hogg-Dube syndrome. Am J Surg Pathol 2002;26:1542–1552.

96. Theones W, Storkel ST, Rumpelt JH. Human chromophobe cell renal carcinoma and its variants. Report on 32 cases. J Pathol 1988;155:277–287.

97. Birt Ar, Hogg GR, Dube WJ. Hereditary multiple fibrofilliculomas with trichodiscomas and acrochordomas. Arch Dermatol 1977;113:1674–1677.

98. Zbar B, Alvord G, Glenn G, Turner M, Pavlovich C, Schmidt L. Risk of renal and colonic neoplasm and spontaneous pneumothorax in the Birt-Hogg-Dube syndrome. Cancer Epidemiol Biomarkers Prev 2002;11:393.

99. Nickerson ML, Warren MB, Toro JR, Matrosova V, et al. Mutations in a novel gene lead to kidney tumors, lung wall defects, and benign tumors of the hair follicle in patients with the Birt-Hogg-Dube syndrome. Cancer Cell 2002;2:157.

100. Leiber MM, Tomera KM, Farrow GM. Renal oncocytoma. J Urol 1981;125:481–485.

101. Amin R, Anthony R. Metastatic renal oncocytoma: a case report and review of the literature. Clin Oncol (R Coll Radiol) 1999;11:277–279.

102. Van den Berg E, Dijkhuizen T, Storkel S, et al. Chromosomal changes in renal oncocytomas: evidence that t(5;11)(q35;q13) may characterize a second subgroup of oncocytomas. Cancer Genet Cytogenet 1995;79:164–168.

103. Thrash-Bingham CA, Salazar H, Greenberg RE, Tartof KD. Loss of heterozygosity studies indicate that chromosome arm 1p harbors a tumor suppressor gene for renal oncocytomas. Genes Chromosomes Cancer 1996;16:64–67.

104. Presti JC Jr, Rao PH, Chen Q, et al. Histopathological, cytogenetic and molecular characterization of renal cortical tumors. Cancer Res 1991; 51:1544–1552.

105. Sinke RJ, Dijkhuizen T, Janssen B, et al. Fine mapping of human renal oncocytoma-associated translocation (5;11)(q35;q13) breakpoint. Cancer Genet Cytogenet 1997;96:95–101.

106. Walter TA, Pennington RD, Decker H-J, Sandberg AA. Translocation t(9;11) (p23;q12): a primary chromosomal change in renal oncocytoma. J Urol 1989;142:117–119.

107. Fuzesi L, Gunawan B, Braun S, Boeckman W. Renal oncocytoma with a translocation t(9;11) (p23;q13). J Urol 1994;152:471–472.

108. Neuhaus C, Dijkhuizen T, van den Berg E, et al. Involvement of the chromosomal region 11q13 in renal oncocytoma: a case report and literature review. Cancer Genet Cytogenet 1997;94:95–98.

109. Weirich G, Glenn G, Junker K, et al. Familial renal oncocytoma: clinicopathological study of 5 families. J Urol 1998;160:335–340.

110. Kuoda N, Toi M, Hiroi M, Enzman H. Review of collecting duct carcinoma with focus on clinical and pathobiological aspects. Histopathology 2002;17:1329–1334.

111. Chao D, Zisman A, Pantuck AJ, et al. Collecting duct carcinoma: a clinical study of a rare tumor. J Urol 2002;167: 71–74.

112. Antonellli A, Portesi E, Cozzot A, et al. The collecting duct carcinoma of the kidney: a cytogenetical study. Eur Urol 203;43:680–685.

113. Suartz MA, Kanta J, Schneider DT, et al. Renal medullary carcinoma: clinical, pathologic, immunohistochemical, and genetic analysis with pathogenetic implications. Urology 2002;60: 1083–1089.

114. Fuhrman SA, Lasky LC, Limas C. Prognostic significance of morphologic parameters in renal cell carcinoma. Am J Surg Pathol 1982;6:655–663.

115. Thrasher JB, Paulson DF. Prognostic factors in renal cancer. Urol Clin North Am 1993;20: 247–262.

116. Medeiros LJ, Gelb AB, Weiss LM. Renal cell carcinoma: prognostic significance of morphologic parameters in 121 cases. Cancer 1988;61:1639–1651.

117. Helpap B. Grading and prognostic significance of urologic carcinomas. J Urol 1992;48:245–257.

118. Moch H, Sauter G, Buchholz N, et al. Epidermal growth factor receptor expression is associated with rapid tumor cell proliferation in renal cell carcinoma. Hum Pathol 1997;28:1255–1259.

119. Flint A, Grossman HB, Liebert M, Lloyd RV, Bromberg J. DNA and PCNA content of renal cell carcinoma and prognosis. Am J Clin Pathol 1995;103:14–19.

120. Grignon DG, Abdel-Malak M, Mertens W. Prognostic significance of cellular proliferation in renal cell carcinoma: a comparison of synthesis-phase fraction and proliferating cell nuclear antigen index. Mod Pathol 1995;8:18.

121. Gelb AB, Sudilowsky D, Wu CD, Weiss LM, Meideros LJ. Appraisal of intratumoral microvessel density, MIB-1 score, DNA content and p53 protein expression as prognostic indicators in patients with locally confined renal cell carcinoma. Cancer 1997;80:1768–1775.

122. Hofmockel G, Tsatalpas P, Muller H, et al. Significance of conventional and new prognostic

factors for locally confined renal cell carcinoma. Cancer 1995;76:296–306.

123. Menke A, McInnes L, Hastie ND, Schedl A. The Wilms' tumor suppressor WT1: approaches to gene function. Kidney Int 1998;53:1512–1518.

124. Bove KE. Wilms' tumor and related abnormalities in the fetus and newborn. Semin Perinatol 1999;23:310–318.

125. Call KM, Glaser T, Ito CY, et al. Isolation and characterization of a zinc finger polypeptide gene at the human chromosome 11 Wilms' tumor locus. Cell 1990;60:509–520.

126. Gessler M, Konig A, Bruns GA. The genomic organization and expression of the WT1 gene. Genomics 1992;12:807–813.

127. Kreidberg JA, Sariola H, Loring JM, et al. WT-1 is required for early kidney development. Cell 1993; 74:679–691.

128. Grundy P, Telzerow P, Moksness JM, Breslow NE. clinicopathologic correlates of loss of heterozygosity in Wilms' tumor patients: preliminary results. Med Pediatr Oncol 1996;27:429–433.

129. Knudson AG, Strong LC. Mutation and cancer: a model for Wilms' tumor of the kidney. J Natl Cancer Inst 1976;48:313–324.

130. Haber DA, Sohn RL, Buckler AJ, Pelleteir J, Call KM, Housman DE. Alternative splicing and genomic structure of the Wilms' tumor gene WT1. Proc Natl Acad Sci USA 1991;88:9618–9622.

131. Tadokoro K, Oki N, Fujhi H, Oshima A, Inque T, Yamada M. Genomic organisation of the human WT1 gene. Jpn J Cancer Res 1992;83:1198–1203.

132. Haber D, Englert C, Maheswaran S. Functional properties of WT1. Med Pediatr Oncol 1996;27: 453–455.

133. Englert C, Hou X, Maheswaran S, et al. WT1 suppresses synthesis of the epidermal growth factor receptor and induces apoptosis. EMBO J 1995; 14:4662.

17

Cytokine and Angiogenesis Inhibitors

Simon Chowdhury, Timothy G. Eisen, and Martin Gore

Renal cell carcinoma is an important malignancy accounting for approximately 3% of all adult cancers [1]. The incidence of renal cell carcinoma has been steadily and significantly increasing over the past two decades, with worldwide mortality expected to exceed 100,000 [2]. A significant proportion of patients with localized disease can be cured by nephrectomy; however, at presentation approximately 50% of patients have locally advanced or metastatic disease [3]. The outlook for these patients remains poor, with a 5-year survival of less than 10% [2].

Renal cell carcinoma is an inherently chemoresistant tumor. There have been many trials of single agent and combination chemotherapy regimens; however, response rates are low and characteristically of short duration. Yagoda and colleagues [4], in a review of 4093 adequately treated patients in 83 phase II chemotherapy trials published between 1983 and 1993, showed an overall response rate of only 6%. Thus, there is no role for chemotherapy alone in the treatment of renal cell carcinoma, but there have been improvements in survival as a result of the development of cytokine therapy.

Prognostic Factors

Metastatic renal cell carcinoma encompasses a heterogeneous group of patients, and it is important to identify prognostic factors that predict survival. Assessment of these factors can assist in decisions regarding patient management as well as categorizing patients in clinical studies, thus aiding trial interpretation. The initial analysis of these factors was carried out by Elson and colleagues [5]. This retrospective study looked at 610 patients treated in the Eastern Cooperative Group (ECOG) phase II trials for advanced renal cell carcinoma between 1975 and 1984. They identified the following risk factors (see below), which enabled them to stratify patients into appropriate risk groups (Table 17.1):

1. ECOG performance status (performance status 1, 2, and 3 counting as one, two, and three risk factors respectively)
2. Recent diagnosis (<1 year)
3. More than one metastatic site
4. Recent weight loss
5. Prior cytotoxic chemotherapy

Other studies analyzing prognostic factors in patients with metastatic renal cell carcinoma have defined different parameters, but consistently performance status and a measure of disease extent appear to be important indicators of survival [6–8].

A retrospective study by Motzer and colleagues [9] looked at the relationship between pretreatment clinical features and survival in 670 patients with advanced renal cell carcinoma treated in Memorial Sloan-Kettering Cancer Center clinical trials between 1975 and 1996. The

Table 17.1. Prognostic groups and their impact on survival

Risk group	No. of risk factors	No. of patients	Median survival (months)
1	0–1	113	12.8
2	2	141	7.7
3	3	151	5.3
4	4	123	3.4
5	5	82	2.1

From Elson et al. [5].

following five pretreatment features were associated with a shorter survival in the multivariate analysis:

1. Low Karnofsky performance status (<80%)
2. High serum lactate dehydrogenase (>1.5 times upper limit of normal)
3. Low hemoglobin (less than the lower limit of normal)
4. High corrected serum calcium (≥10 mg/dL)
5. Absence of prior nephrectomy

Using these factors the authors stratified patients into three separate risk groups (Table 17.2). A recent study from the same group has analyzed prognostic factors in previously treated patients with metastatic renal cell carcinoma [10]. More patients are entering second-line trials of therapy, and thus stratification of these patients is becoming increasingly important. A total of 251 patients treated in 29 consecutive trials between 1975 and 2002 were analyzed. Median survival for the 251 patients was 10.2 months and differed according to the year of treatment, with patients treated after 1990 showing longer survival. The median overall survival for this group was 12.7 months.

The purpose of this study was to establish prognostic factors for this group of patients, who had all received prior cytokine therapy (interferon and/or interleukin-2), and thus establish prognostic factors for current clinical trial design. Pretreatment features associated with a poorer prognosis in the multivariate analysis were low Karnofsky performance status (<80%), low hemoglobin (less than the lower limit of normal), and high corrected serum calcium (≥10 mg/dL). Although these and the previously mentioned prognostic factors are useful in aiding management decisions and subsequently in interpreting trial results, they are not prescriptive, and each patient should be assessed individually.

It is also important to be aware that histologically renal cell carcinoma is a diverse group of tumors, including clear cell, papillary, chromophobe, collecting duct and unclassified cell types. Of these, clear cell is the most common subtype, accounting for approximately 70% of cases. The importance of distinguishing between these different histologies is shown by the fact that metastatic non–clear cell carcinoma is characterized by an increased resistance to systemic therapy and poorer survival [11].

Immunotherapy

The immune system has evolved to detect and destroy molecules or pathogens that are recognized as "non-self" but not to react to host tissues. Manipulation of the immune system for cancer treatment attempts either to make the tumor appear more foreign when compared to normal tissues or to magnify host immune responses to tumors. The variable natural history of metastatic renal cell carcinoma, and occasional observed spontaneous regression

Table 17.2. Prognostic groups and their impact on survival

Risk group	Risk factors	Percent of patients	Median survival (months)
Favorable	0	25	20
Intermediate	1–2	53	10
Poor	3 or more	22	4

From Motzer et al. [9].

Table 17.3. The impact of interferon-alpha on survival in renal cancer

Prognostic group	Median survival ECOG (months)	Median survival IFN-α (months)	p value
Good	11.4	23.3	<.001
Moderate	8.1	11.3	.1014
Poor	5.0	6.9	NS

ECOG, Eastern Cooperative Oncology Group; NS, nonsignificant.
From Fossa et al. [8].

suggest a role for the immune system in control of tumor progression and provide a rationale for the use of immunotherapy. To improve on the current rate of success seen with immunotherapy, some important issues need to be addressed:

- Why are certain cancers more susceptible?
- Are there factors that predict responsiveness?
- What mechanisms underlie resistance and development of resistance?

Studies addressing some of these points are already underway and have already demonstrated T cell [12,13] and dendritic cell dysfunction [14] in this patient group.

Further evidence of an innate antitumor response is provided by the fact that tumor-infiltrating lymphocytes can be detected in renal cell carcinoma tissue [15]. In addition, the presence of cytotoxic T lymphocytes (CTLs) within this population suggests the presence of antigens for their development, and analysis of CTLs has revealed four separate antigens defined in renal cell carcinoma [16]. The ways in which these discoveries can be harnessed to improve current therapies are under investigation.

Cytokine Therapy

Cytokines are soluble proteins produced by mononuclear cells of the immune system that act as messengers between cells. They have a wide range of biological effects, particularly on cells of the immune system and hemopoietic lineage. The cytokine network is complicated, and this complexity makes it difficult to know how intervention with one cytokine will affect the production of others. Cytokines may act antagonistically, and thus an intervention planned to enhance a particular branch of the immune response could actually lead to suppression. Another difficulty is in providing adequate dose levels and maintaining them over a clinically significant period.

Despite these difficulties, cytokine therapy has become an integral part of biological therapy for metastatic renal cell carcinoma. Their activity is shown in separate survival analyzes by Fossa et al. [8] (Table 17.3), Jones et al. [7] (Table 17.4), and Motzer et al. [9]. In the analysis by Motzer et al., cytokine therapy (interferon-α [IFN-α] and/or interleukin-2 [IL-2]) was shown to have a statistically significant survival advantage: 12.9 months versus 6.3 months for chemotherapy; $p < .0001$). The benefit of cytokine therapy appeared to be greatest in those with more favor-

Table 17.4. The impact of interleukin-2 (IL-2) on survival in renal cancer

Prognostic group	Median survival ECOG (months)	Median survival IL-2 (months)	p value
Good	12.6	20.4	.0001
Moderate	7.2	11.4	.0013
Poor	5.6	6.3	NS

From Jones et al. [7].

able prognostic disease. The median survival times for favorable-risk, intermediate-risk and poor-risk patients were 27, 12, and 6 months for those treated with cytokines and 15, 7, and 3 months for those treated with chemotherapy, respectively [17].

Negrier and colleagues [18] have identified factors predictive of rapid progression of patients with metastatic renal cell carcinoma treated by cytokines. They looked at the records of 782 patients enrolled in trials using cytokine regimens by the Groupe Francais d'Immunotherapie. Four independent factors predictive of rapid progression under cytokine treatment were identified: hepatic metastases, short interval from primary to metastases (<1 year), more than one metastatic site, and elevated neutrophil counts. Patients who had at least three of these factors have ≥80% probability of rapid progression despite treatment, and this may well influence treatment choices.

The Role of Nephrectomy Before Cytokine Therapy

The role of nephrectomy in metastatic renal cell carcinoma remains controversial. Distant metastases may regress after nephrectomy. However, because the rate of regression is low (<1%) [19], the theory that nephrectomy causes regression is unproven, and morbidity is associated with nephrectomy, it is not indicated for this purpose. Historically there was a role for nephrectomy under the following circumstances:

1. Large symptomatic primary tumor associated with small to moderate volume metastatic disease. Local symptoms such as pain and hemorrhage are well palliated by nephrectomy. Nephrectomy has a lower morbidity than radiotherapy or embolization and may also improve or completely reverse systemic constitutional symptoms by substantially reducing the tumor burden.

2. Large asymptomatic primary tumor associated with small metastatic disease, where it is likely that the patient will develop local symptoms before symptoms related to metastases occur. We have called this "prophylactic palliation."

3. Patients with a solitary metastasis, where prolonged survival can occur following a combination of nephrectomy and resection of the metastasis [20].

These clinical scenarios in our view are still valid reasons to perform a nephrectomy in the presence of metastatic disease. However, recently randomized trials have provided us with data that argues more strongly for nephrectomy prior to cytokine therapy in the setting of metastatic disease. Certain immunotherapy trials have required patients to have a nephrectomy prior to trial entry. The rationale for this approach is that reduction of tumor burden may increase the likelihood of response. This biological argument is supported by animal data showing that the large bulk of primary tumor is either immunosuppressive or acts as an "immunological sink" with suppression of cell-mediated immunity that is reversed upon removal of the primary tumor [21,22]. Improvements in human immune responses have also been demonstrated postnephrectomy [23]. Removal of the primary also gives the possibility of harvesting tumor infiltrating lymphocytes and tumor cells for use in experimental therapies.

The role of cytoreductive surgery in relation to cytokine therapy for metastatic renal cell carcinoma has been addressed by three studies. In the first of these studies Pantuck and colleagues [24] conducted a retrospective analysis of patients with renal cell carcinoma treated with nephrectomy at UCLA. Patients with metastatic disease treated with nephrectomy prior to IL-2 therapy had significantly improved survival compared to patients treated with IL-2 alone (IL-2 alone; 1- and 2-year survival 29% and 4%, nephrectomy followed by IL-2 67% and 44%, respectively). Like any retrospective analysis there is a concern about selection bias, and patients who are not offered nephrectomy are often those with worse prognostic factors.

However, these results have been supported by two randomized phase III trials. In the larger of these studies, the Southwest Oncology Group (SWOG) trial 8949 assessed whether nephrectomy prior to treatment with IFN-α prolonged survival. A total of 246 patients with metastatic renal cell carcinoma were randomized to radical nephrectomy followed by IFN-α or to IFN-α alone. This trial showed that nephrectomy prior to systemic IFN-α gave a significant survival benefit (median survival: IFN-α alone: 8.1

months; nephrectomy followed by IFN-α 11.1 months, $p = .05$) [25].

A similar positive result was obtained in a simultaneous phase III trial conducted by the European Organization for Research and Treatment of Cancer (EORTC) that randomized 85 patients into the same treatment arms as SWOG 8949 [26]. Again nephrectomy preceding treatment with IFN-α significantly improved survival (median survival: IFN-α alone: 7 months; nephrectomy followed by IFN-α 17 months, hazard ratio 0.54, 95% confidence interval [CI] 0.31–0.94). This confirmatory result, even in a smaller study, strengthens the results from the SWOG trial and increases the likelihood that the differences seen in survival are due to nephrectomy.

The combined updated analysis of these two trials has just been published, and yielded a median survival of 13.6 months for nephrectomy followed by IFN-α versus 7.8 months for IFN-α alone [27]. This represents a 31% reduction in the risk of death ($p = .002$). Thus, cytoreductive nephrectomy appears to significantly improve overall survival in patients with metastatic renal cell carcinoma treated with IFN-α. This effect was independent of performance status, the site of metastases, and the presence of measurable disease. Although the result is statistically significant, the overall survival advantage is only 5.8 months, and as the authors state, emphasizes the need for more potent immunotherapy in the setting of cytoreductive nephrectomy.

It is important to stress that in both trials patients were highly selected initially by high performance status (0 or 1). The EORTC also excluded patients whose responses they felt would not be improved by removal of the primary tumor. This included disease distribution (bone, liver, contralateral kidney), extent of metastases, non–clear cell histology, and patients at risk of rapid worsening of symptoms after surgery. Although the Flanigan et al. [27] study does not comment on such additional exclusion factors, it would appear likely that further selection occurred, as it took 7 years to accrue 246 patients from 80 institutions at an average of one patient recruited every 2 years from each institution. Authors from both studies recommend nephrectomy before immunotherapy as a standard treatment for patients with metastatic renal cell carcinoma. Although we would concur with this conclusion, it is important to stress that these results are not applicable to the overall population of patients with metastatic renal cell carcinoma especially those of lower performance statuses and other negative prognostic features.

A concern especially when considering post-nephrectomy systemic therapies is the morbidity associated with surgery. Improved surgical techniques mean that a high proportion of patients will proceed to systemic therapies postoperatively. For example, in the EORTC study only one patient randomized to surgery failed to receive postoperative IFN-α. A report from Naitoh and colleagues [28] suggests that even patients with locally advanced disease (T3 with vena caval thrombi) can safely undergo nephrectomy, with 80% subsequently receiving immunotherapy. Improvements in operative technique are likely to further decrease operative morbidity and improve the number of patients eligible for systemic therapies as well as the time to commencement of such therapies.

Interferons

Interferons were the first cytokines to be identified as a family of proteins produced by cells in response to viral infection or stimulation with double-stranded RNA, antigens, or mitogens [29]. They have a wide range of actions including immunomodulatory activity, antiviral activity, antiproliferative effects on normal and malignant cells, inhibition of angiogenesis, and enhancement of expression of a variety of cell surface antigens. Their direct antiproliferative activity is thought to play a major part in their antitumor effects, but other actions may prove important. No definitive mechanism has been identified to explain how interferons inhibit the growth of tumors, except that they prolong the G0/G1 phase of the cell cycle. This heterogeneous group of glycoproteins are classified into α, β, and γ types.

The majority of clinical research has centered on IFN-α, as it appears to have the greatest activity. Most studies have reported response rates of 15% to 20% with IFN-α and median response durations of 6 to 10 months [29]. A dosing range of 5 to 10 million IU/m^2 given intramuscularly or subcutaneously has been most commonly used, although an optimum treatment regimen or duration has not been defined. An alternative form is pegylated interferon (PEG-IFN) where IFN-α is modified by the addition of a branched polyethylene-glycol (PEG) molecule. This results in sustained absorption and prolonged half-life after subcutaneous administration, allowing weekly administration, although it may cause longer duration side effects. Two recent multi-center phase II trials have reported comparable results. Motzer and colleagues [30] reported a response rate of 13% (five of 40 previously untreated patients; one complete response [CR], and four partial responses [PRs]) [30]. Bukowski and colleagues [31] reported a response rate of 14% in 44 previously untreated patients.

Despite numerous clinical trials, it was not known until recently whether therapy with IFN-α improved survival. A Medical Research Council (MRC) study addressed this issue by comparing subcutaneous IFN-α (10 mU sub-cutaneously [sc] three times per week for 12 weeks; $n = 174$) with oral medroxyprogesterone acetate (MPA) (300 mg daily for 12 weeks; $n = 176$) [32]. The trial was stopped in November 1997 when data were available for 335 patients. There was a 28% reduction in the risk of death in the IFN-α group (hazard ratio 0.72; 95% CI, 0.55–0.94; $p = .017$). Interferon-α gave an improvement in 1 year survival of 12% (MPA 31%, IFN-α 43%) and an improvement in median survival of 2.5 months (MPA 6 moths, IFN-α 8.5 months). A reanalysis of the mature data confirms the survival advantage in patients treated with IFN-α (2-year survival improvement 9%; 13% MPA and 22% with IFN-α) [33]. As the authors suggest, the small benefit of IFN-α should be weighed against potential toxicity. However, IFN-α should become the standard control arm in future trials for advanced renal cell carcinoma.

Support for this view comes from the Cochrane Review of immunotherapy for advanced renal cell carcinoma [34]. The results from six studies (involving 963 patients) showed that IFN-α is superior to controls (odds ratio for death at 1 year = 0.67; 95% CI, 0.5–0.89). The weighted average median improvement in sur-vival was 2.6 months. The reviewers concluded that IFN-α provides a survival benefit when compared to other commonly used treatments, and that it should be considered as the control arm in future studies of systemic agents.

Unlike chemotherapy, the time taken to respond to interferons may be prolonged and varies widely. Most patients who are going to respond will have done so by 3 to 4 months, and it is unusual for patients who progress on inter-ferons to subsequently respond. However, there are reports of responses only starting to occur at 6 and 9 months. There is also the question of treatment duration in patients with either stabilization of disease or a partial or complete remission. Our current practice is to continue treatment indefinitely for those patients with stable disease or in remission, provided they are able to tolerate the side effects and treatment is stopped as soon as progressive disease occurs. Toxicity associated with interferon therapy includes flu-like symptoms, rashes, gastroin-testinal complaints, liver dysfunction, neurolog-ical complaints, and fatigue, and are highly dose and schedule dependent. It is possible to allevi-ate some symptoms by administration at night and by the use of paracetamol and/or nonsteroidal antiinflammatory drugs prior to administration.

The benefit observed with IFN-α appears to be greatest in patients with good or moderate prognostic disease [17]. Table 17. 3 shows the impact of IFN α on survival in renal cancer; it is derived from a case-control study involving 231 patients. Controls were obtained from an ECOG database of patients treated in nonbiological therapy trials.

Attempts have been made to augment the activity of IFN-α with 13-cis-retinoic acid (13-CRA). The rationale for this approach was the observation that 13-CRA increased the antipro-liferative effects of IFN-α in several interferon-sensitive renal carcinoma cell lines [35]. An initial phase II trial showed a promising response rate of 30% [36], and so a randomized phase III study was conducted to see whether the addition of 13-CRA to IFN-α was superior to IFN-α alone [37]. Response proportion and sur-vival did not increase with the combination, and so this cannot be recommended in the treatment of metastatic renal cell carcinoma.

A trial of IFN-γ versus placebo in metastatic renal cell carcinoma showed similar response rates in both groups (4.4% interferon versus 6.6% placebo; $p = .54$) [38]. The median time to progression was 1.9 months in both arms of the study ($p = .49$), and there was no significant dif-ference in median survival (12.2 months with interferon versus 15.7 months with placebo; $p = .52$). The addition IFN-γ to IFN-α has also been

cause tumor regression. In a pilot study by Figlin and colleagues [47] involving 55 patients treated with nephrectomy followed by TILs plus low-dose IL-2, 19/55 patients (34.5%) responded and 5 (9%) achieved a complete response. In the sub-group of 23 patients, who received CD8$^+$ TILs, the overall response rate was 43.5%. In view of this encouraging single-institution study, a randomized multicenter study was conducted to compare CD8$^+$ TILs plus low-dose IL-2 versus low-dose IL-2 alone [48]. All patients underwent nephrectomy from which tissue was obtained to generate CD8$^+$ TILs. In the intention-to-treat analysis, there was no significant difference in response rate (9.4% vs. 11.4%) and 1-year survival rate (55% vs. 47%) in the TIL/IL-2 and IL-2 groups, respectively. However, it is difficult to draw meaningful conclusions from this study, as only 48% of patients who were randomized to the TIL/IL-2 arm actually received TIL therapy. The major cause for this was cell-processing failures with insufficient yield of viable cells, although in the pilot study 96% of intended patients were treated with CD8$^+$ TILs (23 of 24).

In patients who have initially responded to IL-2, there remains the possibility to re-treat with IL-2 at relapse. In a study from Rosenberg's group [49], 48 patients with either metastatic renal cell carcinoma or melanoma who had initially achieved a partial or complete response to IL-2–based immunotherapy were re-treated at relapse. Only two of the 48 patients responded, and so it seems that re-treatment rarely produces a second response, and alternative approaches should be considered in these patients.

Interleukin-2 and Interferon-α

Synergistic antitumor effects of combining IL-2 and IFN-α are seen in murine tumor models and provide a rationale for their use in the clinical setting. The exact mechanisms of synergy are unknown, but it is possible that administration of IFN-α may increase the immunogenicity of tumor cells via an enhancement of their histocompatibility and tumor-associated antigens, thus increasing their lysis by CTLs, the number of which are increased by IL-2.

Clinical trials investigating IFN-α and IL-2 combination therapy have used different routes of administration, treatment schedules, cytokine doses, patient selection and response criteria. Thus comparisons are difficult; however, an overview of phase I and II trials showed a response rate of 20% in over 1400 patients with metastatic renal cell carcinoma [44], with approximately 25% of responders achieving a complete response.

A French multicenter randomized trial investigated the efficacy of single-agent versus combination IL-2 and IFN-α [50]. A total of 425 patients were randomized to receive either IL-2 alone (18 mU/m^2/day CVI on days 1 to 5 and days 12 to 15, as two induction cycles followed by four maintenance cycles), IFN-α alone (18 mU sc 3 times/week for 10 weeks), or a combination of IL-2 and IFN-α (same dose IL-2, but only 6 mU IFN-α three times/week, during the two induction and subsequent maintenance periods). Intention-to-treat analysis showed a significantly improved response rate after 10 weeks (IL-2: 6.5%; IFN-α: 7.5%; IL-2 and IFN-α: 20%; $p < .01$) and 1-year event-free survival (IL-2: 15%; IFN-α: 12%; IL-2 and IFN-α: 20%; $p = .01$) for patients receiving combination therapy. However, there was no significant difference in overall survival between the three groups (IL-2: 12 months; IFN-α: 13 months; IL-2 and IFN-α: 17 months; $p = .55$). Importantly, as with the case-control studies of IFN-α and IL-2, this study identified a subgroup of patients who had little chance of benefiting from treatment. These patients had more than one metastatic site, liver involvement, an interval between diagnosis of the primary tumor and development of metastases of less than 1 year, or a performance status of $\geqslant 1$.

This study also assessed the benefit of crossover therapy after failure of IL-2 or IFN-α [51]. A total of 113 patients with progressive disease after first-line treatment received either IFN-α ($n = 48$) or IL-2 ($n = 65$) as second-line treatment. Only four patients achieved a PR (one with IFN-α; three with IL-2); of these patients, three had stable disease or had responded to first-line treatment. All partial responders had a performance status of 0 and pulmonary metastases. Only one patient with confirmed disease progression after IL-2 subsequently responded to IFN-α. Thus in patients who progress rapidly during first-line treatment, additional benefit from further cytokine treatment is unlikely. Further studies are needed to see whether crossing over from one cytokine to another is able to increase survival in selected patients who have experienced a long period of stabilization or have relapsed after an initial response.

Other Cytokines

Several other interleukins (for example IL-1, -4, and -6) have been tested in phase I and II trials in renal cell carcinoma, but antitumor activity has been low, with response rates of less than 5%. One of the more promising new agents is IL-12, which promotes cell-mediated immunity through its regulatory effects on T and natural killer (NK) cells. In a randomized phase II trial of IL-12 versus IFN-α in advanced renal cell carcinoma, 30 patients were treated with IL-12 and 2 (7%) achieved a partial response, whereas no responses were seen in the IFN-α arm [52].

Although the activity of IL-12 alone appears low, animal models have noted a synergy between IL-2 and IL-12. This interaction has been shown in a study that assessed in vivo stimulation of IL-12 secretion by subcutaneous low-dose IL-2 in metastatic renal cell carcinoma [53]. By evaluating IL-12 variations in relation to clinical response, a marked significant increase in IL-12 values occurred in patients with disease response or stabilization of disease, whereas progressing patients showed a significant decline in IL-12 levels during IL-2 administration. Thus, IL-2 may stimulate release of IL-12, and this is possibly associated with a favorable prognosis. Further studies of IL-12 as part of combination therapy with IL-2 are needed to see if this synergy can be exploited.

Biochemotherapy

The lack of cross-resistance, nonoverlapping toxicity, and potential synergy between chemotherapy and biological therapy has led to several trials combining cytokines and chemotherapeutic agents (so-called biochemotherapy) in metastatic renal cell carcinoma. One rationale for this approach is that by causing cytotoxicity chemotherapy will release tumor antigens, which are processed by IFN-α–stimulated antigen-presenting cells that in turn activate IL-2–stimulated CTLs. The counterargument would be that chemotherapy may downregulate immunological responses.

A phase III study involving 160 patients has compared IFN-α plus vinblastine (VLB) with vinblastine alone [54]. This study showed a significant benefit for biochemotherapy both in terms of median survival (IFN-α + VLB: 67.6 weeks; VLB: 37.8 weeks; $p = .0049$) and response rate (IFN-α + VLB: 16.5%; VLB: 2.5%; $p = .0025$). The increase in survival is both clinically and statistically significant, and long-term survivors who remained in remission after 4 to 5 years were noted.

This study did not address the role of vinblastine in the combination, and it could be argued that the benefit seen is solely due to IFN-α. A phase III study by Fossa and colleagues [55] compared IFN-α with or without vinblastine. They found no statistically significant differences in activity or survival between the two regimens, although combination treatment was associated with a higher response rate (24% versus 11%) and a trend to longer median survival (55 versus 47 weeks). The role of vinblastine in combination with cytokines requires further investigation; it may contribute only modestly to antitumor activity.

The most extensively studied chemotherapeutic agent used in combination with cytokines in the treatment of renal cell carcinoma is 5-fluorouracil (5-FU). The administration of IFN-α with 5-FU modulates the effects of 5-FU, resulting in synergy due to the blocking of thymidine incorporation into DNA. Although in vitro models demonstrated augmentation of cytotoxicity, this was not reflected in the results of a phase II trial where there were no objective clinical responses when IFN-α and 5-FU were given to patients and median survival was only 5 months [56].

The highest response rates in metastatic renal cell carcinoma are obtained using a combination of IFN-α, IL-2, and 5-FU (bolus). This was first described by Atzpodien and colleagues [57] and is an outpatient-based regimen of subcutaneous IFN-α, IL-2, and bolus intravenous 5-FU. Their initial study demonstrated a response rate of 48.6% (four CR and 13 PR out of 35 patients). They went on to confirm the activity of this regimen in a randomized trial comparing IFN-α, IL-2, and 5-FU with oral tamoxifen [58]. There was a response rate of 39% in the IFN-α, IL-2, and 5-FU arm, whereas no responses occurred in patients treated with tamoxifen. Furthermore, overall and progression-free survivals were both significantly improved in the biochemotherapy arm (overall survival: IFN-α, IL-2, and 5-FU median not reached after 42 months versus 14 months for tamoxifen; $p < .04$; progression-free survival: 13 vs. 4 months, $p < .01$).

Several other groups have tested this combination and response rates vary widely (Table 17.5). This is probably due to differences in patient characteristics between study groups and/or altered dose intensity and scheduling of the drugs [59–63]. A study by Ravaud and colleagues [64], which gave a response rate of only 1.8%, highlights the second of these points. In their study the dose and scheduling of all three agents differed from that used by Atzpodien et al. [57], and the result suggests that scheduling of cytokines, perhaps particularly in the context of 5-FU, may be important.

The importance of dose, schedule, and patient selection is again shown in a study from the Groupe Francais d'Immunotherapie [65]. Here Negrier and colleagues randomized 131 patients with metastatic renal cell carcinoma to receive subcutaneous IL-2 and IFN-α with or without 5-FU. The dose and schedule was the same as that used by Ravaud and colleagues. There was one PR in the IL-2 and IFN-α arm and five PRs in the IL-2, IFN-α, and 5-FU arm ($p = .1$). Overall survival rates at 1 year were 53% in the IL-2 and IFN-α arm and 52% in the IL-2, IFN-α, and 5-FU arm.

The optimal method of scheduling and delivery of these agents has yet to be established. Our group has explored an alternative way of delivering 5-FU within this combination. 5-Fluorouracil is principally active in the S phase of the cell cycle, and this may be more effective when given as a protracted venous infusion (PVI). Protracted venous infusion 5-FU–containing regimens have given high response rates in neoadjuvant treatment of breast cancer [66] and relapsed ovarian cancer [67]. Our study using IFN-α, IL-2, and 5-FU (PVI) showed an overall response rate of 31% in 55 patients (CR: three patients; PR: 14 patients) [68]. Interestingly, there was a trend toward higher response rates and longer survival in the poorer prognosis group, although this did not reach statistical significance. Again this supports the inclusion of fit patients even if they have poor prognostic features in future studies.

Despite high response rates seen with the IFN-α, IL-2, and 5-FU combination, the majority of patients relapse. The concept of continuing immune stimulation in responders is an attractive one and our own group and Atzpodien's are investigating the feasibility of this approach.

Capecitabine, which as stated earlier is selectively activated to 5-FU, has been substituted for 5-FU in this regimen. Atzpodien's group [69] used oral capecitabine with subcutaneous IFN-α and IL-2 and oral 13-cis-retinoic acid to treat 30 patients with metastatic renal cell carcinoma. There were two complete responses and eight partial responses for an overall response rate of 33%. These results are comparable to other 5-FU–based biochemotherapy regimens, with the advantage of oral administration of capecitabine and low toxicity. Without randomized data the

Table 17.5. Treatment of renal cell carcinoma with interferon-α (IFN-α) + interleukin-2 (IL-2) + 5-fluorouracil (5-FU)

Author, year [reference]	No. of patients	Response rate (%)	Median survival
Atzpodien 1993 [57]	35	49	Not reported
Hofmockel 1996 [59]	34	38	Not reported
Joffe 1996 [60]	55	16	12 months
Ellerhorst 1997 [61]	55	31	23 months
Ravaud 1998 [64]	111	2	12 months
Tourani 1998 [62]	62	19	33% at 2 years
Allen 2000 [68]	55	31	10.7 months
Elias 2000 [63]	38	11	Not reported
Atzpodien 2001 [58]	41	39.1	2.1

contribution of capecitabine and its potential improvement in toxicity cannot be assessed and so Atzpodien's group has initiated a phase III study to investigate its role.

Adjuvant Therapy

The only curative treatment for renal cell carcinoma is complete surgical excision of the primary lesion. As stated earlier, 20% to 30% of patients who initially present with localized disease subsequently relapse after nephrectomy, usually with metastatic disease . Thus there is a need for an effective adjuvant therapy.

Three large randomized trials totaling 250 patients have compared adjuvant interferon with observation in resected Robson stages II (perinephric fat involved) and III (tumor extension into renal vein or inferior vena cava; resected lymph node metastases) [70–72]. None of these studies showed an improvement in survival for adjuvant interferon over observation.

The role of adjuvant high-dose bolus IL-2 for patients with high-risk renal cell carcinoma has recently been addressed in a randomized trial [73]. The authors randomized patients with locally advanced (T3b–4 or N1–3) or postmetastasectomy to one course of high-dose IL-2 or to observation. The study was designed and powered to show an improvement in predicted 2-year disease-free survival from 40% in the observation group to 70% in the treatment group. The accrual goal was 68 patients with locally advanced disease, with 34 patients per treatment arm. Patients who underwent metastasectomy were to be analyzed separately because of their different natural history.

Sixty-nine patients were entered into the study, 44 with locally advanced disease and 25 postmetastasectomy. The study was closed early when an interim analysis determined that the 30% improvement in 2-year disease-free survival could not be achieved despite full accrual. Sixteen of the 21 locally advanced patients receiving IL-2 relapsed compared with 15 of 23 in the observation arm ($p = .73$). Extension of the analysis to include metastasectomy patients made no difference in disease-free survival or overall survival. As the authors concede, a study powered for an improvement in disease-free survival as large as 30% was highly ambitious, considering that high-dose IL-2 is associated with

an objective overall response rate of only 15% to 20% in good performance status patients with advanced renal cell carcinoma.

The high response rates seen with the IFN-α, IL-2, and 5-FU combination in metastatic disease has led the EORTC to undertake a randomized trial to assess whether a single cycle of biochemotherapy (IFN-α, IL-2, and 5-FU) is beneficial after resection of high-risk renal cell carcinoma. Standard therapy for fully resected renal cell carcinoma outside of clinical trials remains observation.

Angiogenesis Inhibitors

Angiogenesis is the growth of new microvessels. The growth of tumors beyond 1 to 2 mm^3 depends on angiogenesis, which is necessary for the supply of nutrients and also provides a route for metastasis. In adults the vascular endothelium is a quiescent tissue with a low cell division rate, and thus pathological angiogenesis must occur to allow tumor development. A number of proangiogenic factors (e.g., basic fibroblast growth factor and vascular endothelial growth factor [VEGF]) have been identified, as well as antiangiogenic factors (e.g., angiostatin and endostatin). The balance between these factors is important in tumor dormancy and control of micrometastases, where the apoptotic rate remains high until angiogenesis occurs. This shift in balance is termed the "angiogenic switch," which is a complex process resulting in a shift in the balance between stimulators and inhibitors of angiogenesis, during which inhibitors are downregulated [74].

Neovascularization provides not only a perfusion stimulus for tumor growth, but also a paracrine effect, which results from endothelial-derived growth factors and cytokines that stimulate growth and migration of tumor cells. This paracrine effect is thought to operate in both directions; that is, endothelial cell survival and growth are driven by tumor-derived endothelial factors. This two-cell compartment model of tumor growth may influence the design of clinical trials; for instance, angiogenesis inhibitors can be combined with conventional cytotoxic therapy.

The close relationship between angiogenesis and tumor growth and metastasis make it an attractive target for cancer therapy. Also the amplification factor seen in the relationship between tumor and vascular endothelial cells means that suppression of one endothelial cell could inhibit the growth of approximately 100 tumor cells [75]. Initial experience with angiogenesis inhibitors in animal models and from early clinical trials in advanced cancer has led to general guidelines about their use [74]:

1. Long-term therapy is necessary. Antiangiogenic therapy is a relatively slower process than cytotoxic therapy.

2. Antiangiogenic therapy should not be interrupted because of the ability of microvessels to regrow quickly.

3. Resistance does not appear to be a problem with long-term use. The theoretical basis for this is that endothelial cells, unlike tumor cells, are not considered to be mutating and thus are unlikely to generate resistant clones.

4. Combination of antioangiogenic agents with different mechanisms of action and/or with cytotoxic agents appears to be more effective [76]. Such combinations in animal models have been curative, whereas either agent alone is merely inhibitory [77].

Angiogenesis Inhibitors Used in Clinical Trials to Treat Renal Cell Carcinoma

TNP-470 is a fumagillin analogue and is one of the first angiogenesis inhibitors to undergo clinical testing. Fumagillin was originally isolated from *Aspergillus fumigatus* contaminating endothelial cell cultures [78] and is a potent inhibitor of endothelial growth in vitro and in vivo. A number of analogues of fumagillin were synthesized, and TNP-470 was selected as the least toxic compound with the greatest antiangiogenic effect [78].

A phase II trial of TNP-470 was carried out in 33 patients with metastatic renal cell carcinoma [79]. There was only one partial response of short duration (response rate 3%), but six patients (18%) had stabilization of disease for 6 months or longer. At a median follow-up of 14 months, median survival is 56 weeks. Therapy was reasonably tolerated, although neurocortical toxicities were common (67% of patients) and

led to withdrawal of five patients. Fatigue and asthenia were also common and were seen in 60% of patients.

This patient group had been heavily pretreated, and it is unclear whether this resulted in accrual of patients with indolent disease (median interval from diagnosis of metastatic disease to study initiation was 14 months). Thus, was the prolonged overall and progression-free survival in several patients due to TNP-470, or was it merely a reflection of the natural history of their disease? Further studies using TNP-470 are warranted, and combination with other angiogenesis inhibitors, cytotoxic drugs, and cytokines is indicated.

An attractive option would be the combination of TNP-470 with IFN-α, which is known to have both antiangiogenic and direct antitumor activity. Future studies should also address ways of increasing exposure to TNP-470, which animal studies suggest is necessary to maximize its antiangiogenic properties. In this study exposure was likely to be suboptimal, as the half-life of TNP-470 and its active metabolite are only 2 and 6 minutes, respectively. It may also be that the greatest benefit in using TNP-470 and other antiangiogenics to delay progression in renal cell carcinoma is seen in the adjuvant or minimal disease setting.

The likelihood of successfully introducing a new drug increases when the mechanisms of both the drug and the disease are well understood and linked in a biologically coherent fashion. This has been shown to a degree by the use of bevacizumab in the treatment of metastatic renal cancer. Studies of the hereditary form of clear-cell renal carcinoma, which occurs in the von Hippel–Lindau tumor syndrome, led to the identification of the von Hippel–Lindau tumor-suppressor gene *(VHL)* [80]. An inactivated *VHL* gene inherited from either parent causes von Hippel–Lindau disease, in which tumors with multiple blood vessels develop in the central nervous system and the risk of clear cell carcinoma of the kidney is increased. The development of tumors in von Hippel–Lindau disease is linked to loss of the remaining normal *VHL* allele, thus eliminating the *VHL* gene product. The gene is also mutated in most sporadic cases of clear cell renal carcinoma, where both alleles have acquired mutations or deletions [80]. Tumors caused by the inactivation of the *VHL* tumor-suppressor gene should be an ideal testing ground for VEGF inhibition because there is a close relationship between *VHL* inactivation and VEGF overproduction through a mechanism involving hypoxia-inducible factor α.

Bevacizumab is a humanized version of a murine monoclonal antibody against VEGF. Yang and colleagues [81] conducted a randomized phase II trial comparing placebo with bevacizumab at low or high dose in patients with metastatic clear cell renal carcinoma. The trial was stopped after the interim analysis met the criteria for early stopping based on the difference in time to progression between the placebo and high-dose bevacizumab arms. A total of 116 patients were randomly assigned to placebo (40 patients), low-dose bevacizumab (37 patients), or high-dose bevacizumab (39 patients). There was a significant prolongation of the time to progression in the high-dose antibody group as compared to placebo (hazard ratio 2.55; $p < .001$). The probability of being progression-free for patients given high-dose antibody, low-dose antibody, or placebo was 64%, 39%, and 20%, respectively, at 4 months and 30%, 14%, and 5% at 8 months. Only four patients achieved objective responses (all partial responses), all of whom received high-dose bevacizumab. Thus the response rate for high-dose antibody was 10%. There were no significant differences in survival between the treatment groups. However, time to disease progression and overall response rate were the primary end points. Survival was a secondary end point, as patients whose disease progressed on placebo were offered crossover to either low-dose bevacizumab or low-dose bevacizumab and thalidomide.

There were no significant associations between detectable pretreatment levels of VEGF and clinical response or time to progression in either bevacizumab group. However, the authors note the limited sensitivity of the assay used. After antibody treatment is started, plasma levels of VEGF are difficult to interpret, as the assay measures both free and antibody-bound VEGF, but the levels rose steadily. This study is encouraging and could serve as a platform for the integration of antioangiogenic agents into the treatment of renal cell cancer. Phase III studies are needed to address the true clinical benefits of VEGF inhibition. A crucial question is whether status of expression of the *VHL* gene product affects response to treatment. Knowl-

edge of the function of the *VHL* gene product and its intimate association with hypoxia-inducible factor α support combination with agents that interrupt other hypoxia-inducible genes such as platelet-derived growth factor.

Several other antiangiogenic agents have shown potential activity in phase I/II trials, some of which are discussed below.

Vascular endothelial growth factor (VEGF) is abnormally expressed in up to 70% of renal cell carcinomas and is thus a rational therapeutic target. SU5416 inhibits VEGF-mediated signaling through Flk-1, a transmembrane tyrosine kinase, resulting in decreased angiogenesis. In a phase I trial of 63 patients, stabilization of disease for greater than 6 months was seen in several tumor types including renal cell carcinoma [82]. A recent study assessed the activity of SU5416 in 29 patients with renal cell carcinoma. A low response rate was seen with one minor response and five patients achieving stable disease (3 months or longer) [83].

AE-941 (Neovastat) is a naturally occurring product extracted from cartilage that has antiangiogenic properties [84]. It inhibits several steps of the angiogenesis process, including matrix metalloproteinase activities and VEGF signaling pathways. Also, AE-941 induces endothelial cell apoptosis and tissue-type plasminogen activator activity, suggesting that it is a multifunctional antiangiogenic drug. Twenty-two patients with refractory renal cell carcinoma were treated as part of a larger phase II study assessing two dosing levels of neovastat [85]. Median survival time was significantly longer (16.3 versus 7.1 months; $p = .01$) in patients treated with Neovastat 240 mL/day ($n = 14$) compared with patients receiving 60 mL/day ($n = 8$). This difference in survival was not explained by any significant differences in major prognostic factors between the two groups. Neovastat is administered orally and has low toxicity. It is now being evaluated in a phase III trial in patients who have failed immunotherapy.

There is currently considerable interest in antiangiogenesis, with several new agents in development, many of which have entered clinical trials. Two of the most interesting compounds are angiostatin and endostatin, both of which were isolated by Folkman and colleagues. Angiostatin is a proteolytic degradation product of plasminogen and is a specific inhibitor of endothelial proliferation [86]. It is the first angiogenesis inhibitor that can cause regression of human cancer xenografts in mice. A microscopic dormant state in which virtually all neovascularization has been blocked is achieved by prolonged blockade of angiogenesis [87].

Endostatin, a proteolytic degradation product of collagen type XVIII, has also been shown to cause tumor regression in murine carcinoma models. Tumors recurred when treatment was stopped but regressed again when endostatin therapy was recommenced. Interestingly, when therapy was withdrawn for a second time, no tumor recurrence was observed [88]. Both angiostatin and endostatin have entered clinical trials that will determine their efficacy. Initial phase I trials with endostatin have shown it is well tolerated when treating several malignancies, but little clinical activity has been demonstrated [89].

The integration of antiangiogenic drugs into current practice may represent an important advance. New therapeutic end points, such as disease stabilization, may be required during the evaluation of these compounds. Imaging techniques, such as Doppler (measuring blood flow) and positron emission tomography (PET) scanning (measuring tumor metabolism) may aid in assessing response to antiangiogenic treatment. Other useful indicators of response may be angiogenic factors such as VEGF and fibroblast growth factor (FGF) in plasma and urine.

Thalidomide

Thalidomide has been discovered to have powerful antiangiogenic activity. Its mechanism of action is complex including breakdown of messenger RNA (mRNA) of a number of molecules such as FGF and tumor necrosis factor-α (TNF-α). Our group's phase II study tested low-dose thalidomide (100 mg orally every night) in 66 patients with metastatic cancer, including several with renal cell carcinoma [90]. There were three partial responses and 13 stabilizations of previously progressive disease (3 for more than 3 months) in the 18 patients with renal cell carcinoma who were treated. Treatment was well tolerated and no World Health Organization (WHO) grade 3 or 4 toxicities were seen. The main toxicity was lethargy (38 patients grade 1, eight patients grade 2), but conversely,

several patients experienced improvement in sleep and appetite. In a further study using thalidomide, 600 mg orally every night, there were two partial responses. Seven patients had stable disease for greater than 6 months and five had stable disease for between 3 and 6 months out of the 25 patients treated [91]. In patients who achieved a partial response or who had stable disease for at least 3 months. a statistically significant decrease in serum TNF-α levels was seen ($p = .05$).

Several other groups have now published studies of thalidomide in renal cell carcinoma. Overall response rate in these trials was 6%. with 10 partial responses out of 158 patients [90–95]. The low response rates do not support the use of thalidomide to induce responses in patients with metastatic renal cell carcinoma. However, its actions may only be able to achieve disease stabilization by cytostatic inhibition of further tumor growth, and so this may be a more appropriate treatment end point than objective responses. Stabilization of disease is recognized as part of the natural history of renal cell carcinoma, although this is unlikely to occur in patients who have progressed through cytokine therapy. To address whether thalidomide can extend time to progression and improve survival, a phase III randomized trial has been initiated by ECOG that compares low-dose interferon with or without thalidomide.

The exact mechanism of action of thalidomide is unknown and this requires further investigation. A possible mechanism in renal cell carcinoma is inhibition of TNF-α, which is known to be secreted by renal cell carcinomas. This cytokine enhances neoangiogenesis and stimulation of renal carcinoma cells by IL-6, and contributes to many systemic features of advanced malignancy, for example, cachexia and malaise. Two new classes of thalidomide have been developed: one class of compounds are potent phosphodiesterase 4 inhibitors that inhibit TNF-α but have little effect on T-cell activation [96]. The other class of compounds, similar to thalidomide, are not phosphodiesterase 4 inhibitors, but inhibit TNF-α and IL-6, and stimulate T-cell proliferation and IL-2 and IFN-γ production. One of the new immunomodulatory analogues, CC-5013, has shown impressive activity in refractory multiple myeloma [97]. The use of these novel compounds will help to elucidate the mechanisms that underlie thalidomide's activity in renal cell carcinoma.

The combination of thalidomide with immunotherapy is an attractive one. Our group commenced a phase II study of IFN-α (9 MU 3 times/week subcutaneously) and thalidomide (400 mg). Unfortunately, unexpected neurological toxicity was seen in four of 13 patients treated with this regimen and the study has been closed [98]. The authors recommended that caution be used when combining these agents and lower doses of IFN-α.

A recent study has confirmed the feasibility of combining thalidomide with lower doses of IFN-α [99]. Thirty patients were given IFN-α (0.9 MU 3 times/day subcutaneously for 1 month and subsequently 1.2 MU 3 times/day) and thalidomide (100 mg/day for 1 week and 300 mg/day thereafter). The response rate was 20%, all responses were partial, and median survival was 14.9 months. The most common toxicity was sensory neuropathy, causing 19 patients (63%) to discontinue thalidomide. Median duration of thalidomide treatment was 6.5 months and that of IFN-α was 7.2 months. Interestingly, serum VEGF levels decreased more in patients who responded to therapy compared to those who had stable or progressive disease ($p = .036$). This combination is undoubtedly neurotoxic, and careful follow-up of patients is needed. Results of an ongoing ECOG phase III trial comparing IFN-α with or without thalidomide are awaited with interest.

The combination of thalidomide with IL-2 has also been addressed in a recent phase II study [100]. Out of 37 patients there was one complete response, 14 partial responses, and 11 patients with stable disease. Time on therapy ranged from 3 to 15 months. Twenty-six patients continue on therapy with either objective response or stable disease. Treatment was generally well tolerated with mainly grade 1 to 2 toxicities. This therefore appears to be a promising new regimen, and a phase III trial of IL-2 plus thalidomide versus IL-2 versus thalidomide is planned.

Conclusion

Patients with metastatic renal cell still have a very poor prognosis and there remains the continued need for research. It should be noted that patients entering clinical trials are often highly selected, particularly where protocols of intensive treatments are involved. Entry criteria to most studies are often those that predict response and good survival, such as good performance status and nephrectomy. Results therefore may not be applicable to an unselected population of patients.

It is important to remember that many of the treatments discussed here are still in their infancy, compared to conventional cancer treatments. It is likely that over the next few years some of these therapies will become important management options. Of the newer agents, cytokines have been shown to improve overall survival as demonstrated by three randomized controlled studies.

Our knowledge of the molecular biology of renal cell carcinoma is ever increasing, allowing new therapeutic options such as signal transduction inhibitors, antiangiogenesis agents, tumor vaccines, dendritic cell vaccines, monoclonal antibodies, antisense oligonucleotides, and gene therapy to be developed. The translation of targeted biological therapy into a frontline treatment, as exemplified by the use of trastuzumab in breast cancer, remains the ultimate goal for future trials.

Other aims include:

- The identification of patients most likely to respond to treatment
- The development of methods to maintain response
- A decrease in the toxicity of treatment
- Integration of new agents into currently active regimens

Whenever possible patients undergoing systemic treatment should be entered into appropriate clinical trials. Standard therapy for fit patients is single-agent interferon-α or single-agent interleukin-2.

References

1. Jemal A, et al. Cancer statistics, 2002. CA Cancer J Clin 2002;52(1):23–47.
2. Motzer RJ, Bander NH, Nanus DM. Renal-cell carcinoma. N Engl J Med 1996;335(12):865–875.
3. Dhote R, et al. Risk factors for adult renal cell carcinoma: a systematic review and implications for prevention. BJU Int 2000;86(1):20–27.

4. Yagoda A, Abi-Rached B, Petrylak D. Chemotherapy for advanced renal-cell carcinoma: 1983–1993. Semin Oncol 1995;22(1):42–60.

5. Elson PJ, Witte RS, Trump DL. Prognostic factors for survival in patients with recurrent or metastatic renal cell carcinoma. Cancer Res 1988;48(24 pt 1):7310–7313.

6. Palmer PA, et al. Prognostic factors for survival in patients with advanced renal cell carcinoma treated with recombinant interleukin-2. Ann Oncol 1992;3(6):475–480.

7. Jones M, et al. The impact of interleukin-2 on survival in renal cancer: a multivariate analysis. Cancer Biother 1993;8(4):275–288.

8. Fossa SD, Kramar A, Droz JP. Prognostic factors and survival in patients with metastatic renal cell carcinoma treated with chemotherapy or interferon-alpha. Eur J Cancer 1994;30A(9):1310–1314.

9. Motzer RJ, et al. Survival and prognostic stratification of 670 patients with advanced renal cell carcinoma. J Clin Oncol 1999;17(8):2530–2540.

10. Motzer RJ, et al. Prognostic factors for survival in previously treated patients with metastatic renal cell carcinoma. J Clin Oncol 2004;22(3):454–463.

11. Motzer RJ, et al. Treatment outcome and survival associated with metastatic renal cell carcinoma of non-clear-cell histology. J Clin Oncol 2002; 20(9):2376–2381.

12. Kudoh S, et al. Defective granzyme B gene expression and lytic response in T lymphocytes infiltrating human renal cell carcinoma. J Immunother 1997;20(6):479–487.

13. Ulchaker J, et al. Interferon-gamma production by T lymphocytes from renal cell carcinoma patients: evidence of impaired secretion in response to interleukin-12. J Immunother 1999; 22(1):71–79.

14. Almand B, et al. Increased production of immature myeloid cells in cancer patients: a mechanism of immunosuppression in cancer. J Immunol 2001;166(1):678–689.

15. Finke JH, et al. Tumor-infiltrating lymphocytes in patients with renal-cell carcinoma. Ann N Y Acad Sci 1988;532:387–394.

16. Van Den Eynde BJ, et al. A new antigen recognized by cytolytic T lymphocytes on a human kidney tumor results from reverse strand transcription. J Exp Med 1999;190(12):1793–1800.

17. Motzer RJ, et al. Effect of cytokine therapy on survival for patients with advanced renal cell carcinoma. J Clin Oncol 2000;18(9):1928–1935.

18. Negrier S, et al. Prognostic factors of survival and rapid progression in 782 patients with metastatic renal carcinomas treated by cytokines: a report from the Groupe Francais d'Immunotherapie. Ann Oncol 2002;13(9):1460–1468.

19. Van Poppel H, Baert L. Nephrectomy for metastatic renal cell carcinoma and surgery for distant metastases. Acta Urol Belg 1996;64(2):11–17.

20. Piltz S, et al. Long-term results after pulmonary resection of renal cell carcinoma metastases. Ann Thorac Surg 2002;73(4):1082–1087.

21. Le Francois D, et al. Evolution of cell-mediated immunity in mice bearing tumors produced by a mammary carcinoma cell line. Influence of tumor growth, surgical removal, and treatment with irradiated tumor cells. J Natl Cancer Inst 1971;46(5):981–987.

22. Whitney RB, Levy JG, Smith AG. Influence of tumor size and surgical resection on cell-mediated immunity in mice. J Natl Cancer Inst 1974;53(1):111–116.

23. Dadian G, et al. Immunological parameters in peripheral blood of patients with renal cell carcinoma before and after nephrectomy. Br J Urol 1994;74(1):15–22.

24. Pantuck AZA, Shvarts O, Gitlitz B, deKernion J, Figlin R, Belldegrun A. Natural history and the role of nephrectomy in the biology of RCC: the UCLA experience. Proc Am Soc Clin Oncol 2000; 19:1348.

25. Flanigan RC, et al. Nephrectomy followed by interferon alfa-2b compared with interferon alfa-2b alone for metastatic renal-cell cancer. N Engl J Med 2001;345(23):1655–1659.

26. Mickisch GH, et al. Radical nephrectomy plus interferon-alfa-based immunotherapy compared with interferon alfa alone in metastatic renal-cell carcinoma: a randomised trial. Lancet 2001; 358(9286):966–970.

27. Flanigan RC, et al. Cytoreductive nephrectomy in patients with metastatic renal cancer: a combined analysis. J Urol 2004;171(3):1071–1076.

28. Naitoh J, et al. Metastatic renal cell carcinoma with concurrent inferior vena caval invasion: long-term survival after combination therapy with radical nephrectomy, vena caval thrombectomy and postoperative immunotherapy. J Urol 1999;162(1):46–50.

29. Lineham WM, et al. Cancer of the kidney and ureter. In: Devita VT, ed. Cancer: Principles and Practice of Oncology. Philadephia: Lippincott Williams and Wilkins, 1997:1271–1300.

30. Motzer RJ, et al. Phase II trial of branched peg interferon-alpha 2a (40 kDa) for patients with advanced renal cell carcinoma. Ann Oncol 2002;13(11):1799–1805.

31. Bukowski, R, et al. Pegylated interferon alfa-2b treatment for patients with solid tumors: a phase I/II study. J Clin Oncol 2002;20(18):3841–3849.

32. Interferon-alpha and survival in metastatic renal carcinoma: early results of a randomised controlled trial. Medical Research Council Renal

Cancer Collaborators. Lancet 1999;353(9146): 14–17.

33. Hancock B, Griffiths G, Ritchie A, et al., on behalf of the MRC Renal Cancer Collaborators. Updated results of the MRC randomised controlled trial of alpha interferon vs. MPA in patients with metastatic renal carcinoma. Proc Am Soc Clin Oncol 2000;abstract 1336.

34. Coppin C, et al. Immunotherapy for advanced renal cell cancer. Cochrane Database Syst Rev 2000(3):CD001425.

35. Hoffman AD, et al. Expression of retinoic acid receptor beta in human renal cell carcinomas correlates with sensitivity to the antiproliferative effects of 13–cis-retinoic acid. Clin Cancer Res 1996;2(6):1077–1082.

36. Motzer RJ, et al. Interferon alfa-2a and 13–cis-retinoic acid in renal cell carcinoma: antitumor activity in a phase II trial and interactions in vitro. J Clin Oncol 1995;13(8):1950–1957.

37. Motzer RJ, et al. Phase III trial of interferon alfa-2a with or without 13–cis-retinoic acid for patients with advanced renal cell carcinoma. J Clin Oncol 2000;18(16):2972–2980.

38. Gleave ME, et al. Interferon gamma-1b compared with placebo in metastatic renal-cell carcinoma. Canadian Urologic Oncology Group. N Engl J Med 1998;338(18):1265–1271.

39. De Mulder PH, et al. EORTC (30885) randomised phase III study with recombinant interferon alpha and recombinant interferon alpha and gamma in patients with advanced renal cell carcinoma. The EORTC Genitourinary Group. Br J Cancer 1995;71(2):371–375.

40. Fyfe G, et al. Results of treatment of 255 patients with metastatic renal cell carcinoma who received high-dose recombinant interleukin-2 therapy. J Clin Oncol 1995;13(3):688–696.

41. Fisher RI, Rosenberg SA, Fyfe G. Long-term survival update for high-dose recombinant interleukin-2 in patients with renal cell carcinoma. Cancer J Sci Am 2000;6(suppl 1):S55–57.

42. Yang JC, et al. Randomized comparison of high-dose and low-dose intravenous interleukin-2 for the therapy of metastatic renal cell carcinoma: an interim report. J Clin Oncol 1994;12(8):1572–1576.

43. Yang JC, et al. Randomized study of high-dose and low-dose interleukin-2 in patients with metastatic renal cancer. J Clin Oncol 2003; 21(16):3127–3132.

44. Bukowski RM. Natural history and therapy of metastatic renal cell carcinoma: the role of interleukin-2. Cancer 1997;80(7):1198–1220.

45. Lindsey KR, Rosenberg SA, Sherry RM. Impact of the number of treatment courses on the clinical response of patients who receive high-dose bolus interleukin-2. J Clin Oncol 2000;18(9):1954–1959.

46. Rosenberg SA, et al. Prospective randomized trial of high-dose interleukin-2 alone or in conjunction with lymphokine-activated killer cells for the treatment of patients with advanced cancer. J Natl Cancer Inst 1993;85(8):622–632.

47. Figlin RA, et al. Treatment of metastatic renal cell carcinoma with nephrectomy, interleukin-2 and cytokine-primed or CD8(+) selected tumor infiltrating lymphocytes from primary tumor. J Urol 1997;158(3 Pt 1):740–745.

48. Figlin RA, et al. Multicenter, randomized, phase III trial of CD8(+) tumor-infiltrating lymphocytes in combination with recombinant interleukin-2 in metastatic renal cell carcinoma. J Clin Oncol 1999;17(8):2521–2529.

49. Sherry RM, Rosenberg SA, Yang JC. Relapse after response to interleukin-2–based immunotherapy: patterns of progression and response to retreatment. J Immunother 1991;10(5):371–375.

50. Negrier S, et al. Recombinant human interleukin-2, recombinant human interferon alfa-2a, or both in metastatic renal-cell carcinoma. Groupe Francais d'Immunotherapie. N Engl J Med 1998; 338(18):1272–1278.

51. Escudier B, et al. Cytokines in metastatic renal cell carcinoma: is it useful to switch to interleukin-2 or interferon after failure of a first treatment? Groupe Francais d'Immunotherape. J Clin Oncol 1999;17(7):2039–2043.

52. Motzer RJ, et al. Randomized multicenter phase II trial of subcutaneous recombinant human interleukin-12 versus interferon-alpha 2a for patients with advanced renal cell carcinoma. J Interferon Cytokine Res 2001;21(4):257–263.

53. Lissoni P, et al. In vivo stimulation of IL-12 secretion by subcutaneous low-dose IL-2 in metastatic cancer patients. Br J Cancer 1998; 77(11):1957–1960.

54. Pyrhonen S, et al. Prospective randomized trial of interferon alfa-2a plus vinblastine versus vinblastine alone in patients with advanced renal cell cancer. J Clin Oncol 1999;17(9):2859–2867.

55. Fossa SD, et al. Recombinant interferon alfa-2a with or without vinblastine in metastatic renal cell carcinoma: results of a European multicenter phase III study. Ann Oncol 1992;3(4): 301–305.

56. Murphy BR, et al. A phase II trial of interferon alpha-2A plus fluorouracil in advanced renal cell carcinoma. A Hoosier Oncology Group study. Invest New Drugs 1992;10(3):225–230.

57. Atzpodien J, et al. Interleukin-2 in combination with interferon-alpha and 5–fluorouracil for metastatic renal cell cancer. Eur J Cancer 1993;29A(suppl 5):S6–8.

58. Atzpodien J, et al. IL-2 in combination with IFN-alpha and 5–FU versus tamoxifen in metastatic

renal cell carcinoma: long-term results of a controlled randomized clinical trial. Br J Cancer 2001;85(8):1130–1136.

59. Hofmockel G, et al. Immunochemotherapy for metastatic renal cell carcinoma using a regimen of interleukin-2, interferon-alpha and 5–fluorouracil. J Urol 1996;156(1):18–21.

60. Joffe JK, et al. A phase II study of interferon-alpha, interleukin-2 and 5–fluorouracil in advanced renal carcinoma: clinical data and laboratory evidence of protease activation. Br J Urol 1996;77(5):638–649.

61. Ellerhorst JA, et al. Phase II trial of 5–fluorouracil, interferon-alpha and continuous infusion interleukin-2 for patients with metastatic renal cell carcinoma. Cancer 1997;80(11): 2128–2132.

62. Tourani JM, et al. Outpatient treatment with subcutaneous interleukin-2 and interferon alfa administration in combination with fluorouracil in patients with metastatic renal cell carcinoma: results of a sequential nonrandomized phase II study. Subcutaneous Administration Proleukin Program Cooperative Group. J Clin Oncol 1998;16(7):2505–2513.

63. Elias L, et al. Infusional interleukin-2 and 5–fluorouracil with subcutaneous interferon-alpha for the treatment of patients with advanced renal cell carcinoma: a southwest oncology group Phase II study. Cancer 2000; 89(3):597–603.

64. Ravaud A, et al. Subcutaneous interleukin-2, interferon alfa-2a, and continuous infusion of fluorouracil in metastatic renal cell carcinoma: a multicenter phase II trial. Groupe Francais d'Immunotherapie. J Clin Oncol 1998;16(8):2728–2732.

65. Negrier S, et al. Treatment of patients with metastatic renal carcinoma with a combination of subcutaneous interleukin-2 and interferon alfa with or without fluorouracil. Groupe Francais d'Immunotherapie, Federation Nationale des Centres de Lutte Contre le Cancer. J Clin Oncol 2000;18(24):4009–4015.

66. Smith IE, et al. High complete remission rates with primary neoadjuvant infusional chemotherapy for large early breast cancer. J Clin Oncol 1995;13(2):424–429.

67. Ahmed FMP, Macfarlane V, Gore M. Infusional chemotherapy (cisplatin, epirubicin, 5–FU: ECF) for patients with epithelial ovarian carcinoma. In: 9th NCI-EORTC Symposium on New Drug Therapy, 1996, Amsterdam.

68. Allen MJ, et al. Protracted venous infusion 5–fluorouracil in combination with subcutaneous interleukin-2 and alpha-interferon in patients with metastatic renal cell cancer: a phase II study. Br J Cancer 2000;83(8):980–985.

69. Oevermann K, et al. Capecitabine in the treatment of metastatic renal cell carcinoma. Br J Cancer 2000;83(5):583–587.

70. Porzsolt F. Adjuvant therapy of renal cell carcinoma with interferon alpha-2a. Proc Am Soc Clin Oncol 1992;11:622.

71. Trump DL, Elson P, Propert K, et al. Randomized, controlled trial of adjuvant therapy with lymphoblastoid interferon (L-IFN) in resected, high-risk renal cell carcinoma (HR-RCC) Proc Am Soc Clin Oncol 1966;15:253.

72. Pizzocaro G, et al. Interferon adjuvant to radical nephrectomy in Robson stages II and III renal cell carcinoma: a multicentric randomized study. J Clin Oncol 2001;19(2):425–431.

73. Clark JI, et al. Adjuvant high-dose bolus interleukin-2 for patients with high-risk renal cell carcinoma: a cytokine working group randomized trial. J Clin Oncol 2003;21(16):3133–3140.

74. Folkman J. Antiangiogenic therapy. In: Devita VT, ed. Cancer: Principles and Practice of Oncology. Philadephia: Lippincott Williams and Wilkins, 1997.

75. Modzelewski RA, et al. Isolation and identification of fresh tumor-derived endothelial cells from a murine RIF-1 fibrosarcoma. Cancer Res 1994;54(2):336–339.

76. Kato T, et al. Enhanced suppression of tumor growth by combination of angiogenesis inhibitor O-(chloroacetyl-carbamoyl)fumagillol (TNP-470) and cytotoxic agents in mice. Cancer Res 1994;54(19):5143–5147.

77. Teicher BA, et al. Potentiation of cytotoxic cancer therapies by TNP-470 alone and with other anti-angiogenic agents. Int J Cancer 1994;57(6): 920–925.

78. Ingber D, et al. Synthetic analogues of fumagillin that inhibit angiogenesis and suppress tumour growth. Nature 1990;348(6301):555–557.

79. Stadler WM, et al. Multi-institutional study of the angiogenesis inhibitor TNP-470 in metastatic renal carcinoma. J Clin Oncol 1999;17(8): 2541–2545.

80. George DJ, Kaelin WG Jr. The von Hippel-Lindau protein, vascular endothelial growth factor, and kidney cancer. N Engl J Med 2003;349(5): 419–421.

81. Yang JC, et al. A randomized trial of bevacizumab, an anti-vascular endothelial growth factor antibody, for metastatic renal cancer. N Engl J Med 2003;349(5):427–434.

82. Rosen L, Mulay M, Mayers A, et al. Phase I dose-escalating trial of SU5416, a novel angiogenesis inhibitor in patients with advanced malignancies (meeting abstract). Proc Am Soc Clin Oncol 1999;18:618.

83. Kuenen BC, et al. Efficacy and toxicity of the angiogenesis inhibitor SU5416 as a single agent

in patients with advanced renal cell carcinoma, melanoma, and soft tissue sarcoma. Clin Cancer Res 2003;9(5):1648–1655.

84. Gingras D, et al. Matrix proteinase inhibition by AE-941, a multifunctional antiangiogenic compound. Anticancer Res 2001;21(1A):145–155.

85. Batist G, et al. Neovastat (AE-941) in refractory renal cell carcinoma patients: report of a phase II trial with two dose levels. Ann Oncol 2002; 13(8):1259–1263.

86. O'Reilly MS, et al. Angiostatin: a novel angiogenesis inhibitor that mediates the suppression of metastases by a Lewis lung carcinoma. Cell 1994; 79(2):315–328.

87. O'Reilly MS, et al. Angiostatin induces and sustains dormancy of human primary tumors in mice. Nat Med 1996;2(6):689–692.

88. O'Reilly MS, et al. Endostatin: an endogenous inhibitor of angiogenesis and tumor growth. Cell 1997;88(2):277–285.

89. Herbst RS, et al. Phase I study of recombinant human endostatin in patients with advanced solid tumors. J Clin Oncol 2002;20(18):3792–3803.

90. Eisen T, et al. Continuous low dose thalidomide: a phase II study in advanced melanoma, renal cell, ovarian and breast cancer. Br J Cancer 2000; 82(4):812–817.

91. Stebbing J, et al. The treatment of advanced renal cell cancer with high-dose oral thalidomide. Br J Cancer 2001;85(7):953–958.

92. Motzer RJ, et al. Phase II trial of thalidomide for patients with advanced renal cell carcinoma. J Clin Oncol 2002;20(1):302–306.

93. Minor DR, et al. A phase II study of thalidomide in advanced metastatic renal cell carcinoma. Invest New Drugs 2002;20(4):389–393.

94. Escudier B, et al. Phase II trial of thalidomide in renal-cell carcinoma. Ann Oncol 2002;13(7): 1029–1035.

95. Daliani DD, et al. A pilot study of thalidomide in patients with progressive metastatic renal cell carcinoma. Cancer 2002;95(4):758–765.

96. Corral LG, et al. Differential cytokine modulation and T cell activation by two distinct classes of thalidomide analogues that are potent inhibitors of TNF-alpha. J Immunol 1999;163(1): 380–386.

97. Richardson PG, et al. Immunomodulatory drug CC-5013 overcomes drug resistance and is well tolerated in patients with relapsed multiple myeloma. Blood 2002;100(9):3063–3067.

98. Nathan PD, Gore ME, Eisen TG. Unexpected toxicity of combination thalidomide and interferon alpha-2a treatment in metastatic renal cell carcinoma. J Clin Oncol 2002;20(5):1429–1430.

99. Hernberg M, et al. Interferon alfa-2b three times daily and thalidomide in the treatment of metastatic renal cell carcinoma. J Clin Oncol 2003;21(20):3770–3776.

100. Amato R, Schell J, Thompson N, Moore R, Miles B. Phase II study of thalidomide and interleukin-2 in patients with metastatic renal cell carcinoma. Proc Am Soc Clin Oncol 2003;abstract 1556.

define a stable point for building a chemotherapy-based approach to renal cancer.

As for single-agent capecitabine and capecitabine in combination with interferon, Wenzel and colleagues [9] in Austria reported that of 23 patients, two had a major response, five had a minor response, and 13 had stable disease, so that a total of 87% of patients had at least stable disease. A U.S. series had a lower response rate, with only 32% stable disease, a result that may have been attributable to selection of a heavily pretreated, refractory population [10]. A newer series from Austria shows a high frequency of stable disease when capecitabine was combined with low-dose IL-2 (4.5 mIU) *or* with interferon-α (6 mIU three times a week) [11]. This series also showed several patients with major response (5/52), minor response (5/52), and again a high frequency of stable disease (32/52).

Although platinum-containing drugs are among the conventional cytotoxic identified to have low activity in renal cancer (see citations [1]), theoretical synergism with gemcitabine is a basis for an open trial using this gemcitabine plus cisplatin combination in kidney cancer (cancer.gov).

Gemcitabine is also part of a two-drug combination with doxorubicin that is to be tested in a single-arm phase II study in sarcomatoid renal cancer. The Eastern Cooperative Oncology Group (ECOG) study will focus on a subtype routinely identified as refractory to medical therapy and as a prognostically unfavorable outlier, even within the general renal cancer group [12].

The novel antimetabolite troxacitabine was tested in a National Cancer Institute (NCI)–Canada phase II study for renal cancer; of 33 patients, two were major responders, and 21 had stable disease, eight of whom were for over 6 months. The mechanism of action of troxacitabine, a stereochemically nonnatural nucleoside analogue, is chain termination, interfering with the function of mammalian DNA polymerases [13]. Additional testing with this compound may yield a more favorable way to extend the duration of stable disease, or increase the frequency of major responses.

Among drugs directed at the microtubule, vinblastine is notable for having been the single agent on the inferior arm of the most favorable randomized phase III trial of interferon plus vinblastine versus vinblastine [14]. A similarly pessimistic conclusion was reached in single-arm trials of the taxane docetaxel [15–17]. The epothilone compounds are derived from a soil bacterium, *Sorangium cellulosum*, instead of plant parent compounds. The site of contact with tubulin is the same as that of taxanes, and point mutations (not identified to be common in kidney cancer) inhibit responsiveness to either drug [18]. However, non–cross-resistance has been observed in some early testing. The difference may be related to drug efflux or to a nonmicrotubule target. Patupilone (EP0906, Novartis East Hanover, NJ) and Ixabepilone (BMS247550, Bristol-Myers Squib, Princeton, NJ). The latter is the treatment plan in a single-arm phase II renal cell cancer (RCC) trial at the NCI, and 10% partial responses in kidney cancer were reported in June 2004 [19]. Additional microtubule targeting drugs are discussed below (see Vascular Targeting).

Key determinants of renal cancer resistance to conventional cytotoxic drugs remain to be identified and circumvented. Teleologically, the kidney is an organ that must resist and expel toxic substances, and this may be part of the basis for the recalcitrance of renal cancer to conventional cytotoxic treatment. Drugs directed at the adenosine triphosphate (ATP)-binding cassette (ABC) transporter drugs, such as P-glycoprotein (Pgp), multidrug resistance-related protein (MRP), and breast cancer resistance protein (BCRP) are another category of compounds that may ultimately have relevance for improving the outcomes for conventional cytotoxic drugs in renal cancer.

Targeted Drugs

Targeted drug therapy has become the watchword of the pharmaceutical industry in the new millennium. Isolated successes such as rituximab for non-Hodgkin's lymphoma or imatinib mesylate in chronic myelogenous leukemia are a basis for hope that each cancer will have a pharmacogenomically discoverable Achilles' heel, susceptible to the right target/targeted drug combination, with inconsequential toxicity. The targets of renal cancer remain elusive. Pathophysiological studies highlight the pathway related to von Hippel–Lindau protein (pVHL), mutated or silent in over half of cases [20].

Within this pathway, the impaired degradation of the hypoxia-inducible factor 1α (HIF1α) protein and the consequent dysregulated (increased) transcription of genes bearing the hypoxia response element (HRE) sequence in their promoter are leading candidates to be a major contributor to the pathological phenotype of clear cell renal cancer. The dysregulated activity of HIF1α- and HRE-bearing genes is found in other kidney cancer and many other malignancies. Many investigational approaches in preclinical testing that target HIF directly include, small interfering siRNA and others, such as small molecules and novel agents already in clinical testing [21,22]. Vascular endothelial growth factor (VEGF) is a gene product with HRE regulation. VEGF-depleting drugs and VEGF receptor (VEGFR1 or Flt-1 and VEGFR2 or Flk-1/KDR) in tyrosine kinase enzyme inhibitors are discussed below (see Angiogenic Targeting), although the pathology caused by VEGF likely extends beyond the recruitment of blood vessel growth and lymphatic vessel growth into the tumor, and may include immune impairment or direct tumor stimulation.

Receptor tyrosine kinase inhibitors and antibodies or other drugs that block the external domains of these receptors are in broad development in oncology. The epidermal growth factor receptor (EGFR) is targeted by small molecule drugs gefitinib (ZD1839, Iressa™), erlotinib (Tarceva™), and CI-1033 (also blocks Her2/neu, EGFR3, and EGFR4 tyrosine kinases), and by antibodies such as cetuximab (Erbitux™, Bristol Myers Squib, C225). Diverse trials of gefitinib monotherapy and in combination with cytotoxic drugs have led to its approval for non–small-cell lung cancer. Two single-agent gefitinib trials in renal cancer have been reported; one trial of 16 patients demonstrated a response in none, with only three patients not progressing at 4 months [23], and the other trial of 21 patients reported a major response in none and stable disease in eight (38%) [24]. The SD patients had significantly better survival [24]. Although these gefitinib trials suggest that chronic oral EGFR tyrosine kinase inhibition is a blockade and is not relevant in renal cancer, the chemically related drug erlotinib (Tarceva™) is in active trials as well. Two of these are a second-line therapy of renal cancer (NCI Web site), and essentially the only phase II trial directed exclusively at therapy of the papillary histology subset

(Southwest Oncology Group [SWOG] trial 0317). Another trial testing the combination of erlotinib and the anti-VEGF antibody bevacizumab was presented positively at the June 2004 American Society of Clinical Oncology (ASCO) meeting [25]. Among 58 evaluable patients reported, 12 (21%) had partial response and 38 (66%) had stable disease or minor response, 26 of whom had at least 6 months of treatment. Rash, diarrhea, and nausea were the most frequent side effects. A randomized trial of bevacizumab with or without erlotinib has completed accrual.

The small molecule inhibitor Su11248 (also called Su011248, Pfizer, New York, NY) is an orally available tyrosine kinase inhibitor of VEGFR2, PDGFR, flt3, and c-kit. It will be studied a phase III study with randomization versus interferon. The first phase II single-agent trial, for second-line therapy, was sponsored by the manufacturer and open at several centers. Favorable data were presented at the June 2004 ASCO meeting. The presentation reported that 63 evaluable patients progressed after prior treatment with a single line of immunotherapy; 21 of them (33%) had a partial response (PR), and 23 (37%) had stable disease at least 3 months [26]. A confirmatory single-arm study and a randomized phase III study comparing the single agent to interferon are accruing patients.

The proteasome inhibitor bortezimib has also been tested for renal cancer. The proteasome is the site of degradation of ubiquitylated proteins, many of which are involved in the cell cycle. Proteasome inhibition may have impact on HIF1α levels. In one single-agent phase II series there was one objective response in 21 patients [27]. In an independent series, there were three responses among 24 clear cell subtype patients, which may be encouraging for exploring further development of this unique class of agents [28].

The drug CCI-779 (Wyeth) is an inhibitor of the mammalian target of rapamycin (mTOR) protein. Several intracellular signaling processes function through mTOR, which interacts with HIF1α, the PI3K/Akt pathway, and cell cycle proteins including cyclin D1 (leading to a late-G1 arrest from mTOR inhibition). This point of cytoplasmic interference is not just a new target protein but a new point of attack in the growth and survival of the malignant cell cycle. A randomized phase II study in renal cancer, using dose levels of 25 mg/m^2, 75 mg/m^2, or 250 mg/m^2

was reported by Atkins et al. [29]. There were no differences identified across dose levels, and the $25\,mg/m^2$ dose has been selected for further study in renal cancer. Among 111 patients, the observed response rate was 7%, with an additional 26% minor responses. Most frequent toxicities were rash and mucositis. The median time to progression and overall survival were 5.8 months and 15 months, respectively. The prognostic criteria of Motzer et al. [30] identified intermediate and poor subsets, which appeared to have a better improvement of progression-free survival. Atkins et al. [29] speculate that a relationship to the Akt pathway in these patients may be basis for this observation. A randomized phase III study of CCI-779, interferon, and CCI-779 plus interferon is open at international centers, restricted to worse-prognosis patients [30]. A single-arm phase I study of CCI-779 plus interferon in renal cancer has also been presented [31].

Finally, an exciting development in 2003 that was reported at the ASCO 2004 meeting was the single-agent phase II study of sorafenib (previously called Bay 43-9006) [32]. The small-molecule inhibits (at different levels) b-*raf*, c-*raf*, PDGFR, c-*kit*, flt-3, and VEGF-R2 (KDR). The Raf proteins are involved in signal transduction from cell surface receptor molecules, in the widely present RAS/RAF/MEK/MAPK pathway.

The Bay43-9006 study design originally emphasized colon cancer until it was evident that RCC appears as the most responsive of the histological types tested. The design has a three-part plan at the 12-week evaluation: subjects with ≥25% improvement are continued on treatment, those with >25% worsening are discontinued for progression, and those with stable disease are offered randomization between placebo and continued treatment. In all, at the time of the June 2004 presentation, 203 renal cancer patients had been accrued, 106 by September 2003, and 89 of these were evaluable. At the 12-week evaluation, seven continued without randomization, 45 were in the middle category, and 37 were discontinued because of a >25% increase. Side effects of hypertension, rash, and hand–foot syndrome were observed, but were not a major problem. A study of second-line (progression after one line of immunotherapy) patients, compared to placebo, has opened for accrual in a multinational phase III format.

These drugs reach their molecular targets, and as reported, only a minority of patients progress at 3 to 6 months in the respective single-arm trials. It is reasonable to view these targeted results optimistically. The best way to bring this to bear for longer, complete responses in renal cancer is a task for subsequent empiric experience, in the hopeful context of several active non–cross-resistant drugs. Combination with other drugs affecting cell surface receptor tyrosine kinase, RAS/RAF/MEK/MAP pathway, and common points such as the proteasome or mTOR can be anticipated to be of interest in renal and other cancers. Complex interactions, such as VEGFR-mediated resistance to EGFR blockade [25] may be important and only revealed in combination applications.

General Immunity

Although sometimes stereotyped as "the chemotherapy nonresponder," kidney cancer, particularly the clear cell subtype, is also considered to be "immune-sensitive." Partly on this basis, and notwithstanding that many cancer types are immune-sensitive in murine models, it is kidney cancer that is a frequent focus of the translational effort of immunotherapy. Some of these novel treatments build on IL-2 or interferon therapy. Specific immunity vaccine approaches are discussed in the next section. The mechanisms of immune evasion by renal cancers, and by cancers in general, are undoubtedly complex. Some of the cytokines elaborated by tumors are known to have anergy-favoring effects on the immune systems, include transforming growth factor-β (TGF-β), IL-10, and VEGF. The ultimate therapeutic attack may involve directly negating this effect, or circumventing it through a different immune-enhancing maneuver.

The cytokine IL-12 influences dendritic cell function, favoring promotion of cellular immunity, including possibly useful antitumor immunity. Striking synergy of IL-12 plus IL-2 in murine models [33] has been encouraging. Practical synergy is yet to be demonstrated. A phase I trial using six doses of high-dose bolus IL-2, given in groups of three with IL-12 on intervening days, is open at NCI, and a phase I trial using IL-12 with interferon has been reported [34]. Hematological and hepatic toxicity were observed. Two of 18 kidney cancer patients in the trial had responses, a preliminary efficacy assessment.

Antibody drugs that suppress the CTLA4+ (CD152) cell subset (corresponding to the suppressors lymphocytes, also identified as Treg) had good success in some murine tumor models [35,36], and an immunologically detectable effect in vaccinated cancer patients [37]. A phase II single-arm study of MDX 010 (Medarex, Princeton, NY), for IL-2 refractory or ineligible patients is open at the National Institutes of Health (NIH). The optimal use of this type of manipulation of the immune system will undoubtedly be in combination with other available immune maneuvers and treatments. One may anticipate that combination development will be contingent on the single-agent experience.

Thalidomide is a drug with many proposed mechanisms of action. The relevant mechanism of action is unknown, but may be immune modulation or downregulation of cytokines, including tumor necrosis factor-α (TNF-α), VEGF, basic fibroblast growth factor (bFGF), or IL-12, as well as interfering with some step of angiogenesis. The antiangiogenic and immune-modulation mechanisms were the key rationales for application testing in several series of RCC clinical trials. The dominant response reported was disease stabilization, although some series identified some partial responders [38–42]. A safe conclusion across these series appears to be that at best the impact of the drug is on a minority of patients, the observed disease stabilization is not of conclusive survival benefit, and further single-agent testing is unlikely to show an impact on median survival.

Disparate results were identified in two single-arm trials combining the drug with IL-2. Amato et al. [43] reported a major response frequency of 39% (two complete responses [CR] and 11 PR among 37 evaluable patients) using a regimen of 4 weeks of 5-day-a-week IL-2 at 7 million IU/m^2 plus thalidomide 200 mg/d. Additionally, 10 patients had stable disease. Formal publication is awaited; a trial using the same two agents with the addition of granulocyte-macrophage colony-stimulating factor (GM-CSF) as an antigen presentation enhancing drug has been opened [44]. In contrast, Olenoki et al. [45] found three responders in 33 patients with a regimen of thalidomide 100 mg/d and IL-2 at 250,000 IU/kg during week 1 and 125,000 IU/kg

during weeks 2 to 6. Two related drugs, Actimid™ (CC4017) and (CC5013, Revimid™ and lenolidomide celgene, summit, NJ) have potent in vitro effects on lymphocytes as well as on TNF-α. These newer analogs appear to lack the teratogenicity risk and neuropathy problem that have been pervasive in efforts to expand the oncological application of thalidomide. One may anticipate the potential for testing in kidney cancer; a single-agent phase II renal cancer study with lenolidomide is open at Baylor University [46] and other centers.

A cooperative group phase III randomized trial of low-dose interferon-α2b (3 million units three times a week versus interferon plus thalidomide) has been presented (E2898). It addressed the issue of whether the thalidomide plus interferon combination is active in renal cancer, by antiangiogenesis or another mechanism. The results presented in June 2004 revealed an extremely low response in the control arm (2.2%), and a response of 6.5% in the combination arm. There were more thrombotic events (12 vs. 4) in the combination arm, the median progression-free survival favored the combination (2.8 vs. 3.8 months, $p = .04$), and the overall survival favored (nonsignificantly) the control arm (12.2 vs. 10.8 months) [47].

Finally, pharmacokinetic modifications of IL-2 and interferon have been developed. The Bayer compound BAY 50-4798 is an analogue of natural IL-2, but with modification to activate T cells but not natural killer (NK) cells. This may have a favorable effect on toxicity. Considering that the relevant mechanism of action of IL-2 remains a subject of controversy—one view is that for renal cancer it is the NK cells that are more relevant than CD8+ T cells (as may be the case in melanoma)—further disease-specific clinical testing will certainly be warranted. Subcutaneous pegylated interferons have a longer half-life and a higher molecular weight compared to unmodified interferon (molecular weight 19,000 to 20,000 dalton). Available pegylated interferons, with indications for treatment of infectious hepatitis, used in combination with Ribavirin include Pegasys™ (interferon-α2a, molecular weight 60,000, manufactured by Roche, Basel, Switzerland) and Pegintron™ (interferon-α2b, molecular weight 31,000, manufactured by Schering-Plough, Kenilworth, NJ) [48,49]. Anticancer testing of interferon-α2a for renal cancer showed five PR (19%) among 27 patients treated in the phase I testing, [50]; the recommended dose for further testing was 450 µg once a week. There was one CR and four PRs (overall 13%) among 40 previously untreated renal cancer patients in the phase II experience [51]. The report of phase I to II testing of the trial of pegylated interferon-α2b in renal cancer determined a dose of 6µg/kg/week, with the observation that some patients could tolerate 7.5µg/kg/week. Thirty-five previously untreated renal cell cancer patients were in the phase II part of the trial; 23 of 57 had at least stable disease at week 12. Objective response was observed in six of the 44 evaluable previously untreated renal cancer patients. At 1 year, two CRs and four PRs (overall 11% of the 57) were ongoing [52], and a total of 44 previously untreated renal cell cancer patients were evaluable for response.

Leukocyte Products

In the preclinical experience, nucleated blood cells have enormous potential for therapeutic immune manipulation. Ex vivo isolation, sorting, expansion, and activation seem to define an untenable matrix of testable approaches. Historically tested methods, including tumor infiltrating lymphocytes (TIL) [53,54] and autologous lymphocyte infusion (ALT) [55], offer ready contexts for new variations, such as cell sorting and ex vivo cytokine application. The open single-arm trial in St. Luke's Medical Center (Milwaukee, WI) uses IL-2 and anti-CD3 activating antibodies on the apheresis-derived lymphocytes, which are reinfused to subjects [56].

A special case of leukocyte-derived novel therapies involve use of dendritic cells (DCs), the major antigen-presenting cell type. Monocyte-derived DCs may be prepared from the apheresis product by culture of adherent mononuclear cells, which are then exposed to GM-CSF and IL-4. These autologous, human leukocyte antigen (HLA)-matched DCs may then be loaded with antigen in a variety of ways, and then reintroduced.

Vieweg's group [57] has explored the use of nucleic acid material to load DCs. The messenger RNA (mRNA) of tumor cells may encompass tumor-specific antigens, with advantages over protein-based approaches in that it may be non-

specifically amplified as needed using standard techniques. Similarly, RNA coding for selected antigens, such as telomerase protein (TERT), present in the whole-tumor derived mRNA, can be used to load DCs, offering both the advantage of emphasizing specific tumor antigens, as well as a specific strategy for monitoring response to a single protein. The acquisition of cytotoxic T lymphocyte (CTL) with this specificity was identified with the acquisition of polyclonal CTL, in six of seven evaluated patients in a 10-patient clinical trial. The clinical implication of the immune changes remain uncertain, as most subjects took other therapy after the study treatment.

Dendritic cells physiologically take up apoptotic bodies. Another vaccine approach, recently reported in non–small-cell lung cancer patients, is with allogeneic tumor cells, treated with ultraviolet (UV) radiation to induce apoptosis and admixed with autologous DCs. Acquisition of T cells with antitumor specificity was detectable by, enzyme linked immunospot (ELISPOT) assay [58]. The ex vivo fusion of dendritic cells with autologous tumor cells is a way to introduce cells bearing both the in situ particular antigen and the HLA repertoire of the tumor and competent antigen-presentation cell surface molecules. Avigan and colleagues [59] described a clinical trial applying this technique. Among 13 renal cancer patients treated, five had disease stabilization for 3 to 9 months; two breast cancer patients had responses, one durable for more than 24 months. Practical drawbacks include the need for three separate ex vivo cellular manipulations: single-cell suspension of autologous tumor, apheresis of peripheral blood mononuclear cells for DC culture, and cell fusion with verification of presence of biphenotypic (tumor and DC) cells for vaccine administration. In the cited report, 32 subjects had successful product preparation, and 23 of 58 enrolled subjects were actually treated, with products having 28% to 71% fusion efficiency.

A groundbreaking investigational clear cell renal cancer therapy is based on transfer of stem cells is the nonmyeloablative allogeneic stem cell transplant. The seminal publication in 2000 showed nine of 19 patients (who had disease refractory to IL-2) demonstrating at least partial responses, attributable to the graft versus tumor (GVT) effect. Three had complete responses [60]. Additional experience including from

Europe and from other centers will be critical in defining the best patient selection criteria and graft-versus-host management [61,62].

In the nonmyeloablative transplant technique, the path to the therapeutic outcome can be considered as separate steps. The first is selection of a suitable patient and suitable donor. In the initial experience at NCI, favorable responses were seen essentially only in the clear cell subtype, and the worldwide experience emphasizes this subtype. (Treatment of individuals with a histological type that is not clear cell, an even more heterogeneous group, remains an area for exploration, as the current series emphasize or require the clear cell type.)

Since the time until therapeutic effect may be long, a further requirement is that the patient will be able to survive until the therapeutic effect becomes apparent. The ideal donor is most frequently defined as an HLA-identical (nonidentical twin) full sibling, who is an individual with mismatches of other alleles (minor antigens). Alternative donors, such as partial mismatch siblings or matched unrelated donors, are another area in active exploration, because it appears that the frequency of patients who have donors meeting the first criterion is limited; for example, only 84 of 284 (29.6%) at University of Chicago had donors that could be screened [63]. Besides the limitations on donors, limitations on histological subtype, rate of growth of the tumor, sites of tumor, and comorbidities can be anticipated to continue to limit applicability of the method.

A next step is manipulation of the graft material obtained by apheresis. For example, this can include depletion of lymphocytes to a defined dose. Preparative chemotherapy for the host is directed at host lymphocytes, and of lower intensity than in a traditional myeloablative stem cell transplant, such as for a hematological malignancy. Fludarabine and cyclophosphamide combinations have been used, with an emphasis on marrow ablation, not antitumor effect. Following graft infusion, the extent of engraftment may be monitored. Complete donor chimerism may be a necessary intermediate goal. Subsequently, discontinuation of immune suppression, as well as donor lymphocyte infusions (DLIs) to support the graft, can be used, titrated against observed graft-versus-host disease. General immune-function deficits may require antibacterial, antiviral, and antifungal support. Finally, hands-on management of graft-versus-host disease,

with a variety of immune suppressive drugs including steroids, cyclosporine, methotrexate, and others, is requisite.

Tumor Products

Cellular material for therapeutic use can also be obtained directly from the tumor. As mentioned above, tumor material can be used to obtain peptide, nucleic acid, or other material for loading into dendritic cells. Tumor cell material may also be used without ex vivo dendritic cell loading. Presumably antigen presentation can occur in vivo with either the modified tumor cell acting as substitute antigen-presenting cell, or attracting autologous dendritic cells that then take up the relevant antigen and process and present it effectively.

The Oncophage™ product, in phase III RCC testing, uses heat shock protein and the associated peptides obtained from fresh tumor (HSPPC-96) as the material for the loading of DCs. This set of peptides has the feature that it contains peptides that will be loaded onto cell surface major histocompatibility complex (MHC) molecules, and so may represent an immunogenically useful panel to which to stimulate a response. The mixture may be particularly well acquired for processing by dendritic cells [64,65]. Some published studies indicate that this strategy is sufficient to induce measurable, apparently useful antitumor immunity, even in the context of a cancer that had been metastatic [66]. Two randomized studies using Oncophage seek to enroll either patients having nephrectomy in the face of metastatic disease or patients having nephrectomy for cure, but for whom tumor, node, metastasis (TNM) staging is consistent with a high recurrence risk [67].

Our group has worked with B7.1 transduced autologous tumor cell vaccine that is irradiated and then given sequentially before an outpatient schedule of subcutaneous IL-2. Upon resection of tumor material, often primary tumor but also metastasis, short-term tissue culture is used and then the dendritic cell surface co-stimulatory protein B7.1 is introduced with a viral vector. Theoretically this would allow naive lymphocytes with antitumor specificity to encounter tumor antigens in the context of this "second signal" (B7.1 on the antigen-presenting cell, CD28 on the lymphocyte) that would promote activation over anergy or deletion [68]. A different cytokine that tumor cells can be modified to release is GM-CSF. This localized secretion of GM-CSF should recruit dendritic cells that will process the antigen [69]. The GVAX® products (cell Genesys, South San Francisco, CA) are in trial in several cancer subtypes, uses this strategy [70].

The autologous tumor lysate (aTL) product was the subject of a randomized phase III adjuvant trial in Germany for which progression-free survival results were reported in 2004. For this vaccine, the tumor cells are in culture for several hours in media containing interferon-γ and tocopherol, and then devitalized with freeze/thaw cycling. The former should induce higher expression of MHC cell surface molecules, causing an enhanced immunogenicity. The reported results—the only large, randomized vaccine renal cancer trial conducted in Europe—are consistent with an improvement in time-to-detected progression [71]. An apparent imbalance of the attrition in patients randomized to active treatment, and the unreported overall survival data, among other factors, may limit interpretation of the clinical outcome data [72].

In common across all of these tumor cell–derived therapeutic products is a product safety infrastructure. This includes the need for product characterization, irradiation of potentially live tumor cell material, monitoring for bacterial or other contaminants, and explicit vaccine material/patient matching. The decision about which aspects of the product must be monitored may be a difficult one. A continued reference to the huge theoretical potency of specific anticancer immunotherapy is required to justify this significant infrastructure and expense.

Angiogenic Targeting

Renal cancer specimens are often observed to be densely vascularized; reports of difficult-to-control bleeding during surgery on metastases (as opposed to nephrectomy, where the renal vascular stalk is a point of control) are common. The concept of targeting the blood vessels of the cancer is appealing for several reasons: low toxicity, conversion of the disease to a chronic pattern, and an independent attack at a fundamental vulnerability of the growing tumor. The

genotype of the targeted cell type is theoretically stable and comparable across cancer subtypes. A variety of drugs have been validated as members of the antiangiogenic class, using in vitro and murine models. The transition to clinical application has been slow, but includes some testing in kidney cancer, in addition to renal cancer patients who have participated in phase I studies. In contrast to conventional cytotoxic drugs, an emphasis could be on nontoxic disease stabilization rather than on regression. Thalidomide and related compounds and Su11248 are discussed above [73,74].

Vascular endothelial growth factor A (VEGF-A), which is present in several isoforms [75], is the ligand of cell surface receptors [VEGF-R1, (flt-1), VEGF-R2, and (flk)]. The VEGF levels may be high in RCC, relating to HRE in the gene promoter. Other VEGF gene family members (VEGF-B, VEGF-C, VEGF-D, VEGF-E) may have other diverse roles in cancer [76]. The presence of the (receptors) in tumor blood vessels identifies blocking of the VEGF/VEGFR pathway as an appealing target. Depletion of free VEGF occurs with bevacizumab (Avastin™, Genentech, South San Francisco, CA), a 93% humanized antibody, approved for colorectal cancer [77]. The VEGF-TRAP drug, a synthetic protein composed of domains of the immunoglobulin Fc, and extracellular domains of flt-1 and flk, appears to have the same general mechanism of action [78].

In a randomized phase II trial of bevacizumab for progressive, refractory renal cancer, a high frequency of stable disease was identified in the high-dose arm (64% at 4 months, versus 20% for the placebo group). Major responses were observed in four of 40 patients (10%), and multiyear stabilizations were identified as well [79]. Clinical testing of combinations with interferon and IL-2 will be of interest, as the optimal use of bevacizumab for renal cancer is developed. A cooperative group trial of interferon with or without bevacizumab is open [80]. Side effects observed in the experience to this point include risk of bleeding and hypertension. The bevacizumab plus erlotinib trial is cited above.

Vascular Targeting

Vascular targeting drugs employ a different strategy. A transient direct attack on the tumor endothelium may result in tumor infarction. Combretastatin is one member of this group that targets endothelial cell microtubules, for which phase I trials have been completed [81,82]. Measurement of tumor blood flow, for example by dynamic contrast magnetic resonance imaging (DC-MRI), may provide a method to identify the occurrence of vascular blockade by this class of drugs. Another member of the class for which phase I testing was completed is ZD6126 (AstraZeneca, Wilmington, DE), and ABT-751 (Abbott, Chicago, IL), which is orally available, was tested in a phase II company-sponsored renal cancer trial. A review of many of these agents suggests that one may anticipate their development for renal cancer [83]. The vascular targeting drugs remain in an early stage of development.

A natural product drug, Neovastat (AE-941, Aeterna Laboratories, Quebec city, Quebec, Canada) may affect VEGF-related signaling and inhibit matrix metalloproteases. For classification purposes, the mechanism of action for this cartilage-derived substance can be considered as a multifunctional antiangiogenesis. A favorable subset analysis from a multidiagnosis trial that had 22 evaluable renal cancer patients suggested that a higher dose was consistent with a survival benefit. [84,85]. A randomized phase III Kidney cancer trial has completed accrual and was negative, but again a subject for which favorable outcome from the drug was identified.

Conclusion

The process of developing a concept, translational testing, verification of targets, and clinical trials takes years. The complex intracellular and immunological targets and numerous classes of drugs seem to define an unending array of testable strategies. Development strategies depend both on conceptual priorities and on practical (economic) realization issues of pharmaceutical companies. Renal cancer, therefore, is often not the initial development target, and a significant amount of experience in other histologies with a particular strategy may accrue before any formal testing is done in renal cancer. Conversely, early responses observed in renal cancer have been met with enthusiastic, significant trial infrastructure investment, includ-

ing for CCI-779, sorafenib, bevacizumab, and Su-111248. Besides biological theory, there will be the relevance of this other experience, obviously more appealing in the case of positive trials, weighing on the decision process.

For patients seeking to decide on a treatment trial, the absence of a nontoxic, frequently effective standard therapy puts investigational vaccines, compounds, and combinations in the forefront. A practical approach is to canvas available treatments, using Web sites and personal contacts, and to then try to reach a rapid decision. Despite an understandable ambition to get a chance at access to every promising drug, the therapeutic plan must integrate logistic issues and the uncertain appeal of theoretical mechanisms of action. Patients, even those with slowly progressing disease, may have relatively limited realistic options for participation in clinical trials.

Among isolated pharmaceutical compounds, key compounds in later phase trials in 2005 include sorafenib, CCI-779, Su11248, and bevacizumab. Some immune manipulations are similarly centered on single drugs, such as the MDX-010 antibody or IL-12. Older drugs, such as high-dose IL-2 (still the only regimen with occasional long-term disease-free survivors), IL-2 and interferon combinations, and phase I drugs, are typically part of the discussion as well.

Many immune manipulations are more complex, such as nonmyeloablative transplant or combinations of vaccines or immune modulators with IL-2 or interferon. Trials frequently focus on never-treated or once-treated/now-progressing subsets. Conversely, the prevalent patient population interested in new therapy is a group more heterogeneous for comorbidities, extent of pretreatment, and distribution of metastatic disease, especially brain metastasis.

From where will the next breakthrough treatment for renal cancer come? Notwithstanding the uncertainty of enthusiasm derived from single-arm trials, the targeted drugs appear to be a frontrunner category. Any one additional drug with an indication for renal cancer will almost certainly have a toxicity profile better than cytokine (IL-2, interferon) approaches and may change the face of therapeutic planning for metastatic RCC. One may remain hopeful that the paradigm shift toward targeted, tolerated, durable metastatic RCC management can

2a for patients with advanced renal cell carcinoma. J Clin Oncol 2001;19(5):1312–1319.

52. Bukowski R, Ernstoff MS, Gore ME, et al. Pegylated interferon alfa-2b treatment for patients with solid tumors: a phase I/II study. J Clin Oncol 2002;20(18):3841–3849.

53. Rosenberg SA, Lotze MT, Yang JC, et al. Prospective randomized trial of high-dose interleukin-2 alone or in conjunction with lymphokine-activated killer cells for the treatment of patients with advanced cancer. J Natl Cancer Inst 1993; 85(8):622–632.

54. Law TM, Motzer RJ, Mazumdar M, et al. Phase III randomized trial of interleukin-2 with or without lymphokine-activated killer cells in the treatment of patients with advanced renal cell carcinoma. Cancer 1995;76(5):824–832.

55. Figlin RA, Thompson JA, Bukowski RM, et al. Multicenter, randomized, phase III trial of CD8(+) tumor-infiltrating lymphocytes in combination with recombinant interleukin-2 in metastatic renal cell carcinoma. J Clin Oncol 1999;17(8): 2521–2529.

56. http://www.nci.nih.gov/search/clinical_trials/ (Search kidney cancer: STLMC-BRM-9401, NCI-V94-0514; John Hanson, P.I.).

57. Su Z, Dannull J, Heiser A, et al. Immunological and clinical responses in metastatic renal cancer patients vaccinated with tumor RNA-transfected dendritic cells. Cancer Res 2003;63(9):2127–2133.

58. Hirschowitz EA, Foody T, Kryscio R, Dickson L, Sturgill J, Yannelli J. Autologous dendritic cell vaccines for non-small-cell lung cancer. J Clin Oncol 2004;22(14):2808–2815.

59. Avigan D, Vasir B, Gong J, et al. Fusion cell vaccination of patients with metastatic breast and renal cancer induces immunological and clinical responses. Clin Cancer Res 2004;10(14):4699–4708.

60. Childs R, Chernoff A, Contentin N, et al. Regression of metastatic renal-cell carcinoma after nonmyeloablative allogeneic peripheral-blood stem-cell transplantation. N Engl J Med 2000; 343(11):750–758.

61. Ueno NT, Cheng YC, Rondon G, et al. Rapid induction of complete donor chimerism by the use of a reduced-intensity conditioning regimen composed of fludarabine and melphalan in allogeneic stem cell transplantation for metastatic solid tumors. Blood 2003;102(10):3829–3836.

62. Blaise D, Bay JO, Faucher C, et al. Reduced-intensity preparative regimen and allogeneic stem cell transplantation for advanced solid tumors. Blood 2004;103(2):435–441.

63. Rini BI, Zimmerman TM, Gajewski TF, Stadler WM, Vogelzang NJ. Allogeneic peripheral blood stem cell transplantation for metastatic renal cell carcinoma. J Urol 2001;165(4):1208–1209.

64. Dai J, Liu B, Caudill MM, et al. Cell surface expression of heat shock protein gp96 enhances cross-presentation of cellular antigens and the generation of tumor-specific T cell memory. Cancer Immunol 2003;3:1.

65. Graner MW, Zeng Y, Feng H, Katsanis E. Tumor-derived chaperone-rich cell lysates are effective therapeutic vaccines against a variety of cancers. Cancer Immunol Immunother 2003;52(4):226–234.

66. Mazzaferro V, Coppa J, Carrabba MG, et al. Vaccination with autologous tumor-derived heat-shock protein gp96 after liver resection for metastatic colorectal cancer. Clin Cancer Res 2003;9(9): 3235–3245.

67. http://www.antigenics.com/products/cancer/ oncophage/ and http://www.antigenics.com/.

68. Antonia SJ, Seigne J, Diaz J, et al. Phase I trial of a B7–1 (CD80) gene modified autologous tumor cell vaccine in combination with systemic interleukin-2 in patients with metastatic renal cell carcinoma. J Urol 2002;167(5):1995–2000.

69. Borrello I, Sotomayor EM, Cooke S, Levitsky HI. A universal granulocyte-macrophage colony-stimulating factor-producing bystander cell line for use in the formulation of autologous tumor cell-based vaccines. Hum Gene Ther 1999;10(12): 1983–1991.

70. http://www.gvax.com/home.shtml.

71. Jocham D, Richter A, Hoffmann L, et al. Adjuvant autologous renal tumour cell vaccine and risk of tumour progression in patients with renal-cell carcinoma after radical nephrectomy: phase III, randomised controlled trial. Lancet 2004; 363(9409):594–599.

72. Fishman M, Antonia S. Specific antitumour vaccine for renal cancer. Lancet 2004;363(9409): 583–584.

73. Folkman J, Kalluri R. Cancer without disease. Nature 2004;427(6977):787.

74. Folkman J. Angiogenesis inhibitors: a new class of drugs. Cancer Biol Ther 2003;2(4 suppl 1): S127–133.

75. Nakamura M, Abe Y, Tokunaga T. Pathological significance of vascular endothelial growth factor A isoform expression in human cancer. Pathol Int 2002;52(5–6):331–339.

76. Clauss M. Molecular biology of the VEGF and the VEGF receptor family. Semin Thromb Hemost 2000;26(5):561–569.

77. Hurwitz H, Fehrenbacher L, Novotny W, et al. Bevacizumab plus irinotecan, fluorouracil, and leucovorin for metastatic colorectal cancer. N Engl J Med 2004;350(23):2335–2342.

78. Holash J, Davis S, Papadopoulos N, et al. VEGF-Trap: a VEGF blocker with potent antitumor effects. Proc Natl Acad Sci USA 2002;99(17):11393–11398.

79. Yang JC, Haworth L, Sherry RM, et al. A randomized trial of bevacizumab, an anti-vascular endothelial growth factor antibody, for metastatic renal cancer. N Engl J Med 2003;349(5):427–434.

80. Rini BI, Halabi S, Taylor J, Small EJ, Schilsky RL. Cancer and Leukemia Group B 90206: a randomized phase III trial of interferon-alpha or interferon-alpha plus anti-vascular endothelial growth factor antibody (bevacizumab) in metastatic renal cell carcinoma. Clin Cancer Res 2004;10(8):2584–2586.

81. www.oxigene.com.

82. Stevenson JP, Rosen M, Sun W, et al. Phase I trial of the antivascular agent combretastatin A4 phosphate on a 5–day schedule to patients with cancer: magnetic resonance imaging evidence for altered tumor blood flow. J Clin Oncol 2003;21(23): 4428–4438.

83. Thorpe PE. Vascular targeting agents as cancer therapeutics. Clin Cancer Res 2004;10(2):415–427.

84. Gingras D, Renaud A, Mousseau N, Beaulieu E, Kachra Z, Beliveau R. Matrix proteinase inhibition by AE-941, a multifunctional antiangiogenic compound. Anticancer Res 2001;21(1A):145–155.

85. Beliveau R, Gingras D, Kruger EA, et al. The antiangiogenic agent neovastat (AE-941) inhibits vascular endothelial growth factor-mediated biological effects. Clin Cancer Res 2002;8(4):1242–1250.

19

Genetics and Biology of Adult Male Germ Cell Tumors

Jane Houldsworth, George J. Bosl, and R.S.K. Chaganti

Germ cell tumors (GCTs) are the most common malignancy in young adult males between the ages of 15 and 40 presenting predominantly in the testis [1]. They arise by transformation of a germ cell (GC) that during its normal life span undergoes series of proliferative and differentiation events that culminate in the formation of gametes [2]. Transformed GCs uniquely exhibit the potential to initiate molecular pathways in part resembling those occurring during normal human development, as evidenced by the array of histologies observed within tumor specimens [3]. Occasionally within well-differentiated components, further malignant transformation occurs. leading to the appearance of a non-GC malignancy [3]. More than 90% of newly diagnosed patients are cured, with 70% to 80% of advanced cases being cured with cisplatin-based chemotherapy [1]. Thus, GCTs are an ideal system in which the molecular mechanisms underlying this exquisite sensitivity can be studied. This chapter discusses the current state of knowledge of the genetics and biology of GC transformation, differentiation, and response to cisplatin.

Pathobiology of Male Germ Cell Tumors

Adult GCTs are broadly classified into two morphologically distinct groups: seminomas and nonseminomas [3]. The first recognizable lesion in the testis is intratubular germ cell neoplasia (ITGCN), where transformed GCs are evident within the seminiferous tubules. Although it morphologically more closely resembles seminomas than nonseminomas, ITGCN is generally accepted as the precursor of all invasive GCTs [3]. Seminomatous GCTs frequently express protein markers of GCs early in development such as placental alkaline phosphatase, KIT, RET (GDNF receptor), and POU5F1 (OCT3/OCT4), and retain the morphology of undifferentiated spermatogonial GCs [4–6]. They exhibit low mitotic and apoptotic indices, low metastatic potential, and are generally cured by a combination of orchiectomy and radiation therapy [1,3]. Nonseminomas display an array of histologies mimicking different patterns of embryonic and extraembryonic differentiation that normally occur during human development. Embryonal carcinoma (EC) resembles zygotic cells early in embryonic development and display the highest mitotic and apoptotic indices of all GCT histological components [3,7]. Teratomas exhibit somatic differentiation normally seen in the developing three germ layers of the embryo proper resembling incomplete differentiation (immature teratoma) or well-differentiated tissues (mature teratoma), and tend to have both low mitotic and apoptotic indices [3,7]. On occasion, mature teratomas undergo malignant transformation of one of the histological components, necessitating similar treatment to that of the malignant tissue counterpart [8]. α-Fetoprotein (AFP) and human chorionic

[46,47]. These studies identified distinct stages in the transition from an EC cell to neuroprogenitor cells expressing patterning markers compatible with posterior hindbrain fates, and to immature postmitotic neurons with an evolving synaptic apparatus [46]. Comparison of this transcriptional program with that induced in the same cell line by other morphogens along other pathways such as bone morphogenetic proteins-2 and -4 along an epithelial pathway, should yield molecular clues as to how both agents effect a decrease in proliferation but two different somatic cell fates. Thus, EC cell lines represent an in vitro system wherein the functional involvement of candidate genes in human cell fate/lineage decisions can be studied.

Genetic and Biologic Basis of Chemoresistance

Germ cell tumors are a good model for a curable malignancy. Over 90% of newly diagnosed GCT cases are cured, and in patients with advanced disease requiring initial cisplatin-based chemotherapy, 70% to 80% are cured. The molecular basis for this exquisite sensitivity probably resides in the inherent biological features of GCs involved in cell growth, cell death, differentiation pathways, and cellular response to DNA damage. Immunohistochemical analyses of GCTs for the expression of markers of cell proliferation, of susceptibility to apoptosis and resistance, and for the evaluation of spontaneous apoptotic cell death have indicated a clear difference in the balance of cell growth and death between histological subtypes of GCTs [7,48,49]. However, excluding one recent study of ECs [50], these analyses have not led to the identification of specific markers or combinations of markers that predict response to treatment. As evidenced both in vivo and in vitro, the process of cellular differentiation in GCTs is associated with the acquisition of a resistant phenotype. Teratomas are relatively unresponsive to chemotherapy, and surgical resection is often required to remove this component [1]. Likewise, induction of differentiation of pluripotent EC cell lines in vitro is accompanied by loss of a cisplatin-sensitive phenotype [51]. Differences in response to treatment within nonseminomas are clinically known and may reflect the inherent sensitivity of the normal tissue counterparts. The mole-

cular determinants of these differences are unknown, and must be taken into consideration when using global screening expression methods to look for molecular markers of resistance.

A number of molecular clues involved in the sensitive phenotype and acquisition of resistance by GCTs has come from examination of the response of GCT-derived cell lines to DNA-damaging agents. Few reports have attributed the sensitivity of GCTs to the reduced ability to repair DNA lesions induced by cisplatin resulting from either shielding lesions in DNA by high-mobility group domain proteins unique to GCs [52] or decreased levels of XPA involved in DNA damage recognition and facilitation of the DNA repair complex assembly [53]. Unlike other tumor systems, the tumor-suppressor gene TP53 is rarely mutated in GCTs, but mutations and deletions were found in a subset of clinically resistant GCTs [54–56]. A cell line derived from a resistant GCT contained the same TP53 mutation as the original specimen and was unable to activate an apoptotic response to cisplatin treatment compared with a GCT cell line with wild-type TP53 [56]. Thus, inactivating mutations within TP53 may comprise one molecular means by which GCTs circumvent the usually rapid apoptotic response to DNA-damaging agents exhibited by most transformed GCs and normal GCs. In another study, one GCT cell line with mutant TP53 did not display a resistance to cisplatin in culture, indicating that perhaps in a minority of GCTs, TP53 mutation may not lead to a resistant phenotype [57]. Other studies have implicated failure to activate caspase-9 [58] or failure to induce expression of FAS and recruitment of FADD and caspase-8 to FAS [59] as other possible means by which GCTs subvert the inherent capacity of these cells to rapidly activate cell death pathways [reviewed in ref. 60]. Through such studies, identification of the biological factors that predispose GCs and consequently GCTs to apoptosis are being identified and ultimately may have relevance in understanding the poorer responses of other tumor types to the same agents.

Clinically, patients are risk-stratified according to criteria established by the International Germ Cell Consensus Cancer Group (IGCCCG), based on primary site, serum tumor marker levels, histology, and sites of metastasis [1]. Few genetic markers predicting resistance have been reported. As discussed above, mutation/deletion of *TP53* is one. Another reported by us is high-level gene amplification, a genetic feature often associated in other tumor types with a poorer prognosis [17]. Comparative genomic hybridization, (CGH) analysis revealed amplification of genetic material at multiple sites other than 12p, in five of 17 GCTs not cured by cisplatin-based therapy, but not in 17 cured GCTs. Follow-up studies are currently being performed to identify candidate target genes of the amplification events using a combination of array-CGH and expression array analyses. Additional expression studies aim at identifying markers of resistance not restricted to regions identified by molecular genetic studies and provide an exciting prospect of utilizing a group of expression identifiers together with clinical parameters for risk-stratification of patients.

Genetic Basis of Malignant Transformation

Occasionally, teratomas exhibit histological evidence of a non-GC malignancy, whose GCT clonal origin has been confirmed by the presence of i(12p). Such "malignant transformation" of teratomas leads to aggressive malignancies displaying histological differentiation along mesenchymal lineages such as sarcoma (in particular, rhabdomyosarcoma), hematopoietic lineages such as myeloid leukemia, epithelial lineages such as carcinoma, and neurogenic lineages such as primitive neuroectodermal tumor (PNET) [1]. In addition to the cytogenetic/genetic abnormalities displayed by the original GCT, the transformed malignancy contains abnormalities characteristic of the differentiated malignant phenotype [61,62]. Sarcomatous transformation is the most common form exemplified by one case described by us where a posttreatment mediastinal mass comprised a teratomatous cystic region and an embryonal rhabdomyosarcoma solid region [62]. Upon karyotypic analysis, both regions exhibited i(12p), with the embryonal rhabdomyosarcoma component exhibiting additional chromosomal abnormalities including a translocation involving 2q37 and a deleted 6q [62]. Of note, breakpoints in 2q have frequently been reported for de novo embryonal rhabdomyosarcomas. Both tumor regions exhibited a common *TP53* deletion, implying acquisition of

this genetic lesion prior to malignant transformation [56]. Comparative genomic hybridization, (CGH) analysis revealed high-level amplification only in the transformed component, implying acquisition of this genetic lesion during or after malignant transformation [17]. For one of the sites (7q31), follow-up array-CGH and Southern hybridization has implicated *MET* as the candidate amplified target gene, for which a role in metastasis and response of rhabdomyosarcoma to radiochemotherapy has recently been described [63]. Molecular interrogation of these tumors has overall been limited, and future studies will yield information regarding GCT biology as well as transforming events of other non-GC malignancies.

Acknowledgments

The reported studies were supported by the Byrne Fund and the Lance Armstrong Foundation.

References

1. Bosl GJ, Motzer RJ. Testicular germ-cell cancer. N Engl J Med 1997;337:242–253.
2. Chaganti RSK, Houldsworth J. Genetics and biology of adult human male germ cell tumors. Cancer Res 2000;60:1475–1482.
3. Mostofi FK, Sesterhenn IA, Davis CJ Jr. Anatomy and pathology of testis cancer. In: Vogelzang NJ, Scardino PT, Shipley WU, Coffey DS, eds. Comprehensive Textbook of Genitourinary Urology, 2nd ed. Philadelphia: Lippincott Williams & Wilkins, 2000:909–926.
4. Rajpert-De Meyts E, Skakkebaek NE. Expression of the c-kit protein product in carcinoma-in-situ and invasive testicular germ cell tumours. Int J Androl 1994;17:85–92.
5. Tezel G, Nagasaka T, Shimono Y, et al. Differential expression of RET finger protein in testicular germ cell tumors. Pathol Int 2002;52:623–627.
6. Looijenga LH, Stoop H, de Leeuw HP, et al. POU5F1 (OCT3/4) identifies cells with pluripotent potential in human germ cell tumors. Cancer Res 2003;63:2244–2250.
7. Soini Y, Paakko P. Extent of apoptosis in relation to p53 and bcl-2 expression in germ cell tumors. Hum Pathol 1996;27:1221–1226.
8. Motzer RJ, Amsterdam A, Prieto V, et al. Teratoma with malignant transformation: diverse malignant histologies arising in men with germ cell tumors. J Urol 1988;159:133–138.

20

Chemotherapy for Testicular Cancer

Thomas R. Geldart and Graham M. Mead

The last 30 years have seen extraordinary advances in the management of metastatic germ cell cancer of the testis. Prior to the advent of cisplatin-containing chemotherapy in the mid-1970s, chemotherapy was highly toxic, and gave poor results, with cure unusual in those with advanced disease. Following the introduction of cisplatin, and subsequently etoposide, progress has been rapid, not least in the development of ancillary drugs (e.g., 5-hydroxytryptamine [5-HT$_3$] antagonists and growth factors). Modern therapy is now usually curative, tolerable, and has few long-term side effects. Indeed, the current dearth of randomized trials for most subgroups of these patients is largely a testimony to the advances taking place during this period.

This chapter describes the evolution of this therapy to the present, virtually worldwide consensus, emphasizing data derived from randomized trials. It is assumed throughout that patients with nonseminomatous germ cell cancer and residual masses postchemotherapy will, wherever possible, have these resected surgically. The emphasis is on failure-free survival and survival, the preferred trial end points in these diseases.

Prognostic Factors

Since the publication of the International Germ Cell Consensus Classification (IGCCC) data in 1997 [1], there has been virtually complete acceptance that patient management and clinical trials should be derived from the three prognostic groups of good, intermediate, and poor that were described in this study. Prior to this period, a wide variety of often conflicting parameters were used to allocate patients to two or three prognostic groups. It is beyond the scope of this text to describe each of these classifications in detail, and readers are referred to the original publications in each of the references for further detail.

In most modern studies, patients with seminoma requiring chemotherapy (a minority group) are combined with those with nonseminoma. Patients with seminoma are a median of 10 years older than patients with nonseminoma, which may have important implications for therapy. Those few studies specifically design for seminoma are considered separately.

Bleomycin, Etoposide, and Cisplatin (BEP): The Evolution of a Standard Therapy

The first effective steps in the development of effective chemotherapy for metastatic testicular cancer were the combination of vinblastine with infusional bleomycin and then incorporation of cisplatin to form the PVB regimen [2]. The Royal Marsden Hospital substituted etoposide (at a dose of 360 mg/m^2 given over 3 days per course) for vinblastine, resulting in the "European BEP" or BEP[360] regimen given for four courses at 3 weekly intervals, resulting in a highly effective regimen that became widely adopted in the United Kingdom [3]. International acceptance of BEP was to come when the Indiana Group, in a seminal study across all prognostic groups, compared four cycles of PVB and BEP[500] (etoposide and cisplatin given over 5 days with etoposide at a total dose of 500 mg/m^2) [4]. A total of 244 evaluable patients were randomized, and BEP[500] was found to improve survival in the poor prognostic group and to be associated with much improved tolerance. Bleomycin, given to a total dose of 360,000 IU in both arms resulted in five toxic deaths from bleomycin lung, and six patients died of infectious complications. Since this study was published, BEP, in many guises, has dominated the international therapy of metastatic germ cell cancer. Multiple attempts have been made to reduce its toxicity in patients with a good prognosis, and many studies have used BEP as a comparison against more intensive regimens in patients with a poor prognosis. These studies will now be described.

Treatment of Metastatic Disease

Good Prognosis Disease

Substitution of Carboplatin for Cisplatin

Platinum analogues have been one of the key elements in the successful evolution of germ cell cancer chemotherapy. Cisplatin is highly effec-

tive in combination, but universally associated with emesis, neurotoxicity, auditory toxicity, and renal toxicity. Carboplatin, although more myelotoxic, is associated with none of these problems and can be delivered easily on an outpatient basis. Initial studies suggested a high efficacy for this drug, particularly in seminoma (where it was widely adopted in Europe as a single agent for metastatic disease [5,6], but also in combination in nonseminoma [7], where comparative studies were designed to evaluate its role.

Seminoma

Two series from the Royal Marsden Hospital [5] and Germany [6] evaluated single-agent carboplatin in metastatic seminoma, both using a dose calculated from body surface area, rather than the more widely accepted area under the curve (AUC) dosing, giving 400 mg/m^2 of this drug every 3 to 4 weeks. The results from these two studies were remarkably similar, with failure-free survival rates of 71% and 77% and survival rates of 91% and 93%, respectively.

These two studies prompted two randomized trials (Table 20.1). The Medical Research Council (MRC) randomized 130 patients with metastatic seminoma between intravenous carboplatin and cisplatin/etoposide [8]. The trial was closed prematurely as recruitment had slowed following a negative assessment of carboplatin in metastatic nonseminoma in another trial. Carboplatin was associated with a 10% inferior progression-free survival (71% vs. 81%) with a nonsignificant survival difference favoring the cisplatin combination (84% vs. 89%).

Table 20.1. Randomized trials in seminoma comparing carboplatin against cisplatin combinations

Author	Number	Median follow-up (months)	FFS (%)			Survival (%)			Comment
			Carbo	PEI	EP	Carbo	PEI	EP	
Horwich et al. (8)	130	54	71	—	81	84	—	89	Trial closed prematurely; NS differences; EC recommended
Clemm et al. (9)	280	52	74	95	—	87	95	—	Significant FFS benefit ($p = .01$); NS overall survival difference

FFS, failure-free survival; NS, nonsignificant; Carbo, carboplatin; PEI, cisplatin, etoposide, and ifosfamide; EC, etoposide and cisplatin.

para-aortic strip radiotherapy. A total of 1477 patients were recruited into this trial, which closed to recruitment in March 2001. A median follow-up of 3 years has now elapsed, and preliminary results were presented in abstract form at the American Society of Clinical Oncology (ASCO) 2004 meeting. This trial has shown that adjuvant radiotherapy and carboplatin are of equivalent efficacy. Carboplatin can thereby be regarded as an equivalent (and probably preferred) management approach.

Long-Term Toxicities of Chemotherapy for Germ Cell Cancers

The majority of patients with testicular germ cell cancer are cured by surgery alone or surgery in combination with cisplatin-based chemotherapy and/or radiotherapy. In general, patients cured of their disease have a long life expectancy, and therefore the potential long-term toxicities of treatment are of considerable importance. A number of studies have evaluated the long-term toxicities of platinum-based chemotherapy.

Fertility and Gonadal Function

Spermatogenesis is impaired in a substantial proportion of patients presenting with germ cell cancer. In normospermic men who undergo combination BEP chemotherapy, a reduction in fertility is apparent postchemotherapy, although for most individuals sperm counts will recover over a period of years [50]. Of note, a good prechemotherapy sperm count is associated with a increased likelihood of recovery of spermatogenesis. With regard to hormonal function, a comparison of patients treated with surgery alone or surgery plus chemotherapy suggests that standard-dose BEP chemotherapy does not seem to contribute additionally to a significant impairment in Leydig cell function [51]. In contrast, higher doses ($\geq 400 \, \text{mg/m}^2$ cisplatin) may be associated with a significant and persistent impact in Leydig cell function with a consequent reduction in mean testosterone levels.

Pulmonary Function

As discussed earlier, the use of bleomycin has long been associated with pulmonary toxicity, with studies recording a 4% to 6% incidence of demonstrable lung toxicity with a 1% to 2% mortality rate. Toxicity is predominantly fibrotic in nature. Standard lung function tests are generally unhelpful in predicting toxicity and treatments (such as steroids) for established toxicity of unproven benefit. A number of pretreatment parameters do predict for bleomycin-induced toxicity, and these include poor renal function, age greater than 40, cumulative bleomycin dose greater than 300,000 units, and stage IV disease [52]. Careful consideration of bleomycin dose and close monitoring of patients presenting with one or more of these risk factors is of considerable importance.

Cardiovascular Morbidity

A number of studies have suggested a higher than expected incidence of cardiovascular disease (CVD) in patients receiving chemotherapy for metastatic disease. The largest of these studies has suggested that after a median of 10 years' follow-up, there may be a twofold or greater risk of developing CVD in such patients when compared to (stage I) matched patients followed by surveillance alone; the absolute risk is 6.7%, and the age-adjusted relative risk is 2.59 (95% confidence interval [CI], 1.1 to 5.8) [53]. A variety of potential mechanisms could account for an increased risk of CVD following chemotherapy, including vascular endothelial damage, renal impairment, hypertension, hyperlipidemia, and an increase in body mass index. Although no clear relationship was established for any of these risk factors in this study, other studies have demonstrated a relationship between chemotherapy and an increased incidence of classical CVD risk factors such as plasma lipid profiles and raised blood pressure [54].

Secondary Malignancies

Large population-based studies have suggested a small but significant increase in the subsequent risk of acute leukemia in patients who have received cisplatin/etoposide-based chemotherapy for metastatic testicular cancer. The risk appears to be dose related, but for conventional dose treatment (three to four cycles of BEP), the relative risk may be increased by approximately threefold or more [55]. However, it is noteworthy that in absolute values, this translates to an extremely small increase in incidence in the region of 1.6 per 1000 patients treated. Clearly, the huge survival advantage provided by chemotherapy far outweighs this small absolute risk of a secondary leukemia.

Neuropathy

Cisplatin-induced sensory neuropathy is commonly encountered following BEP chemotherapy. Approximately 15% to 20% of individuals experience persisting neuropathy following treatment, with prevalence, severity, and duration of neuropathy being related to increasing cisplatin dose [56]. Additionally, persistent symptomatic ototoxicity (manifested by high-tone hearing loss and tinnitus) may been seen in approximately 20% receiving standard-dose BEP chemotherapy with prevalence increasing to around 60% in those patients receiving higher ($\geq$600 mg) cumulative doses of cisplatin [57]. Following completion of chemotherapy, cisplatin-induced neuropathy and ototoxicity generally improve over time and may resolve completely for a substantial number of individuals. However, severe neuropathy related to high cumulative doses of cisplatin may persist long term.

Conclusion

The last 30 years has seen a revolution in the chemotherapy treatment of germ cell cancer, and the vast majority of patients with metastatic disease can now expect to be cured. Worldwide, BEP remains the gold standard chemotherapy treatment for all groups of patients presenting with metastatic germ cell cancer. For patients presenting with good prognosis metastatic disease, cure rates now approach 98% and the research focus has switched from improving outcome to reducing treatment-related morbidity. For patients with intermediate and poor prognosis metastatic disease, further improvements in treatment outcomes remain a research priority through the use of novel agents or the safe delivery of dose-intensified treatments. In the adjuvant setting, short-course BEP has established itself as a treatment option for high-risk stage I nonseminoma; for seminoma, the use of single-agent carboplatin seems likely to replace para-aortic nodal strip radiotherapy as the standard adjuvant treatment for stage I disease. The long-term morbidities of BEP chemotherapy are now more clearly defined and allow for an informed discussion with patients about to embark on chemotherapy and appropriate surveillance of individuals thereafter. It would be optimistic to predict that the next 30 years will yield as many advances in the treatment of this disease as have been witnessed since the mid-1970s; however, with our ever-increasing understanding about the natural history and biology of this disease, we should remain determined in our efforts to maximize cure and minimize morbidity in all patients presenting with germ cell cancer.

References

1. International Germ Cell Cancer Collaborative Group. International Germ Cell Consensus Classification: a prognostic factor-based staging system for metastatic germ cell cancers. J Clin Oncol 1997;15(2):594–603.
2. Einhorn LH, Donohue J. Cis-diamminedichloroplatinum, vinblastine, and bleomycin combination chemotherapy in disseminated testicular cancer. Ann Intern Med 1977;87(3):293–298.
3. Peckham MJ, Barrett A, Liew KH, et al. The treatment of metastatic germ-cell testicular tumours with bleomycin, etoposide and cis-platin (BEP). Br J Cancer 1983;47(5):613–619.
4. Williams SD, Birch R, Einhorn LH, Irwin L, Greco FA, Loehrer PJ. Treatment of disseminated germ-cell tumors with cisplatin, bleomycin, and either vinblastine or etoposide. N Engl J Med 1987; 316(23):1435–1440.
5. Horwich A, Dearnaley DP, A'Hern R, et al. The activity of single-agent carboplatin in advanced seminoma. Eur J Cancer 1992;28A(8–9):1307–1310.
6. Schmoll HJ, Harstrick A, Bokemeyer C, et al. Single-agent carboplatinum for advanced seminoma. A phase II study. Cancer 1993;72(1):237–243.
7. Childs WJ, Nicholls EJ, Horwich A. The optimisation of carboplatin dose in carboplatin, etoposide and bleomycin combination chemotherapy for good prognosis metastatic nonseminomatous

germ cell tumours of the testis. Ann Oncol 1992; 3(4):291–296.

8. Horwich A, Oliver RT, Wilkinson PM, et al. A medical research council randomized trial of single agent carboplatin versus etoposide and cisplatin for advanced metastatic seminoma. MRC Testicular Tumour Working Party. Br J Cancer 2000;83(12):1623–1629.

9. Clemm C, Bokemeyer C, Gerl A, et al. Randomized trial comparing cisplatin/etoposide/ifosfamide with carboplatin monotherapy in patients with advanced metastatic seminoma. Proc Am Soc Clin Oncol 2000:326a.

10. Bokemeyer C, Kollmannsberger C, Flechon A, et al. Prognostic factors in patients (pts) with advanced metastatic seminoma (SEM) treated with either single agent carboplatin (CP) or cisplatin based (DDP) combination chemotherapy (CTX): a meta-analysis of prospective European trials. Proc Am Soc Clin Oncol 2002;19:186a.

11. Bajorin DF, Sarosdy MF, Pfister DG, et al. Randomized trial of etoposide and cisplatin versus etoposide and carboplatin in patients with good-risk germ cell tumors: a multiinstitutional study. J Clin Oncol 1993;11(4):598–606.

12. Horwich A, Sleijfer DT, Fossa SD, et al. Randomized trial of bleomycin, etoposide, and cisplatin compared with bleomycin, etoposide, and carboplatin in good-prognosis metastatic nonseminomatous germ cell cancer: a Multiinstitutional Medical Research Council/European Organization for Research and Treatment of Cancer Trial. J Clin Oncol 1997;15(5):1844–1852.

13. Xiao H, Mazumdar M, Bajorin DF, et al. Long-term follow-up of patients with good-risk germ cell tumors treated with etoposide and cisplatin. J Clin Oncol 1997;15(7):2553–2558.

14. de Wit R, Stoter G, Kaye SB, et al. Importance of bleomycin in combination chemotherapy for good-prognosis testicular nonseminoma: a randomized study of the European Organization for Research and Treatment of Cancer Genitourinary Tract Cancer Cooperative Group. J Clin Oncol 1997;15(5):1837–1843.

15. Loehrer PJ Sr, Johnson D, Elson P, Einhorn LH, Trump D. Importance of bleomycin in favorable-prognosis disseminated germ cell tumors: an Eastern Cooperative Oncology Group trial. J Clin Oncol 1995;13(2):470–476.

16. Einhorn LH, Williams SD, Loehrer PJ, et al. Evaluation of optimal duration of chemotherapy in favorable-prognosis disseminated germ cell tumors: a Southeastern Cancer Study Group protocol. J Clin Oncol 1989;7(3):387–391.

17. Saxman SB, Finch D, Gonin R, Einhorn LH. Long-term follow-up of a phase III study of three versus four cycles of bleomycin, etoposide, and cisplatin in favorable-prognosis germ-cell tumors: the Indian University experience. J Clin Oncol 1998; 16(2):702–706.

18. de Wit R, Roberts JT, Wilkinson PM, et al. Equivalence of three or four cycles of bleomycin, etoposide, and cisplatin chemotherapy and of a 3- or 5-day schedule in good-prognosis germ cell cancer: a randomized study of the European Organization for Research and Treatment of Cancer Genitourinary Tract Cancer Cooperative Group and the Medical Research Council. J Clin Oncol 2001;19(6):1629–1640.

19. Fossa SD, de Wit R, Roberts JT, et al. Quality of life in good prognosis patients with metastatic germ cell cancer: a prospective study of the European Organization for Research and Treatment of Cancer Genitourinary Group/Medical Research Council Testicular Cancer Study Group (30941/TE20). J Clin Oncol 2003;21(6):1107–1118.

20. Toner GC, Stockler MR, Boyer MJ, et al. Comparison of two standard chemotherapy regimens for good-prognosis germ-cell tumours: a randomised trial. Australian and New Zealand Germ Cell Trial Group. Lancet 2001;357(9258):739–745.

21. Culine S, Kerbrat P, Bouzy J, et al. The optimal chemotherapy regimen for good-risk metastatic non seminomatous germ cell tumours (MSNGCT) is 3 cycles of bleomycin, etoposide and cisplatin. Mature results of a randomized trial. Proc Am Soc Clin Oncol 2003;22:382.

22. Nichols CR, Williams SD, Loehrer PJ, et al. Randomized study of cisplatin dose intensity in poor-risk germ cell tumors: a Southeastern Cancer Study Group and Southwest Oncology Group protocol. J Clin Oncol 1991;9(7):1163–1172.

23. Nichols CR, Catalano PJ, Crawford ED, Vogelzang NJ, Einhorn LH, Loehrer PJ. Randomized comparison of cisplatin and etoposide and either bleomycin or ifosfamide in treatment of advanced disseminated germ cell tumors: an Eastern Cooperative Oncology Group, Southwest Oncology Group, and Cancer and Leukemia Group B Study. J Clin Oncol 1998;16(4):1287–1293.

24. Hinton S, Catalano PJ, Einhorn LH, et al. Cisplatin, etoposide and either bleomycin or ifosfamide in the treatment of disseminated germ cell tumors: final analysis of an intergroup trial. Cancer 2003; 97(8):1869–1875.

25. Kaye SB, Mead GM, Fossa S, et al. Intensive induction-sequential chemotherapy with BOP/VIP-B compared with treatment with BEP/EP for poor-prognosis metastatic nonseminomatous germ cell tumor: a randomized Medical Research Council/European Organization for Research and Treatment of Cancer study. J Clin Oncol 1998; 16(2):692–701.

26. Fossa SD, Kaye SB, Mead GM, et al. Filgrastim during combination chemotherapy of patients

with poor-prognosis metastatic germ cell malignancy. European Organization for Research and Treatment of Cancer, Genito-Urinary Group, and the Medical Research Council Testicular Cancer Working Party, Cambridge, United Kingdom. J Clin Oncol 1998;16(2):716–724.

27. Collette L, Sylvester RJ, Stenning SP, et al. Impact of the treating institution on survival of patients with "poor-prognosis" metastatic nonseminoma. European Organization for Research and Treatment of Cancer Genito-Urinary Tract Cancer Collaborative Group and the Medical Research Council Testicular Cancer Working Party. J Natl Cancer Inst 1999;91(10):839–846.

28. Motzer RJ, Mazumdar M, Bajorin DF, Bosl GJ, Lyn P, Vlamis V. High-dose carboplatin, etoposide, and cyclophosphamide with autologous bone marrow transplantation in first-line therapy for patients with poor-risk germ cell tumors. J Clin Oncol 1997;15(7):2546–2552.

29. Bokemeyer C, Schmoll HJ, Harstrick A, et al. A phase I/II study of a stepwise dose-escalated regimen of cisplatin, etoposide and ifosfamide plus granulocyte-macrophage colony-stimulating factor (GM-CSF) in patients with advanced germ cell tumours. Eur J Cancer 1993;29A(16):2225–2231.

30. Schmoll HJ, Kollmannsberger C, Metzner B, et al. Long-term results of first-line sequential high-dose etoposide, ifosfamide, and cisplatin chemotherapy plus autologous stem cell support for patients with advanced metastatic germ cell cancer: an extended phase I/II study of the German Testicular Cancer Study Group. J Clin Oncol 2003;21(22):4083–4091.

31. Bower M, Newlands ES, Holden L, Rustin GJ, Begent RH. Treatment of men with metastatic non-seminomatous germ cell tumours with cyclical POMB/ACE chemotherapy. Ann Oncol 1997; 8(5):477–483.

32. Christian JA, Huddart RA, Norman A, et al. Intensive induction chemotherapy with CBOP/BEP in patients with poor prognosis germ cell tumors. J Clin Oncol 2003;21(5):871–877.

33. Freedman LS, Parkinson MC, Jones WG, et al. Histopathology in the prediction of relapse of patients with stage I testicular teratoma treated by orchidectomy alone. Lancet 1987;2(8554):294–298.

34. Read G, Stenning SP, Cullen MH, et al. Medical Research Council prospective study of surveillance for stage I testicular teratoma. Medical Research Council Testicular Tumors Working Party. J Clin Oncol 1992;10(11):1762–1768.

35. Bohlen D, Borner M, Sonntag RW, Fey MF, Studer UE. Long-term results following adjuvant chemotherapy in patients with clinical stage I testicular nonseminomatous malignant germ cell

tumors with high risk factors. J Urol 1999;161(4): 1148–1152.

36. Oliver RT, Raja MA, Ong J, Gallagher CJ. Pilot study to evaluate impact of a policy of adjuvant chemotherapy for high risk stage 1 malignant teratoma on overall relapse rate of stage 1 cancer patients. J Urol 1992;148(5):1453–1455; discussion 1455–1456.

37. Pont J, Albrecht W, Postner G, Sellner F, Angel K, Holtl W. Adjuvant chemotherapy for high-risk clinical stage I nonseminomatous testicular germ cell cancer: long-term results of a prospective trial. J Clin Oncol 1996;14(2):441–448.

38. Cullen MH, Stenning SP, Parkinson MC, et al. Short-course adjuvant chemotherapy in high-risk stage I nonseminomatous germ cell tumors of the testis: a Medical Research Council report. J Clin Oncol 1996;14(4):1106–1113.

39. Abratt RP, Pontin AR, Barnes RD, Reddi BV. Adjuvant chemotherapy for stage I non-seminomatous testicular cancer. S Afr Med J 1994;84(9):605–607.

40. Studer UE, Burkhard FC, Sonntag RW. Risk adapted management with adjuvant chemotherapy in patients with high risk clinical stage I nonseminomatous germ cell tumor. J Urol 2000; 163(6):1785–1787.

41. Warde P, Gospodarowicz MK, Banerjee D, et al. Prognostic factors for relapse in stage I testicular seminoma treated with surveillance. J Urol 1997; 157(5):1705–1709; discussion 1709–1710.

42. Fossa SD, Horwich A, Russell JM, et al. Optimal planning target volume for stage I testicular seminoma: A Medical Research Council randomized trial. Medical Research Council Testicular Tumor Working Group. J Clin Oncol 1999;17(4):1146.

43. Jones WG, Fossa SD, Mead GM, et al. A randomised trial of two radiotherapy schedules in the adjuvant treatment of stage I seminoma (MRC TE18). Eur J Cancer 2001;37(suppl 6):S157.

44. van Leeuwen FE, Stiggelbout AM, van den Belt-Dusebout AW, et al. Second cancer risk following testicular cancer: a follow-up study of 1,909 patients. J Clin Oncol 1993;11(3):415–424.

45. Wanderas EH, Fossa SD, Tretli S. Risk of subsequent non-germ cell cancer after treatment of germ cell cancer in 2006 Norwegian male patients. Eur J Cancer 1997;33(2):253–262.

46. Dieckmann KP, Bruggeboes B, Pichlmeier U, Kuster J, Mullerleile U, Bartels H. Adjuvant treatment of clinical stage I seminoma: is a single course of carboplatin sufficient? Urology 2000; 55(1):102–106.

47. Aparicio J, Garcia del Muro X, Maroto P, et al. Multicenter study evaluating a dual policy of postorchiectomy surveillance and selective adjuvant single-agent carboplatin for patients with clinical stage I seminoma. Ann Oncol 2003;14(6): 867–872.

48. Krege S, Kalund G, Otto T, Goepel M, Rubben H. Phase II study: adjuvant single-agent carboplatin therapy for clinical stage I seminoma. Eur Urol 1997;31(4):405–407.

49. Oliver RT, Edmonds PM, Ong JY, et al. Pilot studies of 2 and 1 course carboplatin as adjuvant for stage I seminoma: should it be tested in a randomized trial against radiotherapy? Int J Radiat Oncol Biol Phys 1994;29(1):3–8.

50. Lampe H, Horwich A, Norman A, Nicholls J, Dearnaley DP. Fertility after chemotherapy for testicular germ cell cancers. J Clin Oncol 1997; 15(1):239–245.

51. Gerl A, Muhlbayer D, Hansmann G, Mraz W, Hiddemann W. The impact of chemotherapy on Leydig cell function in long term survivors of germ cell tumors. Cancer 2001;91(7):1297–1303.

52. O'Sullivan JM, Huddart RA, Norman AR, Nicholls J, Dearnaley DP, Horwich A. Predicting the risk of bleomycin lung toxicity in patients with germ-cell tumours. Ann Oncol 2003;14(1):91–96.

53. Huddart RA, Norman A, Shahidi M, et al. Cardio-vascular disease as a long-term complication of treatment for testicular cancer. J Clin Oncol 2003; 21(8):1513–1523.

54. Meinardi MT, Gietema JA, van der Graaf WT, et al. Cardiovascular morbidity in long-term survivors of metastatic testicular cancer. J Clin Oncol 2000; 18(8):1725–1732.

55. Travis LB, Andersson M, Gospodarowicz M, et al. Treatment-associated leukemia following testicular cancer. J Natl Cancer Inst 2000;92(14):1165–1171.

56. Bokemeyer C, Berger CC, Kuczyk MA, Schmoll HJ. Evaluation of long-term toxicity after chemotherapy for testicular cancer. J Clin Oncol 1996;14(11): 2923–2932.

57. Bokemeyer C, Berger CC, Hartmann JT, et al. Analysis of risk factors for cisplatin-induced ototoxicity in patients with testicular cancer. Br J Cancer 1998;77(8):1355–1362.

21

Surgery for Testicular Cancer

Gillian L. Smith and Timothy J. Christmas

Testicular germ cell tumors are highly curable, even when metastatic at presentation. Although this is largely because of their sensitivity to platinum-based chemotherapy, well-timed surgical intervention is also crucial in achieving a high cure rate. The diagnosis is usually established by inguinal orchidectomy, and orchidectomy alone represents adequate treatment for many patients. Operative removal of metastatic disease, usually after chemotherapy, is also highly effective and may be curative. Thus the importance of surgical treatment for testicular cancer should not be underestimated.

Inguinal Orchidectomy

Timing of Orchidectomy

Inguinal orchidectomy is the first step in the management and staging of most patients presenting with testicular cancer. Certainly, well patients presenting with a solid testicular mass, the most common presentation, should undergo inguinal orchidectomy as soon as possible followed by radiological staging and referral to an oncologist. In the less common situation of an ill patient with metastases typical of a germ cell tumor and elevated β-human chorionic gonadotropin (βHCG), α-fetoprotein (α-FP), or lactate dehydrogenase (LDH), orchidectomy can be scheduled for after completion of chemotherapy as prognosis may be adversely affected by delaying chemotherapy. Orchidectomy of the

affected testis should be performed even if the tumor appears to resolve after chemotherapy, as the testis can be a sanctuary site for persistent active tumor.

Surgical Approach

An inguinal, rather than scrotal, incision should be employed to avoid tumor contamination of the scrotal skin and exposure of the inguinal lymph nodes to the risk of metastasis. In a meta-analysis, scrotal violation increased the risk of local recurrence from 0.4% to 2.9% [1]. The excess risk applied mainly in cases where gross tumor spillage had occurred.

Surgery may be carried out under general or regional anesthesia. A skin crease incision is made over the external inguinal ring, the size depending on the size of the tumor. For a very large tumor, the medial end of the incision can be curved down onto the scrotum allowing resection of a tumor of any size.

The subcutaneous tissues are divided and the external oblique opened to the external ring. A self-retaining retractor aids exposure. The ilioinguinal nerve should be preserved if possible. The cord is mobilized in the inguinal canal. If there is uncertainty about the diagnosis of tumor, a noncrushing bowel clamp or a soft Penrose drain may be used to clamp the cord at this stage. In most cases, however, the preoperative diagnosis of tumor is effectively certain and the cord may be clamped with an artery forceps or ligated at this stage. The cord should be mobilized up to the internal ring, where it should be both ligated and transfixed with nonabsorbable suture material. This ensures clearance of all distal cord structures so that if later retroperitoneal lymph node dissection (RPLND) is required the inguinal canal is already empty and does not require further clearance. The use of a non-absorbable suture (e.g., Prolene) to transfix or ligate the cut end of the divided cord facilitates identification of the distal end of the cord at RPLND. The testis is then mobilized from the scrotum. Gentle pressure from below and traction on the cord deliver the testis into the incision. The gubernacular attachments can then be divided using the hand-held diathermy spatula with careful attention to hemostasis. Intraoperative local anesthetic infiltration of wound edges and nerves aids postoperative analgesia. Wound lavage with water may be tumoricidal. An inguinal orchidectomy specimen is shown in Figure 21.1.

Complications

Inguinal orchidectomy is generally well tolerated by patients and can be performed as a day case procedure. The most serious complication is scrotal or retroperitoneal hematoma. The risk can be minimized by careful attention to hemostasis and meticulous transfixion and ligation of the divided cord at the internal inguinal ring.

Testicular Prostheses

A testicular prosthesis can be inserted at the time of orchidectomy if the patient wishes. Testicular prostheses were previously manufactured using a solid shell containing a silicon gel core. Concerns were expressed in the early 1990s about such designs in breast prostheses, and a possible association with autoimmune diseases. No causal relationship has been established, although histological and serological evidence of silicone shedding has been identified [2,3]. Currently manufacturers employ either (solid) silicone elastomer or a saline filled silicone shell.

Strict asepsis is essential during insertion and many surgeons administer prophylactic broad-spectrum antibiotics during the procedure. The prosthesis is placed in the scrotum via the inguinal incision. An anchoring suture may be employed, but care should be taken to ensure an

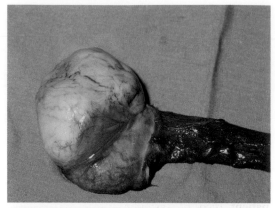

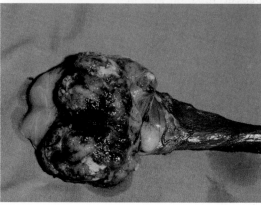

Fig. 21.1. A: Inguinal orchidectomy specimen. B: Inguinal orchidectomy specimen bivalved to demonstrate tumor.

appropriate lie and position, and symmetry of size selection. An inguinal approach should be used for delayed as well as immediate insertion of a prosthesis, as erosion through scrotal incisions is well recognized.

The most troublesome complication is infection, which often necessitates removal of the prosthesis. In the long term, satisfaction with testicular prostheses is variable. Encapsulation resulting in hardening can occur with time, resulting in a less natural texture. In one series 27% of men were dissatisfied and felt that they had an average or poor cosmetic result [4]. In another series, 20% of patients felt uncomfortable in sexual encounters and only 58% were happy with their sex life [5]. Patients therefore should be counseled appropriately preoperatively and many will opt simply to have an orchidectomy without prosthesis.

Partial Orchidectomy

Partial orchidectomy may be considered in patients with a tumor in a solitary testis or bilateral tumors. The advantage is that it may allow the patient to avoid hormone replacement therapy and, in some cases, to preserve fertility. In a series of 73 men who underwent partial orchidectomy for testicular cancer (primarily seminoma), 85% avoided the need for subsequent hormone replacement. In 82% of patients there was associated carcinoma in situ (CIS) treated with local irradiation (18 Gy). One patient died of systemic tumor progression. There were no local recurrences in the men with CIS who received radiotherapy. There were four local recurrences in patients not irradiated, but all were treated successfully with inguinal orchidectomy. Of 10 men who postponed radiotherapy for fertility reasons, five fathered a child after organ-sparing surgery [6]. The procedure does require specialist expertise, and patients should be referred to a center with experience with partial orchidectomy. Specialist techniques that may be involved are preoperative scrotal magnetic resonance imaging (MRI), intraoperative ultrasound, and frozen section. Intraoperative cooling can be helpful, as Sertoli cells will be morphologically altered after 30 minutes of warm ischemia. Preoperative counseling is vital regarding the potential need for completion orchidectomy, the risk of local recurrence, and the possibility of requiring hormone replacement therapy. Preoperative semen storage should be offered, and patients must be able to comply with intensive follow-up.

Contralateral Testicular Biopsy

Carcinoma in situ (intratubular germ cell neoplasia [ITGCN]) consists of atypical cells located in a single row at the basement membrane of seminiferous tubules. It is universally detected in the tissue surrounding germ cell tumors [7]. These cells are the uniform precursor of all germ cell neoplasms of the testis (other than spermatocytic seminoma) and develop during embryogenesis. Cellular proliferation then probably occurs during and after puberty [8]. Usually all spermatogenic cells are replaced as the CIS cells spread longitudinally along the tubules, leaving only CIS cells and Sertoli cells in a multifocal distribution. Fifty percent of men with ITGCN progress to invasive cancer in 5 years [9,10]. It is unknown whether nonseminomatous tumors develop via a stage of seminoma or progress directly. In view of the high progression rate to invasive tumors, it is desirable to detect CIS by biopsy so that it can be treated before progression occurs.

The following are risk factors for CIS of the residual testis in men with germ cell tumors:

- Age less than 30 years
- Small volume testes (<12 mL)
- Gonadal dysgenesis syndromes
- History of cryptorchid testis (2–3% have CIS)
- Extragonadal germ cell tumor (42% men with primary retroperitoneal disease have CIS)
- Abnormal spermatogenesis (oligozoospermia on semen analysis) (0.4–1.1% of infertile men have CIS)
- Microcalcification (remains controversial)

The potential drawbacks of contralateral testicular biopsy include a 15% to 20% complication rate, with the possibility of impaired hormone production or fertility as a consequence. If CIS is confirmed, radiotherapy does result in irreversible infertility. Most patients who do develop metachronous tumors can be cured with inguinal orchidectomy at the time of recurrence. Thus the potential advantages of preventing second tumors in those with CIS have to be weighed against the possibility of damaging residual testicular function in patients without CIS who have nothing to gain from a biopsy. Most units, therefore, adopt a selective approach to biopsies of the contralateral testis carrying out biopsies in the groups at increased risk. Patients with negative biopsies do require follow-up despite the negative result, as there is a small false-negative rate (0.3%).

Surgical open (stab) biopsy should be undertaken laterally in the upper pole to avoid intratesticular vasculature. The sample should be fixed immediately to preserve architecture ideally in Bouin's solution although formalin suffices. A 3 × 3 × 3 mm biopsy will almost certainly detect CIS if it is present in at least 10% of the tubules. Eighteen-gauge core needle biopsies are probably comparable and take deeper cores [11]. The biopsy may be synchronous with the initial orchidectomy or deferred depending on the clinical scenario.

Retroperitoneal Lymph Node Dissection for Testicular Tumors

Germ Cell Tumors

For a long time it has been recognized that the primary location for the spread of nonseminomatous germ cell of the testis (NSGCT) is the chain of lymph nodes in the retroperitoneum surrounding the aorta and inferior vena cava (IVC). Back in 1897 removal of inguinal lymph nodes at the time radical orchidectomy was recommended [12]. However, when surgeons subsequently became more aware of the lymphatic drainage of the testis, RPLND was advocated and was performed at the same time as radical orchidectomy for testis cancer [13,14]. The location of nodal metastases from the testis was later mapped out in precise detail in men undergoing RPLND for metastatic testis cancer. The most common location for nodal metastases emanating from the right-sided tumors was found to be the aortocaval groove area, whereas left-sided tumors initially spread to the left para-aortic region [15,16]. The RPLND procedure has been a popular treatment for clinical stage II NSGCT and also as a staging procedure (and sometimes of therapeutic benefit) for clinical stage I NSGCT. However, in the modern era the major role for surgery in the treatment of testis cancer has been to establish the diagnosis by radical orchidectomy. Since the advent of platinum-based chemotherapy, many patients with metastatic testis cancer have been cured after orchidectomy by chemotherapy alone. About 25% of men with stage II to IV NSGCT have a residual mass after an intensive course of platinum-based chemotherapy [17]. When the residual mass is greater than 1 to 2 cm in diameter, then postchemotherapy RPLND (PC-RPLND) is indicated as well as excision of residual masses from other sites such as the chest, liver, and brain. When an active tumor recurrence develops after PC-RPLND, further chemotherapy is warranted, and in certain circumstances autologous bone marrow transplantation may be necessary to allow further high-dose chemotherapy. In a few cases further relapse may occur when the disease becomes resistant to chemotherapy,

and then "desperation" RPLND (D-RPLND) may be indicated [18].

RPLND for Stage I NSGCT

There has been a trans-Atlantic division of opinion on the role of RPLND for clinical stage I NSGCT. It is usual practice to perform RPLND for clinical stage I NSGCT in some centers in the United States [19]. The rationale behind this is that approximately 30% to 35% of clinical stage I patients are in fact pathological stage II [20]. In men with tumor within the nodes, up to 60% may be cured by RPLND alone, and those who do relapse do so away from the retroperitoneum. Furthermore, because the sympathetic nerve fibers that subserve ejaculation are now identifiable and the anatomy well recognized [21], it is possible to perform nerve-sparing RPLND in men with such low-volume lymph nodes, hence preserving ejaculation. The alternatives to RPLND for stage I disease are long-term surveillance or adjuvant chemotherapy. Chemotherapy would normally be considered only in high risk patients with malignant teratoma undifferentiated (MTU) in the primary tumor and vascular invasion within the testis/cord. Surveillance is the most popular option in most countries; in a survey of 273 urologists in the United Kingdom all patients with clinical stage I NSGCT were referred to major cancer centers for surveillance [22]. Comparison between surveillance and RPLND for stage I disease reveals similar mortality figures. However, it has been argued that primary RPLND is more likely to preserve fertility because fewer patients require chemotherapy, and retroperitoneal relapse in the surveillance group may also necessitate PC-RPLND, which may compromise ejaculation if the sympathetic nerves cannot be preserved [23].

RPLND for Stage II NSGCT

Since the advent of the platinum-based chemotherapy era, most men with clinical stage II NSGCT are treated with chemotherapy. However, the Indiana University group has advocated primary RPLND for stage II NSGCT and has compared the results with similar patients treated with platinum-based chemotherapy. Both treatments were curative as monotherapy in 67%; survival was 98% in those treated by RPLND and 96% who had primary chemotherapy. Late relapse and toxicity rates were greater in the chemotherapy group [24,25]. However, in spite of the findings in Indianapolis, the favored primary treatment for stage II testicular NSGCT is chemotherapy.

Postchemotherapy RPLND

After an intensive course of platinum-based chemotherapy for stage II to IV NSGCT of the testis, a residual mass will be apparent within the retroperitoneum on computed tomography (CT) or MRI scans (Fig. 21.2) in 25% or more cases [26]. It is now established practice to excise such residual masses in order to increase the chance of cure [27]. However, when the mass is <1 cm in diameter, it most likely contains necrotic tissue only [28] and can be safely observed [29]. Patients with malignant teratoma intermediate that contains differentiated teratoma (MTI) are at risk of the tumor masses becoming cystic and enlarging during chemotherapy. Enlarging masses with falling tumor markers are characteristic of "growing teratoma syndrome," which requires surgical removal of all tumor masses. All patients with MTI should have a CT scan after two or three courses of chemotherapy as masses in "growing teratoma syndrome" can become inoperable and there may be only a limited window of opportunity in which to plan successful surgery. Patients who relapse after an

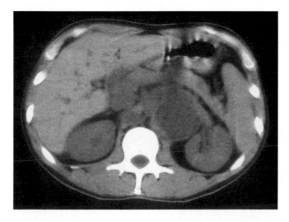

Fig. 21.2. Computed tomography (CT) scan showing residual retroperitoneal nodal mass after chemotherapy for stage II germ cell tumor of the testis.

initial response to chemotherapy should always be worked up to locate any tumor masses that might be resectable. Development of new masses, enlargement of previously known masses, or positivity on positron emission tomography (PET) scan can indicate the masses most likely to contain active tumor. Resection of all apparent disease with subsequent fall of tumor markers to normal can avoid further chemotherapy in a proportion of patients.

The objective of PC-RPLND in men with residual masses is to excise all the remaining tissue. Incomplete excision is associated with a considerably worse prognosis [27]. After PC-RPLND, decision making regarding follow-up and further therapy depends on the result of histological examination of the resected tissue. In the authors' personal series of 303 cases of PC-RPLND for NSGCT performed between 1993 and 2004, the overall survival rate is over 90%. This series includes a number of patients who had recurred after previous PC-RPLND performed at other hospitals; this has been shown to worsen the long-term chance of survival [30]. Approximately half of the resected specimens contained differentiated teratoma (TD); just over one fifth contained necrosis/fibrosis only; and the remainder contained active malignancy (MTU, yolk sac tumor, choriocarcinoma, sarcoma, neuroectodermal tumor, or carcinoma). These findings are similar to those of other large series of PC-RPLND [27]. Factors that increase the chance of finding active tumor in the resected specimen are persistent elevation of tumor markers, large size, failure to serially decrease in size, and history of relapse. Factors that increase the chance of finding differentiated teratoma are presence of MTI initially and heterogeneous or cystic masses on CT scans.

Nearly all patients with necrosis/fibrosis in the specimen are cured but should be followed up in the long-term (Fig. 21.3). Those men with TD in the specimen have a >95% chance of cure, provided that all residual tissue has been removed. Malignant tissue within the PC-RPLND specimen confers a worse prognosis. The majority of these patients are best treated with further chemotherapy, sometimes a high-dose regimen including Taxol with autologous bone marrow transplantation. When a further recurrence occurs after a second course of chemotherapy, then desperation RPLND can be considered and is likely to be of benefit in up to 50% [31]. All

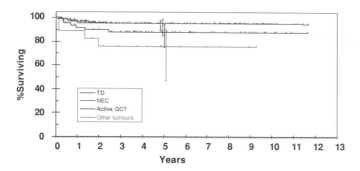

Fig. 21.3. Cause specific survival after postchemotherapy retroperitoneal lymph node dissection (RPLND) for nonseminomatous germ cell of the testis (NSGCT) of the testis according to histology of the resected specimen. TD, differentiated teratoma; NEC, necrosis; GCT, germ cell tumors.

men who have undergone PC-RPLND should remain under follow-up because there is a 2% risk of developing a contralateral tumor, and recurrence can occur beyond 15 years after PC-RPLND [32].

Seminoma

Patients with seminoma may have residual masses following chemotherapy. These masses are often associated with a fibrous reaction that makes retroperitoneal surgery more difficult. In the majority of cases, these masses are best observed due to the difficulty of removing them and the high chance that they will not contain active tumor. Patients with a seminomatous element in their germ cell tumors do have a higher rate of intra- and postoperative complications than patients with pure NSGCT undergoing postchemotherapy RPLND. Additional procedures such as nephrectomy and vascular interventions are more commonly required [33].

Stromal Tumors

Stromal tumors of the testis (e.g., Leydig, Sertoli, and granulosa cell tumors) are uncommon, accounting for about 2% of adult testicular tumors. Most do not behave in a malignant fashion and can be cured by orchidectomy, but approximately 10% have metastatic potential. In contrast with treatment for germ cell tumors, treatment for metastatic stromal tumors is not very effective. Patients with a malignant stromal tumor that metastasizes survive on average only 3 years from diagnosis. In addition, it is difficult to identify high-risk patients who might benefit from more intensive treatment or surveillance,

as there are no consistently reliable histological indicators of malignant potential. Although several adverse features have been described, accurate prediction of aggressive tumor behavior in individual cases remains difficult. Experience with these tumors and the potential for clinical trials are limited by the small numbers of patients and there is therefore no consensus on the best treatment. A number of studies have suggested that there is a role for prophylactic RPLND in stage I stromal tumors [34–36]. Early results suggest that the procedure is safe in this group of patients, although the long-term effect on survival is not yet known.

Surgical Technique

In all stage I cases it is possible to perform RPLND through a midline abdominal incision, and the same applies to men undergoing low volume PC-RPLND. A thoracoabdominal approach (Fig. 21.4) affords excellent exposure

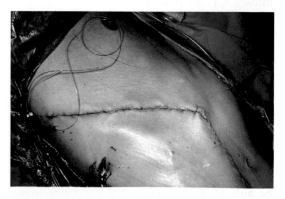

Fig. 21.4. Thoracoabdominal incision for postchemotherapy RPLND.

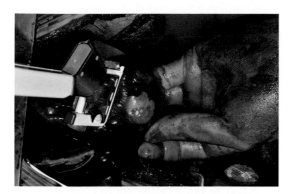

Fig. 21.5. Resection of a small lung metastasis using a stapling device at thoracoabdominal postchemotherapy RPLND.

for resection of large-volume disease. The thoracoabdominal incision is also advantageous when there is residual disease within both the retroperitoneum and thoracic cavity, as it allows synchronous excision of pulmonary metastases (Fig. 21.5) [37] and intrathoracic lymph nodes [38].

Complete bilateral RPLND has in the past been shown to lead to loss of ejaculation due to excision of sympathetic nerve fibers surrounding the aorta and IVC [39]. We now know much more about the distribution of nodal metastases from testis cancer [16] and the anatomy of the sympathetic nerves [21], which together have resulted in the development of modified templates for RPLND. In the case of left-sided tumors, a template nodal excision is performed in an area bounded by the left renal vein, aorta, left common iliac artery, and the left ureter. The midaorta, right common iliac artery, right ureter, and right renal vein bound the right-sided template. Although it may not be possible to preserve all sympathetic nerve fibers during RPLND, the use of a modified template should reduce damage to contralateral sympathetic fibers and hence prevent anejaculation after surgery [40].

The objective in PC-RPLND is to remove all the residual mass, and this may also necessitate excision of adjacent structures such as the kidney [41], the aorta, and the IVC [42]. Hence, it advisable that the surgeon performing RPLND be able to undertake such procedures or call for assistance from another surgeon at short notice.

Complications

The operative mortality of RPLND is low at less than 1% [43]. In one large series of primary nerve sparing RPLND for stage I NSGCT, only 5.4% of patients developed complications that prolonged hospital stay by more than 2 days. Antegrade ejaculation was preserved in most patients (93.3%) [44]. The postoperative complication rate of postchemotherapy RPLND is reported as around 7%, with most patients tolerating surgery well and recovering uneventfully [45]. Postchemotherapy patients may have diminished pulmonary, renal, and nutritional reserves, and are more likely to have a large disease burden necessitating longer and more extensive surgery with a higher risk of additional procedures such as nephrectomy, bowel resection, and vascular repair. The most common perioperative complications are wound infection and prolonged ileus. Acute renal failure, pancreatitis, ascites, and pulmonary complications are also recognized. Ejaculatory dysfunction is the main long-term complication.

Conclusion

The ability to cure the great majority of men with testis cancer has generally been attributed to platinum-based chemotherapy. However, the role of RPLND should not be underestimated. In low-stage NSGCT, surveillance (stage I) and primary chemotherapy (stage II) have in most centers replaced primary RPLND, and PC-RPLND is a crucial adjunct to chemotherapy, enabling a very high cure rate for more advanced stages of NSGCT. The best chance of cure is when complete excision of the residual masses after chemotherapy is achieved, and this is most likely to be the case in a specialized cancer center [27,30].

References

1. Capelouto CC, Clark PE, Ransil BJ, Loughlin KR. A review of scrotal violation in testicular cancer: is adjuvant local therapy necessary? J Urol 1995; 153:981–985.
2. Barrett DM, O'Sullivan DC, Malizia AA, et al. Particle shedding and migration from silicone

genitourinary prosthetic devices. J Urol 1991;146:
319–322.

3. Henderson J, Culkin D, Mata J, Wilson M, Venable
D. Analysis of immunological alterations associated with testicular prostheses. J Urol 1995;154:
1748–1751.

4. Adshead J, Khoubehi B, Wood J, Rustin G. Testicular implants and patient satisfaction: a question-
naire-based study of men after orchidectomy for
testicular cancer. BJU Int 2001;88(6):559–562.

5. Incrocci L, Bosch JL, Slob AK. Testicular prostheses: body image and sexual functioning. BJU Int
1999;84(9):1043–1045.

6. Heidenreich A, Albers P, Hartmann M, Kliesch S,
Kohrmann KU, Dieckmann KP, German Testicular Cancer Study Group. Organ sparing surgery
for malignant germ cell tumor of the testis. J Urol
2001;166:2161–2165.

7. Skakkebaek NE. Possible carcinoma-in-situ of
testis. Lancet 1992;2(7776):516–517.

8. Skakkebaek NE, Rajpert-De Meyts E, Jorgensen N,
et al. Germ cell cancer and disorders of spermatogenesis: an environmental connection? Acta
Pathol Microbial Scand 1998;106:3–11.

9. Bettocchi C, Coker CB, Deacon J, Parkinson C,
Pryor JP. A review of testicular intratubular germ
cell neoplasia in infertile men. J Androl 1994;
15(suppl):14S-16S.

10. Montironi R. Intratubular germ cell neoplasia of
the testis: testicular intraepithelial neoplasia. Eur
Urol 2002;41:651–654.

11. Harland S, Cook PA, Fossa SD, et al. Intratubular
germ cell neoplasia of the contralateral testis in
testicular cancer: defining a high risk group. J Urol
1998;16:1353–1357.

12. Stimson JC. A new operation for malignant
tumors of the testicle. The necessity of a more
extensive operation than castration for carcinoma, sarcoma of the testicle. Medical Record
1897;52:623.

13. Roberts JB. Excision of the lumbar lymph nodes
and spermatic vein in malignant tumors of the
testicle. Am J Surg 1902;36:539.

14. Bland-Sutton J. An operation for lumbar gland
removal in cases of testis tumour. Lancet 1909;
1:1406.

15. Ray B, Hajdu SI, Whitmore WF. Distribution of
retroperitoneal lymph node metastases in testicular germinal tumors. Cancer 1973;33:340–348.

16. Donohue JP, Zachary JM, Maynard BR. Distribution of nodal metastases in nonseminomatous
testis cancer. J Urol 1982;128:315–320.

17. Hendry WF. Decision making in abdominal
surgery following chemotherapy for testicular
cancer. Eur J Cancer 1995;5:649–650.

18. Nichols CR, Saxman S. Primary salvage treatment
of recurrent germ cell tumors: experience at
Indiana University. Semin Oncol 1998;25:210–214.

19. Donohue JP, Thornhill JA, Foster RS, et al.
Retroperitoneal lymphadenectomy for clinical
stage A testis cancer (1965 to 1989): modifications
of technique and impact on ejaculation. J Urol
1993;149:237–243.

20. Foster RS, Donohue JP. Surgical treatment of
clinical stage A nonseminomatous testis cancer.
Semin Oncol 1992;19:166–170.

21. Foster RS, Donohue JP. Nerve-sparing retroperitoneal lymphadenectomy. Urol Clin North Am
1993;20:117–125.

22. Bower M, Ma R, Savage P, et al. British urological
surgery practice: 2. Renal, bladder and testis
cancer. Br J Urol 1998;81:513–517.

23. Foster RS, McNulty A, Rubin LR, et al. The fertility of patients with clinical stage I testis cancer
managed by nerve sparing retroperitoneal lymph
node dissection [see comments]. J Urol 1994;152:
1139–1142.

24. Donohue JP, Thornhill JA, Foster RS, et al. The role
of retroperitoneal lymphadenectomy in clinical
stage B testis cancer: the Indiana University experience (1965 to 1989). J Urol 1995;153:85–89.

25. Baniel J, Sella A. Complications of retroperitoneal
lymph node dissection in testicular cancer:
primary and post-chemotherapy. Semin Surg
Oncol 1999;17(4):263–267.

26. Tait D, Peckham MJ, Hendry WF, Goldstraw P.
Post-chemotherapy surgery in advanced nonseminomatous germ cell testicular tumours: the
significance of histology with particular reference
to differentiated (mature) teratoma. Br J Cancer
1984;50:601–609.

27. Hendry WF, A'Hern RP, Hetherington JW, et al.
Para-aortic lymphadenectomy after chemotherapy for metastatic non-seminomatous germ cell
tumours: prognostic value and therapeutic
benefit. Br J Urol 1993;71:208–213.

28. Janetschek G, Hobisch A, Hittmair A, et al. Laparoscopic retroperitoneal lymphadenectomy after
chemotherapy for stage IIB nonseminomatous
testicular carcinoma. J Urol 1999;161:477–481.

29. Napier MP, Naraghi A, Christmas TJ, Rustin GJ.
Long-term follow-up of residual masses after
chemotherapy in patients with non-seminomatous germ cell tumours. Br J Cancer 2000;83:1274–
1280.

30. Christmas TJ, Smith GL, Kooner RS. Reoperation
for metastatic testis cancer after chemotherapy.
J Urol 1998;159(suppl):49.

31. Ravi R, Ong J, Oiver RT, et al. Surgery as salvage
therapy in chemotherapy-resistant nonseminomatous germ cell tumours. Br J Urol 1998;81:884–
888.

32. Elkabir JJ, Christmas TJ, Ellamushi H, Mendoza N.
Late relapse of metastatic teratoma invading a
vertebral body: a combined surgical approach. Br
J Urol 1997;79:999–1000.

33. Mosharafa AA, Foster RS, Leibovich BC, Bihrle R, Johnson C, Donohue JP. Is post-chemotherapy resection of seminomatous elements associated with higher acute morbidity? J Urol 2003;169: 2126–2128.

34. Mosharafa AA, Foster RS, Bihrle R, et al. Does retroperitoneal lymph node dissection have a curative role for patients with sex cord-stromal testicular tumors? Cancer 2003;98(4):753–757.

35. Smith GL, Christmas TJ, Seckl MJ, Rustin GJS. The role of retroperitoneal lymph node dissection in the management of stromal tumours of the testis. BJU Int 2003;91(suppl):61.

36. Peschel R, Gettman MT, Steiner H, Neururer R, Bartsch G. Management of adult Leydig-cell testicular tumors: assessing the role of laparoscopic retroperitoneal lymph node dissection. J Endourol 2003;17:777–780.

37. Christmas TJ, Smith GL, Kooner RS. Wedge resection of pulmonary metastases from cancer of the testis or kidney using a vascular staple device. Br J Urol 1998;81(6):911–912.

38. Christmas TJ, Doherty AP, Bower M. Retrocrural lymph node metastases from testis germ cell tumours: removal via a thoraco-abdominal extra-peritoneal approach after chemotherapy. Br J Urol 1997;79(3):468–470.

39. Leiter E, Brendler H. Loss of ejaculation following bilateral retroperitoneal lymphadenectomy. J Urol 1967;98:375–378.

40. Donohue JP, Foster RS, Rowland RG, et al. Nerve-sparing retroperitoneal lymphadenectomy with preservation of ejaculation. J Urol 1990;144:287–291.

41. Nash PA, Leibovitch I, Foster RS, et al. En bloc nephrectomy in patients undergoing post-chemotherapy retroperitoneal lymph node dissection for nonseminomatous testis cancer: indications, implications and outcomes. J Urol 1998;159:707–710.

42. Christmas TJ, Smith GL, Kooner R. Vascular interventions during post-chemotherapy retroperitoneal lymph-node dissection for metastatic testis cancer. Eur J Surg Oncol 1998;24(4):292–297.

43. Baniel J, Foster RS, Rowland RG, et al. Complications of post-chemotherapy retroperitoneal lymph node dissection. J Urol 1995;153:976–980.

44. Heidenreich, A, Albers P, Hartmann M, et al., German Testicular Cancer Study Group. Complications of primary nerve sparing retroperitoneal lymph node dissection for clinical stage I nonseminomatous germ cell tumors of the testis: experience of the German Testicular Cancer Study Group. J Urol 2003;169:1710–1714.

45. Mosharafa AA, Foster RS, Koch MO, Bihrle R, Donohue JP. Complications of post-chemotherapy retroperitoneal lymph node dissection for testis cancer. J Urol 2004;171:1839–1841.

46. Christmas TJ, Doherty AP, Rustin IIJ, et al. Excision of residual masses of metastatic germ cell tumours after chemotherapy: the role of extra-peritoneal surgical approaches. Br J Urol 1998;81: 301–308.

22

Pathobiological Basis of Treatment Strategies of Germ Cell Tumors

J. Wolter Oosterhuis, Friedemann Honecker, Frank Mayer, Carsten Bokemeyer, and L.H.J. Looijenga

Human germ cell tumors (GCTs) are at the crossroads of developmental and tumor biology. Therefore, they are an interesting target for investigation, both from a pathobiological as well as a developmental point of view. However, with regard to some aspects, this can also be a limiting factor, because the observed findings can be either due to the process of tumorigenesis, or just a reflection of normal development. This is, for example, highlighted by the finding of overall sensitivity of GCTs for DNA damaging agents, and the specific resistance of the mature teratomas, with or without malignant transformation (see below). Most likely, this also accounts for the telomerase activity, as found in a selection of these tumors [1,2]. Often, this distinction is not easy to make. Therefore, understanding of the pathobiology of GCTs is required for proper understanding of clinical and experimental findings. This chapter discusses the current knowledge of the pathobiology in the context of the biological basis for treatment strategies in GCTs.

Pathobiology of Human Germ Cell Tumors

Germ cell tumors can be found along the midline of the body, possibly related to the migration route of the primordial germ cells (PGCs) from the yolk sac to the genital ridge during intrauterine development [3]. In some of these tumors the germ cell origin is supported by their VASA staining [4]. This protein is specific for the germline [5]. Histologically, GCTs mimic intrauterine development to a certain extent, including both somatic and extraembryonic tissues [6, for review]. Based on histology, GCTs can be subdivided in a limited number of variants. These are the seminoma-like tumors (i.e., classic seminoma of the testis and the mediastinum, in the ovary known as dysgerminomas, in the brain known as germinomas; and spermatocytic seminoma of the testis), and the different variants of nonseminomatous GCTs. The nonseminomas can be composed of somatic tissue: mature and immature teratomas, as well as extraembryonic tissues (i.e., yolk sac tumors and choriocarcinomas). Within this group of histological variants, a number of pathologically and clinically relevant entities can be identified. The most obvious group includes the spermatocytic seminomas. These tumors are rare, and relatively benign, affecting predominantly elderly males [7,8]. Spermatocytic seminoma can specifically be distinguished from classic seminoma based on morphology, and more recently also using (immuno)histochemistry [9–11] and chromosomal constitution [12]. They originate most likely from a spermatogonial germ cell/spermatocyte. In the latest World Health Organization (WHO) classification system, these tumors are therefore distinguished from classical seminomas and are referred to as type III tumors. The second, more complex distinction concerns the various types of nonseminomatous

GCTs. Although histologically correct, the subdivision of the nonseminomas into embryonal carcinomas, teratomas, yolk sac tumors, and choriocarcinomas ignores the existence of a clinical and pathobiological heterogeneity. In fact, the nonseminomas include two entities: type I, the teratomas and yolk sac tumors of neonates and infants; and type II, the nonseminomatous GCTs of adolescents and young adults. The latter entity also encompasses the seminomas/dysgerminomas/germinomas, which resemble PGCs/gonocytes. The type I and II GCTs are characterized by the histology of the tumor, age of the patient at clinical presentation, clinical behavior, as well as chromosomal constitution [13–16]. The type I teratomas and yolk sac tumors can be found in the gonads, the sacrococcygeal region, neck, and the hypothalamic/hypophyseal region. No consistent chromosomal anomalies have been found so far in the type I teratomas [17], with the exception of an isochromosome 1q [18]. In contrast, the type I yolk sac tumors are aneuploid, with recurrent chromosomal changes [17,19,20]. They consistently lack the characteristic overrepresentation of the short arm of chromosome 12p, most often as an isochromosome 12p as found in the type II GCTs (see below and Chapter 19), supporting a separate pathogenesis of these tumors [21,22, for review]. The precursor lesion of the teratomas and yolk sac tumors is not yet identified, although it is reported in the representative mouse model, giving rise to teratocarcinoma [23]. Clinically, teratomas show a benign behavior without metastasizing, but they can progress, when incompletely surgically removed, to yolk

sac tumors, which have the potential to disseminate and therefore must be treated with chemotherapy [14,24].

The type II GCTs include the seminomas/dysgerminomas/germinomas and the nonseminomatous elements—embryonal carcinomas, teratomas, yolk sac tumors, and choriocarcinomas. Note that a pure or mixed teratoma–yolk sac tumor can also be a type I GCT. The type II GCTs of the adult testis, here referred to as TGCTs, are consistently aneuploid [20,25], with the characteristic gain of 12p, mostly as isochromosomes [i[12p]] [26] (see also Chapter 19). Pure seminomas are seen in about 50% of cases and occur at a median age of 37 years. Nonseminomas develop earlier (median age 27 years) and account for 40% of cases. The rest are so-called combined tumors, according to the British Classification system [27], which contain both seminoma and nonseminoma components, and occur in patients aged somewhere in between those with seminomas and nonseminomas. Embryonal carcinoma cells are pluripotent stem cells of nonseminomas, which can differentiate into the other histologies [28,29]. Pluripotency of embryonal carcinoma is also demonstrated by the expression of OCT3/4, a factor exclusively expressed by potentially pluripotent cells [30,31].

No representative animal model has been reported for TGCTs, significantly hampering pathobiological and preclinical studies. The classification system for GCTs distinguishing type I, II, and III (spermatocytic seminomas) was recently accepted by the WHO, and is summarized in Table 22.1.

Table 22.1. Overview of the three types of testicular germ cell tumors, including age at clinical diagnosis (years), histology, supposed cell or origin, and chromosomal anomalies

Age	Histology	Cell of origin	Chromosomal anomalies
0–5	Teratoma Yolk sac tumor	Embryonic germ cell	Unknown Aneuploidy Gain 1q,20q,22 Loss 6q
15–45	Seminoma/nonseminoma	Primordial germ cell or gonocyte	Aneuploidy: Gain 7,8,12p, Loss 4,5,11,13,18,Y
50 and older	Spermatocytic seminoma	Spermatogonia or spermatocyte	Diploid/aneuploid: Gain 9

Diagnosis and Treatment of Carcinoma in Situ/Intratubular Germ Cell Neoplasia Unclassified

Carcinoma in situ (CIS) [32], also known as intratubular germ cell neoplasia unclassified (ITGCNU) [33] or testicular intratubular neoplasia (TIN) [34], is the common precursor of all histological types of TGCTs, both the seminomas and type II nonseminomatous tumors. The gonadoblastoma is the counterpart of CIS/ITGCNU of the dysgenetic gonad [35]. The precursor lesion of the normal ovary, mediastinum, and brain has not yet been identified. The incidence of CIS/ITGCNU in the general male Caucasian population is similar to the lifetime risk to develop a TGCT [36], being up to about 1% in, for example, Switzerland and Denmark [37]. This indicates that CIS/ITGCNU does not regress spontaneously, and that eventually all patients with CIS/ITGCNU develop an invasive TGCT. In about 50% of the patients this happens within 5 years, and after 7 years the incidence is 70% [38]. Because of the sensitivity of TGCT to the available treatment strategies and presence of defined risk-populations (see below), development of strategies for early (molecular) diagnosis is of clinical interest. This might help to prevent overtreatment and undertreatment with the risk of progression of the tumor to treatment resistance (see below).

Carcinoma in situ/ITGCNU resembles early germ cells, most likely PGCs/gonocytes [39, for review]. This is illustrated by various phenotypical and ultrastructural characteristics [40–42, for review], as well as the presence of glycogen [43], placental/germ cell alkaline phosphatase (PLAP) [44,45], the stem cell factor receptor c-KIT [46–48], and most recently, the transcription factor OCT3/4 (POU5F1) (Fig. 22.1) [30,31, 49]. This suggests an intrauterine initiation of TGCTs, of which a maturation block of PGCs/gonocytes to more differentiated gametes is a hallmark. This model is also supported by epidemiological data [50], as well as specific risk factors (see below).

The aforementioned (immuno)histochemical markers are informative for the diagnosis of CIS/ITGCNU, although they may result in false-positive findings in early neonatal life [51], as well as in the case of disturbed germ cell maturation [Friedemann et al., J Path, 2004] and gonadal dysgenesis [52]. Various risk factors for CIS/ITGCNU have been identified, including familial predisposition, cryptorchidism, infertility, a previous TGCT, and various forms of gonadal dysgenesis (in particular related to the Y chromosome) [53, for review]. Early diagnosis of CIS/ITGCNU is clinically relevant. Currently, a surgical biopsy is the method of choice [54, for review]. This policy is applied to all patients with unilateral TGCT in Germany and Denmark. A negative biopsy finding, however, does not completely exclude development of an invasive TGCT [55–57]. Because of possible complications, a biopsy is currently not recommended for all patients with unilateral disease [58]. Therefore, better selective parameters are needed to identify individuals with an increased risk for the presence of CIS/ITGCNU, both initially, and after diagnosis of a unilateral TGCT. Some improvement has been made recently in this context.

Although 1% out of the general subfertile population has CIS/ITGCNU, we demonstrated that if bilateral microlithiasis, diagnosed using scrotal ultrasound, is present, the risk for the presence of CIS/ITGCNU is 20 times higher, reaching up to 20% of this population [59]. This finding has recently been supported by the higher incidence of microlithiasis in patients with a proven unilateral TGCT, and contralateral CIS/ITGCNU [60], and this knowledge can help to reduce the number of unnecessary biopsies in the future.

Another population suitable for CIS/ITGCNU screening are patients with unilateral TGCTs; about 2.5% to 5% of these patients develop bilateral disease [55,61]. About 50% of patients with CIS/ITGCNU in the contralateral testis develop an invasive TGCT within 5 years after diagnosis [62]. Testicular atrophy has been found to be a strong indicator for contralateral CIS/ITGCNU, although still 60% of CIS/ITGCNU occurs without atrophy [55]. Development of a second invasive TGCT leads to castration of the majority of patients, resulting in the need for hormone supplementation and psychological burden. About half of the contralateral tumors are diagnosed within the first 5 years after the initial diagnosis, although 25% of patients present with the second tumor 10 years after diagnosis of the first, and the latency period can be up to 20 years

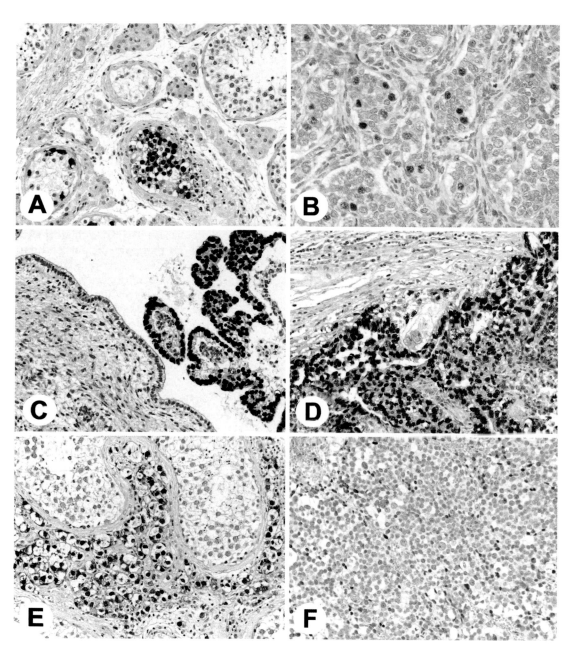

Fig. 22.1. OCT3/4 in germ cell tumors (GCTs). The transcription factor and marker for pluripotency OCT3/4 is a useful diagnostic tool for GCTs and offers insights in the histological heterogeneity of this cancer. OCT3/4 protein is visualized as a brown nuclear signal by immunohistochemistry on formalin-fixed, paraffin-embedded tissue sections. A: Parenchyma of a patient with a GCT showing, normal spermatogenesis, carcinoma in situ (CIS)/intratubular germ cell neoplasia unclassified (ITGCNU), and intratubular seminoma. Note that tubules containing normal spermatogenesis are negative, whereas tubules containing CIS/ITGCNU (left lower corner) and intratubular seminoma (center) are positive. B: Fetal testis, 15 weeks of gestational age. Note OCT3/4 signal in normal immature germ cells (gonocytes) in a number of tubules. In contrast to CIS/ITGCNU, which are almost exclusively found in close contact to the basal membrane (A), these immature germ cells are also seen in a central localization within the tubules (arrow). C: Nonseminoma showing mixed histology: tumor areas showing teratomatous differentiation to the left are negative, embryonal carcinoma cells to the right are positive for OCT3/4. D: Nonseminoma showing embryonal carcinoma cells positive for OCT3/4. Note the centrally located trophoblastic giant cell that is negative for OCT3/4. E: Seminoma cells positive for OCT3/4 surrounding a tubule containing normal spermatogenesis (negative for OCT3/4). F: Spermatocytic seminoma (type III tumor, according to WHO classification), negative for OCT3/4.

[61,63,64]. This means that surveillance must sometimes be continued for decades.

Early diagnosis allows low-dose irradiation (18 Gy) to eradicate CIS/ITGCNU while at the same time preserving the hormonal function in most patients [54, for review]. However, this inevitably results in infertility. In contrast, platin-based chemotherapy has only a temporal effect on spermatogenesis [65]. The risk of development of an invasive TGCT from CIS/ITGCNU is only reduced, not excluded [64].

We demonstrated recently that bilateral TGCTs are associated with a mutation within codon 816 of c-*KIT* [66]. This allows accurate identification of patients with a unilateral TGCT who are at risk to develop contralateral disease. These patients have to undergo a surgical biopsy for confirmation of the presence of CIS/ITGCNU. Moreover, the presence of specific mutations within c-*KIT* might allow development of alternative treatment strategies using small molecules, specifically interacting with the mutated receptor, as has been reported for gastrointestinal stromal tumors (GIST) and the specific tyrosine kinase inhibitor STK 571 [67, for review]. This treatment option might also be of interest for patients with extragonadal GCTs, whose tumors have activating c-*KIT* mutations in a significant proportion of the cases [68]. However, it is highly unlikely that this approach will benefit patients with nonseminomatous disease, either primary or as a late recurrence (see below).

Patients with extragonadal GCT, in particular localized in the retroperitoneal area, have an increased risk for development of a metachronous TGCT [69]. Therefore, thorough investigation for the presence of CIS/ITGCNU is mandatory. On the other hand, patients with extragonadal GCTs not localized in the retroperitoneum, are not at risk to have CIS/ITGCNU [70]. These data support the contention that retroperitoneal GCTs usually are metastases from an occult or burned-out TGCT.

Treatment of Invasive Germ Cell Tumors

Overall, type II GCTs are highly curable malignancies. Important improvements in the staging and treatment of this disease have significantly altered overall cure rates. Risk-adapted therapeutic strategies, related to known prognostic variables, are of importance in the treatment of GCTs, as therapeutic options are highly variable and include surveillance, irradiation, high-dose chemotherapy, and surgery. Therefore, a thorough knowledge of the underlying pathology and patterns of spread of disease is required.

Clinically, the consensus classification of the International Germ Cell Cancer Collaborative Group (IGCCCG), applicable to both seminoma and nonseminoma, has proven useful and should form the basis for treatment decisions and the design of clinical trials in patients with metastatic disease [71]. With the introduction of cisplatin (*cis*-diamminedichloroplatinum [CDDP]) in the early 1970s, cure rates of patients with metastatic of TGCTs dramatically improved [72]. Today, approximately 70% of metastatic TGCT patients are cured after initial CDDP-based combination chemotherapy and possibly secondary surgery. With effective salvage therapy, including high-dose chemotherapy, a significant proportion of poor-risk patients can be cured in a relapse situation, resulting in longtime survival of more than 80% of patients with metastatic disease. In the following section, pathologic findings found to have a prognostic importance are discussed. In addition, the current knowledge on the underlying pathobiological basis of overall high sensitivity to chemotherapy, and the infrequent but mostly lethal occurrence of resistant phenotypes are described.

Biological Basis for Treatment

Histopathology

The pathological findings play a central role in patient management, as different histologies not only show different sensitivity to treatment modalities like radiation and chemotherapy, but also correlate with prognosis. Therefore, a central review by a pathologist with experience in GCT pathology is advised [73]. Seminomas are highly sensitive to both radiation and chemotherapy. Nonseminomas are less susceptible to radiation but show an overall high sensitivity to combination chemotherapy. Combined tumors must be treated as nonseminomas, and in fact, in contrast to the British Classification, are diagnosed as nonseminoma by the WHO classification system [33]. Pathological findings in the primary tumor do not necessarily predict those at metastatic sites, although they often do correlate [74].

The pluripotency of embryonal carcinoma, as indicated by OCT3/4 (see above) does not seem to be linked to treatment sensitivity, as no difference in expression was found between chemosensitive and chemoresistant type II GCTs [30]. Mature teratoma elements (either as a component of type II or as part of the type I GCTs) do not share the general chemosensitivity of GCTs to cisplatin-based chemotherapy (see also below). Therefore, residual mature teratoma is found in about 30% to 40% of remnants of initial metastases after chemotherapy. A predictive model for the histology of a residual retroperitoneal mass, based on primary tumor histology, prechemotherapy markers, mass size, and size reduction under chemotherapy, has been developed [75]. Absence of teratoma elements in the primary tumor has been identified as the most powerful predictor for benign residual tissue (i.e., absence of teratoma or viable cancer cells) [74,76]. Nevertheless, some caution is warranted because small teratoma areas may be missed in the primary tumor, and absence of teratoma elements does not exclude occurrence of malignant cells in residual masses. As type II teratomas show a similar genetic constitution as other vari-

ants of type II GCTs [77,78], most likely other mechanisms, for example, epigenetic phenomena, are underlying the intrinsic chemotherapy resistance of this histology. Regardless of their relatively benign behavior, radical resection of residual lesions containing teratomas after chemotherapy of a nonseminoma is warranted, and may be more critical than postoperative chemotherapy in the setting of viable malignant nonseminoma (Fig. 22.2) [79–81].

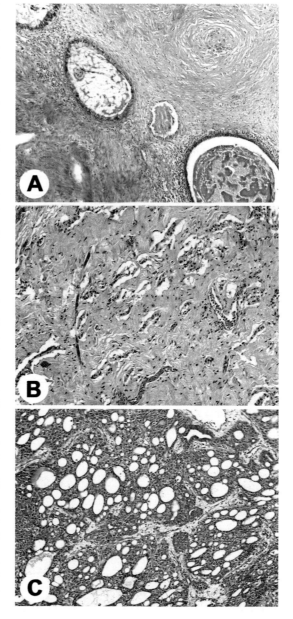

Fig. 22.2. Histologies of patients showing relapse of a TGCT. A: Tumor tissue of a 41-year-old patient with TGCT with a nonseminoma including teratoma at primary diagnosis. The illustration shows the histology of the resection of a residual lesion (para-aortic localization) after completion of chemotherapy. The lesion shows vital tumor, mostly mature teratoma, with epithelial and mesenchymal components. B: Same patient, tumor at relapse (retrocarinal lymph node) 6 months later. Apart from mature teratoma (not present in this section), areas showing neural differentiation were detectable. The tumor was therefore diagnosed as a secondary non–germ cell malignancy. The strands of epithelioid cells were immunohistochemically positive for neural markers like S100, neurofilament, and NSE (not shown). C: Third relapse of a TGCT in a 44-year-old patient, showing a nonseminoma of mixed histology at primary diagnosis. The illustration shows histology of the resection of a tumor mass (paravertebral localization) more than 5 years after first diagnosis. The lesion shows yolk sac tumor differentiation with a micro- and macrocystic pattern, and was immunohistochemically strongly positive for α-fetoprotein (AFP; not shown). Other areas of the tumor (not included in this section) show a more solid, hepatoid differentiation.

Based on these considerations, the pathology report must include all histological subtypes encountered in the tumor, including the observation of CIS/ITGCNU if present. Any secondary non–germ cell malignancy, mostly developing within mature teratoma, should be noted. Particular attention must be given to the presence or absence of vascular invasion, as a predictor of metastatic spread and occult metastases [82]. The distinction between venous or lymphatic does not add information to the risk of occult metastasis. Besides vascular invasion, high proliferative activity (assessed with the MIB-1 monoclonal antibody), and to a lesser extent the presence of embryonal carcinoma in the primary tumor and a high pathologic stage, were predictors of systemic spread in clinical stage I nonseminoma [83, for review]. Nevertheless, the predictive value of the present model is still somewhat limited, as the group defined as high risk in fact has a risk of approximately 50% for occult metastasis, and the low-risk group a risk of approximately 16%, which means gross overestimation of risk for the first and some underestimation for the latter group. Furthermore, for clinical stage I nonseminomas, risk factors for relapse have been assessed prospectively [84]. Again, vascular invasion was most predictive of stage in multifactorial analysis. With the addition of two other risk parameters (MIB-1 score >70% and embryonal carcinoma ≥50%) the positive predictive value could be improved to 63.6%. However, this means that even with an optimal combination of prognostic factors and reference pathology, more than one third of patients predicted to have pathologic stage II or relapse during follow-up will not have metastatic disease and will be overtreated with adjuvant therapy. On the other hand, patients at low risk can be predicted with more accuracy (86.5%), suggesting that surveillance for highly compliant patients of this cohort may be a valuable option. Recently, cluster analysis was used to discover a prognostic subgroup within a particular histology of GCT, namely embryonal carcinoma [85]. One subgroup with a specific tumor biology profile (high proliferation, assessed with Ki-67, low apoptosis, and low TP53) showed better survival than the overall patient group. This illustrates the potential usefulness of multivariate cluster analysis to identify subgroups within the existing prognostic categories.

Tumor Localization

In about 5% of type II GCTs, the tumor develops at extragonadal locations along the midline of the body [86]. The recent finding of the presence of activating mutations affecting the c-*KIT* both in bilateral TGCTs and extragonadal GCTs suggests a common pathogenetic mechanism, possibly related to an altered survival and proliferation of migrating germ cells during the intrauterine period [66,68]. Whereas patients with extragonadal GCTs showing pure seminoma histology have a long-term chance of cure similar to patients with a testicular primary tumor, patients with a mediastinal nonseminoma show a significantly inferior outcome. In fact they constitute the group with the poorest prognosis of all "poor prognosis" patients (IGCCCG classification), and outcome is even worse than in patients with multiple metastases [87].

Relapses

Another relatively rare but clinically meaningful phenomenon is the occurrence of relapses of GCTs after CDDP-based therapy. A number of predictive variables, both clinical and histological, such as platinum or absolute platinum refractoriness, primary mediastinal nonseminomatous histology, progressive disease before high-dose chemotherapy, and high levels of human chorionic gonadotropin (HCG), have been described in this group and allowed the formulation of a prognostic score [88]. This score not only can help to identify factors that influence outcome after high-dose chemotherapy, but also allows an estimation of the risk of relapse. With an overall incidence of about 10%, relapse occurs within 2 years after initial therapy, and long-term disease-free survival can be achieved in approximately 30% to 50% of cases with salvage treatment, preferably high-dose chemotherapy and stem cell support [89–92]. Late relapses occurring more than 2 years after an initial diagnosis of seminoma or nonseminoma have been reported in 1% to 5% of patients [93]. Cytogenetic comparison of a primary nonseminoma and a late relapse showing yolk sac differentiation revealed that these tumors were related, but the progression was accompanied by net loss of chromosomal material [94]. Whereas isolated mature teratoma can usually be cured by complete excision, a high proportion of patients with marker-positive findings seem to suffer from chemotherapy-resistant disease and show a less favorable response to additional chemotherapy [95,96]. Historically, in late relapses response rates to chemotherapy have been reported to be less than 30%, with an even lower long-term survival [93], yet more recent data seem to indicate that chemotherapy may have a role to play in the management of this disease [97,98]. Furthermore, late relapses can present as secondary non–germ cell malignancies (also called teratoma with malignant transformation), which develop from nonseminomatous histology, mostly teratomas (Fig. 22.2) [98]. These components often show adenocarcinoma-histology and are characterized by relative resistance to CDDP-based chemotherapy and an adverse prognosis (see below). Currently, the underlying pathobiological changes leading to the occurrence of relapse and the mechanisms involved in refractoriness to chemotherapy in this particular group of patients are poorly understood and need further investigation.

Biological Basis of Drug Response

Notwithstanding the overall good prognosis, 10% to 30% of patients diagnosed with metastatic nonseminomatous GCT do not achieve a durable complete remission after initial treatment, either due to incomplete response or relapse. Based on this clinical background, understanding of the mechanisms of chemosensitivity and resistance of GCTs is becoming more important to further improve therapeutic outcome. An improved prediction of treatment outcome could help to avoid both under- and overtreatment. The rapid development of targeted therapy with the aim of influencing specific cellular pathways may potentially facilitate reversing or overcoming individual resistance mechanisms and help to cure more patients in the future. Recently, a number of reviews have been dedicated to sensitivity and refractoriness of GCTs [99–101]. The currently available data on the molecular basis of chemotherapy response in these tumors is reviewed below. Special attention is given to cisplatin (CDDP), presumably the most active drug in the treatment of this disease, as the introduction of this

agent into combination treatment has yielded unprecedented improvement in survival of patients with metastatic disease. The course of the drug from entering the cell to the execution of apoptosis is followed (summarized in Fig. 22.3). Furthermore, different models that have been put forward to explain the unusual overall chemosensitivity of GCTs and findings in refractoriness are discussed, including a brief section on possible explanations for the intrinsic resistance observed in mature teratoma and secondary non–germ cell malignancies.

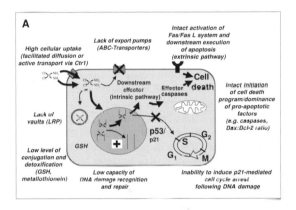

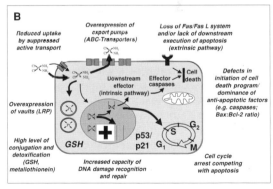

Fig. 22.3. Schematic representation of mechanisms potentially involved in cisplatin (CDDP) resistance in GCT cells. A: Model of a CDDP-sensitive tumor cell. Lack of potential resistance mechanisms leads to initiation and execution of apoptosis. B: Model of a CDDP-resistant cell. Note that multiple factors can potentially be involved in drug resistance, ranging from mechanisms that lower free intracellular CDDP levels to increased DNA repair, failure to execute apoptosis, and induction of cell cycle arrest rather than cell death after DNA damage. ABC, ATP binding cassette; Ctr1, copper transporter; FAS L, FAS ligand; GSH, glutathione; LRP, lung resistance protein. (Modified from Mayer et al. [107].)

Factors Involved in Drug Sensitivity

Cisplatin (CDDP) exerts its effect by damaging DNA. In principle, different processes leading to binding of a drug to DNA can be distinguished: whereas mechanisms such as influx and efflux of a drug across the cell membrane can affect intracellular concentration, other factors influence drug activation, detoxification, or DNA binding itself. Most findings, however, suggest that crucial determinators of drug sensitivity in GCTs lie downstream of DNA binding, for example, in the intrinsic or extrinsic pathways of apoptosis or DNA repair.

Drug Influx, efflux, and DNA Binding

The mechanism by which CDDP enters a cell are not fully understood yet, and different models, including a passive or facilitated diffusion, have been described [102]. In the latter case, reduced uptake could hardly play a role in drug resistance. Recent data suggest a role of the copper transporter CTR1 in cellular CDDP uptake, which might be responsible for at least a part of the CDDP entering the cell [103]. No differences were observed in the intracellular accumulation of CDDP in different cell lines, including those derived from GCTs, which makes a critical role of active membrane transport an unlikely factor for sensitivity [104]. Members of the adenosine triphosphate (ATP)-binding cassette (ABC) superfamily of transporters show affinity for CDDP, in particular when conjugated to glutathione. Overexpression of these pumps can result in resistance to the drug, as has been demonstrated for different tumor cell lines [105]. Exerting a comparable effect by unrelated means, overexpression of the lung resistance protein (LRP) can also lead to elimination of CDDP [106]. For GCTs, data on export pumps are scarce. In one small series, GCTs were found to rarely express LRP [107]. In a second study comparing GCT specimens from patients with resistant or sensitive disease, multidrug resistance (MDR)-related protein (MRP2) and LRP were hardly detectable in invasive components, with the exception of sporadic refractory cases [108]. However, the differences found between chemosensitive and refractory tumors did not reach statistical significance. The ABC transporters were not found to be involved in induced

CDDP resistance of the GCT-derived cell line GCT27, in contrast to an ovarian cancer and a colon cancer derived cell line [109].

In addition to the facilitation of drug export by ABC transporters, conjugation to glutathione limits the toxic effect of CDDP [110]. For GCT cell lines, a correlation between loss of CDDP activity and an increased glutathione [111] or metallothionein [112] content has been described.

However, conflicting data have been reported regarding an inverse correlation between resistance and metallothionein or total amount of sulfhydryl groups both in cell lines and clinical samples of GCTs [104,113]. In GCTs, different isoforms of glutathione-S-transferase (GST)—the enzyme transferring glutathione to toxins—have been investigated, demonstrating a clear dominance of the isoform π, covering over 80% of the total GST activity, and a low enzyme activity of all isoforms together [114]. The authors suggested that the chemosensitivity of GCTs could be related to these findings. In a different study, GST π was detected only in mature teratomas, but hardly in other histological tumor components. A clear staining was only seen in a few of the refractory cases; however, the differences between refractory and responsive tumors were not significant [108].

In conclusion, most invasive GCTs lack export pumps with affinity for CDDP and show low levels of GST activity. It is conceivable that these features contribute to their chemosensitivity. On the other hand, even though it is probably not a common resistance mechanism, overexpression of selected transporters or GST π and/or an increased content of glutathione may contribute to chemotherapy resistance in individual cases of GCTs.

Some data are available on the binding of CDDP to DNA in different cell lines, including GCTs [115–117]. A wide range of CDDP-DNA adducts is seen in cancer cells of different origin following exposure to the drug. As GCT cell lines do not show higher numbers of DNA adducts compared to other cell lines, it can be concluded that none of the steps described above is particularly more effective in GCTs than in other tumors.

Therefore, explanations for the unique sensitivity of GCTs are more likely to be found in the response to DNA damage than in factors affecting DNA binding.

DNA Repair Pathways

Nucleotide Excision Repair

It has been suggested that embryonic stem cells are equipped with efficient defense mechanisms to cope with damaged DNA, either by removal of damage by repair mechanisms, or by elimination of irreparably damaged cells via apoptosis [118,119]. Similar importance of this control mechanism can be expected for germ cells, which share many properties of embryonic stem cells, in order to limit the risk that mutations are being passed on to the next generation. The role of DNA repair pathways in sensitivity and resistance of GCTs has been addressed in different studies. Of the various DNA repair mechanisms, the nucleotide excision repair (NER) pathway is supposed to be of major importance when CDDP exposure has resulted in covalent DNA lesions that distort the DNA helix [120]. The CDDP is removed slowly from the genomic DNA in different GCT-derived cell lines, indicating a low capacity of the respective DNA repair pathway (i.e., NER) [116]. However, in two CDDP-resistant sublines the DNA repair capacity was unchanged compared to their parental line [121]. The low intrinsic capacity of the NER demonstrated in GCT cell lines has been attributed to low levels of xeroderma pigmentosum complementation group A protein (XPA) [122]. Yet, in another study, the XPA levels found in GCT cell lines were not substantially lower than in other tumor cell lines investigated, and no correlation between XPA and sensitivity to CDDP was seen in three GCT cell lines [123]. Furthermore, with regard to the clinical situation, data from experiments with cell lines must be interpreted with some caution, as has been shown by the study cited above, as no differences in XPA expression in tumors were found by immunohistochemistry between samples of GCTs refractory or sensitive to chemotherapy [123]. Therefore, low XPA levels cannot serve as a universal explanation for the sensitivity to chemotherapy, and XPA has no predictive value in these tumors. Alternatively, it has been proposed that the DNA adducts could be concealed by testis-specific high mobility group (HMG)-box proteins preventing damage detection and repair by NER factors [124]. Given the circumstance that many factors are involved in NER, it is conceivable that factors other than XPA can contribute to the overall low repair activity, thereby influencing the chemosensitivity of GCTs [100].

Base Excision Repair

Small base alterations that do not distort the DNA helix are eliminated by the base excision repair (BER) pathway. In the treatment of GCT, this type of damage is found after use of ionizing radiation or bleomycin [125]. In vitro overexpression of Ape1/ref1 in GCT-derived cell lines resulted in a twofold resistance to bleomycin [126]. Again, these data from in vitro experiments are difficult to interpret with regard to their clinical value, as the majority of GCTs investigated displayed a strong immunohistochemical staining for this factor, and bleomycin is never used as a single agent in the therapy of metastatic disease. Therefore, a major effect of mere protein levels of Ape1/ref1 in determining chemotherapy resistance is unlikely.

Mismatch Repair

The DNA mismatch repair (MMR) pathway seems to act as a link between damage recognition and initiation of apoptosis after cisplatin treatment [127]. Defects of MMR factors lead to instability of short repetitive DNA sequences called microsatellite instability (MSI), which can provide information about the functional capacity of the MMR system. Losses or defects of MMR factors can confer resistance to a whole range of cytotoxic agents, including CDDP, alkylating agents, methotrexate, and the topoisomerase II inhibitor doxorubicin [128,129]. Possibly, resistance can be explained by the acquisition of secondary mutations (e.g., in effectors of apoptosis due to genetic instability). Alternatively, assuming a critical role of the MMR in linking the detection of damage to apoptosis, respective defects would directly result in failure to initiate the apoptotic cascade. On the other hand, patients with colorectal cancer showing MSI did not only have a better prognosis, but also showed better treatment response to 5-fluorouracil–based chemotherapy, indicating that MSI can have different effects in different tumor entities [130]. Interestingly, MMR-deficient cells have shown an abrogated G2/M cell cycle checkpoint and decreased apoptosis following DNA damage [131,132]. Germ cell tumors have been found to be microsatellite stable in previous studies [128,133]. This was confirmed in a series of 100 unselected GCTs, where only 6% of the cases showed MSI in at most one out of eight investigated loci. In contrast, five of 11 (45%) tumor samples from patients with refractory disease had unstable microsatellites, four of them in at least two loci. This suggests that failure to initiate apoptosis due to defects in MMR might contribute to resistance in a significant number of GCT [134]. Interestingly, yeast knockout cells for *sky1*, a serine/arginine-rich protein-specific kinase, shown to be a cisplatin-sensitivity gene [135], also show this mutator phenotype. Indeed, cisplatin-resistant GCT show a significant lower SRPK1 (the human counterpart of *sky*) compared to sensitive GCTs [136]. Yet, further investigations of this topic are warranted to validate this finding in a larger number of refractory cases and to confirm the clinical relevance and the potential predictive value of these findings.

The Role of TP53 in Germ Cell Tumors

TP53 is known to play a dual role in stress response. On the one hand, it mediates a G1/S-phase cell cycle arrest via transactivation of p21, allowing time for DNA repair. Furthermore, TP53 can lead to apoptosis via the mitochondrial (intrinsic) pathway, for example, by induction of BAX [137, for review]. In contrast to other solid tumors, *p53* is hardly ever found to be mutated in GCTs, even though GCT cell lines do not have an overall lower frequency of mutations, both spontaneous and induced, compared with other cell lines [138]. At the same time, TP53 can be detected immunohistochemically in most GCTs. Therefore, a high level of wild-type TP53 in GCTs has commonly been regarded as the biological explanation for the chemosensitivity of this entity. However, experimental evidence supporting this idea is partly based on studies in mouse teratocarcinoma cell lines [125,139], whereas data on human cell lines are conflicting [117,140].

In two studies, the TP53 status in tumor samples from refractory patients was analyzed. In relapsed GCTs, *p53* mutations were detected in four of 28 tumors; three of them were mature teratomas, and the remaining one a secondary non–germ cell malignancy derived from a teratoma [141]. All mutation-containing tumors, therefore, belonged to intrinsically chemother-

apy resistant histological subgroups, making it difficult to assess the contribution of the TP53 status to the clinical behavior. In another study, no *p53* mutations were found in a group of 18 refractory cases, except in one sensitive case, and TP53 levels were comparable to those of sensitive and unselected cases [142]. For the majority of refractory GCT patients *p53* mutations are unlikely to be the cause of treatment failure. In conclusion, the level of TP53 alone cannot explain the chemotherapy sensitivity of GCTs and has no predictive value with regard to chemotherapy resistance. Another level of complexity is introduced by the fact that the TP53 pathway can be influenced by a number of other factors, such as phosphorylation, acetylation, sumoylation, and binding to other proteins [143]. Therefore, inactivation of TP53 might occur at different levels. For example, a specific role of *p73*, a family member of the *p53* gene family interacting with TP53, has been reported in the response to ionizing radiation of the testis, and *p63*, another member of the same family, has been found in GCT of a certain histological subtype [144]. Future research has to elucidate the importance of these factors for chemotherapy response of GCTs.

Execution of Apoptosis

The rapid induction of apoptosis following exposure to CDDP has been interpreted as an inherent property of the cell of origin (i.e., an early germ cell) to undergo programmed cell death [101]. In view of the potentially disastrous consequences of passing on genetic defects to the next generation, it is tempting to speculate that the extreme sensitivity of germ cells to apoptotic stimuli serves as a kind of quality control. Although this might be one of the factors explaining the overall sensitivity of GCT, it is conceivable that resistance can emerge from failure to execute apoptosis in the rare case of refractoriness. A number of findings point to different levels of disruption of the apoptotic pathway, including the BCL2/BAX family, the CD95 death pathway, and downstream effectors like caspases.

In GCT-derived cell lines the sensitivity for etoposide—after CDDP the second most commonly used drug for GCTs—was ascribed to a high ratio of proapoptotic BAX to antiapoptotic BCL-2, both members of the BCL-2 family acting downstream of *p53* [145]. No such correlation was found in four different GCT cell lines treated with CDDP. After exposure to the drug, no induction of BCL2 and BAX was observed [146]. Two studies on GCT samples have confirmed the high BAX/BCL2 ratio in invasive components. However, in both studies, no correlation of BAX or BCL2 with clinical outcome was evident [108,147]. When BCL2 was overexpressed in GCT cells, the somewhat unexpected finding of increased sensitivity to cytotoxic drugs was explained by the reciprocal downregulation of another proapoptotic protein, BCL-XL [148].

A role for the "extrinsic" death pathway involving FAS/FAS-L has been described in paracrine signaling regulating apoptosis of germ cells [149,150]. However, data on expression of FAS and FASL in GCT is controversial [151,152]. The fact that treatment with CDDP results in activation of this system, and the observation that the CD95 apoptotic pathway is lost in a CDDP-resistant GCT cell lines indicates a potential role in CDDP sensitivity in GCT [153]. A high frequency of *FAS* inactivating mutations has been observed in TGCTs, and has been interpreted as an early step in the pathogenesis of this cancer [154]. Using direct sequencing of multiple TGCTs, we have not been able to confirm this finding (unpublished observations).

Finally, CDDP resistance in a GCT cell line has been shown to be mediated by a failure to activate caspase-9 [155]. This indicates that alterations of downstream effects in the mitochondrial, "intrinsic" pathway can also lead to a resistant phenotype. The importance of these findings has yet to be confirmed in samples from patients with GCTs to assess their relevance in clinical resistance.

Extracellular Factors Influencing the Efficacy of Chemotherapy

So far, only cellular factors affecting platinum activity have been discussed. Yet, as a drug first has to reach the tumor cell in order to exert its action, a number of extracellular factors are likely to be involved in therapy resistance. An increased diffusion distance from vessels to tumor cells by changes in the extracellular matrix may cause reduced intracellular CDDP concentration. Microvessel density or the composition of the extracellular matrix will addi-

tionally determine the efficacy of treatment. Large metastases in patients with GCTs will at least be partly hypoxic as indicated by extensive necrotic areas in many of these tumor masses. A range of cytotoxic agents have recently been tested under hypoxic conditions in GCT cell lines [156]. The relative effect of hypoxia in decreasing apoptosis was mainly dependent on the cell line and to a lesser extent on the drug, but without exception, all drugs were less effective under hypoxic conditions. This indicates that hypoxia, either due to poorly perfused tumors, or lowered oxygen concentration in the blood, for example, as a consequence of anemia, could contribute to the occurrence of resistance in GCTs. In the clinical setting, this model has led to the design of treatment strategies that aim at preventing anemia by the concomitant use of erythropoietin, a hematopoietic growth factor, with chemotherapy (C. Bokemeyer, personal communication).

Cell Cycle Arrest and the Intrinsic Cisplatin-Resistance of Mature Teratoma and Secondary Non–Germ Cell Malignancies

Teratomas

Mature teratomas are clinically resistant to effects of chemotherapy. This is somewhat surprising, as no genetic differences between mature teratoma and the invasive components of GCTs could be demonstrated so far [157]. Therefore, their resistant phenotype must be due to subtle or so far unidentified genetic changes. Alternatively, and more likely, intrinsic resistance of somatic tissue, possibly related to epigenetic gene-expression regulatory events, is underlying the resistance of these tumors. In contrast to invasive GCT components, epithelial tissues of mature teratomas were found to express MDR, MRP2, BCRP, and LRP by immunohistochemistry. Furthermore, the presence of GST π has been demonstrated in tissue of mature teratoma. A further difference can be observed in the expression of the cell cycle–associated proteins p21 and RB. In contrast to other invasive components of GCTs, mature teratomas have been found to express RB and p21, suggesting the ability of these components to go into G1/S cycle arrest [108]. In fact, several studies have reported on a deregulated G1/S checkpoint in GCTs. For example, a significant lack of the cell cycle regulator RB has been described for both seminomas and nonseminomas [158]. Interestingly, cells lacking p21 were found to have a reduced ability to repair CDDP-induced DNA damages and showed an increased sensitivity to this agent [159]. Because embryonal carcinoma is the precursor of the more differentiated nonseminomatous elements, this phenomenon is most likely not due to a genetic inactivation of the cell cycle checkpoint. Alternatively, this could be related to the embryonic origin of these tumors: expression of RB and p19ink4d, a cyclin-dependent kinase inhibitor, is lacking both in human fetal gonocytes and CIS/ITGCNU [160]. This finding has been interpreted as yet another indicator that the precursor lesion of TGCTs arises from an early, developmentally arrested germ cell [42]. In addition, unlike the other invasive GCT components, mature teratomas show a low BAX/BCL2 ratio [108]. Further evidence that induction of differentiation plays a role in treatment resistance of GCTs comes from in vitro analyses of the embryonal carcinoma cell line Tera-2 [161]. Using all-*trans*-retinoic acid, increased differentiation of these cells was accompanied by reduced sensitivity to CDDP due to reduced apoptotic susceptibility. Taken together, these findings suggest that mature teratomas may respond to CDDP-induced DNA damage by upregulating p21 and induction of cell cycle arrest rather than undergoing BAX-mediated apoptosis, possibly related to their loss of embryonic characteristics.

Teratomas with Malignant Transformation or Secondary Non–Germ Cell Malignancies

This rare but clinically significant occurrence in GCTs refers to the transformation of a somatic teratomatous component in a nonseminoma to histologies resembling tumors of a primary somatic origin [162]. The clonal GCT origin of these lesions can be confirmed by the identification of isochromosome 12p or excess 12p copy numbers, the genetic hallmark of type II GCTs [77,98]. Most frequently found histologies are rhabdomyosarcomas, primitive neurectodermal tumors, enteric adenocarcinomas, and leukemias. The latter occur virtually only after mediastinal nonseminomas. If the malignant transformation is confined to lesions that are resectable by radical surgery, this treatment approach can offer definitive cure. However, if complete resection is not possible, for example, due to disseminated disease or infiltration of vital organs, prognosis is poor, with a median survival of less than 3 years [163]. Recently, a chart review of a series of more than 60 patients with secondary non–germ cell malignancies from one single institution has been published [98]. It was reported that with chemotherapy, dictated by the transformed histology, some responses could be achieved, indicating that systemic treatment might confer benefit for a minority of these patients. Limited by the small size of this study, this analysis shows that the histological subtypes primitive neuroectodermal tumor and rhabdomyosarcoma seem to respond better to chemotherapy than malignancies in patients presenting with adenocarcinoma or leukemias as transformed histology of their GCT. It is an interesting observation that chemotherapy strategies adapted from somatic tumors for these malignant transformations (e.g., 5-fluorouracil treatment for adenocarcinoma), showed some effect, whereas CDDP-based therapy (usually the most effective treatment in GCTs) has no role in this situation [98]. Given that clonality with GCT was cytogenetically proven in a number of these tumors, it is tempting to speculate on epigenetic changes occurring during somatic differentiation decrease sensitivity to DNA damage and could be a major factor explaining cisplatin-resistance in GCTs.

In summary, the available data indicate that the chemotherapy-resistant phenotype of mature teratomas and secondary non–germ cell malignancies results from the concerted expression of different resistance factors in the line of somatic differentiation, affecting multiple cellular functions like drug export, cell cycle control, and regulation of apoptosis.

Conclusions and Perspectives

In recent years significant progress has been made regarding our knowledge about different factors and pathways involved in GCT sensitivity and resistance. Yet the overall picture is just beginning to evolve. The exquisite chemosensitivity of GCTs seems to be the consequence of an inherent property of germ cells and embryonal cells to readily undergo cell death upon apoptotic stimulation. This might be due to a favorable combination of factors including a lack of drug export and detoxification mechanisms, low DNA repair capacity, and sensitive DNA damage detection systems with effective subsequent initiation and execution of apoptotic pathways in the vast majority of cases.

As the phenotype of mature teratomas is most likely a consequence of somatic differentiation rather than a tumor specific alteration, it is conceivable that it will be difficult to develop a systemic treatment approach that is able to eliminate mature teratomas without at the same time affecting regular somatic tissues showing identical histological differentiation. Any such treatment will elicit unacceptable toxicities. Complete surgical resection of residual teratoma after chemotherapy therefore remains the adequate treatment approach to date.

No uniform explanation for the development of a resistant phenotype in invasive GCT components can be offered yet. A significant proportion of these cases may be caused by defects in the MMR system resulting in microsatellite instability. Whether the observed resistance is the direct consequence of failure to detect DNA damage caused by CDDP and to subsequently initiate apoptotic pathways, or an indirect consequence of the accumulation of mutations affecting apoptotic effectors remains to be determined. On the other hand, overexpression of export pumps or enzymes detoxifying drugs might confer resistance in only a small number of cases, but does not account for the majority of patients suffering from chemotherapy resistant GCTs.

In view of the variety and complex interactions of pathways resulting in or preventing cell death, methods with the ability to investigate multiple factors at the same time are probably necessary to further elucidate the mechanisms of resistance and possibly be able to predict the response to chemotherapy in the future.

Acknowledgments

Freidemann Honecker is supported by a personal grant of the Dr. Mildred Scheel Stiftung für Krebsforschung. J. Wolter Oosterhuis and L.H.J. Looijenga are supported by the Dutch Cancer Society.

References

1. Albanell J, Bosl GJ, Reuter VE, et al. Telomerase activity in germ cell cancers and mature teratomas. J Natl Cancer Inst 1999;91(15):1321–1326.
2. Delgado R, Rathi A, Albores-Saavedra J, Gazdar AF. Expression of the RNA component of human telomerase in adult testicular germ cell neoplasia. Cancer 1999;86(9):1802–1811.
3. Wylie C. Germ cells. Cell 1999;96(2):165–174.
4. Zeeman AM, Stoop H, Boter M, et al. VASA is a specific marker for both normal and malignant human germ cells. Lab Invest 2002;82:159–166.
5. Castrillon DH, Quade BJ, Wang TY, Quigley C, Crum CP. The human VASA gene is specifically expressed in the germ cell lineage. Proc Natl Acad Sci USA 2000;97(17):9585–9590.
6. Mostofi FK, Sesterhenn IA. Histological Typing of Testis Tumours, 2nd ed. Berlin: Springer, 1998.
7. Cummings OW, Ulbright TM, Eble JN, Roth LM. Spermatocytic seminoma: an immunohistochemical study. Hum Pathol 1994;25:54–59.
8. Eble JN. Spermatocytic seminoma. Hum Pathol 1994;25:1035–1042.
9. Dekker I, Rozeboom T, Delemarre J, Dam A, Oosterhuis JW. Placental-like alkaline phosphatase and DNA flow cytometry in spermatocytic seminoma. Cancer 1992;69:993–996.
10. Stoop H, Van Gurp RHJLM, De Krijger R, et al. Reactivity of germ cell maturation stage-specific markers in spermatocytic seminoma: diagnostic and etiological implications. Lab Invest 2001;81:919–928.
11. Rajpert-De Meyts E, Jacobsen GK, Bartkova J, et al. The immunohistochemical expression pattern of Chk2, p53, p19INK4d, MAGE-A4 and other selected antigens provides new evidence for the premeiotic origin of spermatocytic seminoma. Histopathology 2003;42(3):217–226.
12. Rosenberg C, Mostert MC, Bakker Schut T, et al. Chromosomal constitution of human spermatocytic seminomas: comparative genomic hybridization supported by conventional and interphase cytogenetics. Genes Chromosome Cancer 1998;23:286–291.
13. Oosterhuis JW, Looijenga LHJ, Van Echten-Arends J, De Jong B. Chromosomal constitution and developmental potential of human germ cell tumors and teratomas. Cancer Genet Cytogenet 1997;95:96–102.
14. Gobel U, Schneider DT, Calaminus G, Haas RJ, Schmidt P, Harms D. Germ-cell tumors in childhood and adolescence. GPOH MAKEI and the MAHO study groups. Ann Oncol 2000;11(3):263–271.

15. Looijenga LHJ, Oosterhuis JW. Pathobiology of testicular germ cell tumors: views and news. Anal Quant Cytol Histol 2002;24:263–279.

16. Calaminus G, Schneider DT, Bokkerink JP, et al. Prognostic value of tumor size, metastases, extension into bone, and increased tumor marker in children with malignant sacrococcygeal germ cell tumors: a prospective evaluation of 71 patients treated in the German cooperative protocols Maligne Keimzelltumoren (MAKEI) 83/86 and MAKEI 89. J Clin Oncol 2003;21(5): 781–786.

17. Mostert MC, Rosenberg C, Stoop H, et al. Comparative genomic and in situ hybridization of germ cell tumors of the infantile testis. Lab Invest 2000;80:1055–1064.

18. Scheres JM, de Pater JM, Stoutenbeek P, Wijmenga C, Rosenberg C, Pearson PL. Isochromosome 1q as the sole chromosomal abnormality in two fetal teratomas. Possible trisomic or tetrasomic zygote rescue in fetal teratoma with an additional isochromosome 1q. Cancer Genet Cytogenet 1999;115(1):1–10.

19. Perlman EJ, Hu J, Ho D, Cushing B, Lauer S, Castleberry RP. Genetic analysis of childhood endodermal sinus tumors by comparative genomic hybridization. J Pediatr Hematol Oncol 2000;22(2):100–105.

20. Mayer F, Stoop H, Sen S, Bokemeyer C, Oosterhuis JW, Looijenga LHJ. Aneuploidy of human testicular germ cell tumors is associated with amplification of centrosomes. Oncogene 2003;22: 3859–3866.

21. van Echten J, Timmer A, van der Veen AY, Molenaar WM, de Jong B. Infantile and adult testicular germ cell tumors. a different pathogenesis? Cancer Genet Cytogenet 2002;135(1): 57–62.

22. Veltman I, Schepens MT, Looijenga LHJ, Strong LC, Geurts van Kessel A. Germ cell tumours in neonates and infants: a distinct subgroup. APMIS 2003;111:152–160.

23. Walt H, Oosterhuis JW, Stevens LC. Experimental testicular germ cell tumorigenesis in mouse strains with and without spontaneous tumours differs from development of germ cell tumours of the adult human testis. Int J Androl 1993;16: 267–271.

24. Van Berlo RJ, Oosterhuis JW, Schrijnemakers E, Schoots CJ, de Jong B, Damjanov I. Yolk-sac carcinoma develops spontaneously as a late occurrence in slow- growing teratoid tumors produced from transplanted 7–day mouse embryos. Int J Cancer 1990;45(1):153–155.

25. Oosterhuis JW, Castedo SMMJ, De Jong B, et al. Ploidy of primary germ cell tumors of the testis. Pathogenetic and clinical relevance. Lab Invest 1989;60:14–20.

26. Looijenga LHJ, Zafarana G, Grygalewicz B, et al. Role of gain of 12p in germ cell tumour development. APMIS 2003;111:161–173.

27. Pugh RCB. Combined tumours. In: Pugh RCB, ed. Pathology of the Testis. Oxford: Blackwell, 1976: 245–258.

28. Andrews PW, Casper J, Damjanov I, et al. A comparative analysis of cell surface antigens expressed by cell lines derived from human germ cell tumors. Int J Cancer 1996;66:806–816.

29. Looijenga LHJ, Gillis AJM, Van Gurp RJHLM, Verkerk AJMH, Oosterhuis JW. X inactivation in human testicular tumors. XIST expression and androgen receptor methylation status. Am J Pathol 1997;151:581–590.

30. Looijenga LHJ, Stoop H, De Leeuw PJC, et al. POU5F1 (OCT3/4) identifies cells with pluripotent potential in human germ cell tumors. Cancer Res 2003;63:2244–2250.

31. Sperger JM, Chen X, Draper JS, et al. Gene expression patterns in human embryonic stem cells and human pluripotent germ cell tumors. Proc Natl Acad Sci USA 2003;100:13350–13355.

32. Skakkebæk NE. Possible carcinoma-in-situ of the testis. Lancet 1972:516–517.

33. Mostofi FK, Sesterhenn IA, Davis CJJ. Immunopathology of germ cell tumors of the testis. Semin Diagn Pathol 1987;4:320–341.

34. Loy V, Dieckmann KP. Carcinoma in situ of the testis: intratubular germ cell neoplasia or testicular intraepithelial neoplasia? [letter; comment]. Hum Pathol 1990;21:457–458.

35. Scully RE. Gonadoblastoma: a review of 74 cases. Cancer 1970;25:1340–1356.

36. Giwercman A, Müller J, Skakkebæk NE. Prevalence of carcinoma-in situ and other histopathological abnormalities in testes from 399 men who died suddenly and unexpectedly. J Urol 1991;145:77–80.

37. Adami HO, Bergström R, Möhner M, et al. Testicular cancer in nine northern European countries. Int J Cancer 1994;59:33–38.

38. Giwercman A, Skakkebæk NE. Carcinoma in situ of the testis: Biology, screening and management. Eur Urol 1993;23:19–21.

39. Rajpert-De Meyts E, Jorgensen N, Brondum-Nielsen K, Muller J, Skakkebæk NE. Developmental arrest of germ cells in the pathogenesis of germ cell neoplasia. APMIS 1998;106(1):198–204; discussion 204–206.

40. Gondos B. Ultrastructure of developing and malignant germ cells. Eur Urol 1993;23:68–75.

41. Jørgensen N, Rajpert-De Meyts E, Graem N, Müller J, Giwercman A, Skakkebæk NE. Expression of immunohistochemical markers for testicular carcinoma in situ by normal fetal germ cells. Lab Invest 1995;72:223–231.

42. Rajpert-De Meyts E, Bartkova J, Samson M, et al. The emerging phenotype of the testicular carcinoma in situ germ cell. APMIS 2003;111(1):267–278.

43. Nielsen SW, Lein DH. Tumours of the testis. Bulletin Word Health Organization 1974;50:71–78.

44. Jacobsen GK, Norgaard-Pedersen B. Placental alkaline phosphatase in testicular germ cell tumours and in carcinoma-in-situ of the testis. An immunohistochemical study. Acta Pathol Microbiol Immunol Scand [A] 1984;92(5):323–329.

45. Roelofs H, Manes T, Millan JL, Oosterhuis JW, Looijenga LHJ. Heterogeneity in alkaline phosphatase isozyme expression in human testicular germ cell tumors. An enzyme-/immunohistochemical and molecular analysis. J Pathol 1999;189:236–244.

46. Rajpert-De Meyts E, Skakkebæk NE. Expression of the c-kit protein product in carcinoma-in-situ and invasive testicular germ cell tumours. Int J Androl 1994;17:85–92.

47. Bokemeyer C, Kuczyk MA, Dunn T, et al. Expression of stem-cell factor and its receptor c-kit protein in normal testicular tissue and malignant germ-cell tumors. J Cancer Res Clin Oncol 1996;122:301–306.

48. Strohmeyer T, Peter S, Hartmann M, et al. Expression of the hst 1 and c-kit protooncogenes in human testicular germ cell tumors. Cancer Res 1991;51:1811–1816.

49. Gidekel S, Pizov G, Bergman Y, Pikarsky E. Oct-3/4 is a dose-dependent oncogenic fate determinant. Cancer Cell 2003;4:361–370.

50. Møller H. Decreased testicular cancer risk in men born in wartime. J Natl Cancer Inst 1989;81(21):1668–1669.

51. Jørgensen N, Giwercman A, Müller J, Skakkebæk NE. Immunohistochemical markers of carcinoma in situ of the testis also expressed in normal infantile germ cells. Histopathology 1993;22:373–378.

52. Skakkebæk NE, Holm M, Hoei-Hansen C, Jørgensen N, Rajpert-De Meyts E. Association between testicular dysgenesis syndrome (TDS) and testicular neoplasia: evidence from 20 adult patients with signs of maldevelopment of the testis. APMIS 2003;111(1):1–11.

53. Skakkebæk NE, Raipert-de Meyts E, Jærgensen N, et al. Germ cell cancer and disorders of spermatogenesis: an environmental connection? APMIS 1998;106:3–12.

54. Rorth M, Rajpert-de Meyts E, Skakkebæk NE, et al. Carcinoma in situ of the testis. Scand J Urol 2000;205:166–186.

55. Dieckmann KP, Loy V. Prevalence of contralateral testicular intraepithelial neoplasia in patients

with testicular germ cell neoplasms. J Clin Oncol 1996;14:3126–3132.

56. Dieckmann KP, Loy V. False-negative biopsies for the diagnosis of testicular intraepithelial neoplasia (TIN)—an update. Eur Urol 2003;43(5):516–521.

57. Dieckmann KP, Classen J, Loy V. Diagnosis and management of testicular intraepithelial neoplasia (carcinoma in situ)—surgical aspects. APMIS 2003;111(1):64–68; discussion 68–69.

58. Heidenreich A, Moul JW. Contralateral testicular biopsy procedure in patients with unilateral testis cancer: Is it indicated? Semin Urol Oncol 2002;20(4):234–238.

59. De Gouveia Brazao CA, Pierik FH, Oosterhuis JW, Dohle GR, Looijenga LHJ, Weber RFA. Bilateral testicular microlithiasis predicts development of malignant testicular germ cell tumours in subfertile men. J Urol 2004;171:158–160.

60. Holm M, Hoei-Hansen CE, Rajpert-De Meyts E, Skakkebaek NE. Increased risk of carcinoma in situ in patients with testicular germ cell cancer with ultrasonic microlithiasis in the contralateral testicle. J Urol 2003;170(4):1163–1167.

61. Che M, Tamboli P, Ro JY, et al. Bilateral testicular germ cell tumors: twenty-year experience at M.D. Anderson Cancer Center. Cancer 2002;95(6):1228–1233.

62. Berthelsen JG, Skakkebæk NE, von der Maase H, Sorensen BL, Mogensen P. Screening for carcinoma in situ of the contralateral testis in patients with germinal testicular cancer. Br Med J (Clin Res Ed) 1982;285(6356):1683–1686.

63. Holzbeierlein JM, Sogani PC, Sheinfeld J. Histology and clinical outcomes in patients with bilateral testicular germ cell tumors: the Memorial Sloan Kettering cancer center experience 1950 to 2001. J Urol 2003;169(6):2122–2125.

64. Lajos G, Gomez F, Mihaly B, Istvan B. The incidence, prognosis, clinical and histological characteristics, treatment and outcome of patients with bilateral germ cell testicular cancer in Hungary. J Cancer Res Clin Oncol 2003;129:309–315.

65. Gaffan J, Holden L, Newlands ES, et al. Infertility rates following POMB/ACE chemotherapy for male and female germ cell tumours—a retrospective long-term follow-up study. Br J Cancer 2003;89(10):1849–1854.

66. Looijenga LHJ, De Leeuw PJC, Van Oorschot M, et al. Stem cell factor receptor (c-KIT) codon 816 mutations predict development of bilateral testicular germ cell tumors. Cancer Res 2003;63:7674–7678.

67. van Oosterom AT, Judson I, Verweij J, et al. Safety and efficacy of imatinib (STI571) in metastatic gastrointestinal stromal tumours: a phase I study. Lancet 2001;358(9291):1421–1423.

68. Przygodzki RM, Hubbs AE, Zhao FQ, O'Leary TJ. Primary mediastinal seminomas: evidence of single and multiple KIT mutations. Lab Invest 2002;82(10):1369–1375.

69. Hartmann JT, Fossa SD, Nichols CR, et al. Incidence of metachronous testicular cancer in patients with extragonadal germ cell tumors. J Natl Cancer Inst 2001;93(22):1733–1738.

70. Fossa SD, Aass N, Heilo A, et al. Testicular carcinoma in situ in patients with extragonadal germ-cell tumours: the clinical role of pretreatment biopsy. Ann Oncol 2003;14(9):1412–1418.

71. International Germ Cell Consensus Classification: a prognostic factor-based staging system for metastatic germ cell cancers. International Germ Cell Cancer Collaborative Group [see comments]. J Clin Oncol 1997;15(2):594–603.

72. Einhorn LH. Curing metastatic testicular cancer. Proc Natl Acad Sci USA 2002;99(7):4592–4595.

73. Lee AH, Mead GM, Theaker JM. The value of central histopathological review of testicular tumours before treatment. BJU Int 1999;84(1): 75–78.

74. Oosterhuis JW. The metastasis of human teratomas. In: Damjanov I, Knowles B, Solter D, eds. The Human Teratomas, 1st ed. Clifton, NJ: Humana Press, 1983:137–171.

75. Steyerberg EW, Keizer HJ, Habbema JD. Prediction models for the histology of residual masses after chemotherapy for metastatic testicular cancer. ReHiT Study Group. Int J Cancer 1999; 83(6):856–859.

76. Oosterhuis JW, Suurmeijer AJH, Sleijfer DTh, Schraffordt Koops H, Oldhoff J, Fleuren GJ. Effects of multiple drug chemotherapy (CIS-diammine-dichloro-platinum, bleomycin and vinblastine) on the maturation of retroperitoneal lymph node metastases of non-seminomatous germ cell tumors of the testis: no evidence for the novo induction of differentiation. Cancer 1983; 51:408–416.

77. Oosterhuis JW, De Jong B, Cornelisse CJ, et al. Karyotyping and DNA-flow cytometry of mature residual teratoma after intensive chemotherapy of disseminated non-seminomatous germ cell tumor of the testis: a report of two cases. Cancer Genet Cytogenet 1986;22:149–157.

78. Van Echten-Arends J, Van der Vloedt WS, Van de Pol M, et al. Comparison of the chromosomal pattern of primary testicular nonseminomas and residual mature teratomas after chemotherapy. Cancer Genet Cytogenet 1997;99:59–67.

79. Andre F, Fizazi K, Culine S, et al. The growing teratoma syndrome: results of therapy and long-term follow-up of 33 patients. Eur J Cancer 2000; 36(11):1389–1394.

80. Fizazi K, Tjulandin S, Salvioni R, et al. Viable malignant cells after primary chemotherapy for disseminated nonseminomatous germ cell tumors: prognostic factors and role of post-surgery chemotherapy-results from an international study group. J Clin Oncol 2001;19(10): 2647–2657.

81. Oldenburg J, Alfsen GC, Lien HH, Aass N, Waehre H, Fossa SD. Postchemotherapy retroperitoneal surgery remains necessary in patients with non-seminomatous testicular cancer and minimal residual tumor masses. J Clin Oncol 2003;21(17): 3310–3317.

82. Freedman LS, Jones WG, Peckham MJ, et al. Histopathology in the prediction of relapse of patients with stage I testicular teratoma treated by orchidectomy alone. Lancet 1987:294–298.

83. Vergouwe Y, Steyerberg EW, Eijkemans MJ, Albers P, Habbema JD. Predictors of occult metastasis in clinical stage I nonseminoma: a systematic review. J Clin Oncol 2003;21(22): 4092–4099.

84. Albers P, Siener R, Kliesch S, et al. Risk factors for relapse in clinical stage I nonseminomatous testicular germ cell tumors: results of the German Testicular Cancer Study Group Trial. J Clin Oncol 2003;21(8):1505–1512.

85. Mazumdar M, Bacik J, Tickoo SK, et al. Cluster analysis of p53 and Ki67 expression, apoptosis, alpha-fetoprotein, and human chorionic gonadotrophin indicates a favorable prognostic subgroup within the embryonal carcinoma germ cell tumor. J Clin Oncol 2003;21(14):2679–2688.

86. Mostofi FK. Testicular tumors: epidemiologic, etiologic and pathologic features. Cancer 1973; 32:1186–1201.

87. Bokemeyer C, Kollmannsberger C, Oechsle K, et al. Early prediction of treatment response to high-dose salvage chemotherapy in patients with relapsed germ cell cancer using [(18)F]FDG PET. Br J Cancer 2002;86(4):506–511.

88. Beyer J, Kramar A, Mandanas R, et al. High-dose chemotherapy as salvage treatment in germ cell tumors: a multivariate analysis of prognostic variables. J Clin Oncol 1996;14:2638–2645.

89. Miller KD, Loehrer PJ, Gonin R, Einhorn LH. Salvage chemotherapy with vinblastine, ifosfamide, and cisplatin in recurrent seminoma. J Clin Oncol 1997;15(4):1427–1431.

90. Loehrer PJ, Sr., Gonin R, Nichols CR, Weathers T, Einhorn LH. Vinblastine plus ifosfamide plus cisplatin as initial salvage therapy in recurrent germ cell tumor. J Clin Oncol 1998;16(7): 2500–2504.

91. Bhatia S, Abonour R, Porcu P, et al. High-dose chemotherapy as initial salvage chemotherapy in patients with relapsed testicular cancer. J Clin Oncol 2000;18(19):3346–3351.

92. Vaena DA, Abonour R, Einhorn LH. Long-term survival after high-dose salvage chemotherapy

for germ cell malignancies with adverse prognostic variables. J Clin Oncol 2003;21(22):4100–4104.

93. Baniel J, Foster RS, Gonin R, Messemer JE, Donohue JP, Einhorn LH. Late relapse of testicular cancer. J Clin Oncol 1995;13(5):1170–1176.

94. van Echten J, Timmer B, Dam A, Sleijfer DT, Schraffordt Koops H, de Jong B. Cytogenetic analysis of a mature teratoma and a yolk sac tumor component of a late relapse of a disseminated testicular nonseminoma. Cancer Genet Cytogenet 1999;111(1):49–54.

95. Nichols CR. Treatment of recurrent germ cell tumors. Semin Surg Oncol 1999;17(4):268–274.

96. George DW, Foster RS, Hromas RA, et al. Update on late relapse of germ cell tumor: a clinical and molecular analysis. J Clin Oncol 2003;21(1):113–122.

97. Kuczyk MA, Bokemeyer C, Kollmannsberger C, et al. Late relapse after treatment for nonseminomatous testicular germ cell tumors according to a single center-based experience. World J Urol 2003.

98. Donadio AC, Motzer RJ, Bajorin DF, et al. Chemotherapy for teratoma with malignant transformation. J Clin Oncol 2003;21(23):4285–4291.

99. Mayer F, Honecker F, Looijenga LHJ, Bokemeyer C. Towards understanding the biological basis of the response to cisplatin-based chemotherapy in germ cell tumors. Ann Oncol 2003;9:825–832.

100. Masters JR, Koberle B. Curing metastatic cancer: lessons from testicular germ-cell tumours. Nat Rev Cancer 2003;3(7):517–525.

101. Spierings DC, de Vries EG, Vellenga E, de Jong S. The attractive Achilles heel of germ cell tumours: an inherent sensitivity to apoptosis-inducing stimuli. J Pathol 2003;200(2):137–148.

102. Kartalou M, Essigmann JM. Mechanisms of resistance to cisplatin. Mutat Res 2001;478(1–2):23–43.

103. Ishida S, Lee J, Thiele DJ, Herskowitz I. Uptake of the anticancer drug cisplatin mediated by the copper transporter Ctr1 in yeast and mammals. Proc Natl Acad Sci USA 2002;99(22):14298–14302.

104. Sark MW, Timmer-Bosscha H, Meijer C, et al. Cellular basis for differential sensitivity to cisplatin in human germ cell tumour and colon carcinoma cell lines. Br J Cancer 1995;71(4):684–690.

105. Borst P, Evers R, Kool M, Wijnholds J. A family of drug transporters: the multidrug resistance-associated proteins. J Natl Cancer Inst 2000;92(16):1295–1302.

106. Scheffer GL, Kool M, Heijn M, et al. Specific detection of multidrug resistance proteins MRP1, MRP2, MRP3, MRP5, and MDR3 P-glyco-protein with a panel of monoclonal antibodies. Cancer Res 2000;60(18):5269–5277.

107. Izquierdo MA, Shoemaker RH, Flens MJ, et al. Overlapping phenotypes of multidrug resistance among panels of human cancer-cell lines. Int J Cancer 1996;65(2):230–237.

108. Mayer F, Stoop H, Scheffer GL, et al. Molecular determinants of treatment response in human germ cell tumors. Clin Cancer Res 2003;9(2):767–773.

109. Kool M, de Haas M, Scheffer GL, et al. Analysis of expression of cMOAT (MRP2), MRP3, MRP4, and MRP5, homologues of the multidrug resistance-associated protein gene (MRP1), in human cancer cell lines. Cancer Res 1997;57(16):3537–3547.

110. Jansen BA, Brouwer J, Reedijk J. Glutathione induces cellular resistance against cationic dinuclear platinum anticancer drugs. J Inorg Biochem 2002;89(3–4):197–202.

111. Masters JR, Thomas R, Hall AG, et al. Sensitivity of testis tumour cells to chemotherapeutic drugs: role of detoxifying pathways. Eur J Cancer 1996;32A(7):1248–1253.

112. Koropatnick J, Kloth DM, Kadhim S, Chin JL, Cherian MG. Metallothionein expression and resistance to cisplatin in a human germ cell tumor cell line. J Pharmacol Exp Ther 1995;275:1681–1687.

113. Meijer C, Timmer A, De Vries EG, et al. Role of metallothionein in cisplatin sensitivity of germ-cell tumours. Int J Cancer 2000;85(6):777–781.

114. Strohmeyer T, Klone A, Wagner G, Hartmann M, Sies H. Glutathione S-transferases in human testicular germ cell tumors: changes of expression and activity. J Urol 1992;147:1424–1428.

115. Pera MF, Blasco Lafita MJ, Mills J. Cultured stem cells from human testicular teratomas: the nature of human embryonal carcinoma, and its comparison with two types of yolk-sac carcinoma. Int J Cancer 1987;40:334–343.

116. Koberle B, Grimaldi KA, Sunters A, Hartley JA, Kelland LR, Masters JR. DNA repair capacity and cisplatin sensitivity of human testis tumour cells. Int J Cancer 1997;70(5):551–555.

117. Burger H, Nooter K, Boersma AWM, Kortland CJ, Stoter G. Lack of correlation between cisplatin-induced apoptosis, p53 status, and expression of bcl-2 family proteins in testicular germ cell tumor cell lines. Int J Cancer 1997;73:592–599.

118. Cairns J. Somatic stem cells and the kinetics of mutagenesis and carcinogenesis. Proc Natl Acad Sci USA 2002;99(16):10567–10570.

119. Van Sloun PP, Jansen JG, Weeda G, et al. The role of nucleotide excision repair in protecting embryonic stem cells from genotoxic effects of UV-induced DNA damage. Nucleic Acids Res 1999;27(16):3276–3282.

120. Reed E. Platinum-DNA adduct, nucleotide excision repair and platinum based anti-cancer chemotherapy. Cancer Treat Rev 1998;24(5):331–344.

121. Koberle B, Payne J, Grimaldi KA, Hartley JA, Masters JR. DNA repair in cisplatin-sensitive and resistant human cell lines measured in specific genes by quantitative polymerase chain reaction. Biochem Pharmacol 1996;52(11):1729–1734.

122. Koberle B, Masters JR, Hartley JA, Wood RD. Defective repair of cisplatin-induced DNA damage caused by reduced XPA protein in testicular germ cell tumours. Curr Biol 1999;9(5):273–276.

123. Honecker F, Mayer F, Stoop H, et al. Xeroderma pigmentosum group A protein and chemotherapy-resistance in human germ cell tumors. Lab Invest 2003;83:1489–1495.

124. Zamble DB, Mikata Y, Eng CH, Sandman KE, Lippard SJ. Testis-specific HMG-domain protein alters the responses of cells to cisplatin. J Inorg Biochem 2002;91(3):451–462.

125. Lutzker SG, Mathew R, Taller DR. A p53 dose-response relationship for sensitivity to DNA damage in isogenic teratocarcinoma cells. Oncogene 2001;20(23):2982–2986.

126. Robertson KA, Bullock HA, Xu Y, et al. Altered expression of Ape1/ref-1 in germ cell tumors and overexpression in NT2 cells confers resistance to bleomycin and radiation. Cancer Res 2001;61(5):2220–2225.

127. Zhou BB, Elledge SJ. The DNA damage response: putting checkpoints in perspective. Nature 2000;408(6811):433–439.

128. Lothe RA, Peltomaeki P, Tommerup N, et al. Molecular genetic changes in human male germ cell tumors. Lab Invest 1995;73:606–614.

129. Lage H, Dietel M. Involvement of the DNA mismatch repair system in antineoplastic drug resistance. J Cancer Res Clin Oncol 1999;125(3–4):156–165.

130. Van Rijnsoever M, Elsaleh H, Joseph D, McCaul K, Iacopetta B. CpG island methylator phenotype is an independent predictor of survival benefit from 5–fluorouracil in stage III colorectal cancer. Clin Cancer Res 2003;9(8):2898–2903.

131. Hawn MT, Umar A, Carethers JM, et al. Evidence for a connection between the mismatch repair system and the G2 cell cycle checkpoint. Cancer Res 1995;55(17):3721–3725.

132. Davis TW, Wilson-Van Patten C, Meyers M, et al. Defective expression of the DNA mismatch repair protein, MLH1, alters G2–M cell cycle checkpoint arrest following ionizing radiation. Cancer Res 1998;58(4):767–778.

133. Devouassoux-Shisheboran M, Mauduit C, Bouvier R, et al. Expression of hMLH1 and hMSH2 and assessment of microsatellite instability in testicular and mediastinal germ cell tumours. Mol Hum Reprod 2001;7(12):1099–1105.

134. Mayer F, Gillis AJM, Dinjens W, Oosterhuis JW, Bokemeyer C, Looijenga LHJ. Microsatellite instability of germ cell tumors is associated with resistance to systemic treatment. Cancer Res 2002;62:2758–2760.

135. Schenk PW, Boersma AW, Brandsma JA, et al. SKY1 is involved in cisplatin-induced cell kill in Saccharomyces cerevisiae, and inactivation of its human homologue, SRPK1, induces cisplatin resistance in a human ovarian carcinoma cell line. Cancer Res 2001;61(19):6982–6986.

136. Schenk PW, Stoop H, Mayer F, et al. Resistance to platinum-containing chemotherapy in testicular germ cell tumours is associated with downregulation of the protein kinase SRPK1. Neoplasia 2004;6:297–301.

137. Levine AJ. p53, the cellular gatekeeper for growth and division. Cell 1997;88:323–331.

138. Parris CN, Walker MC, Masters JR, Arlett CF. Inherent sensitivity and induced resistance to chemotherapeutic drugs and irradiation in human cancer cell lines: relationship to mutation frequencies. Cancer Res 1990;50(23):7513–7518.

139. Lutzker SG, Levine AJ. A functionally inactive p53 protein in teratocarcinoma cells is activated by either DNA damage or cellular differentiation. Nature Med 1996;2:804–810.

140. Burger H, Nooter K, Boersma AW, et al. Distinct p53–independent apoptotic cell death signalling pathways in testicular germ cell tumour cell lines. Int J Cancer 1999;81(4):620–628.

141. Houldsworth J, Xiao H, Murty VV, et al. Human male germ cell tumor resistance to cisplatin is linked to TP53 gene mutation. Oncogene 1998;16(18):2345–2349.

142. Kersemaekers AMF, Mayer F, Molier M, et al. Role of P53 and MDM2 in treatment response of human germ cell tumors. J Clin Oncol 2002;20:1551–1561.

143. Woods DB, Vousden KH. Regulation of p53 function. Exp Cell Res 2001;264(1):56–66.

144. Di Como CJ, Urist MJ, Babayan I, et al. p63 expression profiles in human normal and tumor tissues. Clin Cancer Res 2002;8(2):494–501.

145. Chresta CM, Masters JRW, Hickman JA. Hypersensitivity of human testicular tumors to etoposide-induced apoptosis is associated with functional p53 and a high Bax:Bcl-2 ratio. Cancer Res 1996;56:1834–1841.

146. Burger H, Nooter K, Boersma AWM, Kortland CJ, Van den Berg A, Stoter G. Expression of p53, p21/waf/cip, bcl2, bax, bcl-x, and bak in radiation-induced apoptosis in testicular germ cell tumor lines. Int J Radiat Oncol Biol Phys 1998;41(2):415–424.

147. Baltaci S, Orhan D, Turkolmez K, Yesilli C, Beduk Y, Tulunay O. P53, bcl-2 and bax immunoreactivity as predictors of response and outcome after chemotherapy for metastatic germ cell testicular tumours. BJU Int 2001;87(7):661–666.

148. Arriola EL, Rodriguez-Lopez AM, Hickman JA, Chresta CM. Bcl-2 overexpression results in reciprocal downregulation of Bcl-X(L) and sensitizes human testicular germ cell tumours to chemotherapy-induced apoptosis. Oncogene 1999;18(7):1457–1464.

149. Lee J, Richburg JH, Younkin SC, Boekelheide K. The Fas system is a key regulator of germ cell apoptosis in the testis. Endocrinology 1997; 138(5):2081–2088.

150. Francavilla S, D'Abrizio P, Cordeschi G, et al. Fas expression correlates with human germ cell degeneration in meiotic and post-meiotic arrest of spermatogenesis. Mol Hum Reprod 2002;8(3): 213–220.

151. Kersemaekers AM, van Weeren PC, Oosterhuis JW, Looijenga LH. Involvement of the Fas/FasL pathway in the pathogenesis of germ cell tumours of the adult testis. J Pathol 2002;196(4): 423–429.

152. Sugihara A, Saiki S, Tsuji M, et al. Expression of fas and fas ligand in the testis and testicular germ cell tumors: an immunohistochemical study. Anticancer Res 1997;17:3861–3865.

153. Spierings DC, de Vries EG, Vellenga E, de Jong S. Loss of drug-induced activation of the CD95 apoptotic pathway in a cisplatin-resistant testicular germ cell tumor cell line. Cell Death Differ 2003;10(7):808–822.

154. Takayama H, Takakuwa T, Tsujimoto Y, et al. Frequent Fas gene mutations in testicular germ cell tumors. Am J Pathol 2002;161:635–641.

155. Mueller T, Voigt W, Simon H, et al. Failure of activation of caspase-9 induces a higher threshold for apoptosis and Cisplatin resistance in testicular cancer. Cancer Res 2003;63(2):513–521.

156. Koch S, Mayer F, Honecker F, Schittenhelm M, Bokemeyer C. Efficacy of cytotoxic agents used in the treatment of testicular germ cell tumours under normoxic and hypoxic conditions in vitro. Br J Cancer 2003;89(11):2133–2139.

157. De Graaff WE, Oosterhuis JW, De Jong B, et al. Cytogenetic analysis of the mature teratoma and the choriocarcinoma component of a testicular mixed nonseminomatous germ cell tumor. Cancer Genet Cytogenet 1992;61:67–73.

158. Strohmeyer T, Reissmann P, Cordon-Cardo C, Hartmann M, Ackermann R, Slamon D. Correlation between retinoblastoma gene expression and differentiation in human testicular tumors. Proc Natl Acad Sci USA 1991;88:6662–6666.

159. Fan S, Chang JK, Smith ML, Duba D, Fornace AJ Jr, O'Connor PM. Cells lacking CIP1/WAF1 genes exhibit preferential sensitivity to cisplatin and nitrogen mustard. Oncogene 1997;14(18):2127–2136.

160. Bartkova J, Rajpert-De Meyts E, Skakkebæk NE, Lukas J, Bartek J. Deregulation of the G1/S-phase control in human testicular germ cell tumours. APMIS 2003;111(1):252–265; discussion 265–266.

161. Timmer-Bosscha H, de Vries EG, Meijer C, Oosterhuis JW, Mulder NH. Differential effects of all-trans-retinoic acid, docosahexaenoic acid, and hexadecylphosphocholine on cisplatin-induced cytotoxicity and apoptosis in a cisplatin-sensitive and resistant human embryonal carcinoma cell line. Cancer Chemother Pharmacol 1998;41(6):469–476.

162. Ulbright TM. Germ cell neoplasms of the testis. Am J Surg Pathol 1993;17:1075–1091.

163. Motzer RJ, Amsterdam A, Prieto V, et al. Teratoma with malignant transformation: diverse malignant histologies arising in men with germ cell tumors. J Urol 1998;159:133–138.

Part V

Penile Cancer

23

A Scientific Understanding of the Development of Penile Tumors

T.R. Leyshon Griffiths and J. Kilian Mellon

Penile cancer is a relatively rare disease in developed countries. The incidence in Europe is 1 per 100,000 men per year with a mean age at diagnosis of 60 years. Higher incidence rates have been reported in Africa, Asia, and in parts of South America [1–3]. Approximately 95% of all penile cancers in developed countries are squamous cell carcinomas (SCCs); the remaining 5% are nonsquamous primary neoplasms such as sarcomas, melanomas, basal cell carcinomas, and lymphomas. Penile carcinomas include several different histological subtypes. The majority are well differentiated keratinizing SCCs; the second most common subtype is verrucous carcinoma, and less prevalent types include basaloid carcinomas and warty carcinomas. A further subtype is the giant condyloma of Buschke-Löwenstein (GCBL). There is confusion in the literature with regard to this tumor, because some investigators believe that GCBL is simply a clinical variant of verrucous carcinoma; in contrast, others regard these lesions as distinct entities. Although the GCBL tumor shows none of the histological criteria for malignancy, it behaves like a carcinoma, with a tendency to compress and displace deeper tissues by downward growth rather than by infiltration or metastasis. Invasive penile cancer initially occurs on the glans (48%), the prepuce (25%), the glans and prepuce (9%), the coronal sulcus (6%) and the penile shaft (2%) [4].

Three preneoplastic lesions of the penis have been described: erythroplasia of Queyrat, Bowen's disease, and bowenoid papulosis. These lesions have also been referred to as high-grade penile intraepithelial neoplasia (PIN), dysplasia, and carcinoma in situ. However, the minor histological differences between bowenoid papulosis and Bowen's disease and erythroplasia of Queyrat do not allow for an accurate diagnosis on the basis of histological findings alone. Essentially, they are distinguished on the basis of clinical features. Bowenoid papulosis and Bowen's disease both occur on the penile shaft, whereas erythroplasia is found on the glans or prepuce. Characteristic features include papules in bowenoid papulosis, crusted and scaly plaques in Bowen's disease, and erythematous plaques in erythroplasia of Queyrat. Bowenoid papulosis usually presents in men aged 20 to 40 years, Bowen's disease at 30 to 50 years, and erythroplasia of Queyrat at 40 to 60 years. The incidence of progression to invasive SCC is more common for erythroplasia of Queyrat than for Bowen's disease, with an incidence varying from 10% to 33% [5,6]. Patients with carcinoma in situ of the penis are usually uncircumcised.

Etiology

The development of penile cancer is most likely a stepwise chain of events over a period of years, from preneoplastic lesions to SCC. The etiology of penile SCC is probably multifactorial [7]; poor personal hygiene associated with smegma retention, and phimosis are the most commonly incriminated. Other factors that have been associated with this tumor include balanitis xerotica obliterans (BXO), a history of smoking, and human papillomavirus (HPV) infection. Men exposed to psoralens and ultraviolet irradiation for psoriasis are also at higher risk of developing penile cancer.

Personal Hygiene and Circumcision

Although there are data suggesting that circumcision at birth provides excellent protection against penile cancer, equally low incidence rates can be achieved in uncircumcised males who practice good hygiene. Indeed, the incidence of penile cancer has been reported to be falling in uncircumcised men. In one study, a decreasing penile cancer rate of 0.82/100,000 was found in Denmark (where circumcision is uncommon) compared with an incidence of 1/100,000 in the United States [8].

Phimosis and Balanitis Xerotica Obliterans

Phimosis has been reported to be present in 44% to 85% of men with penile SCC [7]. Balanitis xerotica obliterans (BXO) of the penis is a well-recognized inflammatory dermatosis that causes atrophic and sclerotic changes; this may lead to secondary problems with phimosis and meatal strictures. The association of SCC arising on a background of BXO has not been examined as fully in males as has lichen sclerosus for vulvar SCC in females. It is known that about 40% of

penile SCC also have histological changes of BXO [9,10]. However, the pathogenesis of penile SCC developing in BXO has never been described. One study described 86 patients with penile BXO, three of whom (3%) subsequently developed SCC [11]. However, phimosis often accompanies BXO. It therefore remains unclear whether phimosis is a more important etiological factor than BXO itself.

Smoking

A consistent association has been found between penile cancer and smoking that is dose dependent [7]. In a multivariate analysis of risk factors in 503 patients with penile cancer and age-matched controls, phimosis (odds ratio 7.2), smoking (odds ratio 1.7), chewing tobacco (odds ratio 4.1), or the use of snuff (odds ratio 4.2) were shown to be independent variables [12].

The Human Papillomavirus

Prevalence in Penile Cancer (Table 23.1)

The HPV has been detected in 15% to 80% of penile carcinoma specimens, depending on the sensitivity of the detection method and the selection of the tumor type [13–20]. In studies of more than 100 patients and utilizing polymerase chain reaction (PCR)-based techniques, HPV prevalence in penile carcinoma is 22% to 63% [15,19,20]. In the largest multicenter study of patients with penile cancer to date, of 142

Table 23.1. Prevalence of human papillomavirus (HPV) DNA in penile lesions in Europe and the United States

Genital lesion	Overall HPV-DNA positivity (%)	High-risk HPV-DNA positivity (%)
Penile SCC	40	80–90
Verrucous	20	30
Keratinizing	30	80
Basaloid	80	100
Warty	80	100
Penile carcinoma in situ	90	80
Anogenital condylomas	100	5–10

Low-risk HPVs: −6, −11.
High-risk HPVs: −16, −18, −31, −33, −39, −42, −51, −52, −53, −54.

patients from the United States and Paraguay, HPV-DNA was detected in 40 (42%) patients [19]. DNA amplification was performed using a novel, sensitive, broad-spectrum HPV PCR assay. There was no significant difference between HPV prevalence in tumors from Paraguay and the United States.

A comparison of HPV prevalence rates in penile, cervical and vulvar carcinoma indicate that the etiology and the pathogenetic pathways of penile SCC may parallel the pathogenetic pathways of vulvar, but not cervical, carcinoma. Indeed, the overall prevalence of HPV-DNA in penile carcinoma is lower than in cervical carcinoma (approximately 100%) [21,22] and similar to that reported for vulvar carcinoma (approximately 50%) [23]. Moreover, the correlation between HPV-DNA detection and histological tumor subtypes is similar in vulvar and penile carcinoma. In one study, the basaloid subtype of penile carcinoma was HPV-DNA–positive in 80% (12 of 15) cases and was associated with HPV-16 [19]; in another study, HPV-16 was detected in 82% (nine of 11) cases of the basaloid subtype [24]. With regard to the warty subtype of penile carcinoma, overall HPV-DNA positivity was 100% (five of five) [19] and HPV-16 positivity was 60% (three of five) [24].

The HPV status of verrucous carcinomas of the penis has been assessed in several reports; of 26 cases, only three have been found to be positive for HPV-DNA (12%), and all were positive for low-risk HPVs [13,15,25–28]. Some authors advocate that screening for HPV may be a useful adjunct in differentiating GCBL from verrucous carcinoma. Indeed, published reports suggest that GCBL is always associated with HPV infection. However, in view of our current understanding, the presence or absence of specific HPV types cannot be used to predict malignant transformation.

Prevalence in Carcinoma in Situ

Approximately 90% of carcinoma in situ are HPV-positive, of which around 80% are high-risk HPVs; HPV-16 is the most frequently detected [13,19]. These findings suggest that carcinoma in situ may be a precursor lesion to only a subset of invasive carcinomas, which would include the basaloid and warty subtypes.

Oncogenic Effect of Human Papillomavirus

High-Risk and Low-Risk Human Papillomavirus

The ability of genes to extend the life span of cells in culture indefinitely is termed immortalization. By contrast, transformation requires the acquisition of at least some of the properties characteristic of malignant cells, in particular autonomous proliferation. So-called low-risk HPV subtypes 6 and 11 have a strong tendency to induce anogenital condylomata, but are rarely associated with genital cancer. They do not have immortalizing or transforming properties. In contrast, so-called high-risk HPV subtypes 16, 18, 31, 33, 39, 42, 51, and 54 are linked with genital carcinoma. Immortalizing activities of HPV-16 and HPV-18 DNA have been demonstrated in cultures of primary human keratinocytes, cells that resemble the normal target of the virus [29].

High-risk HPVs exert their oncogenic effect by expressing the oncoproteins E6 and E7, which bind to and inactivate the p53 and retinoblastoma (Rb) tumor-suppressor products, respectively. These activities obviate the need for (epi)genetic alterations, leading to disturbance of the $p14^{ARF}$/MDM2/p53 and $p16^{INK4A}$/cyclin D/Rb pathways. Alteration of these pathways is among the most common alterations seen in human carcinomas, and it has been firmly established that inactivation of these pathways is essential for the genesis of the great majority of human malignancies [30].

HPV-E7 Viral Oncoproteins and $p16^{INK4A}$/Cyclin D/Rb Pathway

The protein product of the Rb tumor-suppressor gene and other Rb family members, including p107 and p130, can block cell cycle progression from the G1 to the S phase. In its active state, Rb is hypophosphorylated and binds to a number of transcription factors, most notably members of the E2F family. Cyclin-dependent kinase (CDK) phosphorylation of Rb inactivates Rb. As a consequence, transcription factors are released from Rb, allowing them to mediate transcriptional activation of S-phase genes. The binding of

HPV-E7 proteins to Rb and Rb-related proteins equates with functional inactivation of Rb; higher affinity binding can be detected for E7 proteins of high-risk HPVs than for those of low-risk HPVs such as HPV-6 and HPV-11. Additionally, the E7-induced ubiquitin-mediated degradation of Rb appears to be essential to efficiently overcome cell cycle arrest. E7 may also degrade Rb family members [31].

There is substantial genetic evidence that only one component in the p16^{INK4A}/cyclinD/Rb pathway needs to be inactivated for neoplastic clonal expansion [32,33]. Evidence from studies in lung cancer suggests that there are important phenotypic differences between cells that have inactive Rb but active p16 function, as compared to cells with active Rb and inactive p16 [32,34]. For example, Rb undergoes mutational inactivation in the genesis of 90% of small cell lung cancers, whereas in non–small-cell lung cancer, the preferential target is p16. In many SCCs that do not reveal viral involvement, the p16^{INK4A}/cyclinD/Rb pathway is commonly disrupted through mutation, deletion, or hypermethylation of the p16 gene, resulting in reduced or absent p16 expression [35,36]. Data from functional studies in mice suggest that overexpression of the polycomb group (PcG) gene BMI-1 can provide a further alternative mechanism to downregulate p16 [37]. In contrast, where the Rb protein is functionally inactive either as a consequence of gene mutation or binding of high-risk HPV-E7 proteins, p16 is released from negative feedback by Rb, and is expressed at enhanced levels in these tumors [38]. P16 is a negative regulator of the cell cycle; its primary action is to inhibit interaction between CDKs 4/6 with cyclin D1. It also simultaneously releases free p27Kip1, which can now transfer to form inhibitory CDK2/cyclinE/p27 complexes.

HPV E6 Viral Oncoproteins and p14^{ARF}/MDM2/p53

The p53 tumor-suppressor gene is located on chromosome 17p13.1 and functions as a negative regulator of cell growth. In response to DNA damage, it can induce G1 arrest or apoptosis. It is known that the p53 protein is a transcription factor that blocks cell proliferation and mediates G1 arrest via the induction of the p21 gene (WAF-1). The 21-kd protein product of this gene

encodes for an inhibitor of the cyclin-dependent kinases, CDK2 and CDK4; consequently, via hypophosphorylation of Rb and subsequent E2F binding, the cell cycle is prolonged in the G1 phase.

Mutations in the p53 gene are very common in almost all solid tumors, with the exception of anogenital carcinomas [39]. This suggests that HPV targeting of p53 protein is an alternative to p53 gene mutation as a mechanism for p53 inactivation. The carcinogenic effect of HPV may be explained, in part, by the transforming viral protein E6, which binds to and induces the degradation of p53 protein through the ubiquitin pathway [40]. It has been proposed that the existence of a common polymorphism of the p53 gene at codon 72, which results in translation to either proline (p53Pro) or arginine (p53Arg), could play a critical role in the development of mucous and cutaneous SCC [41]. One study has shown that the protein E6 from HPV-16 and HPV-18 is more effective at degrading p53Arg than p53Pro in vivo; HPV-11 E6 is less active toward p53Arg and inactive with p53Pro [42].

High-Risk HPV-E6 Viral Oncoprotein and p53-Independent Activities

Activation of Telomerase

The E6 protein has been implicated in the activation of the enzyme telomerase—a potential mechanism for HPV-induced immortalization [43]. Mammalian telomeres are structures at the chromosomal tips consisting of multiple repeats of TTAGG, which shorten as a function of division in vivo as a consequence of an intrinsic inability to replicate the 3' end of DNA. Telomerase replaces the telomeric repeats and is not normally expressed in somatic cells. Activation of telomerase enables cells to escape from the senescence signaled by telomeric shortening. Regulation of telomerase activity has been shown to occur primarily through the level of expression of the human telomerase reverse transcriptase (hTert) gene, encoding the catalytic subunit. The precise mechanism of telomerase activation by E6 protein is unknown; the current favored mechanism is transcriptional activation of the promoter of the hTert gene [44].

Interaction with PDZ Domain-Containing Proteins

High-risk E6 proteins interact with several PDZ domain-containing proteins like hD1g [45], MUPP1 [46], and MAG-1, -2, -3 [47], resulting in their ubiquitin-mediated degradation. PDZ domains consist of approximately 90 amino acid long protein–protein interaction units located at areas of cell–cell contact, such as synaptic junctions in neurons and tight junctions in epithelial cells. It is suggested that PDZ proteins act as molecular scaffolds.

p14^{ARF}/MDM2/p53 and Pathways in Human Squamous Cell Carcinoma of the Penis

In the largest study to date, the frequency of *p53* gene mutations was 33% (seven of 21) in SCC of the penis [48]. This included only 22% (two of nine) HPV-positive tumors, and 42% (five of 12) HPV-negative tumors. In a study of 45 French men with penile SCC, the *p53* Arg/Arg genotype was not a risk factor for the development of SCC, and no correlation was found between *p53* polymorphism at codon 72 and the presence of HPV-DNA [49].

Nuclear immunopositivity for p53 has been detected in 26% to 41% of cases [48,50,51]. This difference could be attributable to the different antibodies used in these series. The simultaneous presence of p53 protein accumulation and DNA of high-risk HPV types appears to be a common finding in cervical and penile lesions. In one study, p53 immunopositivity was detected in 40% (17 of 42) penile carcinomas, most of these being also HPV-DNA positive [50]. P53 immunoreactivity is an independent prognostic factor for lymph node metastasis in penile carcinoma [51].

In contrast, two studies have compared the clinical outcomes of patients with HPV-positive versus HPV-negative penile carcinomas. Both reported no difference in lymph node metastasis rates or survival [52,53].

p16^{INK4A}/Cyclin D/Rb Pathways in Human Squamous Cell Carcinoma of the Penis

In a recent study, alterations pointing to a disturbed p16^{INK4A}/cyclin D1/Rb pathway are commonly present in penile carcinomas [54]. Three alternative mechanisms of disruption were identified (Fig. 23.1); activity of high-risk HPV and the resulting increase in p16^{INK4A} expression was the most frequently detected mechanism, followed by p16^{INK4A} hypermethylation and BMI-1 overexpression. Strong p16 immunostaining was found in 65% of the tumors containing HPV-DNA; this frequency increased to 81% when only the high-risk HPV-positive cases were considered, and 92% when the analysis was restricted to the HPV-16–positive cases with E6/E7 expression. In contrast, in tumors without HPV-DNA, only 6% stained strongly for p16. The

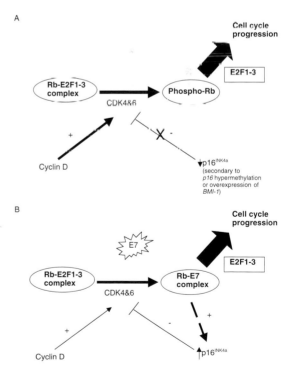

Fig. 23.1. Simplified models depicting effect of alterations in the p16^{INK4A}/cyclin D/Rb pathway on cell cycle progression and p16 protein expression. A: Effect of *p16* gene alteration. B: Effect of HPV-E7 oncoprotein binding to Rb.

frequency of p16^{INK4A} promoter methylation was higher in HPV-DNA–negative tumors (21%) than in HPV-DNA–positive cases (10%). The suggestion again is that penile carcinoma is etiologically heterogeneous, with only a proportion of cases attributable to HPV infection.

Conclusion

The great majority of penile carcinomas diagnosed in Europe and the United States are of a nonbasaloid, nonwarty histological type. At present, an etiological relationship with HPV seems most plausible for penile carcinomas of the basaloid or warty subtypes; the precursor lesion is likely to be carcinoma in situ. In contrast, the precursor lesion for keratinizing SCC or verrucous carcinoma of the penis is not well established. Moreover, a further assessment of BXO in the absence of phimosis, or after circumcision, is needed to determine its role as an independent risk factor for the development of invasive penile cancer. It is also becoming clear that the mere presence of HPV is insufficient to have prognostic implications. Demonstration of HPV-mediated alterations in signaling pathways appears to be necessary. Currently, detection of elevated p16 expression appears to be a potential biomarker of HPV-mediated Rb inactivation in penile SCC.

References

1. Landis SH, Murray T, Bolden S, et al. Cancer statistics, 1999. CA Cancer J Clin 1999;49:8–31.
2. Narayana AS, Olney LE, Loening SA. Carcinoma of the penis: analysis of 219 cases. Cancer 1982;49: 2185–2191.
3. Ornellas AA, Seixax AL, Marota A. Surgical treatment of invasive squamous cell carcinoma of the penis: retrospective analysis of 350 cases. J Urol 1994;151:1244–1249.
4. Burgers JK, Badalement RA, Drago JR. Penile cancer. Clinical presentation, diagnosis and staging. Urol Clin North Am 1992;19:247–256.
5. Graham JH, Helwig EB. Erythroplasia of Queyrat. A clinicopathologic and histological study. Cancer 1973;32:1396–1414.
6. Mikhail GR. Cancers, precancers, and pseudocancers on the male genitalia. A review of clinical appearances, histopathology, and management. J Dermatol Surg Oncol 1980;6:1027–1035.
7. Dillner J, von Krogh G, Horenblas S, et al. Aetiology of squamous cell carcinoma of the penis. Scand J Urol Nephrol Suppl 2000;205:189–193.
8. Frisch M, Friis S, Kjaer SK, et al. Falling incidence of penile cancer in an uncircumcised population. BMJ 1995;311:1471
9. Powell J, Robson A, Cranston D, et al. High incidence of lichen sclerosus in patients with squamous cell carcinoma of the penis. Br J Dermatol 2001;145:85–89.
10. Perceau G, Derancourt C, Clavel C, et al. Lichen sclerosus is frequently present in penile squamous cell carcinomas but is not always associated with oncogenic human papillomavirus. Br J Dermatol 2003;148:934–938.
11. Nasca MR, Innocenzi D, Micali G. Penile cancer among patients with genital lichen sclerosus. J Am Acad Dermatol 1999;41:911–914.
12. Harish K, Ravi R. The role of tobacco in penile carcinoma. Br J Urol 1995;75:375–377.
13. Cupp MR, Malek RS, Goellner JR, et al. The detection of human papillomavirus deoxyribonucleic acid in intraepithelial, in situ, verrucous and invasive carcinoma of the penis. J Urol 1995;154: 1024–1029.
14. Higgins GD, Uzelin DM, Phillips GE, et al. Differing prevalence of human papillomavirus RNA in penile dysplasias and carcinomas may reflect differing aetiologies. Am J Clin Pathol 1992;97: 272–278.
15. Gregoire L, Cubilla AL, Reuter VE, et al. Preferential association of human papillomavirus with high-grade histologic variants of penile-invasive squamous cell carcinoma. J Natl Cancer Inst USA 1995;87:1705–1709.
16. Chan KW, Lam KY, Chan AC, et al. Prevalence of human papillomavirus types 16 and 18 in penile carcinoma: a study of 41 cases using PCR. J Clin Pathol 1994;47:823–826.
17. Ding Q, Zhang Y, Sun S. Role of PCR and dot blot hybridisation in the detection of human papillomavirus of the penile cancer. Chinese J Surg 1996;34:19–21.
18. Sarkar FH, Miles BJ, Plieth DH, et al. Detection of human papillomavirus in squamous neoplasm of penis. J Urol 1992;147:389–392.
19. Rubin MA, Kleter B, Zhou M, et al. Detection and typing of human papillomavirus DNA in penile carcinoma. Am J Pathol 2001;159:1211–1218.
20. Iwasawa A, Kumamoto Y, Fujinaga K. Detection of human papillomavirus deoxyribonucleic acid in penile carcinoma by polymerase chain reaction and in situ hybridisation. J Urol 1993;149:59–63.
21. Bosch FX, Manos MM, Munoz N, et al. Prevalence of human papillomavirus in cervical cancer: a worldwide perspective. International Biological Study on Cervical Cancer (IBSCC) Study Group. J Natl Cancer Inst 1995;87:796–802.

22. Van Muyden RC, ter Harmsel BW, Smedts FM, et al. Detection and typing of human papillomavirus in cervical carcinomas in Russian women: a prognostic study. Cancer 1999;85:2011–2016.

23. Bloss JD, Liao SY, Wilczynski SP, et al. Clinical and histological features of vulvar carcinomas analysed for human papillomavirus status: evidence that squamous cell carcinoma of the vulva has more than one aetiology. Hum Pathol 1991; 22:711–718.

24. Cubilla AL, Reuter VE, Gregoire L, et al. Basaloid squamous cell carcinoma: a distinctive human papilloma-virus related penile neoplasm: a report of 20 cases. Am J Surg Pathol 1998;22:755–761.

25. Noel JC, Vandenbossche M, Peny MO, et al. Verrucous carcinoma of the penis: importance of human papillomavirus typing for diagnosis and therapeutic decision. Eur Urol 1992;22:83–85.

26. Masih AS, Stoler MH, Farrow GM, et al. Penile verrucous carcinoma: a clinicopathologic, human papillomavirus typing and flow cytometric analysis. Mod Pathol 1992;5:48–55.

27. Masih AS, Stoler MH, Farrow GM, et al. Human papillomavirus in penile squamous cell lesions. A comparison of an isotopic RNA and two commercial nonisotopic DNA in situ hybridisation methods. Arch Pathol Lab Med 1993;117:302–307.

28. Dianzani C, Bucci M, Pierangeli A, et al. Association of human papillomavirus type 11 with carcinoma of the penis. Urology 1998;51:1046–1048.

29. Durst M, Dzarlieva-Petrusevska RT, Boukamp P, et al. Molecular and cytogenetic analysis of immortalised human primary keratinocytes obtained after transfection with human papillomavirus type 16 DNA. Oncogene 1987;1:251–256.

30. Scherr CJ. The INK4a/ARF network in tumour suppression. Nature Rev Mol Cell Biol 2001;2: 731–737.

31. Giarre M, Caldeira S, Malanchi I, et al. Induction of pRb degradation by the human papillomavirus type 16 E7 protein is essential to efficiently overcome p16INK4a-imposed G1 cell cycle arrest. J Virol 2001;75:4705–4712.

32. Otterson GA, Kratzke RA, Coxon A, et al. Absence of p16INK4 protein is restricted to the subset of lung cancer lines that retains wildtype RB. Oncogene 1994;9:3375–3378.

33. Weinberg RA. The retinoblastoma protein and cell cycle control. Cell 1995;81:323–330.

34. Kelley MJ, Nakagawa K, Steinberg SM, et al. Differential inactivation of CDKN2 and Rb protein in non-small cell and small-cell lung cancer cell lines. J Natl Cancer Inst 1995;87:756–761.

35. Schutte M, Hruban RH, Geradts J, et al. Abrogation of the Rb/p16 tumour-suppressive pathway in virtually all pancreatic carcinomas. Cancer Res 1997;57:3126–3130.

36. Esteller M, Herman JG. Cancer as an epigenetic disease: DNA methylation and chromatin alterations in human tumours. J Pathol 2002;196: 1–7.

37. Jacobs JJ, Kieborn K, Marino S, et al. The oncogene and Polycomb-group gene bmi-1 regulates cell proliferation and senescence through the ink4a locus. Nature 1999;397:164–168.

38. Li Y, Nichols MA, Shay JW, et al. Transcriptional repression of the D-type cyclin-dependent kinase inhibitor p16 by the retinoblastoma susceptibility gene product pRb. Cancer Res 1994;54: 6078–6082.

39. Scheffner M, Munger K, Byrne JC, et al. The state of the p53 and retinoblastoma genes in human cervical carcinoma cell lines. Proc Natl Acad Sci USA 1991;88:5523–5527.

40. Scheffner M, Werness BA, Huibregtse JM, et al. The E6 oncoprotein encoded by human papillomavirus 16 and 18 promotes the degradation of p53. Cell 1990;63:1129–1136.

41. Bastiaens MT, Struyk L, Tjong-A-Hung SP, et al. Cutaneous squamous cell carcinoma and p53 codon 72 polymorphism: a need for screening? Mol Carcinog 2001;30:56–61.

42. Storey A, Thomas M, Kalita A, et al. Role of a p53 polymorphism in the development of human papillomavirus-associated cancer. Nature 1998; 393:229–234.

43. Klingelhutz AJ, Foster SA, McDougall JK. Telomerase activation by the E6 gene product of human papillomavirus type 16. Nature 1996;380:79–82.

44. Gewin L, Galloway DA. E box-dependent activation of telomerase by human papillomavirus type 16 E6 does not require induction of c-myc. J Virol 2001;75:7198–7201.

45. Kiyono T, Hiraiwa A, Fujita M, et al. Binding of high-risk human papillomavirus E6 oncoproteins to the human homologue of the Drosophila discs large tumor suppressor protein. Proc Natl Acad Sci USA 1997;94:11612–11616.

46. Lee SS, Glaunsinger B, Mantovani F, et al. Multi-PDZ domain protein MUPP1 is a cellular target for both adenovirus E4-ORF1 and high-risk papillomavirus type 18 E6 oncoproteins. J Virol 2000; 74:9680–9693.

47. Glaunsinger BA, Lee SS, Thomas M, et al. Interactions of the PDZ-protein MAGI-1 with adenovirus E4-ORF1 and high-risk papillomavirus E6 oncoproteins. Oncogene 2000;19:5270–5280.

48. Levi JE, Rahal P, Sarkis AS, et al. Human papillomavirus DNA and p53 status in penile carcinomas. Int J Cancer 1998;76:779–783.

49. Humbey O, Cairey-Remonnay S, Guerrini JS, et al. Detection of the human papillomavirus and analysis of the TP53 polymorphism of exon 4 at codon 72 in penile squamous cell carcinomas. Eur J Cancer 2003;39:684–690.

50. Lam KY, Chan ACL, Chan KW, et al. Expression of p53 and its relationship with human papillomavirus in penile carcinomas. Eur J Surg Oncol 1995;21:613–616.
51. Lopes A, Bezerra AL, Pinto CA, et al. P53 as a new prognostic factor for lymph node metastasis in penile carcinoma: Analysis of 82 patients treated with amputation and bilateral lymphadenectomy. J Urol 2002;168:81–86.
52. Wiener JS, Effert PJ, Humphrey PA, et al. Prevalence of human papillomavirus types 16 and 18 in squamous-cell carcinoma of the penis: a retrospective analysis of primary and metastatic lesions by differential polymerase chain reaction. Int J Cancer 1992;50:694–701.
53. Bezerra AL, Lopes A, Santiago GH, et al. Human papillomavirus as a prognostic factor in carcinoma of the penis. Cancer 2001;91:2315–2321.
54. Ferreux E, Lont AP, Horenblas S, et al. Evidence for at least three alternative mechanisms targeting the p16INK4A/cyclin D/Rb pathway in penile carcinoma, one of which is mediated by high-risk human papillomavirus. J Pathol 2003;201:109–118.

24

The Clinical Management of Penile Cancer

Rajiv Sarin, Hemant B. Tongaonkar, and Reena Engineer

Epidemiology and Etiology

Penile malignancies are uncommon in most parts of the world, but there is a striking geographical variation around the world. While the age-adjusted incidence rate is less than 1 per 100,000 in Europe and North America, in parts of South America, Africa, and India, the incidence is as high as 12 per 100,000 men [1]. Even within a country, there are marked regional variations. In Brazil the incidence of penile cancer is as high as 2.8 and 50 per 100,000 men in the cities of Sao Paulo and Recife, respectively [2]. Within Africa, the highest incidence has been reported from Uganda, where it is the most common cancer in males [3]. In India the disease is more common in the rural population with an incidence of 3 per 100,000 people accounting for more than 6% of all cancers in rural men [4].

In a review of risk factors for the development of penile cancers, strong risk factors identified with an odds ratio of more than 10 were phimosis, chronic inflammatory conditions such as balanoposthitis, lichen sclerosis et atrophicus, and treatment with psoralen and ultraviolet A [5]. A three- to fivefold increased risk was found for smoking, sexual history, and condyloma. Circumcision in the neonatal period was associated with a threefold decreased risk of penile cancer. Human papillomavirus (HPV) DNA has been identified in 40% to 50% of invasive penile carcinoma and 70% to 100% of carcinoma in situ [5].

Natural History, Histology, and Clinical Presentation

Penile cancers are diagnosed often in the fifth to seventh decade in the West [3], but in high incidence areas, the disease often manifests one to two decade earlier [2,6,7]. The disease starts from the glans, corona, or prepuce, but in certain parts of the world where delayed presentation is common, the majority of patients have tumor extension to penile shaft or groin nodes at the time of diagnosis [7]. A vast majority of these invasive cancers are squamous carcinomas or their variants such as verrucous or basaloid carcinoma, and other histologies are very rare [3]. The natural history of penile in situ carcinoma has not been studied as extensively as cervical intraepithelial neoplasia. Some reports suggest more aggressive behavior for in situ penile carcinoma with recurrence within 5 years in most cases, with carcinoma in situ at the resection margin [8]. Carcinoma in situ or dysplasia has been reported in one fourth of patients with invasive penile carcinoma [9]. Certain premalignant lesions of the penis have been identified, which may progress to invasive penile cancer over a variable length of time (e.g., leukoplakia, erythroplasia of Queyrat, Bowen's disease, Buschke-Löwenstein tumor, balanitis xerotica obliterans, etc.). The nomenclature of precancerous lesions in this fashion is quite confusing and the use of terms *penile intra-epithelial neoplasia grade I, II, III* or *squamous intraepithelial lesions of low and high grade* are recommended to avoid such confusion [10].

Local Spread

Penile carcinomas arise from the mucosa of the glans or coronal sulcus and sometimes from the foreskin of uncircumcised men. The clinical manifestation depends on the histological type of the tumor and any time lag before the diagnosis. The initial lesion may be warty or verrucous, ulcerative, proliferative, ulceroproliferative, or sometimes like a plaque over the glans. The tumor then invades deeply to involve the corpus cavernosa and spongiosum, urethra, and skin of the shaft, and in very advanced cases it involves the perineum, scrotum, or prostate.

One of the most elegant studies of clinicopathological correlation in penile carcinoma was reported by Cubilla et al. [11] in 1993. On the basis of a detailed examination of whole organ sections of 66 penile resections, they described the following clinicopathological variants: (a) *verrucous carcinoma* (18%): these papillary exophytic tumors of low histological grade are locally aggressive but vascular or perineural invasion and lymph node metastases are rare; (b) *superficially spreading carcinoma* (42%): this commonest variety presented with centrifugal or radial growth to large areas of the epithelial compartments such as the glans, coronal sulcus, and the foreskin; (c) *vertical growth carcinoma* (32%): these unifocal tumors are characteristically aggressive, infiltrating deep anatomical structures, and have a higher histological grade and a higher propensity for lymph node metastases; and (d) *multicentric carcinoma* (8%): an uncommon variety in which there is normal epithelium in between the multiple foci of carcinoma. The pattern of spread of the superficially spreading carcinoma and multicentric carcinomas suggests that glans mucosa, coronal sulcus, and foreskin may be considered as a single field susceptible to malignant transformation.

Nodal Metastasis

Like all squamous carcinomas, penile cancers have a propensity for lymphatic spread to the draining lymph nodes in the superficial and deep inguinal region and later to the iliac chain. Skip metastasis to the iliac nodes is very unusual [12,13]. Lymphatic spread is uncommon in the verrucous cancers of the penis [9,11]. For invasive squamous carcinomas, the risk of nodal metastases increases with increasing depth of invasion [12–14], higher T stage, and histological grade [12,15]. Early cancers without corporal invasion and low or intermediate histological grade have a 6% incidence of nodal metastasis as opposed to 66% risk in tumors with corporal invasion or high grade as shown in Table 24.1. Solsona et al. [13] identified three risk categories for nodal metastases. The frequency of nodal metastasis in low risk (T1 G1) was 0/19; intermediate risk (T1 G2/3 or T2/3 G1) was 8/22 (36%); and high risk (T2/3 G3) was 20/25 (80%). However, tumor infiltration of the corpora cavernosa, urethra, and adjacent structures was not confirmed as a predictor of nodal metastasis in a multivariate analysis of 145 Brazilians [19]. Venous and lymphatic embolization was the only significant predictor of lymph node metastasis in this study.

Metastatic spread to bones, lung, or other organs at presentation is rare. However, during follow up, 5% to 10% of patients may develop distant metastases, generally in the setting of uncontrolled locoregional disease [3].

Table 24.1. Incidence of nodal metastasis for different T stage and histological grades of penile carcinoma

Author [reference]	Nodal metastasis (%) in patients with T1, well or moderately well differentiated tumors	Nodal metastasis (%) in patients with corporal invasion
Solsona et al. [13]	1/17 (6%)	27/42 (64%)
Fraley et al. [16]	1/19 (5%)	26/29 (90%)
Theodorescu et al. [17]	2/18 (11%)	12/18 (67%)
Heyns et al. [18]	5/91 (5%)	15/32 (47%)
Total	9/145 (6%)	80/121 (66%)

Pretreatment Evaluation and Pitfalls in Staging

For optimum management using the most appropriate treatment approach and ensuring best outcome, a simple but systematic pretreatment evaluation is mandatory. A careful history and interview should also include a history of sexual practices, sexually transmitted disease, chronic inflammatory penile conditions, and the likely psychosexual impact of a penectomy if recommended. The location, type, size, and extension of the tumor, presence of any premalignant or inflammatory condition, infection, or phimosis should be documented after examination by a clinician familiar with this disease. Clinical evaluation of the primary tumor may not detect subclinical infiltration in 10% of cases, whereas in 16% of patients tumor edema and infection may be mistaken for infiltration [20]. In small penile tumors, ultrasound was not found accurate enough in distinguishing invasion of subepithelial connective tissue and invasion into the corpus spongiosum [21]. However, in more advanced tumors, ultrasound was found to be more accurate than clinical examination in estimating the extent of penile tumor, thereby allowing preservation of a longer penile stump during partial penectomy [22]. Magnetic resonance imaging (MRI) with its multiplanar imaging and sharp contrast between different penile structures can identify corporal involvement and local extension with more than 80% accuracy [23].

Evaluation of groin nodes is best done by careful palpation of the groin, fine needle aspiration cytology (FNAC) from any palpable nodes, and computed tomography (CT) scan in cases of clinically suspicious nodes or very obese individuals. Clinical examination of the groin may be fallacious, especially in patient populations that frequently have reactive groin nodes due to chronic infections or those with infected fungating tumors. Palpable nodes may be pathologically negative in 60% cases if the clinical node size is <2 cm and in 10% cases if they measure ≥2 cm [12]. In contrast 15% to 20% of patients with clinically negative groin have unsuspected pathological nodal metastases on groin dissection [24]. In a study comparing various methods for evaluation of nodal metastasis, FNAC, CT scan, and lymphangiography all showed 100% specificity but sensitivity was best for FNAC (71%) as opposed to 36% for CT and 31% for lymphangiography [20].

The first widely used staging systems for penile carcinoma was proposed by Jackson [25] in 1966. After the Union Internationale Contre le Cancer (UICC) tumor, node, metastasis (TNM) staging was published in 1978 and subsequently revised in 1987 [26], Jackson's staging system is now going out of favor. Of the three staging systems shown in Table 24.2, the Jackson and UICC 1978 staging is based on clinical examination, whereas the UICC 1987 system is essentially a pathological system. The Jackson staging is based on the involvement of the penile shaft or adjacent structures and the operability of groin nodes. These findings are not only clinically distinguishable but also useful for treatment decision making. However, the main disadvantage of this system is that it groups together tumors with different sizes and different extents of infiltration without considering their prognostic and therapeutic implication. It is also ambiguous about primary tumors confined to the glans but with nodal involvement. In the UICC 1978 system, the T stage is based on tumor size and extent of infiltration and the N stage is based on the laterality and mobility of regional nodes. In the latest revision in the UICC TNM staging of 1987, which has been retained in the 2002 version, the T stage is based on the invasion of the corpus cavernosa and spongiosum, and the N stage is based on the number, laterality, and site (inguinal or iliac) of nodal involvement. Although this provides more refined prognostic information, it is essentially a pathological staging system and not suitable for patients who do not undergo a penectomy. Similarly, although it makes a prognostically very important distinction between inguinal and iliac nodal involvement, it has discarded the previous criteria of node operability, a very important determinant of survival. With inherent limitations of each of the three staging systems, the UICC 1978 system is perhaps most appropriate for the initial staging of all cases and as the only staging of patients not undergoing penectomy or groin dissection. The UICC 1987 version is useful as a pathological staging system for patients who undergo penectomy and ilioinguinal node dissection. Replacing the clinical staging system by a pathology-based staging by the UICC has been criticized by most authorities [26].

Table 24.2. Different staging systems for carcinoma penis

Jackson staging, 1966 [25]

Stage 1: Limited to glans and or prepuce
Stage 2: Extending into the shaft or corpora but without nodal metastases
Stage 3: Confined to the shaft with malignant but operable inguinal nodes
Stage 4: Invasion beyond shaft, inoperable regional nodes or distant metastases

UICC TNM staging, 1978 [26]	
T stage	N stage
T1: Tumor <2 cm, superficial or exophytic	N0: No nodal involvement
T2: Tumor 2–5 cm or minimal extension	N1: Movable unilateral regional nodes
T3: Tumor >5 cm with deep extension or involvement of urethra	N2: Movable bilateral regional nodes
T4: Infiltrates neighboring structures	N3: Fixed regional lymph nodes

UICC TNM staging, 1987 [26] (not changed in the UICC TNM 1997 version and AJCC TNM 2002 version)	
T stage	N stage
T1: Subepithelial connective tissue	N0: No nodal involvement
T2: Corpus spongiosum or cavernosum	N1: One superficial inguinal node
T3: Urethra, prostate	N2: Multiple or bilateral superficial inguinal nodes
T4: Other adjacent structures	N3: Deep inguinal or pelvic nodes

Biopsy

Histological confirmation of malignancy is mandatory before planning definitive treatment. Patients with small lesions restricted to the prepuce or the penile skin may undergo wide excision of the same with a healthy margin all around, which will be both diagnostic and therapeutic in some cases. Lesions involving the glans, however, require a deep punch or incision biopsy to confirm malignancy and its histological subtype, grade, and invasiveness. In case of a phimotic preputial sac, a dorsal slit or circumcision may be required to obtain an adequate biopsy sample.

Treatment Options, Techniques, and Outcome

With a variety of available treatment options for various stages of the disease, there is no evidence-based consensus regarding the best therapeutic approach, especially for early cancers. Although the relative rarity of the disease in the developed countries where most randomized trials are conducted is partly responsible, an equally important reason for the lack of evidence-based consensus is the strong bias among specialists treating this disease. A national survey in the United Kingdom revealed that irrespective of the extent of cancer, the majority of urologists preferred penectomy, whereas clinical oncologists preferred radiotherapy [27].

The management of the primary tumor and nodes has to be considered separately, as the treatment of the primary is always therapeutic but treatment of the nodes may be either prophylactic or therapeutic, sometimes using different treatment modalities for the primary and nodes.

Management of the Penile Primary Tumor

The management of penile primary tumor has gradually evolved in the form of surgery, radiotherapy, and laser excision/ablation. The treatment modality best suited for a patient depends on the patient's age, the size and extension of the tumor, the probability of cure and salvage, and the expected psychosocial impact of amputative surgery. In the absence of any randomized trial or even large comprehensive prospective single-arm studies, and considering the known strong bias for their own specialty among urologists and radiation oncologists [27], one has to exercise great caution in interpreting the available literature. The treatment approach can be broadly categorized as penile conservative therapy (PCT) or penile amputation.

Penile Conservative Therapy

Because amputative surgery for penile cancer may lead to major psychosexual dysfunction, various attempts have been made to devise conservative treatment modalities based on careful oncological, anatomical, and technical considerations. Judicious use of conventional or micrographic surgery, laser ablation, or radiotherapy can allow preservation of a functioning phallus in appropriately selected patients with early cancers. However, there are no comparative studies and no consensus regarding the best modality for PCT. The type of cases suitable for a particular PCT modality depends on the size, site, extent of the tumor, and presence or absence of invasive carcinoma. Circumcision has been reported mostly for cancers limited to the prepuce, conventional/micrographic wide excision for very small superficial invasive carcinoma, laser excision/ablation for in situ or very select superficial invasive carcinoma, and radiotherapy for all variants of early penile cancer. In contrast to 97% to 100% local control rates with partial penectomy for early penile cancer, penile control rate with all these PCT modalities is in the range of 80% to 90% even in appropriately selected cases. Fortunately, almost all penile failures after PCT can be successfully salvaged with a penectomy, thereby allowing preservation of the phallus and better sexual functioning in the vast majority of patients, as shown in Table 24.3.

Wide Excision

For small noninvasive or minimally invasive lesions confined to the prepuce, circumcision may be adequate. Wide excision, with confirmation of an adequate free resection margin by intraoperative frozen section examination, is recommended for small noninvasive or minimally invasive lesions away from the urethra. Strict case selection is imperative because an improper selection of patients for conservative procedures may lead to high local recurrence rates [33–36]. Although Horenblas et al. [37] have reported local recurrence in only two of the 11 patients after wide excision or circumcision, excessive local recurrence rates of 56% for T1 and 100% for T2 tumors was seen after organ-preserving surgical procedures in another study from Heidelberg [38]. Conservative treatments warrant cautious evaluation because of the relatively small number of treated patients and the lack of good-quality comparative data. Besides, the functional and aesthetic results are not always excellent.

Mohs' Micrographic Surgery

This special surgical technique allows for preservation of maximum normal penile tissue and gives results comparable to more radical procedures in patients with small lesions involving distal portion of the glans [38,39]. It entails removal of diseased tissue in thin layers, accurate construction and mapping of excised tissue, and confirmation of negative margins by frozen-section examination of horizontal tissue sections, and it has the capacity to trace out deeper unsuspected extension of the disease. However, when employed for larger lesions, it is rather time-consuming besides resulting in a misshapen glans or meatal stenosis, with an occasional need of correction or reconstruction of the same. Strict case selection is crucial as Mohs reported a 100% local control rate for lesions less than 1 cm but only a 50% local control rate for lesions larger than 3 cm in size.

Laser Therapy

There are many reports of laser therapy, using carbon dioxide and/or neodymium:yttrium-aluminum-garnet (Nd:YAG) lasers for in situ and early invasive penile cancer. In appropriately selected cases laser therapy has the potential for preservation of normal penile tissue and function and local control rates comparable with more radical procedures. Bandiermonte et al. [40] reported CO_2 laser treatment of patients with T1 lesions, with a 15% relapse rate. Subsequently, the Nd:YAG alone or in combination

Urological Cancers: Science and Treatment

Table 24.3. Treatment results of major radiotherapy studies

Author [reference] institute, mean follow-up in years, study period	Treatment modality, median radiation dose (number of patients)	Initial local control	Eventual local control after salvage	Penectomy for necrosis	Urethral stricture rate
Rozan et al. [28], French multicenter, 11.7 years, 1959–1989	Implant alone, 63 Gy (184 patients) Implant, 50 Gy + surgery or external radiotherapy (RT), 40 Gy (75 patients)	218/259 (84%)	16/259 (6%)	19/259 (7%)	79/259 (31%)
Delannes et al. [29], Toulouse, France, 6.9 years, 1971–1989	Implants, 60 Gy (51 patients)	42/51 (82%)	48/51 (94%)	8/51 (16%)	21/51 (41%)
Ravi et al. [30], Cancer Institute, Adyar, India, 11.6 years, 1959–1988	EBRT, 50 to 60 Gy (128 patients) Implants/molds, 60 to 70 Gy (28 patients)	101/156 (65%)	152/156 (97%)	10/156 (6%)	37/156 (24%)
Sarin et al. [31] Royal Marsden, UK, 5.2 years, 1960–1990	EBRT, 60 Gy (56 patients) Implants, 60 Gy (13 patients)	39/69 (57%)	62/69 (90%)	2/69 (3%)	10/69 (14%)
Chaudhary et al. [32], Tata Memorial, India, 2 years, 1988–1996	Implant, 50 Gy	18/23 (78%)	22/23 (96%)	Nil	2/23 (9%)
Present study [unpublished], Tata Memorial, India, 2.5 years, 1996–2003	Accelerated EBRT, 54 to 55 Gy in 16–18 fractions	18/23 (78%)	23/23 (100%)	Nil	Nil

EBRT, external beam radiotherapy.

with CO_2 laser has been successfully used either for complete destruction of the lesion or for laser coagulation of the base after partial excision of the tumor, resulting in satisfactory cosmetic results as well as good local control [37,41–44]. Following laser photocoagulation of the tumor base, healing by secondary intention is usually completed by 8 weeks [37]. However, laser therapy has the disadvantages of having uncontrolled depth of excision, not providing adequate tissue for pathological examination, and entailing the need for close follow-up to identify local relapse. Laser therapy is appropriate initial treatment for carcinoma in situ of the penis and select cases of recurrent carcinoma in situ. However, these patients need to be carefully fol-

lowed to detect local relapse and should also practice self-examination [44].

Radiation Therapy

External beam radiotherapy (EBRT) using megavoltage telecobalt gamma rays or 6 MV photons from linear accelerators or interstitial implantation [28] or surface applicators [45] of radioactive iridium 192 (brachytherapy) has been used successfully in the treatment of early penile cancers for more than 50 years. The type of radiotherapy best suited for a patient depends on the tumor location, size, thickness, and its proximity to the urethra. Small, superficial tumors anywhere over the glans can be treated with surface mold therapy, localized small tumors away from the urethra can be treated with interstitial implant, and any tumor can be adequately treated with EBRT. Although EBRT has universal applicability and can be successfully delivered in all radiotherapy departments, excellent tumor control without severe complications with brachytherapy mandates strict case selection and expertise with the specialized procedure [28]. Thus even for small localized tumors, external radiation may be preferable if the requisite expertise and facilities for penile brachytherapy is not available.

In EBRT, the glans and the distal 2 to 5 cm of penile shaft is irradiated using bilateral megavoltage beams. For immobilization and repositioning of the penis during treatment and for providing surface buildup of radiation dose, a special device such as a wooden jig [30], wax block [45], or transparent Perspex device [31] is used. A transparent device allows visualization of the penis and maximum sparing of the penile shaft in tumors confined to the glans. A variety of fractionation schedules have been described in the literature with variable results. In addition to the conventional fractionation of 60 Gy in 30 daily fractions over 6 weeks [30,31], other hypofractionated accelerated regimens such as 50 to 55 Gy in 16 daily fractions over 3 weeks [46] and 50 to 55 Gy in 20 to 22 daily fractions over 4 weeks [45] have been used. At the Tata Memorial Hospital we traditionally used a hypofractionated accelerated regimen of 55 Gy in 16 daily fractions over 3 weeks. This provided excellent local control in early cancers without any symptomatic late sequelae. However, the acute radiation mucocutaneous reaction over the glans and penile shaft healed after a median period of 12 weeks. After we slightly modified the fractionation to 54 Gy in 18 daily fractions in $3^1/_2$ weeks, the median healing time for acute reaction has been reduced to 6 weeks, without affecting the tumor control rate. This is comparable to the healing time following laser photocoagulation [37]. The main advantage of the accelerated 3- to 4-week regimen over the more protracted 6-week regimen is that it allows the completion of radiotherapy before the onset of the inevitable brisk radiation reaction. Brisk radiation reaction during radiotherapy can cause treatment interruption of a protracted regimen, and this has been shown to adversely affect tumor control due to tumor repopulation [31].

Local tumor control following radiotherapy is largely determined by the tumor stage, with better results for T1 and selected T2 tumors and universally poor local control in more advanced tumors [28,30–32,47]. Results of brachytherapy series [28,32] are superior to external radiotherapy series [30,31], but this may be largely due to the selective use of brachytherapy for smaller and noninfiltrative tumors. Due to successful surgical salvage, the eventual local control rates are comparable between the implant and EBRT series. However, severe complications such as radiation necrosis requiring penectomy or symptomatic urethral strictures are also higher with brachytherapy (Table 24.3). In the ongoing prospective study of accelerated external radiation at our institute, at a median follow-up of 30 months local recurrence has occurred in only one of 17 patients with tumor confined to the glans as compared to four of six patients with signs of shaft infiltration. All five penile recurrences have been successfully salvaged by partial penectomy. Local failure rates as high as 35% to 40% have been reported in the two largest external radiotherapy series using a more protracted 6-week regimen [30,31]. However, in both these studies, the vast majority of penile recurrences were surgically salvaged, thereby achieving local control in 90% to 98% of patients (Table 24.3). These results support the policy of radical radiotherapy, with surgery reserved for salvage in early-stage disease. The European Board of Urology has endorsed this treatment strategy of organ conserving therapy and watchful waiting for early-stage disease [48]. Because the results of radiotherapy alone are poor in more advanced tumors [30,31], initial penectomy is the treatment of choice for such tumors.

Penile Amputation

Amputation of the penis is the most widely used and undoubtedly the safest treatment approach in all stages of the disease. Though it has been considered as the gold standard of local treatment by some [3], due to the associated psychosexual dysfunction amputative surgery should be reserved for patients not suitable for PCT due to tumor infiltration or if sexual dysfunction is unlikely do be of concern to the patient, or due to expected noncompliance with close follow-up after PCT.

Partial penectomy is indicated for lesions involving the glans, corona, and distal shaft, where after adequate surgical excision the residual penile stump ensures upright micturition without scrotal soiling and for sexual function. Traditionally, a 2-cm disease-free margin has been advocated. However, Hoffman et al. [49] reported no recurrence in any of their patients with microscopic margins up to 10 mm. Similar findings have also been reported by Agrawal et al. [50], who feel that a 10-mm margin may be adequate for grade I and II lesions and 15 mm for grade III lesions. This approach would qualify more patients for conservative surgery or partial penectomy rather than total penectomy, and the residual penile length would then be cosmetically and functionally more acceptable. Patients undergoing partial penectomy can be offered penile augmentation or reconstructive surgery at a later date, if they wish to have the normal length of the penis restored.

Total penectomy with perineal urethrostomy is indicated when the lesion extends to involve the proximal shaft or the base of the penis. Sometimes, limited extension to the scrotum or the skin overlying the pubis may also require wide excision of these structures. With local spread and bone invasion, local bone resection may also be required. The risk of local recurrence after an appropriate amputative surgery should be negligible [3,6,31,35,37]. Urethra-sparing total or subtotal penectomy followed by delayed penile reconstruction has been reported for invasive penile lesions involving only the dorsum of the penis [51].

Management of Ilioinguinal Nodes

Lymph node metastasis in patients with penile cancer is the main determinant of survival, and optimal management of regional nodes is challenging as well as controversial. Superficial and deep inguinal nodes are the first-echelon nodes, with skip metastasis in the pelvic lymph nodes being very rare. The diagnostic and therapeutic approach for the ilioinguinal nodes depends on the index of suspicion for nodal metastasis in a clinically negative groin, and the laterality, size, and mobility of any clinically manifest nodes.

Impalpable or Clinically Insignificant Groin Nodes

In patients with impalpable or clinically insignificant groin nodes with a negative FNAC, there is no consensus regarding selection of patients for close surveillance, sentinel node biopsy, or groin node dissection. Because clinical examination, imaging, and FNAC may miss subclinical nodal metastasis in up to 20% patients [3,24], special diagnostic procedures such as sentinel node biopsy or limited surgery to identify occult metastases and prophylactic node dissection have been evaluated by various investigators.

Surveillance

Due to the morbidity of prophylactic node dissection, a procedure that will be an overtreatment in 80% of patients, and pitfalls in special diagnostic procedures such as sentinel node biopsy, a policy of close surveillance with node dissection reserved for clinically manifest nodal metastases seems attractive. However, the safety of such a policy is questionable in patients who are at a high risk of harboring subclinical nodal metastases or those who may not comply with a very strict surveillance program. Various clinical and histological parameters can help to stratify patients at an increased risk of harboring occult inguinal nodal metastasis. Tumor size, histological grade, infiltration of the corpora cavernosa and spongiosum, and lymphovascular emboli have been found as the main predictors of occult nodal metastases in most studies [11,13,16–18]. Of these the most important factors are the T status and histological grade, as shown in Table 24.1 and discussed earlier. Thus patients who are at low risk of occult nodal metastases and reliable for close follow-up are ideal candidates for the policy of surveillance and therapeutic lymphadenectomy for metastatic lymphadenopathy detected at follow-up. Delayed therapeutic lymphadenectomy for clinically positive nodes detected during active surveillance does not seem to jeopardize long-term survival [17]. Because most inguinal node metastases occur within 2 to 3 years following initial therapy, the surveillance must cover this period with repeated examinations at 1- to 3-month intervals. In patients with infiltrating or poorly differentiated tumors, the long-term safety of surveillance is not known.

Sentinel Node Biopsy

This approach, which addresses the concern that delayed node dissection may affect survival, has gained credence due to its potential for significantly reducing the morbidity of ilioinguinal lymphadenectomy. Cabanas [52] described sentinel node biopsy (removal of a node in the superomedial to saphenofemoral junction in the region of the superficial epigastric vein) and advocated formal lymph node dissection if the node was proved metastatic. He hypothesized that in the absence of sentinel node metastasis, metastasis in the inguinofemoral or iliac nodes is not possible. Scappini et al. [53] suggested aspiration cytology under lymphangiographic guidance. However, a significant false-negative rate of sentinel node biopsy manifesting as subsequent nodal relapse has been noted in several studies [54–56]. However, studies have shown that occult lymph node metastases in penile cancer can be detected with a sensitivity of over 80% by dynamic sentinel node biopsy, including preoperative lymphoscintigraphy, vital dye, and a gamma ray detection probe [57–59]. The dynamic sentinel node procedure is a promising staging technique to detect early metastatic dissemination of penile cancer based on individual mapping of lymphatic drainage, and enables identification of patients with clinically node negative disease requiring regional lymph node dissection [57]. Recently, Lont et al. [60] evaluated the clinical outcome of clinically node-negative penile cancers managed by surveillance or further diagnosed by dynamic sentinel node biopsy with subsequent resection of inguinal nodes. They concluded that early detection of lymph node metastases by dynamic sentinel node biopsy and subsequent resection in clinically node negative T2–3 penile cancers improves survival compared with a policy of surveillance (91% vs. 79% at 3 years).

Limited Surgery for Identifying Occult Metastases

Due to significant false-negative rates of sentinel node biopsy noted in a few studies, limited surgery for identifying occult metastases has been evaluated by a number of authors. Senthil

Kumar et al. [61] evaluated the relative value of FNAC, sentinel node biopsy, and medial inguinal node biopsy. They concluded that FNAC is accurate and specific if the nodes are palpable; if the nodes are impalpable, a preliminary medial inguinal node biopsy followed by sentinel node biopsy if medial inguinal node biopsy is negative will accurately select all patients with metastases in the groin nodes. Superficial or modified inguinal lymphadenectomy followed by a deep inguinal and pelvic lymphadenectomy if superficial nodes are positive on frozen section avoids the pitfalls of sentinel node biopsy without significantly increasing the morbidity [19,62].

Prophylactic Lymphadenectomy

Early adjunctive prophylactic lymphadenectomy has been employed in patients who on the basis of the clinical and histological criteria discussed earlier are considered to be at a high risk of harboring occult metastasis. When prophylactic lymphadenectomy is being performed with the aim of curing patients who may have occult metastasis, one has to bear in mind the likely survival benefit and morbidity attributable to the procedure. The cure rates after inguinal lymphadenectomy in the presence of limited nodal metastasis may be as high as 80%. The proponents of lymphadenectomy in patients with clinically nonpalpable inguinal nodes claim that because the curative benefit of lymphadenectomy in the presence of palpable metastatic nodes is well established, it seems logical that lymphadenectomy performed in the setting of occult nodal disease would confer an even greater advantage. Some authors have reported a significant reduction in survival in patients undergoing delayed therapeutic rather than prophylactic lymphadenectomy, thereby suggesting that the best results can be obtained in the presence of a low tumor load [16,63,64] and that delaying lymphadenectomy may be inappropriate [16,17,35,65,66]. Some earlier studies, however, did not find any significant adverse impact on survival of a delayed therapeutic groin node dissection for metastatic nodes on follow-up, with survival rates equivalent to those obtained with initial therapeutic lymphadenectomy for metastatic nodes at presentation [67–69]. These studies, however, reported on lymphadenectomy for clinically palpable nodal disease and do not exclude the possibility that lymphadenectomy for clinically occult nodes may yield a better survival. Randomized trials proving the benefit of prophylactic over delayed therapeutic lymphadenectomy are needed to incorporate routine prophylactic lymphadenectomy into clinical practice. Moreover, the significant early and delayed morbidity of the lymphadenectomy and the lack of therapeutic benefit in nearly 75% of patients undergoing this procedure has prevented routine prophylactic lymphadenectomy from being the standard treatment for all patients with clinically nonpalpable nodes.

Clinically Significant or Cytologically Confirmed Groin Nodes

In patients with operable nodes, surgery is the mainstay of treatment and often curative, especially for those with limited nodal metastasis. In planning the most appropriate treatment, these patients should be evaluated clinically for operability and with a contrast-enhanced CT scan, especially for pelvic nodes. Various authors have reported that 20% to 67% of patients with clinically palpable metastatic inguinal lymph node metastasis will be disease free at 5 years after lymphadenectomy [35,63–67]. The extent and level of lymph node metastases have been shown to be important predictors of survival [16,24,63–67,70].

Extent of Lymphadenectomy

Bilateral ilioinguinal lymphadenectomy is mandatory for patients with bilateral lymph node metastases. Bilateral lymphadenectomy is also recommended for patients with unilateral significant lymphadenopathy at presentation because clinically occult contralateral groin metastases can be present in over 50% of such patients [54,75]. Node dissection on the contralateral side may be limited to superficial node dissection if no histological evidence of metastasis is found in the contralateral superficial nodes. In patients who develop metachronous unilateral lymph node metastasis while on surveillance, it may be sufficient to perform a unilateral lymph node dissection, especially if the metastasis-free interval is longer than 1 year. This is especially so because the patients selected for surveillance have a very low rate (approximately 10%) of metachronous metastasis, and the chance of developing contralateral node metastasis subsequently is extremely low. Enlarged metastatic groin nodes that are adherent to the overlying skin or ulcerating through it require wide excision of the skin around the node mass, with closure of the consequent skin defect using myocutaneous flap.

Modified or extended sentinel node dissection also has been advocated for patients with limited inguinal node disease in order to reduce the morbidity of radical ilioinguinal lymphadenectomy. However, one study reported that five of the 14 patients who underwent a therapeutic modified superficial inguinal dissection relapsed with incurable groin metastases within 2 years [55]. Hence, radical ilioinguinal lymphadenectomy is the procedure of choice in patients with metastatic nodes.

The therapeutic benefit of pelvic lymphadenectomy in the presence of metastatic inguinal nodes is still undetermined. Iliac lymph node metastases are found in approximately 15% to 30% of patients with metastatic inguinal lymph nodes [63,71], the incidence being higher for a greater number of positive inguinal lymph nodes, presence of perinodal extension, and bilaterality of disease [24,63]. Although Srinivas et al. [63] reported that none of their 11 patients with iliac lymph node metastasis survived 3 years, others have reported fair survival with positive pelvic nodes [52], with improvement in survival documented after iliac node dissection [34]. Lopes et al. [19], in their small series, reported that ilioinguinal lymphadenectomy may have a significant role in increasing the survival of patients with metastases to only one iliac lymph node. In view of this, it seems reasonable to extend the lymph node dissection to include the iliac nodes. A laparoscopic approach may also be used to complete the pelvic node dissection [72].

Complications of Ilioinguinal Lymphadenectomy

Although perioperative mortality consequent to ilioinguinal lymphadenectomy is rare, the morbidity of the procedure is quite significant. Skin flap or edge necrosis and wound breakdown along with persistent lymphorrhea are the commonest early complications reported in up to 80% of patients [65,66]. This may lead to prolonged hospitalization or may require secondary reconstruction with skin grafts or pedicled flaps. Routine transposition of the sartorius muscle to cover the femoral vessels has almost completely eliminated the risk of femoral vessel blowout. The commonest delayed complication is debilitating lower extremity or penoscrotal lymphedema seen in nearly one third of patients. In light of this, a lot of attention has recently focused on reduction of morbidity by modification of the surgical procedure.

Modifications of surgical incisions have been explored at a number of centres. Fraley and Hutchens [73] employed two parallel incisions in the groin, one above and one below the inguinal ligament to reduce the skin flap or edge necrosis. Similarly, a technique of a transverse incision below the inguinal ligament for the inguinal lymphadenectomy and a midline infraumbilical incision for bilateral extraperitoneal pelvic node dissection has been described with significant reduction in the skin loss. However, the choice of incision has little or no bearing on the lower extremity edema. The technique of saphenous vein preserving modified inguinal lymphadenectomy was first described by Catalona [74], with consequent reduction in the incidence of debilitating limb edema. He also redefined the lateral boundary of the dissection as the femoral artery and dispensed with the mobilization and transposition of the sartorius muscle. Iliac node dissection was also not carried out in the absence of inguinal nodal metastases. These modifications seemed suitable in patients with negative inguinal nodes and resulted in reduction in the rate of wound breakdown and skin loss to less than 20%. This saphenous vein–sparing approach has gained credibility especially in patients undergoing prophylactic lymphadenectomy. Coblentz and Theodorescu [75] also employed the saphenous vein–sparing approach along with thick skin flaps during prophylactic inguinal lymphadenectomy for high-risk disease. Early follow-up of their patients indicates that the nodal control rates are comparable to those in similar patients reported in the literature treated with classic lymphadenectomy technique. However, the value of these modifications in the context of metastatic lymphadenopathy, which warrants a complete radical lymphadenectomy, is questionable.

Jacobellis [76] described a technique of modified radical inguinal lymphadenectomy, wherein to avoid damage to the vessels of the groin region that run parallel to the inguinal ligament and lie in the fat of the superficial layer of the superficial fascia, dissection is done beneath this layer (deep to Scarpa's fascia), he saphenous nerve is preserved and the sartorius is left in situ so as not to disturb the collateral lymphatic drainage. He reported no skin necrosis, infection, or deep vein thrombosis, and only moderate lymphedema in four patients at a follow up of 6 to 104 months in his series of 10 patients.

At the Tata Memorial Hospital, we practice routine excision of the skin overlying the inguinal nodal area in all patients undergoing radical ilioinguinal lymphadenectomy, even when the skin is not infiltrated by the nodal disease and we perform immediate reconstruction using a tensor fascia lata myocutaneous flap or anterolateral thigh flap [70,77]. We have had no major problems of skin loss or wound breakdown since the time we began employing this procedure. In addition, the incidence of lower extremity lymphedema has also been significantly reduced with a long follow-up in these patients. With the majority of patients having no significant physical impairment and with preservation of a good quality of life, this may represent a significant advance in the reduction of morbidity of ilioinguinal lymphadenectomy. Alternatives to these flaps are the rectus abdominis flap or the gracilis flap.

Chemotherapy

Chemotherapy for penile cancer has been evaluated in two distinct clinical settings. Topical application of 5-fluorouracil cream [78] and more recently imiquimod 5% cream [79] has been found useful in selected patients with carcinoma-in-situ [1]. There are very few studies of systemic chemotherapy in invasive penile cancer. In early invasive T1–2 N0 penile cancer, concurrent daily bleomycin chemotherapy regimen with radiotherapy has been reported to show a local control rate of 80%. However, with good results of modern radiotherapy alone, there is no role for chemotherapy along with radiotherapy in early-stage disease now. Review of the published literature reveals that cisplatin-based chemotherapy is the most commonly used regimen in advanced penile cancer [80], with nearly 70% response rates. It seems to allow approximately 40% patients with regionally disseminated penile cancer to undergo complete inguinal lymphadenectomy and about 23% to achieve a durable long-term disease-free survival [81–85]. In a Southwest Oncology Group study, 45 patients with locally advanced or metastatic penile carcinoma, were treated with cisplatin 75 mg/m^2 day 1, methotrexate 25 mg/m^2 days 1 and 8, and bleomycin 10 U/m^2 on days 1 and 8 with a cycle length of 21 days. Although the response rate was only 32%, five toxic deaths and six life-threatening toxic episodes were seen [83].

Prognosis

In patients with early-stage disease, there are few deaths due to penile cancer and the long-term overall survival rates are often determined by the comorbid conditions in an elderly population [28,31,86]. Depending on the proportion of cases in different stages, 5-year penile cancer–specific survival rates of 66% to 88% have been reported [28,31,86]. Of the few large studies with multivariate analysis of prognostic factors, nodal metastases [9,19,31], higher T stage or invasion [9,31,48], and high histological grade [31,48] were identified as independent adverse prognostic factors for survival. The substratification of nodal status such as three or more nodes, bilateral disease, extranodal extension, and iliac node metastases predict an especially poor prognosis [6,24,34,63,65].

Quality of Life and Psychosexual Issues

These issues, unfortunately, have been entirely neglected in most reports on penile cancer. This is surprising considering the possible major psychosexual impact of a penectomy. There are only a few small, mostly retrospective studies evaluating the quality of life and psychosexual issues (2,88,89). The expected quality of life, particularly sexual functions after treatment, should be specifically discussed with the patient. It is an expansive concept that involves vast and profound evaluation. The Overall Sexual Functioning Questionnaire (OSFQ), first used by

Table 24.4. Overall Sexual Functioning Questionnaire (OSFQ) [2,87]

Parameter	Score
1. Sexual interest	0 (No sexual interest) to 4 (normal)
2. Sexual ability	0 (Lack of ability) to 4 (no problems)
3. Sexual satisfaction	1 (lacking) to 4 (no change)
4. Relationship with partner	1 (very distressed) to 4 (unchanged, good)
5. Sexual identity	2 (very much changed) to 4 (normal)
6. Frequency of coitus	1 (no sexual intercourse) to 4 (no reduction)

Global score of overall sexual function (five categories).
 I No sexual functioning score, 5–8.
 II Severely reduced score, 9–14.
 III Moderately reduced score, 15–19.
 IV Slightly reduced score, 20–22.
 V Normal score, 23–24.

Opjordsmoen et al. [2,87], is a useful tool and should be used to assess sexual quality of life before and after treatment (Table 24.4). This tool can be very useful to compare different treatment modalities like surgery and radiotherapy in deciding the best approach for early cancers. In a Norwegian study [88] moderate to severe sexual dysfunction was observed in only two of 10 patients after radiotherapy compared to four of five after wide excision, seven of nine after partial penectomy, and all four after total penectomy. We have previously reported that of the 29 patients treated with penectomy, one committed suicide and another had a failed suicide attempt [31]. In an Italian study of 17 patients treated with amputative surgery, anxiety was evident in 30% and depression was evident in one patient, and the global sexual function was compromised in 76% [89].

In our ongoing prospective study of accelerated radiotherapy at the Tata Memorial Hospital, of the 18 patients with intact penis (five underwent penectomy for residual/recurrent disease), 16 men have retained their pretreatment erectile function, coital satisfaction, and frequency. The remaining two patients have reported mild sexual dysfunction after radiotherapy.

Conclusion

Penile cancers, though uncommon in developed countries, pose a significant oncological challenge in some parts of the world. With the available treatment options, the aim of treatment should be organ and function preservation whenever possible, without compromising the chances of survival. Early-stage cancers in men who wish to preserve organ and function and are expected to be compliant with a close follow-up program should be offered an appropriate penile conservative therapy. More advanced tumors are difficult to control with radiotherapy; hence initial penectomy is the treatment of choice. Management of the groin still remains controversial, especially regarding the indication, timing, and extent of lymphadenectomy. On the basis of the available evidence, surveillance of a clinically negative groin in an early-stage primary tumor and surgery for the rest seems appropriate. Strong specialty-oriented bias among urologists and clinical oncologists [27] is unfortunate when patients with eminently radiocurable early cancers are subjected to an unnecessary penectomy and is hazardous when patients with advanced disease are treated primarily with ineffective radiotherapy. There is a need for evidence-based guidelines for this disease [90], and outcome reports in the future should incorporate psychosexual impact of various treatment approaches.

References

1. Tomatis L, Aitio A, Day NE, et al (Eds). Cancer: Causes, Occurrence and Control. Lyon: IARC Scientific Publications No. 100, 1990.

2. D'Ancona CAL, Botega NJ, Moraes CD, et al. Quality of life after partial penectomy for penile carcinoma. Adult Urol 1997;50:593–596.

3. Misra S, Chaturvedi A, Misra NC. Penile carcinoma: a challenge for the developing world. Lancet Oncol 2004;5:240–247.

4. Indian Council of Medical Research (ICMR), National Cancer Registry Programme. Consolidated Report of the Population Based Cancer Registries 1990–1996. New Delhi: ICMR, 2001.

5. Dillner J, von Krogh G, Horenblas S, Meijer CJ. Etiology of squamous cell carcinoma of the penis. Scand J Urol Nephrol Suppl 2000;205: 189–193.

6. Kamat MR, Kulkarni JN, Tongaonkar HB. Carcinoma of the penis: the Indian experience. J Surg Oncol 1993;52:50–55.

7. Magoha GA, Ngumi ZW. Cancer of the penis at Kenyatta National Hospital. East Afr Med J 2000; 77:526–530.

8. Sandeman TF. Carcinoma penis. Australas Radiol 1990;34:12–16.

9. Soria JC, Fizazi K, Piron D, et al. Squamous cell carcinoma of the penis: multivariate analysis of prognostic factors and natural history in monocentric study with a conservative policy. Ann Oncol 1997;8:1089–1098.

10. Cubilla AL, Meijer CJ, Young RH. Morphological features of epithelial abnormalities and precancerous lesions of the penis. Scand J Urol Nephrol Suppl 2000;205:215–219.

11. Cubilla AL, Barreto J, Caballero C, Ayala G, Riveros G. Pathological features of epidermoid carcinoma of the penis. Am J Surg Pathol 1993;17:753–763.

12. Ayappan K, Ananthakrishnan N, Sankaran V. Can regional lymph node involvement be predicted in patients with carcinoma of the penis? Br J Urol 1994;73:549–553.

13. Solsona E, Iborra I, Ricos JV, et al. Corpus cavernosum invasion and tumour grade in the prediction of lymph node condition of penile carcinoma. Eur Urol 1992;22:115–118.

14. Villavicencio H, Rubio-Briones J, Regalado R, Chechile G, Algaba F, Palou J. Grade, local stage and growth pattern as prognostic factors in carcinoma of the penis. Eur Urol 1997;32:442–447.

15. Pizzocaro G, Piva L, Nicolai N. Treatment of lymphatic metastasis of squamous cell carcinoma of the penis: experience at the National Tumor Institute of Milan. Arch Ital Urol Androl 1996;68: 169–172.

16. Fraley EE, Zhang G, Manivel C, Niehans GA. The role of ilioinguinal lymphadenectomy and significance of histological differentiation in treatment of carcinoma of the penis. J Urol 1989;142: 1478–1482.

17. Theodorescu D, Russo P, Zhang ZF, Morash C, Fair WR. Outcomes of initial surveillance of invasive squamous cell carcinoma of the penis and negative nodes. J Urol 1996;155:1626–1631.

18. Heyns CF, van Vollenhoven P, Steenkamp JW, Allen FJ, van Velden DJ. Carcinoma of the penis—appraisal of a modified tumour-staging system. Br J Urol 1997;80:307–312.

19. Lopes A, Hidalgo GS, Kowalski LP, Torloni H, Rossi BM, Fonseca FP. Prognostic factors in carcinoma of the penis: multivariate analysis of 145 patients treated with amputation and lymphadenectomy. J Urol 1996;156:1637–1642.

20. Horenblas S, Van Tinteren H, Delemarre JFM, Moonen LMF, Lustig V, Kroger R. Squamous cell

carcinoma of the penis: accuracy of tumour, node and metastases classification system, and role of lymphangiography, computerized tomography scan and fine needle aspiration cytology. J Urol 1991;146:1279–1283.

21. Horenblas S, Kroger R, Gallee MPW, Newling DWW, Van Tinteren H. Ultrasound in squamous cell carcinoma of the penis: a useful addition to clinical staging? A comparison of ultrasound with histopathology. Urology 1994;43:702–707.

22. Agrawal A, Pai D, Ananthakrishnan N, Smile SR, Ratnakar C. Clinical and sonographic findings in carcinoma of the penis. J Clin Ultrasound 2000; 28:399–406.

23. Vapnek JM, Hricak H, Carroll PR. Recent advances in imaging studies for staging of penile and urethral carcinoma. Urol Clin North Am 1992;19: 257–266.

24. Ravi R. Correlation between the extent of nodal involvement and survival following groin dissection for carcinoma of the penis. Br J Urol 1993;72: 817–819.

25. Jackson SM. The treatment of carcinoma of the penis. Br J Surg 1966;53:33–35.

26. Horenblas S, Van Tinteren H. Squamous cell carcinoma of the penis. IV. Prognostic factors of survival: analysis of tumor, nodes and metastasis classification system. J Urol 1994;151:1239–1243.

27. Harden SV, Tan LT. Treatment of localized carcinoma of the penis: a survey of current practice in the UK. Clin Oncol (R Coll Radiol) 2001;13: 284–287.

28. Rozan R, Albuisson E, Giraud B, et al. Interstitial brachytherapy for penile carcinoma: a multicentric survey (259 patients). Radiother Oncol 1995;36:83–93.

29. Delannes M, Malavaud B, Douchez J, Bonnet J, Daly NJ. Iridium-192 interstitial therapy for squamous cell carcinoma of the penis. Int J Radiat Oncol Biol Phys 1992;24:479–483.

30. Ravi R, Chaturvedi HK, Sastry DVLN. Role of radiation therapy in the treatment of carcinoma of the penis. Br J Urol 1994;74:646–651.

31. Sarin R, Norman AR, Steel GG, Horwich A. Treatment results and prognostic factors in 101 men treated for squamous carcinoma of the penis. Int J Radiat Oncol Biol Phys 1997;38:713–722.

32. Chaudhary AJ, Ghosh S, Bhalavat RL, Kulkarni JN, Sequeira BV. Interstitial brachytherapy in carcinoma of the penis. Strahlenther Onkol 1999;175: 17–20.

33. Narayana AS, Olney LE, Loening SA, Weimar G, Culp DA. Carcinoma of the penis: analysis of 219 cases. Cancer 1982;49:2185–2191.

34. Hardner GJ, Bhanalaph T, Murphy GP, Albert DJ, Moore RH. Carcinoma of the penis: analysis of therapy in 100 consecutive cases. J Urol 1972;108: 428–430.

35. McDougal WS, Kirchner FK Jr, Edwards RH, Killon LT. Treatment of carcinoma of the penis: the case of primary lymphadenectomy. J Urol 1986;136:38–41.

36. Jensen MS. Cancer of the penis in Denmark 1942 to 1962 (511 cases). Dan Med Bull 1977;24:66–72.

37. Horenblas S, Van Tinteren H, Delemare JFM. Squamous cell carcinoma of the penis: treatment of the primary tumour. J Urol 1992;147:1533–1538.

38. Mohs FE, Snow SN, Messing EM, Kuglitsch ME. Microscopically controlled surgery in the treatment of carcinoma of the penis. J Urol 1985;133: 961–966.

39. Brown MD, Zachary CB, Grekin RC, Swanson NA. Penile tumors: their management by Mohs micrographic surgery. J Dermatol Surg Oncol 1987;13: 1163–1167.

40. Bandiermonte, Santoro O, Boracchi P, Piva L, Pizzocaro G, DePalo G. Total resection of glans penis surface by CO2 laser microsurgery. Acta Oncol 1988;27:575–578.

41. Rothenberger KH. Value of the neodymium YAG laser in the therapy of penile carcinoma. Eur Urol 1986;12(suppl 1):34–36.

42. Windahl T, Andersson SO. Combined laser treatment for penile carcinoma: results after long-term followup. J Urol 2003;169:2118–2121.

43. Frimberger D, Hungerhuber E, Zaak D, Waidelich R, Hofstetter A, Schneede P. Penile carcinoma. Is Nd:YAG laser therapy radical enough? J Urol 2002; 168:2418–2421.

44. Van Bezooijen BP, Horenblas S, Meinhardt W, Newling DW. Laser therapy for carcinoma in situ of the penis. J Urol 2001;166:670–671.

45. Neave F, Neal AJ, Hoskin PJ, Hope-Stone HF. Carcinoma of the penis: a retrospective review of treatment with iridium mould and external beam irradiation. Clin Oncol 1993;5:207–210.

46. Duncan W, Jackson SM. Treatment of early cancer of penis with megavoltage x-rays. Clin Radiol 1972;23:246–248.

47. Modig H, Duchek M, Sjodin JG. Carcinoma of the penis. Treatment by surgery or combined bleomycin and radiation therapy. Acta Oncol 1993;32:653–655.

48. Lindegaard JC, Nielsen OS, Lundbeck FA, Mamsen A, Studstrup HN, von der Maase H. A retrospective analysis of 82 cases of cancer of the penis. Br J Urol 1996;77:883–890.

49. Hoffman MA, Renshaw AA, Loughlin KR. Squamous cell carcinoma of the penis and microscopic pathologic margins: how much margin is needed for local cure? Cancer. 1999;85:1565–1568.

50. Agrawal A, Pai D, Ananthakrishnan N, Smile SR, Ratnakar C. The histological extent of the local spread of carcinoma of the penis and its therapeutic implications. BJU Int 2000;85:299–301.

51. Bissada NK, Morcos RR, El-Senoussi M. Post-circumcision carcinoma of the penis. I. Clinical aspects. J Urol 1986;135:283–285.

52. Cabanas RM. An approach for the treatment of penile carcinoma. Cancer 1977;39:456–466.

53. Scappini P, Piscioli F, Pusiol T, Hofstetter A, Rothenberger KH, Luciani L. Penile cancer: aspiration biopsy cytology for staging. Cancer 1986; 58:1526–1533.

54. Perinetti EP, Crane DC, Catalona WJ. Unreliability of sentinel node biopsy for staging penile carcinoma. J Urol 1980;124:734–735.

55. Pettaway CA, Pisters LL, Dinney CP, et al. Sentinel lymph node dissection for penile carcinoma: the M. D. Anderson Cancer Center experience. J Urol 1995;154:1999–2003.

56. Valdes Olmos RA, Tanis PJ, Hoefnagel CA, et al. Penile lymphoscintigraphy for sentinel node identification. Eur J Nucl Med 2001;28:581–585.

57. Horenblas S, Jansen L, Meinhardt W, Hoefnagel CA, de Jong D, Nieweg OE. Detection of occult metastasis in squamous cell carcinoma of the penis using a dynamic sentinel node procedure. J Urol 2000;163:100–104.

58. Han KR, Brogle BN, Goydos J, Perrotti M, Cummings KB, Weiss RE. Lymphatic mapping and intraoperative lymphoscintigraphy for identifying the sentinel node in penile tumors. Urology 2000;55:582–585.

59. Tanis PJ, Lont AP, Meinhardt W, Olmos RA, Nieweg OE, Horenblas S. Dynamic sentinel node biopsy for penile cancer: reliability of a staging technique. J Urol 2002;168:76–80.

60. Lont AP, Horenblas S, Tanis PJ, Gallee MP, van Tinteren H, Nieweg OE. Management of clinically node negative penile carcinoma: improved survival after the introduction of dynamic sentinel node biopsy. J Urol 2003;170:783–786.

61. Senthil Kumar MP, Ananthakrishnan N, Prema V. Predicting regional lymph node metastasis in carcinoma of penis: a comparison between fine needle aspiration cytology, sentinel lymph node biopsy and medial inguinal lymph node biopsy. Br J Urol 1998;81:453–457.

62. Sanchez-Oritz RF, Pettaway CA. Natural history, management, and surveillance of recurrent squamous cell penile carcinoma: a risk based approach. Urol Clin North Am 2003;30:853–867.

63. Srinivas V, Morse MJ, Herr HW, Sogani PC, Whitmore WF Jr. Penile cancer: relation of extent of nodal metastasis to survival. J Urol 1987;137: 880–882.

64. Fossa SD, Hall KS, Johannessen NB, Urnes T, Kaalhus O. Cancer of the penis. Experience at the Norwegian Radium Hospital 1974–1985. Eur Urol 1987;13:372–377.

65. Ornellas AA, Seixas LC, Marota A. Surgical treatment of invasive squamous cell carcinoma of the penis: retrospective analysis of 350 cases. J Urol 1994;151:1244–1249.

66. Johnson DE, Lo RK. Management of regional lymph nodes in penile carcinoma: five year results following therapeutic groin dissections. Urology 1984;24:308–311.

67. Beggs JH, Spratt JS. Epidermoid carcinoma of the penis. J Urol 1961;91:166–172.

68. Frew ID, Jefferies JD, Swinney J. Carcinoma of penis. Br J Urol 1967;39:398–404.

69. Baker BH, Spratt JS, Perez-Mesa C. Carcinoma of the penis. J Urol 1976;116:458–461.

70. Tongaonkar HB, Kulkarni JN, Kamat MR. Carcinoma of the penis: relationship of nodal metastases to survival. Indian J Urol 1993;9:54–57.

71. Gursel EO, Georgountzos C, Uson AC, Melicow MM, Veenema RJ. Penile cancer. Urology 1973;1: 569–578.

72. Assimos DG, Jarow JP. Role of laparoscopic pelvic lymph node dissection in the management of patients with penile cancer and inguinal adenopathy. J Endourol 1994;8:365–369.

73. Fraley EE, Hutchens HC. Radical ilio-inguinal node dissection: the skin bridge technique. A new procedure. J Urol 1972;108:279–281.

74. Catalona WJ. Modified inguinal lymphadenectomy for carcinoma of the penis with preservation of saphenous veins: technique and preliminary results. J Urol 1988;140:306–310.

75. Coblentz TR, Theodorescu D. Morbidity of modified prophylactic inguinal lymphadenectomy for squamous cell carcinoma of the penis. J Urol 2002;168:1386–1389.

76. Jacobellis U. Modified radical inguinal lymphadenectomy for carcinoma of the penis: technique and results. J Urol 2003;169:1349–1352.

77. Savant DN, Dalal AV, Patel SG, Bhathena HM, Kavarana NM. Tensor fasciae lata myocutaneous flap reconstruction following ilioinguinal node dissection. Eur J Plast Surg 1996;19:174–177.

78. Goette DK, Carson TE. Erythroplasia of Queyrat: treatment with topical 5–fluorouracil. Cancer 1976;38:1498–1502.

79. Schroeder TL, Sengelmann RD. Squamous cell carcinoma in situ of the penis successfully treated with imiquimod 5% cream. J Am Acad Dermatol 2002;46:545–548.

80. Culkin DJ, Beer TM. Advanced penile carcinoma. J Urol 2003;170:359–365.

81. Hussein AM, Benedetto P, Sridhar KS. Chemotherapy with cisplatin and 5-fluorouracil for penile and urethral squamous cell carcinomas. Cancer 1990; 65:433–438.

82. Shammas FV, Ous S, Fossa SD. Cisplatin and 5-fluorouracil in advanced cancer of the penis. J Urol 1992;147:630–632.

83. Haas GP, Blumenstein BA, Gagliano RG, et al. Cisplatin, methotrexate and bleomycin for the

treatment of carcinoma of the penis: a Southwest Oncology Group study. J Urol 1999;161:1823–1825.

84. Pizzocaro G, Piva L, Bandieramonte G, Tana S. Up-to-date management of carcinoma of the penis. Eur Urol 1997;32:5–15.

85. Kattan J, Culine S, Droz JP, et al. Penile cancer chemotherapy: twelve years' experience at Institut Gustave-Roussy. Urology 1993;42:559–562.

86. Rozan R, Albuisson E, Giraud B, Boiteux JP, Dauplat J. Epithelioma of the penis treated with surgery. Study Group on Urogenital Tumors of the National Federation of the Centers for Cancer Control. Prog Urol 1996;6:926–935.

87. Lindegaard JC, Nielsen OS, Lundbeck FA, Mamsen A, Studstrup HN, von der Maase H. A retrospective analysis of 82 cases of cancer of the penis. Br J Urol 1996;77:883–890.

88. Opjordsmoen S, Waehre H, Aass N, Fossa SD. Sexuality in patients treated for penile cancer: patient's experience and doctor's judgement. Br J Urol 1994;73:554–560.

89. Ficarra V, Mofferdin A, D'Amico A, et al. Comparison of the quality of life of patients treated by surgery or radiotherapy in epidermoid cancer of the penis. Prog Urol 1999;9:715–720.

90. Munro NP, Thomas PJ, Deutsch GP, Hodson NJ. Penile cancer: a case for guidelines. Ann R Coll Surg Engl 2001;83:180–185.

Part VI

Unusual Urological Tumors

25

Oncocytomas and Rare Renal Tumors

Holger Moch

International agreement was reached on the histological classification of renal epithelial neoplasms with the new World Health Organization (WHO) classification of the tumors of the urinary system and male genital organs [1]. This classification defines malignant neoplasms as clear cells renal carcinoma, papillary renal carcinoma, chromophobe renal carcinoma, collecting duct carcinoma, and unclassified renal cell carcinoma. Benign neoplasms are papillary adenoma, renal oncocytoma, and metanephric nephradenoma or adenofibroma. Over the past few years new or rare distinctive kidney tumors have been described. This chapter presents examples of recently recognized tumor entities and discusses molecular alterations, which are important for the differential diagnosis. The following tumors are described and discussed: oncocytoma, mixed epithelial and stromal renal tumors, primary renal synovial sarcomas, renal primitive neuroectodermal tumors (PNETs), and mucinous tubular and spindle cell carcinomas. It is important to distinguish these tumor entities from the well-known frequent renal tumors because of different biological behavior and different therapeutical approaches.

Oncocytoma

Oncocytoma comprises approximately 5% of all neoplasms of renal tubular epithelium and is a benign epithelial tumor [2–4]. The name comes from the predominant cell type, the so-called oncocyte (swollen cell). Oncocytes are round-to-polygonal cells with densely granular cytoplasm. Sporadic oncocytomas have a typical mahogany-brown cut surface and a central stellate scar (Fig. 25.1). Hemorrhage is present in up to 20% of cases [3]. Necrosis is extremely rare. The majority of oncocytomas present by an incidental discovery during a radiographic workup of unrelated conditions. Oncocytomas have a typical ultrastructure with numerous mitochondria in the cytoplasm [5]. Oncocytoma is composed of large cells with mitochondria ridge eosinophilic cytoplasm. It has been suggested that oncocytomas arise from the distal tubular system. Most oncocytomas occur sporadically, although there are several cases that have been reported in the context of inherited tumor syndromes, e.g., the Birt-Hogg-Dubé syndrome. There are also cases with a large number of oncocytic lesions with a spectrum of morphological features, including oncocytic tumors, oncocytic change in benign tubules, microcysts, and a lining of oncocytic cells and clusters of oncocytes within the renal interstitium. Such cases are called oncocytomatosis. The majority of the mitochondria are of normal size and shape. Somatic genetic alterations include translocation of t(5;11)(q35;q13). Some of the cases show loss of chromosome 1 and 14 [6–8].

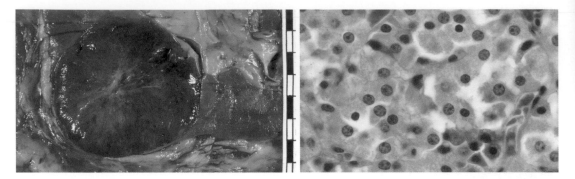

Fig. 25.1. Oncocytoma. Mahogany-brown cut surface with central stellate scar (left). Small eosinophilic cells (oncocytes (right).

Mixed Epithelial and Stromal Renal Tumors

The new WHO classification of tumors includes the entity of mixed epithelial and stromal tumors. This is a complex renal neoplasm composed of a mixture of stromal and epithelial elements. some of these cases have been reported under different names, including cystic hamartoma of the renal pelvis or adult mesoblastic nephroma [9–11]. The new WHO classification accepts the term *mixed epithelial and stromal tumor* [1]. Importantly, there is a 6:1 predominance of women over men, and all of the women are perimenopausal. There are histories of estrogen therapy in most of the reported cases [11]. Surgery has been curative in all cases. The tumors are composed of large cysts, microcysts,

and tubules. The large cysts are lined by columnar epithelium, which forms small papillary tufts (Fig. 25.2). Epithelium with müllerian characteristics has also been described. Areas of myxoid stroma and fascicles of smooth muscle cells may be prominent. By immunohistochemistry, the spindle cells, which look like smooth muscle, have strong reactions with antibodies to actin and desmin. The nuclei of these spindle cells express also estrogen and progesterone receptors (Fig. 25.3). The epithelial elements are positive for antibodies to a variety of cytokeratins [12].

Little is known about the genetics of these tumors. The tumors lack the translocation t(12/15) and trisomies for chromosome 11, which are typical for mesoblastic nephroma [13]. Therefore, there is no genetic relationship between mesoblastic nephroma and mixed

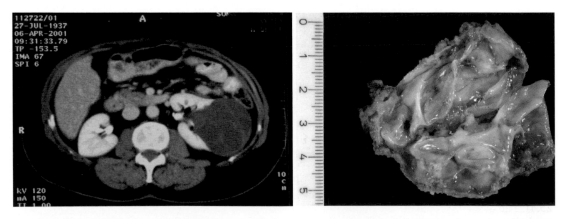

Fig. 25.2. Mixed epithelial-stromal tumor. Large tumor with contact to renal pelvis (left). Not glancing inner surface of the cystic tumor (right).

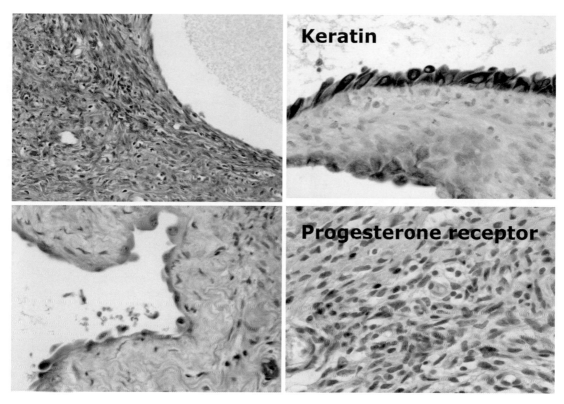

Fig. 25.3. Mixed epithelial and stromal tumor. Spindle cell stroma with smooth muscle differentiation (left). Spindle cells react with antibodies to estrogen and progesterone (right).

epithelial stroma tumors, although the morphology is very similar. The tumors should not be called adult mesoblastic nephroma. It has been suggested that the tumors evolve by long-term hormone exposure.

Primary Renal Synovial Sarcomas

Synovial sarcoma of the kidney is characterized by a specific morphology and specific cytogenetic characteristics [14]. It consists of spindle cells and frequently has large cysts. Many cases show local recurrence after nephrectomy. Most cases are diagnosed between the ages of 20 and 50 years. Microscopically, tumors are characterized by monomorphic plump spindle cells (Fig. 25.4). The cysts are lined by mitotically inactive epithelial cells without striking cellular atypia. The tumors have been previously described as

embryonal sarcoma of the kidney. There is a slight male predilection (1.6:1). No bilateral tumors were identified yet [15,16].

The spindle cells are immune reactive for epithelial membrane antigen (EMA), CD56, and sometimes CD99. They are nonreactive for desmin, actin, S100, and cytokeratins. The cyst epithelium is cytokeratin positive. Synovial sarcoma is cytogenetically characterized by the translocation t(X;18)(p11.2/q11.2), generating a fusion between the *SYT* gene on chromosome 18 and one member of the *SSX* family of genes (*SSX1, SSX2, SSX4*) on chromosome X [17,18]. Molecularly confirmed primary synovial sarcomas of the kidney have demonstrated the characteristic *SYT-SSX* gene fusion (Fig. 25.4). In contrast to soft tissue synovial sarcoma, where the *SYT-SSX* gene fusion is more common than the alternative *SYT-SSX2* form, the majority of renal synovial sarcomas have so far demonstrated the *SYT-SSX2* gene fusion. There is a tendency for a predominance of monophasic

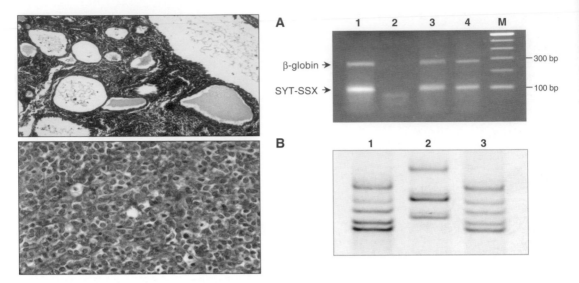

Fig. 25.4. Synovial sarcoma of the kidney. Cystic change (upper left). Monomorphic small spindle cells (lower left). *SYT-SSX* fusion due to translocation t(X;18) (right). A: TaqI-Digestion of PCR-Products (SSX1; SSX2; Positive Control); B: SSCP-Analysis (SSX1; SSX2; Positive Control).

spindle morphology of these tumors in the kidney, and there are more rarely biphasic tumors.

Although prognostic data are limited, there are case reports describing tumors that have responded to chemotherapy. However, recurrence is common.

In summary, primary renal synovial sarcoma is a distinctive tumor entity that should be considered in renal tumors consisting of spindle cells, especially in young adults.

Primitive Neuroectodermal Tumors of the Kidney

Primitive neuroectodermal tumors (PNETs) of the kidney are rare and of highly aggressive malignancy [19–21]. The tumors are composed of small uniform round cells, characterized by a translocation resulting in a fusion transcript of the *EWS* gene and the *ETS*-related family of oncogenes (Fig. 25.5). The neoplasms are rare. The age of the described patients range from 4 to 69 years [22].

The mean age is 27 years. There is a predilection for males. Most patients present with fever, weight loss, and bone pain. The tumors are mostly more than 10 cm in diameter with replacement of the kidney. The weight of some of these tumors is 1 kg or more. The tumor in the kidney is no different from the more common counterpart in the soft tissues. The immunophenotype of PNET is the expression of vimentin and the surface antigen of CD99 or HBA-71.

Some tumors also express pancytokeratin. Virtually all of the reported PNETs of the kidney had the translocation t(11;22)(q24;q12) with the fusion transcript between the *EWS* gene (22q12) and the *ETS*-related oncogene *FLI1* (11q24) (Fig. 25.6). However, there are also other variant translocations [22]. The diagnosis of renal PNETs must be considered in young patients with renal neoplasms, particularly those with advanced disease at presentation. Achieving an exact diagnosis has important clinical consequences because polychemotherapy and high-dose chemotherapy may lead to dramatic tumor reduction or even complete remission. In the past, aggressive multidrug chemotherapy has resulted in an improvement in the clinical outcome [23].

Mucinous Tubular Spindle Cell Carcinoma

Mucinous tubular spindle cell carcinoma are low-grade polymorphic renal epithelial neoplasms with mucinous tubular and spindle cell

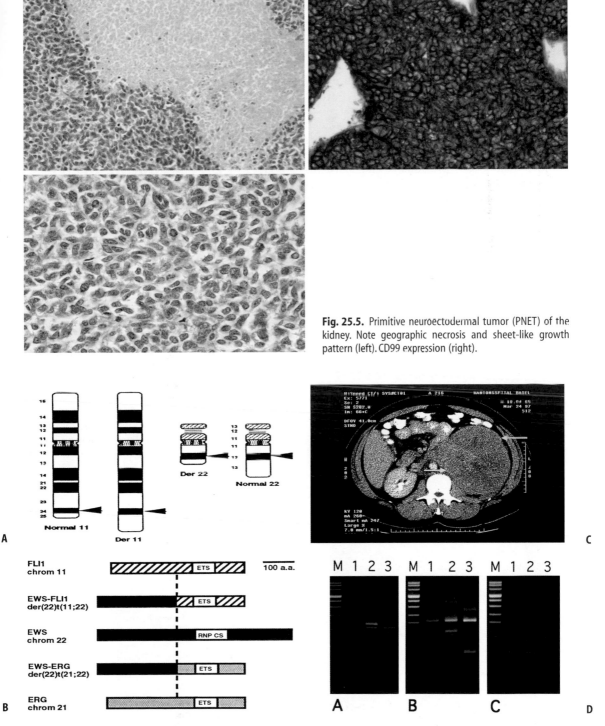

Fig. 25.5. Primitive neuroectodermal tumor (PNET) of the kidney. Note geographic necrosis and sheet-like growth pattern (left). CD99 expression (right).

Fig. 25.6. PNET of the kidney. *EWS-FLI1* translocation. A: Balanced chromosomal translocation t(11;22)(q24;12) in PNET of the kidney (upper left); B: EWS-FLI-1 fusion (t(11;22)(q24,12) or EWS-ERG fusion (t(21;22)(q22;12) (less common) are observed in PNETs; C: CT scan of a young patient showing a renal PNET (upper right); D: Nested PCR with primers that specifically detect EWS/FLI-1 and EWS-ERG chimeric transcripts (lower right).

features. The new WHO classification has included this new tumor subtype [1]. The tumors usually present as a symptomatic masses, often found on ultrasound [24]. There is a wide age range from 17 to 82 years and a male to female rate of 1:4 [25,26]. Macroscopically mucinous tubular and spindle cell carcinomas are well circumscribed and have gray or light tan cut surfaces (Fig. 25.7). The tumors are composed of tightly packed, elongated tubules separated by mucinous stroma. Sometimes the tumors simulate leiomyoma or sarcoma. Many of these tumors had been previously diagnosed as unclassified sarcomatoid carcinomas or as duct Bellini carcinomas. The tumors have a complex immunophenotype and stain for cytokeratin and EMA. Markers of proximal nephron such as CD10 are absent. On comparative genomic hybridization and fluorescence in situ hybridization, there is a characteristic combination of chromosome losses, generally involving chromosome 1, 4, 6, 8, 13, and 14 [27,28]. The prognosis seems to be favorable.

It has been postulated that these tumors are related to the loop of Henle. However, the immunohistochemical and cytogenetic analysis showed complex immunophenotypes, but could not prove a derivation from the loop of Henle. There was no genetic relationship to clear cell renal carcinomas [28].

Renal Cell Carcinoma in Children and Young Adults

In childhood, by far the most common renal neoplasms are nephroblastomas. Renal cell carcinomas are rare in children. The new WHO classification includes new tumor types

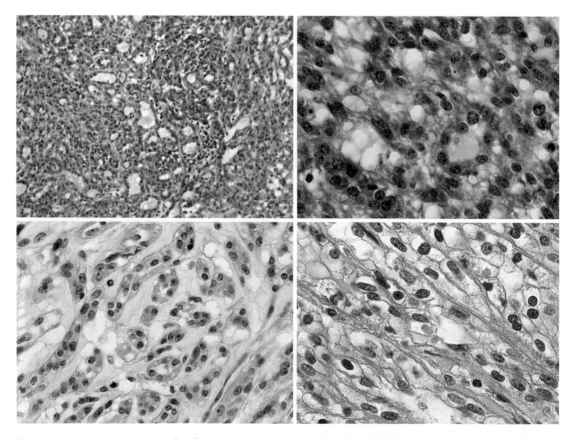

Fig. 25.7. Mucinous tubular and spindle cell carcinoma composed of spindle cells and cuboidal cells forming cords and tubules. Note extracellular mucin.

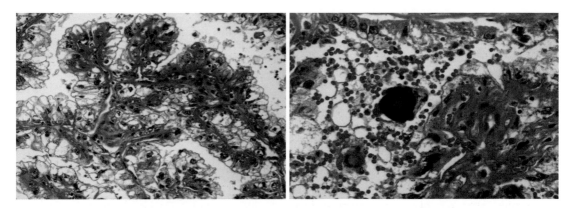

A   B

Fig. 25.8. *ASPL-TFE3* translocation tumor. Note papillary architecture (A) and psammoma bodies (B).

that occur predominantly in children and young adults. Such tumors include renal cell carcinomas with the *ASPL-TFE3* gene fusion and carcinomas with a *PRCC-TFE3* gene fusion. Collectively, these tumors have been termed Xp11.2 or *TFE3* translocation carcinomas [29].

Renal carcinomas associated with Xp11.2 translocations have a distinctive histopathological appearance, which is that of a carcinoma with papillary architecture composed of clear cells. Some tumors have a more nested architecture and often feature cells with granular eosinophilic cytoplasm. The translocation carcinomas are characterized by cells with voluminous clear to eosinophilic cytoplasm and prominent nucleoli [30]. Psammoma bodies are sometimes extensive (Fig. 25.8).

The tumors have the distinctive immunohistochemical feature with nuclear immunoreactivity for TFE3 protein. Only about 50% express epithelial markers such as cytokeratin and EMA.

The carcinomas are defined by several different translocations involving chromosome Xp11.2, all resulting in gene fusions involving the *TFE3* gene, which is a member of the basic helix-loop-helix family of transcription factors. Both the PRCC-TFE3 and ASPL-TFE3 fusion proteins retain the TFE3 DNA-binding domain. This domain localizes to the nucleus and can act as transcription factor [31,32].

Very little is known about the clinical behavior of these carcinomas. They usually present at an advanced stage. However, their clinical course thus far appears to be indolent. Most of these tumors show no virtual mutations [33].

Summary

New tumor entities have been described, which are characteristic for children or young adults. The predominance of *TFE* translocation carcinomas in the first decades of life demonstrates that renal cell carcinomas in young patients contain genetically and phenotypically distinct tumors with further potential for novel renal cell carcinoma subtypes. The far lower frequency of clear cell carcinomas with *VHL* alterations in childhood compared to adults suggests that renal cell carcinomas in young patients have a unique genetic background.

Other tumors with apparent predilection for young age groups include clear cell carcinomas in the context of von Hippel–Lindau disease, carcinomas in combination with nephroblastomas, and renal cell carcinomas associated with neuroblastomas.

References

1. Eble J, et al. World Health Organization classification of tumours. In: Kleihus P, Sobin L, eds. Pathology and Genetics of Tumours of the Urinary System and Male Genital Organs. Lyon: IARC Press, 2004.

2. Moch H, et al. Prognostic utility of the recently recommended histologic classification and revised TNM staging system of renal cell carcinoma: a Swiss experience with 588 tumors. Cancer 2000; 89(3):604–614.

3. Perez-Ordonez B, et al. Renal oncocytoma: a clinicopathologic study of 70 cases. Am J Surg Pathol 1997;21(8):871–883.

4. Kovacs G, et al. The Heidelberg classification of renal cell tumours. J Pathol 1997;183(2):131–133.

5. Tickoo SK, et al. Ultrastructural observations on mitochondria and microvesicles in renal oncocytoma, chromophobe renal cell carcinoma, and eosinophilic variant of conventional (clear cell) renal cell carcinoma. Am J Surg Pathol 2000;24(9): 1247–1256.

6. Fuzesi L, et al. Cytogenetic analysis of 11 renal oncocytomas: further evidence of structural rearrangements of 11q13 as a characteristic chromosomal anomaly. Cancer Genet Cytogenet 1998; 107(1):1–6.

7. Herbers J, et al. Lack of genetic changes at specific genomic sites separates renal oncocytomas from renal cell carcinomas. J Pathol 1998;184(1): 58–62.

8. Sinke RJ, et al. Fine mapping of the human renal oncocytoma-associated translocation (5;11) (q35;q13) breakpoint. Cancer Genet Cytogenet 1997;96(2):95–101.

9. Michal M. Benign mixed epithelial and stromal tumor of the kidney. Pathol Res Pract 2000; 196(4):275–276.

10. Michal M, Syrucek M. Benign mixed epithelial and stromal tumor of the kidney. Pathol Res Pract 1998;194:445–448.

11. Adsay NV, et al. Mixed epithelial and stromal tumor of the kidney. Am J Surg Pathol 2000;24(7): 958–970.

12. Moch H, et al. Mixed epithelial and stromal tumor of the kidney. Pathologe, 2004;25:356–361.

13. Pierson CR, et al. Mixed epithelial and stromal tumor of the kidney lacks the genetic alterations of cellular congenital mesoblastic nephroma. Hum Pathol 2001;32(5):513–520.

14. Argani P, et al. Primary renal synovial sarcoma: molecular and morphologic delineation of an entity previously included among embryonal sarcomas of the kidney. Am J Surg Pathol 2000; 24(8):1087–1096.

15. Kim DH, et al. Primary synovial sarcoma of the kidney. Am J Surg Pathol 2000;24(8):1097–1104.

16. Moch H, et al. Primary renal synovial sarcoma. A new entity in the morphological spectrum of spindle cell tumors. Der Pathologe 2003;24(6): 466–472.

17. Mezzelani A, et al. SYT-SSX fusion transcripts and epithelial differentiation in synovial sarcoma. Diagn Mol Pathol 2000;9(4):234–235.

18. Fligman I, et al. Molecular diagnosis of synovial sarcoma and characterization of a variant SYT-SSX2 fusion transcript. Am J Pathol 1995;147(6): 1592–1599.

19. Furman J, et al. Primary primitive neuroectodermal tumor of the kidney. Am J Clin Pathol 1996; 106:339–344.

20. Rodriguez-Galindo C, et al. Is primitive neuroectodermal tumor of the kidney a distinct entity? Cancer 1997;79(11):2243–2250.

21. Quezado M, Benjamin DR, Tsokos M. EWS/FLI-1 fusion transcripts in three peripheral primitive neuroectodermal tumors of the kidney. Hum Pathol 1997;28(7):767–771.

22. Jimenez RE, et al. Primary Ewing's sarcoma/primitive neuroectodermal tumor of the kidney: a clinicopathologic and immunohistochemical analysis of 11 cases. Am J Surg Pathol 2002;26(3):320–327.

23. Casella R, et al. Metastatic primitive neuroectodermal tumor of the kidney in adults. Eur Urol 2001;39:613–617.

24. MacLennan GT, Farrow GM, Bostwick DG. Low-grade collecting duct carcinoma of the kidney: report of 13 cases of low-grade mucinous tubulocystic renal carcinoma of possible collecting duct origin. Urology 1997;50(5):679–684.

25. Srigley J, Eble JN, Grignon DJ. Unusual renal cell carcinoma (RCC) with prominent spindle cell change possibly related to the loop of Henle. Mod Pathol 1999;12:107A.

26. Srigley J, et al. Phenotypic, molecular and ultrastructural studies of a novel low grade renal epithelial neoplasm possibly related to the loop of Henle. Mod Pathol 2002;15(1):182A.

27. Rakozy C, et al. Low-grade tubular-mucinous renal neoplasms: morphologic, immunohistochemical, and genetic features. Mod Pathol 2002; 15(11):1162–1171.

28. Weber A, Srigley J, Moch H. Mucinous tubular and spindle cell carcinoma of the kidney. A molecular analysis. Pathologe 2003;24(6):453–459.

29. Argani P, et al. Primary renal neoplasms with the ASPL-TFE3 gene fusion of alveolar soft part sarcoma: a distinctive tumor entity previously included among renal cell carcinomas of children and adolescents. Am J Pathol 2001;159(1):179–192.

30. Renshaw AA, et al. Renal cell carcinomas in children and young adults: increased incidence of papillary architecture and unique subtypes. Am J Surg Pathol 1999;23(7):795–802.

31. Weterman MA, Wilbrink M, Geurts van Kessel A. Fusion of the transcription factor TFE3 gene to a novel gene, PRCC, in t(X;1)(p11;q21)-positive papillary renal cell carcinomas. Proc Natl Acad Sci USA 1996;93(26):15294–15298.

32. Weterman MA, et al. Molecular cloning of the papillary renal cell carcinoma-associated translocation (X;1)(p11;q21) breakpoint. Cytogenet Cell Genet 1996;75(1):2–6.

33. Bruder E, et al. Morphologic and molecular characterization of renal cell carcinoma in children and young adults. Am J Surg Pathol 2004;28(9): 1117–1132.

26

Small Cell Tumors, Lymphomas, and Sertoli Cell and Leydig Cell Tumors of the Bladder, Prostate, and Testis

Chris M. Bacon and Alex Freeman

Lymphomas of the Testis, Bladder, and Prostate

Approximately one third of lymphomas arise at an extranodal site (primary extranodal lymphomas), and both primary nodal lymphomas and leukemias not infrequently infiltrate extranodal tissues secondarily during their course. The genitourinary tract is the site of less than 5% of primary extranodal lymphomas [1]. Among these the testis is the most frequent site. Postmortem studies indicate that the genitourinary tract is secondarily involved by lymphoid neoplasms in up to 50% of patients, and such involvement may be clinically apparent in up to 10% of patients [2].

Lymphoid neoplasms are currently classified according to the World Health Organization (WHO) Classification of Tumors of the Hematopoietic and Lymphoid tissues [3]. In this globally accepted classification, devised by an international panel of pathologists, hematologists, and oncologists, lymphomas and leukemias are categorized into discrete entities according to morphological, immunohistological, genetic, and clinical features. Although some lymphomas are defined by their sites of origin, there are no lymphoid neoplasms that arise only in the genitourinary tract. In the clinical setting, the correct identification and then subclassification of lymphoid neoplasms by urologists and urological pathologists is crucial, as many of the entities defined have distinctive clinico-

pathological features, therapeutic needs, and prognoses, and all require specialist management. Another major determinant of treatment choice and outcome is the stage of lymphoma at presentation. In this regard, lymphomas of the genitourinary tract are, like lymphomas arising elsewhere, staged according to the Ann Arbor staging system.

Lymphoma of the Testis

Clinically apparent lymphoma of the testis is rare, representing only approximately 1% of all lymphomas and 5% of all testicular tumors [4,5]. Unlike germ cell tumors, testicular lymphoma typically occurs in older patients, being the commonest testicular neoplasm in men over 60 years of age [4]. Lymphoma may arise primarily in the testis, or may manifest in the testis secondarily (albeit often early) during the course of systemic disease. It may sometimes be impossible to distinguish these scenarios, even in patients with limited (stage I/II) disease, but in most studies primary testicular lymphoma is defined pragmatically as that in which a testicular mass was the predominant site of clinical disease at presentation [6–9]. There are no established predisposing factors for the development of testicular lymphoma, although there is an increased incidence among men infected with HIV [4].

The majority (approximately 80% to 90%) of primary testicular lymphomas are diffuse large B cell lymphomas (DLBCLs) [10–13]. Other subtypes, including mature T/natural killer (NK) cell lymphomas, follicular lymphomas, Burkitt lymphomas, and plasma cell neoplasms, are rare primary testicular tumors. Most non-Hodgkin lymphomas may secondarily involve the testis, as may chronic lymphocytic leukemia (CLL) and precursor B- or T-cell acute lymphoblastic leukemia (ALL), the latter especially in children. Involvement of the testis by classical Hodgkin lymphoma is exceptional. These different types of lymphoproliferative disorder are biologically and clinically distinct, and are thus considered separately below.

Testicular Diffuse Large B Cell Lymphoma

Clinical Features

Testicular DLBCL typically presents with unilateral painless scrotal swelling in men whose median age is 60 to 70 years [6–9,12]. Both testes are involved at presentation in up to 15% of patients [6–8], and 5% to 15% present with systemic ("B") symptoms [6–9,13]. Approximately 50% of patients present with stage I disease (testes only), 20% with stage II disease (regional lymph node involvement), 5% with stage III disease, and 25% with stage IV disease (disseminated) [6–8,12]. Characteristic sites of distant organ involvement include the central nervous system (CNS) (especially), Waldeyer's ring, skin, bone and bone marrow, kidneys, adrenal glands, and lungs [4,6–8]. Compared to nodal DLBCL, testicular lymphoma is associated with presentation at an earlier stage and a greater propensity for spread to other extranodal sites.

Pathology

Macroscopically, testicular DLBCL usually forms an ill-defined, firm or soft, gray, tan, or pink mass, sometimes with areas of hemorrhage or necrosis [4,10]. The lymphoma extends into paratesticular structures in up to 50% of cases. Microscopically, a diffuse infiltrate of atypical lymphoid cells dissects between seminiferous tubules, or sometimes effaces testicular architecture (Fig 26.1). In many cases lymphoma cells show at least focal intratubular growth, and tubules often show suppressed spermatogenesis, or atrophy. Interstitial sclerosis is present in a third of cases [4,10,11]. Testicular DLBCL is cytologically and immunophenotypically similar to DLBCL arising in lymph nodes. The neoplastic cells are typically medium-sized to large, with vesicular nuclei and prominent nucleoli, although there is variation in morphology between cases [3]. They express pan–B-cell antigens such as CD20, and many express detectable immunoglobulin. In most cases, lymphoma cells express the antiapoptotic protein Bcl-2, and a high proportion of cells (>40%) express the cell cycle protein Ki67, indicating that they are in cell cycle. Similar to nodal DLBCL [14], the germinal center–associated proteins Bcl-6 and CD10 are expressed by approximately 80% and 50% of testicular DLBCL, respectively (unpublished observations).

Biology and Genetics

Although relatively few studies have specifically examined the biomolecular features of testicular DLBCL, available evidence suggests that the pathobiology of testicular DLBCL is similar in many ways to DLBCL arising elsewhere. Both primary testicular DLBCL and DLBCL in general are clonal proliferations of mature B cells whose immunoglobulin genes have undergone VDJ (variable-diversity-joining region) rearrangement and, in most cases, somatic hypermutation [15,16]. Because the latter is a mechanism for diversification of immunoglobulin genes that occurs during the germinal center reaction of an immune response, it is believed that DLBCLs arise from germinal center or postgerminal center B cells. Hyland et al. [15] showed that testicular DLBCLs display ongoing somatic hypermutation, clonal diversification, and a pattern of immunoglobulin gene mutation suggestive of a role for ongoing antigen selection in the evolution of the lymphoma [15]. Pasqualucci et al. [17] demonstrated that more than half of DLBCLs show aberrant somatic hypermutation activity resulting in mutation of several known proto-oncogenes, including *MYC* [17]. Thus, aberrant hypermutation may contribute to genomic instability in DLBCLs.

There is now considerable evidence that DLBCL is both biologically and clinically heterogeneous. In landmark studies, Alizadeh et al. [18] and Rosenwald et al. [19] performed large-scale DNA microarray-based gene expression analyses of DLBCLs and demonstrated that DLBCLs showed diverse gene expression patterns, but could be divided into subgroups with germinal center B-cell–like profiles, *in vitro*

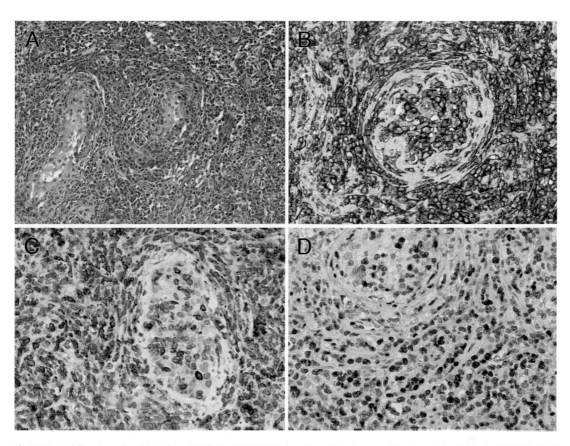

Fig. 26.1. A diffuse large B-cell lymphoma of the testis (A, H&E) showing positive immunohistochemical staining for CD20 (B), Bcl-2 (C) and nuclear BCL-6 (D). Original magnification: A, 100×; B–D, 200×.

activated B-cell–like profiles, or poorly defined heterogeneous type 3 gene expression profiles. Interestingly, these subgroups showed differences in biochemistry and genetics (see below) and in clinical outcome. Patients whose tumors had germinal center B-cell–like gene expression profiles had a significantly better 5-year overall survival than those whose tumors did not. Two studies have used DNA microarray technology to identify genes whose expression correlates with the outcome of DLBCL [19,20]. Many of the genes implicated are associated with cell proliferation, apoptosis, B-cell receptor signaling, germinal center B-cell phenotype, or lymph node stromal and immune cells, or are major histocompatibility complex (MHC) class II genes, highlighting the importance of both intrinsic properties of the lymphoma cells and host–tumor interactions in the behavior of DLBCLs. Some of the differentially expressed

genes were used to successfully formulate prognostic algorithms or outcome predictors for DLBCLs [19,20].

Several studies have used immunohistochemistry to subclassify DLBCLs into those with a germinal center cell phenotype and those with a postgerminal center cell phenotype according to the presence or absence of proteins expressed predominantly by germinal center B cells (Bcl-6 and CD10) or postgerminal center B cells (IRF-4/MUM-1) [21–24]. Some of these studies have shown germinal center–type protein expression to be associated with a favorable overall survival [21,23,24], whereas others have failed to demonstrate any significance [21,22].

Although many DLBCLs exhibit complex cytogenetic abnormalities, several recurrent genetic alterations have been identified. In 15% to 30% of cases, the *BCL2* gene is translocated to the immunoglobulin heavy chain gene locus as a result of a t(14;18)(q32;q21) translocation, with resultant dysregulation of its expression [25–27]. The t(14;18) is seen almost exclusively in DLBCLs with a germinal center cell phenotype [27,28]. However, the Bcl-2 protein is expressed in approximately 50% to 60% of DLBCLs, and is not restricted to those with a germinal center cell phenotype [22–24,28]. In many t(14;18)-negative cases this may result from amplification of the *BCL2* gene locus [29]. Although most studies have failed to show that the presence of a t(14;18) has any prognostic impact [25–27], many have demonstrated that the expression of Bcl-2 protein is associated with an adverse clinical outcome [22–26]. Lambrechts et al. [30] showed that the Bcl-2 protein is consistently expressed by testicular DLBCLs, suggesting that the antiapoptotic functions of Bcl-2 may play an important role in the pathogenesis of these lymphomas. However, t(14;18) was not detected in any of the 29 cases studied [15,30]. The *BCL6* gene at 3q27 is dysregulated by translocation (often to the immunoglobulin heavy chain gene locus) in 25% to 40% of DLBCLs [25,31], and by mutation of its 5′ regulatory region in a further 15% of cases [32]. Because the Bcl-6 protein is a transcriptional repressor that controls the terminal stages of B-cell differentiation, these mutations may promote lymphomagenesis by altering B-cell terminal differentiation. Mutations in the *P53* gene are found in approximately 20% of DLBCLs and are associated in most studies with an adverse clinical outcome [33]. The *MYC* gene is translocated in up to 10% of cases [25]. Amplification of 2p12–16, which includes the *REL* proto-oncogene, a nuclear factor (NF)-κB family member, is observed in approximately 20% of DLBCLs (including one of two testicular DLBCLs studied) [34]. Activation of NF-κB appears important in the pathogenesis of DLBCLs, particularly those with an activated B-cell–like gene expression profile [35].

Differences in host–tumor interactions have been identified between testicular and nodal DLBCL. Although a small subset of nodal DLBCLs is associated with defective expression of human leukocyte antigen (HLA) class I and II molecules, this appears particularly prevalent in testicular DLBCL, in which loss of HLA class I/II molecules was detected in 61% of cases as a result of homozygous and hemizygous deletions in the HLA locus and genetic aberrations in the β$_2$-microglobulin gene [36,37]. This may repre-

sent a mechanism by which testicular DLBCLs can evade a host antitumor immune response. It is interesting that primary DLBCLs of the CNS, a site to which testicular DLBCL characteristically disseminates, show similar defects in HLA molecule expression [36]. The characteristic pattern of extranodal spread displayed by testicular DLBCL may also reflect differences in adhesion molecule expression compared to DLBCL at other sites [38].

Treatment and Outcome

Although the treatment and outcome of testicular DLBCL has varied over the years, most recent studies show 5-year overall survival rates of 37% to 48%, and median survival times of 32 to 58 months [6,12,39]. Stage I/II testicular DLBCL has a considerably worse outcome than stage I/II nodal DLBCL (5-year overall survival approximately 45% to 58% vs. 75% to 80%) [6,40]. The most consistent prognostic factor for testicular DLBCL is Ann Arbor stage [4,7,12,39]. In the large series of Zucca et al. [6], the 5-year overall survival and median survival respectively were as follows: stage I, 58%, 6.1 years; stage II, 46%, 3.9 years; stage III/IV, 22%, 1.1 years. Other prognostic factors identified include age, International Prognostic Index, presence or absence of B symptoms, and presence or absence of microscopic sclerosis within the lymphoma [4,6,10]. Despite exceptional cures (which provide evidence for true primary testicular lymphoma), the vast majority of patients, even with stage I disease, relapse and die of disease after treatment by orchidectomy alone [4,6]. Likewise, although locoregional radiotherapy provides good local control, more than 70% of patients with stage I/II disease treated by orchidectomy and locoregional radiotherapy alone relapse distally and succumb to lymphoma [4]. More recent treatment protocols have employed adjuvant anthracycline-based combined chemotherapy regimens, and several studies have found such chemotherapy to be associated with improved progression-free and overall survival at all stages of disease [4,6–8,41].

Although 70% to 90% of patients achieve an initial complete response, 30% to 80% subsequently relapse [6–9,12,13,39]. It is characteristic of testicular DLBCLs that the majority (approximately 80%) of relapses involve extranodal sites, including the CNS, contralateral testis, bone and bone marrow, skin, lung, and adrenal glands [4,6–8]. Although most relapses occur in the first 2 years after treatment, testicular DLBCL is also unusual in a significant incidence of late relapses—up to 14 years after treatment in some studies [6,8,13]. A CNS relapse occurs in approximately 15% to 30% of patients with testicular DLBCL, including many with stage I/II disease [6,7,12,13,39]. This high rate has led many centers to give intrathecal chemotherapy as CNS prophylaxis to all patients, but the efficacy of such an approach remains unproven [6,8,39]. This may be in part due to the propensity for parenchymal, rather than meningeal, relapse seen in most studies [6,8,13,39]. Another characteristic site of relapse, seen in 5% to 15% of patients, is the contralateral testis [6–8,12,13]. This may be effectively prevented by prophylactic irradiation of the contralateral testis at first treatment [4,6,8]. Thus, current treatment protocols at many centers now include orchidectomy, combination anthracycline-based chemotherapy, prophylactic radiotherapy to the contralateral testis, and CNS prophylaxis, with the possible addition of regional radiotherapy in patients with disease in regional lymph nodes [2]. Addition of the therapeutic anti-CD20 antibody Rituximab, as used successfully against DLBCLs at other sites [42], may also be considered.

Other Lymphoproliferative Disorders Involving the Testis

Testicular Lymphoproliferative Disorders in Childhood

The testis is involved in approximately 5% of childhood lymphomas, most commonly in disseminated Burkitt lymphoma, an aggressive mature B-cell lymphoma associated in all cases with translocation of the *MYC* gene. [43]. With modern combination chemotherapy protocols, testicular involvement at diagnosis does not appear to confer a worse prognosis [43]. The testis is also not infrequently involved during the course of precursor B- or T-cell ALL (more commonly precursor T-cell ALL). It is rarely clinically involved at presentation, although up to 25% of boys have occult testicular disease at diagnosis without adverse prognostic effect [44].

However, 5% to 10% of patients experience overt testicular involvement at relapse, either alone or with simultaneous bone marrow disease [45]. Again, with modern treatment protocols, these patients fare no worse than those without testicular disease at relapse. Rarely, primary follicular lymphomas of the testis arise in children. To date, these have all been stage I tumors, with WHO grade 3 morphology with or without areas of DLBCL, and have shown indolent clinical behavior. Inasmuch as they have been uniformly negative for Bcl-2 protein expression and t(14;18), they may represent a clinicopathological entity distinct from usual adult follicular lymphoma [46].

Plasma Cell Neoplasia

Extraosseous plasmacytomas represent only approximately 0.1% of all testis tumors, and testicular involvement is seen in only approximately 2% of myeloma patients [47,48]. They present as a painless mass at a median age of approximately 55 years. Microscopically, the testis is infiltrated by nodules of atypical monoclonal plasma cells with a predominantly interstitial pattern of infiltration [47]. More than half of these patients have preceding or concurrent plasma cell myeloma, and the vast majority of the remainder develop myeloma in the following 2 to 3 years [48]. Cases of solitary testicular plasmacytoma not followed by myeloma are exceptional, but appear to have a favorable prognosis.

Mature T/NK Cell Lymphomas

Mature T/NK cell lymphomas of the testis are very rare, and have been documented primarily as case reports. The majority are extranodal NK/T cell lymphoma, nasal type, an aggressive angiocentric and angiodestructive Epstein-Barr virus–associated lymphoma of NK-cell or cytotoxic T-cell origin. All have had a rapidly fatal outcome [49]. There have also been occasional reports of peripheral T-cell lymphoma, unspecified, and other subtypes presenting in the testis.

Lymphoma of Paratesticular Tissues

Lymphomas of the epididymis and spermatic cord most often occur as a result of spread from the testis, or sometimes as a site of dissemination of systemic lymphoma. Primary paratesticular lymphoma is very rare [50,51]. Patients with primary lymphoma of the spermatic cord have a mean age of approximately 55 years, and present with hard masses in the groin resembling inguinal hernias. The lymphomas are mostly DLBCLs, and show clinical features and a poor prognosis similar to testicular DLBCLs [50,51]. Primary epididymal lymphoma has been reported in patients with a wide age range (20 to 73 years). Although the older patients mostly developed DLBCL, follicular lymphomas and an extranodal marginal zone lymphoma of mucosa-associated lymphoid tissue (MALT lymphoma), with a more indolent course, were seen in the younger patients [50,51]. Extraosseous plasmacytoma may also occasionally be seen in paratesticular tissues [50].

Lymphoma of the Bladder

The majority of lymphomas affecting the lower urinary tract involve the bladder. Lymphoma arising within, and localized to, the bladder (primary bladder lymphoma, stage I) is very rare, representing only approximately 0.1% to 0.2% of all extranodal lymphomas [1]. More common is secondary involvement of the bladder by previously diagnosed lymphoma arising elsewhere. In a postmortem series, the bladder was involved in 13% of patients who died of advanced lymphoma [52]. A third, rare group of patients presents with urinary tract–related symptoms, but has lymphoma beyond the bladder at diagnosis [53]. A proportion of these patients, in whom the bladder contains the bulk of the disease, may also represent primary bladder lymphoma, stages II to IV.

Clinical Features

Primary lymphoma of the bladder affects predominantly adult women (male/female ratio approximately 1:5), at a median age of approximately 65 years (20 to 85 years) [53–55]. Secondary involvement of the bladder occurs equally in men and women, at a similar age [53,55]. The most common presenting symptoms are painless hematuria, dysuria, urgency, frequency, and nocturia [53,54]. Systemic ("B") symptoms, regional pain, and obstructive features are more frequent in those with advanced disease. The cystoscopic appearance is usually

that of a single or sometimes multiple, submucosal, sessile, or polypoid mass protruding into the lumen, typically without ulceration [53]. Diffuse thickening of the bladder wall may also be seen. Approximately 20% of patients with primary bladder lymphoma have a clinical history of prior chronic cystitis [53,54,56].

Pathology

Studies have shown that almost all low-grade primary lymphomas of the bladder, although rare, are MALT lymphomas [53,55,56]. These tend to remain localized to the bladder (stage 1) [53,56]. A smaller subset of primary bladder lymphomas are DLBCLs, perhaps arising by transformation of MALT lymphoma in some cases [53,55]. Very occasional cases of T-cell lymphoma, plasmacytoma, and Burkitt lymphoma in an HIV-positive person have been reported. Secondary involvement of the bladder is usually by DLBCL, followed by follicular lymphoma, MALT lymphoma, Burkitt lymphoma, mantle cell lymphoma, and classical Hodgkin lymphoma [53,55]. In a postmortem series, 16% of patients who died of CLL and 26% of those who died of ALL had infiltration of the bladder by leukemia [52]; this is usually subclinical.

Microscopically, MALT lymphoma consists of a proliferation of neoplastic small to medium-sized marginal zone cells between and around reactive lymphoid follicles, frequently infiltrating into the muscularis [3,53,55–57] (Fig. 26.2). These cells show variable cytology, often including plasma cell differentiation. In many cases the neoplastic cells infiltrate the epithelium of cystitis glandularis, or sometimes surface transitional epithelium, in small clusters forming characteristic lymphoepithelial lesions. Often a reactive lymphoid infiltrate suggestive of chronic cystitis is seen in the background. The neoplastic cells have an immunophenotype similar to that of normal marginal zone cells (positive for CD20, immunoglobulins [Igs] M and A; negative for CD10, Bcl-6, IgD). The histological features of DLBCLs in the bladder are similar to those in other organs [3].

Biology and Genetics

MALT lymphoma is thought to arise from the marginal zone B cells of MALT, acquired as a

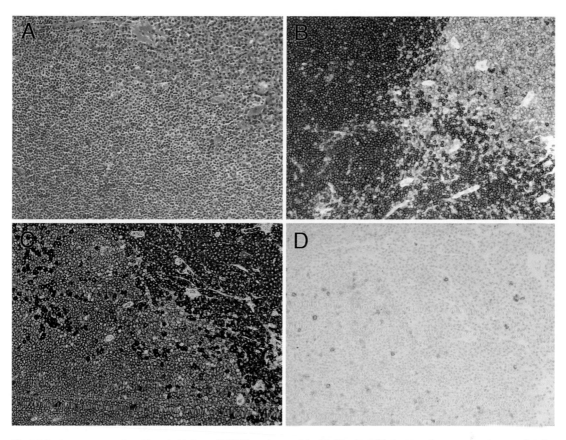

Fig. 26.2. A mucosa associated lymphoid tissue (MALT) lymphoma of the bladder (A, H&E) showing characteristic plasma cell differentiation (top right of each panel). Tumor cells express CD20 (B) and Immunoglobulin M (IgM) (C), but not IgD (D). Original magnification: each 100×.

result of chronic inflammation of a mucosa normally devoid of lymphoid tissue [3,58]. Examples include *Helicobacter pylori*–associated gastritis and Hashimoto thyroiditis. There is evidence to suggest that, at least early in its course, MALT lymphoma may be partially dependent on antigen and T-cell–mediated stimulation occurring in such a microenvironment [58]. Although no studies have specifically investigated the biology of MALT lymphoma arising in the bladder, the lack of convincing native lymphoid tissue in the bladder, the clinical or histological evidence of antecedent chronic cystitis in many patients, and the higher incidence in women than in men of both MALT lymphoma of the bladder and chronic cystitis suggests a similar pathogenesis at this site, in which chronic cystitis is a nonobligate precursor for MALT lymphoma [53,55–57].

A number of recurrent genetic abnormalities have been identified in MALT lymphomas. Thirty to 60% of cases, including one reported case in the bladder, show trisomy 3 [58,59]. Many others contain one of three known recurrent translocations [58,60]: t(11;18)(q21;q21) results in the formation of a chimeric fusion protein between the apoptosis inhibitor API2 and the paracaspase MALT1; t(14;18)(q32;q21) translocates the *MALT1* gene to the immunoglobulin heavy chain gene locus; and t(1;14)(p22;q32) translocates the *BCL10* gene to the immunoglobulin heavy chain gene locus. MALT1 and Bcl10 both function in a biochemical signaling pathway connecting lymphocyte antigen receptor signaling to activation of the transcription factor NF-κB, and dysregulation of this pathway is thought to be important in MALT lymphomagenesis [58]. However, to date, these translocations have not been reported in MALT lymphoma of the bladder.

Treatment and Outcome

Due to its rarity, there is little information regarding the optimal treatment of primary bladder lymphoma. Cases of primary MALT lymphoma of the bladder reported in the literature have been variably treated with transurethral or radical surgery, radiotherapy, or chemotherapy, alone or in combination. In keeping with MALT lymphomas at other sites, the outcome has been favorable in almost all cases, with very few lymphoma-related deaths reported [53–57]. Some have recommended radiotherapy as the treatment of choice for localized cases [2,61]. Interestingly, similar to the ability of antibiotic-mediated *H. pylori* eradication to cure many gastric MALT lymphomas [58], two primary MALT lymphomas of the bladder have resolved after *Helicobacter* eradication therapy or antibiotics for chronic cystitis [62,63]. Several case reports and small series have also reported good outcomes for localized DLBCL treated with radiotherapy or chemotherapy with or without surgical intervention [54,55]. In contrast, in the largest retrospective series published, nonlocalized lymphoma involving the bladder at first diagnosis and lymphoma involving the bladder secondarily in the course of widespread lymphoma had a much worse prognosis (9-year and 0.6-year median survival, respectively) [53].

Lymphoma of the Prostate

Primary lymphoma of the prostate is very rare, representing only approximately 0.2% to 0.8% of extranodal lymphomas and 0.1% of all prostate neoplasms [1,64,65]. Secondary involvement of the prostate by lymphoma or leukemia is more frequent, being found at postmortem in up to 8% of "non-Hodgkin" lymphomas and up to 20% of cases of CLL [66]. However, in most cases this involvement is not clinically apparent. In a series of 62 prostatic lymphomas, Bostwick et al. [67] found 35% to be primary (defined by presenting symptoms of prostatic enlargement, predominant involvement of the prostate, and no involvement of lymph nodes, blood, liver, or spleen within 1 month of diagnosis), 48% to be secondary to known systemic lymphoma/leukemia, and 17% to be unclassifiable as primary or secondary.

Clinical Features

Almost all patients diagnosed with prostatic lymphoma, whether primary or secondary, present with symptoms of lower urinary tract obstruction [64,65,67]. Occasional patients present with pain or hematuria, and some with systemic disease have "B" symptoms. Serum prostate-specific antigen is raised in approximately 20% of patients. On digital rectal examination the prostate appears diffusely enlarged or nodular, and firm. A tissue diagnosis is usually obtained by examination of needle biopsies or tissue obtained by transurethral resection. Occasionally lymphoma/leukemia is diagnosed as an incidental finding in a radical prostatectomy specimen removed for known prostatic adenocarcinoma. Of note, the urologist and pathologist may also encounter lymphoma/leukemia as an incidental finding in approximately 0.2% to 1.2% of the pelvic lymph node resections performed at radical prostatectomy [68,69].

Pathology and Biology

The majority of primary lymphomas of the prostate are DLBCLs, but primary prostatic small lymphocytic lymphomas (SLLs), follicular lymphomas, Burkitt lymphomas, MALT lymphomas, and mantle cell lymphomas have also been reported [64,65,67,70]. A similar spectrum of lymphomas affects the prostate secondarily during the course of disseminated disease, and rare cases of secondary prostatic peripheral T-cell lymphoma, myeloma, and classical "Hodgkin" lymphoma have also been documented [67]. Histologically, lymphomas within the prostate gland show patchy or diffuse stromal infiltration, with compression, but preservation, of ducts and acini. Intraepithelial infiltration of neoplastic cells is seen in some cases. The morphologic and immunophenotypic features of prostatic lymphomas are similar to those of extraprostatic disease [3]. No studies have specifically addressed the genetics of prostatic lymphomas.

As mentioned above, leukemic cells not infrequently infiltrate the prostate, sometimes as the only site of solid tissue involvement [66]. One recent study showed that CLL cells from patients with prostatic infiltration (but not from those without) bound to prostatic epithelial cells via clonally expressed surface IgM [71]. This suggests a mechanism for accumulation of CLL cells in the prostates of some patients.

Treatment and Outcome

Because of the rarity with which lymphoma presents in the prostate, little is known of its prognosis and optimal treatment. In the series of Bostwick et al. [67], 47% of patients with follow-up died of lymphoma, with a lymphoma-specific 5-year survival of only 33%; 73% of patients with primary prostatic lymphoma developed extraprostatic disease 1 to 59 months from diagnosis. There were no significant differences in survival between patients receiving different therapies (chemotherapy, radiotherapy, chemotherapy and radiotherapy, surgery only), between patients with primary or secondary prostatic lymphoma, or between patients with different types of lymphoma. However, patients in this retrospective study were treated over a 58-year period, and it is unlikely that these data reflect the results that would be achieved using current stage and subtype-specific therapeutic regimens. Indeed, a number of more recent case studies have reported good outcomes for patients with high-grade prostatic lymphoma treated with anthracycline-based combination chemotherapy [65,72], and it remains uncertain whether the prognosis of lymphoma presenting in the prostate is significantly worse than that of equivalent lymphomas presenting at most other extranodal sites.

Small Cell Tumors of the Bladder and Prostate

The vast majority of small round blue-cell tumors of the bladder and prostate prove to be either lymphomas or systemic infiltrates in patients with a known history of leukemia. These entities have been covered in detail in the preceding section.

After exclusion of lymphoma, the pathologist must consider a variety of other tumors that may rarely arise at these sites, including tumors of both epithelial and mesenchymal origin. The differential diagnosis greatly relies on the clinical

information provided, and in particular on the age of the patient. In children and adolescents, the most common small round blue-cell tumor of the bladder and prostate, other than leukemia and lymphoma, is embryonal rhabdomyosarcoma. Although there are reports of other rare primary or metastatic tumors occurring in the bladder and prostate, including primitive neuroectodermal tumor (PNET), neuroblastoma, Wilms' tumor, and desmoplastic small round cell tumor [73–78], these should be considered only after exclusion of the more common entities outlined above. In adults, the main differential diagnosis of nonlymphoid small round blue-cell tumors includes poorly differentiated carcinoma and neuroendocrine tumors such as carcinoid and small cell carcinoma. More rarely, neoplasms such as paraganglioma, synovial sarcoma, metastatic lymphoepithelioma-like carcinoma, and small cell melanoma have been reported at these sites [79–84].

The following section outlines a few of the more common and clinically relevant entities in more detail.

Small Cell Carcinoma of the Bladder

Primary small cell carcinoma of the bladder was first reported by Cramer et al. [85] in 1981 as a rare aggressive vesical tumor sharing morphological and ultrastructural features with oat cell (small cell) carcinoma of the lung [85]. Since then, only about 150 cases have been described worldwide [86]. Although they account for less than 1% of bladder tumors, their importance lies in the fact that the tumors have a characteristic histological appearance and are usually associated with a rapidly progressive course, requiring adjuvant treatment with a tailored chemotherapy regimen that often differs from that used to treat high-grade urothelial carcinoma.

Clinical and Radiological Features

The majority of patients present with urinary symptoms, including dysuria and hematuria [87], and over 50% have metastatic deposits at the time of diagnosis in the lymph nodes, bone liver, or lung [88]. In rare cases, the secretion of neuropeptides by the tumor cells may also lead to paraneoplastic symptoms such as peripheral neuropathy and electrolyte abnormalities including hypercalcemia and hypophosphatemia [89,90]. Radiological studies using computed tomography (CT) and magnetic resonance imaging (MRI) have shown that these tumors often are large, broad-based polypoid intramural masses, and are most frequently located on the posterior bladder wall or in the region of the trigone [91,92]. Rare cases are also reported as arising within a bladder diverticulum.

Pathology

Small cell carcinomas are malignant epithelial tumors showing neuroendocrine differentiation, and are composed of small, hyperchromatic cells with a coarse "salt-and-pepper" chromatin pattern, scant cytoplasm, and inconspicuous nucleoli. The tumor cells show characteristic features including the presence of nuclear molding and encrustation of tumor cell DNA within blood vessel walls (Azzopardi phenomenon). Mitoses are frequent and necrosis may be focally present. Specific criteria for diagnosing these tumor cells in cytological preparations have also been described [93]. In a cytological study, from 23 patients with subsequent biopsy and histological confirmation, a combination of cellular and nuclear features were used to correctly diagnose all the tumors as small cell carcinomas on the basis of urine cytology alone [94]. About 50% of vesical small cell carcinomas show focal areas with the morphology of classical urothelial carcinoma, and some may contain small foci of squamous cell or adenocarcinoma [95]. The presence of these elements is still considered compatible with a diagnosis of small cell carcinoma, if the remainder of the tumor shows the characteristic histological features mentioned above.

Ultrastructure and Immunohistochemical Profile

Tumor cells have been shown to contain neurosecretory granules on electron microscopy (1). Immunohistochemistry often shows positive staining for neuroendocrine markers, including CD56 (92%), neuron-specific enolase (87%), and chromogranin A (up to 65%), and shows dot-like positivity with antibodies against cytokeratins such as CAM5.2 (60%) [96,97]. A negative staining pattern for CD45 (leukocyte common antigen) and CD44v6 enables distinction from tumors with a similar morphological appearance, including lymphoma and poorly differentiated urothelial carcinoma, respectively [98]. However, separation of a primary bladder small cell carcinoma from a metastatic small cell carcinoma of pulmonary origin relies more heavily on clinical and radiological findings, as their immunohistochemical profile may be identical.

Biology and Genetics

The exact origin of small cell carcinoma of the bladder is unknown, but it has been postulated that these tumors may arise either from a small population of resident ("Kulchitsky-type") neuroendocrine cells in the vesical mucosa, from neuroendocrine metaplasia of urothelial cells, or from a mucosal stem cell with a capacity for multipotential differentiation [94,99].

Although relatively little is known about the genetic alterations in these tumors, on account of their rarity, studies using comparative genomic hybridization (CGH) have shown that vesical small cell carcinomas contain a high number of genomic alterations (a mean of 11.3 per tumor), including amplification, gains and deletions at specific loci coding for known oncogenes, and tumor-suppressor genes [100]. Elevated telomerase levels have also been identified in exfoliated tumor cells from urine and bladder washings in patients with small cell carcinoma, and may be involved in tumor cell immortalization, although the significance of this finding is unclear [101].

Treatment and Outcome

As mentioned above, these tumors pursue an aggressive clinical course, with early lymphovascular and muscle invasion and are frequently metastatic at the time of presentation. The overall 5-year survival of patients with localized small cell carcinoma may be as low as 8% [88,102]. Predictors of poor survival include age greater than 65 years, tumor stage, and presence of lymphovascular invasion [103]. Treatment options consist of cystectomy and adjuvant chemotherapy or radiotherapy, and a large number of different regimens are in use, showing varying success rates [104,105].

Small Cell Carcinoma of the Prostate

Small cell carcinoma is a rare variant of prostatic carcinoma, accounting for less than 1% of all tumors arising in the gland [106]. It behaves in an aggressive manner, metastasizes early, and is unresponsive to some types of chemotherapeutic regimens [107]. Although pure small cell carcinoma is rare, the presence of neuroendocrine differentiation is not uncommonly seen to some extent in prostatic carcinoma and may take one of three forms:

- Focal neuroendocrine differentiation in a conventional prostatic adenocarcinoma
- Carcinoid tumor (well-differentiated neuroendocrine tumor)
- Small cell carcinoma (poorly differentiated neuroendocrine carcinoma)

Thus, although virtually all prostatic carcinomas show focal neuroendocrine differentiation in terms of scattered neurosecretory cells within the tumor, only about 5% to 10% contain significant groups of cells demonstrating neuroendocrine markers by immunostaining [108].

Clinical Features

A significant proportion of small cell carcinomas of the prostate arise in patients with a previous history of hormonally treated acinar adenocarcinoma [109]. These patients subsequently present with worsening urinary symptoms and increasing tumor load, in the setting of a persistently low serum prostate-specific antigen (PSA) level. As the neuroendocrine component predominates, patients may present with paraneoplastic symptoms associated with elevated levels of adrenocorticotropic hormone (ACTH) or antidiuretic hormone (ADH).

Pathology and Immunohistochemical Profile

The morphology of small cell carcinoma of the prostate is identical to that seen in the bladder (see above) and lung. In about 50% of cases, the tumors are composed of a mixture of small cell carcinoma and acinar adenocarcinoma [110]. The small cell component is positive for CD56, neuron-specific enolase (NSE), and chromogranin A, and shows dot-like positivity using CAM5.2, but is negative for PSA and prostatic acid phosphatase (PSAP). The acinar component shows the reverse immunoprofile. It has been suggested that primary small cell carcinoma of the prostate may be distinguished from a metastasis from the lung by the absence of staining for thyroid transcription factor-1 (TTF-1), but there

have been conflicting results with this marker, and further characterization with this antibody is required [111,112].

Biology

The histogenesis of these tumors is unclear. One hypothesis is that they originate from a multipotential stem cell in the prostatic epithelium, whereas others favor either malignant transformation of normal prostatic neuroendocrine cells or metaplastic change in a conventional acinar adenocarcinoma [107]. There is also evidence to suggest that prostatic tumors with a significant neuroendocrine component may be largely androgen-independent and are thus resistant to conventional forms of treatment, particularly hormonal deprivation, used to treat classical acinar prostatic adenocarcinoma [113].

Treatment and Outcome

The average survival for patients with prostatic small cell carcinoma is less than 1 year. There appears to be no difference in survival between patients with a pure small cell carcinoma and those with a mixed small cell–acinar tumor. Unlike its counterpart in the lung and bladder, studies have reported that small cell carcinoma of the prostate does not appear to respond to treatment with cisplatin-based chemotherapy regimens [103]. However, conflicting studies have suggested that other chemotherapeutic regimens may confer a small survival advantage [114].

Rhabdomyosarcoma of the Bladder

Rhabdomyosarcoma of the bladder is a rare malignant mesenchymal neoplasm composed of tumor cells that recapitulate the morphological features of skeletal muscle. Most commonly seen in childhood and adolescence, the majority of these tumors are of the embryonal subtype in the bladder (and are also known as "sarcoma botryoides"). In contrast, the alveolar subtype, carrying a distinct chromosomal translocation (t2:13), is most commonly seen in the deep soft tissues and rarely arises in the bladder.

Clinical Features

Patients typically present under the age of 10 years, although cases have been reported in adolescents, young adults, and rarely into middle age

[115,116]. In hollow organs such as the bladder or vagina, the tumor grows in a polypoid fashion into the lumen of the viscus, producing a characteristic appearance resembling a bunch of grapes on endoscopic and ultrasonic examination [117]. Vesical rhabdomyosarcoma commonly presents with urinary symptoms, including hematuria, dysuria, and obstruction to urinary flow.

Pathology and Immunohistochemical Profile

Rhabdomyosarcomas are usually composed of a mixture of small round cells with hyperchromatic nuclei and scant cytoplasm, and variable numbers of larger elongated cells with abundant eosinophilic cytoplasm (rhabdomyoblasts). The tumor cells contain intracytoplasmic cross-striations that may be visible on routine hematoxylin and eosin (H&E)-stained sections, but are more clearly identified using special staining techniques. Although classically exophytic, forming papillary structures with a central fibrovascular core, these tumors may show focal accumulation of rhabdomyoblasts under adjacent residual vesical mucosa, resulting in a distinctive subepithelial zone of hypercellularity (cambium layer). This architectural feature may be useful in the distinction of rhabdomyosarcoma from other tumors with a similar morphology such as lymphoma and small cell carcinoma. Tumor cells stain positive for muscle-specific actin, desmin, and nuclear myogenin and myoD1, the latter two being specific markers for skeletal muscle differentiation [118].

Biology and Genetics

Several studies have been performed to elucidate the cytogenetic profile of embryonal rhabdomyosarcomas, using a variety of techniques including CGH and fluorescent in situ hybridization (FISH). These have identified a number of chromosomal abnormalities in these tumors, including gains of regions on chromosomes 2, 7, 8, 11, 12, 13, and 20, and losses of regions on chromosomes 1, 6, 14, and 17 [119,120]. Further work is currently aimed at establishing the exact identity of the oncogenes and tumor-suppressor genes involved at these sites.

Treatment and Outcome

Rhabdomyosarcomas are aggressive neoplasms, usually treated with a combination of surgery, radiotherapy, and chemotherapy [121–123]. The exophytic botryoid subtype, commonly seen in the bladder, has the best prognosis, with an overall 5-year survival of 65% [124].

Sex Cord–Stromal (Mesenchymal) Tumors of the Testis

Sex cord–stromal tumors (SCSTs) are a related group of testicular tumors that are composed of neoplastic cells that recapitulate the primitive sex cord elements and surrounding immature mesenchyme of the fetal testis. They are thus distinct from germ cell tumors of the testis, and only very rare mixed forms occur [125]. The SCSTs account for approximately 3% to 5% of all adult testicular neoplasms and are predominantly either Leydig or Sertoli cell tumors, although a smaller proportion of granulosa cell tumors and rare mixed or indeterminate types may also be seen. They may present at any age from infancy to old age, but are most commonly seen in young children (under the age of 10 years), and account for up to 25% of testicular tumors in this pediatric age group.

Although no specific etiological factors have been established in the majority of patients, case reports note the association of Leydig tumors with tubular atrophy and Leydig cell hyperplasia, for example in Nelson's, Klinefelter's, and adrenogenital and androgen insensitivity syndromes.

In the latter, multiple Leydig-Sertoli hamartomas are found. These underlying conditions, therefore, should be considered as possible predisposing factors, particularly in cases with an unusual clinical presentation or in patients with multiple, bilateral tumors.

As the majority of SCSTs are either of Leydig or Sertoli type, these are discussed in further detail below, with particular reference to their clinical presentation, pathological features, and treatment options.

Leydig Cell Tumors

Leydig cell tumors (LCTs) are a group of sex cord–stromal tumors of the testis composed of neoplastic cells that recapitulate the appearance of Leydig cells.

Clinical Features

Leydig cell tumors account for 2% to 3% of all testicular neoplasms [126], with 20% arising in young children (ages 5 to 10 years), and the remaining 80% seen in young or middle-aged adults (ages 30 to 60 years). These tumors may present with signs of increased androgen and/or estrogen production (most commonly as isosexual pseudoprecocity in children [127] or gynecomastia in adults [128,129]) or as a painless testicular swelling. Around 3% to 5% of tumors occur bilaterally, either synchronously or metachronously [130], and up to 10% display aggressive behavior (malignant LCT) with evidence of subsequent local recurrence or metastatic spread [131,132]. In most instances, ultrasound examination of the testis reveals a well-circumscribed hypoechoic mass, but the radiological appearances are indistinguishable from germ cell tumor. Furthermore, there are no firm radiological criteria to determine whether a particular lesion will behave in a benign or malignant manner.

Pathology

Most LCTs are small (3 to 5 cm), well-circumscribed solid masses, with a yellow/brown cut surface. Commonly, a thin capsule surrounds the tumor, and focal areas of microcalcification and hemorrhage may be seen. Up to 10% cases show extratunical spread, with infiltration of paratesticular soft tissues by tumor.

The tumor may show a variety of patterns, including areas with a solid, pseudoglandular, trabecular, or insular growth pattern. Tumor cells are large and polygonal, with indistinct cell borders. Nuclei are round and vesicular and contain prominent central nucleoli (Fig. 26.3). The cytoplasm is abundant and eosinophilic, and focally may be foamy or vacuolated, and up to 50% of cases contain intracytoplasmic Reinke crystalloids or lipofuscin pigment [133]. Mitoses are scarce, and usually amount to no more than one or two per 10 high power fields. A fine vascularized stroma is present between the tumor cells, but occasionally this may be hyalinized (fibrotic) or edematous (myxoid) in appearance. Rare examples of LCT may show foci of adipocytic differentiation, calcification, ossification, and areas with a spindle cell morphology [134].

Malignant Leydig Cell Tumors

About 10% of LCTs behave in a malignant fashion [132,135]. The following clinical and morphological features have been reported as correlating with an increased risk of malignant behavior: age >60 years, tumor size >5 cm, marked nuclear pleomorphism, increased mitotic activity (>3/10 high power fields) or proliferation rate (>10% with MIB-1), the presence of lymphovascular invasion or coagulative necrosis, infiltrative margins, extension into rete or tunica, and aneuploidy [127,135–138].

Immunophenotype

The tumor cells are positive for vimentin, inhibin [139], calretinin [140], and melan-A [141,142], but negative for placental alkaline phosphatase (PLAP). Focal cytokeratin and S-100 positivity has been reported in some cases [143]. In addition, Leydig cells in the testis are noted to be positive for neuroendocrine markers, such as PGP9.5 [144].

Biology and Genetics

The majority of LCTs are sporadic, and the etiology of these tumors remains largely unknown. In the minority of cases associated with underlying predisposing conditions (mentioned above), there is an increased risk of Leydig or mixed Sertoli-Leydig tumors, and these usually present as multiple lesions bilaterally. It has previously been reported that inactivation of the luteinizing hormone receptor (LHR) gene on chromosome 2p may result in Leydig cell hypoplasia and male hypogonadism [145]. Studies examining a small number of LCTs have reported the presence of activating mutations of the LHR gene in these tumors [146,147]. However, their results have not been confirmed by other studies [148], and thus further validation of these findings in large-scale studies of LCTs is required.

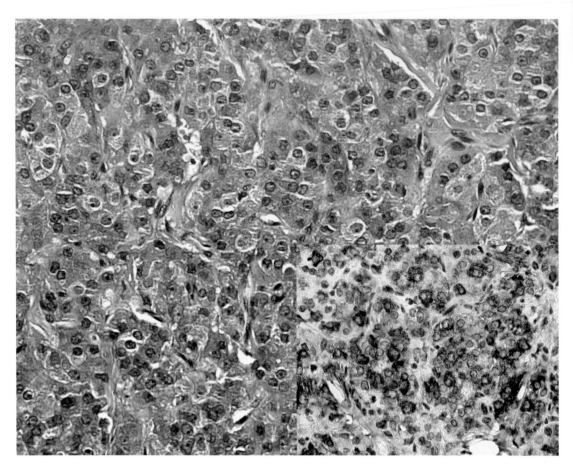

Fig. 26.3. A Leydig cell tumor showing strong cytoplasmic immunohistochemical staining for inhibin (inset) in the majority of tumour cells. Original magnification: H&E, 400×; inhibin, 600×.

Treatment and Outcome

The mainstay of treatment for LCT is surgery. This usually involves radical orchidectomy, but there has been, in recent years, an increasing trend for testis-sparing surgery, particularly in children and younger adults, or those with bilateral tumors. In such instances the diagnosis is made on intraoperative frozen section, allowing planning of conservative surgery rather than orchidectomy. Reports of small series of LCT treated with conservative surgery show a good response to organ-sparing surgery and successful preservation of fertility in the majority of cases, provided that there are no clinical (preoperative) or histopathological (postoperative) features to suggest malignancy and that local resection is complete [149–152].

A role for laparoscopic retroperitoneal lymph node dissection in addition to standard radical orchidectomy has been advocated for selected patient groups (especially those with clinical or histopathological features of malignancy or known small-volume metastatic disease), but its potential utility remains to be proven in clinical terms [153,154]. The vast majority (90%) of LCTs are benign, and potentially cured by local excision of the primary mass. In the remaining 10% cases, there is an increased risk of local recurrence or distant metastasis, and these may require further surgery as well as adjuvant chemotherapy and/or radiotherapy. Although metastatic LCTs are often resistant to chemotherapy [155], there are some cases that appear to respond to cisplatin-based regimens [156].

Sertoli Cell Tumors

Sertoli cell tumors (SCTs) are a group of sex cord–stromal tumors of the testis that are composed of neoplastic cells recapitulating fetal or adult-type Sertoli cells.

Clinical Features

Although rare, accounting for less than 1% of all testicular neoplasms, SCTs may arise at any age (most commonly middle age). They may present with a painless testicular swelling or with symptoms of gynecomastia or impotence. Most are sporadic tumors, but there is an increased risk of SCT in patients with Peutz-Jeghers polyposis, and Carney's and androgen insensitivity syndromes [157,158]. Ultrasound examination shows a well-circumscribed, hypoechoic mass, with a variable amount of cystic change [159]. Most cases show no features enabling distinction from other testicular neoplasms, including germ cell tumors. A rare variant, the large cell calcifying SCT, however, commonly presents in young children and adolescents with bilateral tumors containing large calcified areas, and has a characteristic ultrasound pattern of bright echogenicity and posterior acoustic shadowing [160].

Pathology

Sertoli cell tumors are well-circumscribed lobulated lesions with a variable size (ranging from 2 to 20 cm) and a pale white/yellow solid cut surface. Focal cystic change or hemorrhage may be seen, but necrosis is usually absent [161]. Most cases are unilateral, except for cases in patients with Peutz-Jeghers syndrome or those with a large cell calcifying variant [162,163].

The tumor forms a variety of patterns, commonly including areas with a tubular or glandular pattern of growth. The tubules may show a central lumen or form solid islands. Tumor cells have oval, elongated nuclei with small micronucleoli and pale eosinophilic or vacuolated cytoplasm [161]. The nucleus may show features of indentation or nuclear grooving, especially on cytological preparations [164]. There is minimal nuclear pleomorphism, and mitotic activity is not prominent (usually <5 per 10 high power fields). The surrounding stroma may be focally cellular and fibrotic or show areas of hyalinization.

Immunophenotype and Electron Microscopy

The tumor cells are usually positive for vimentin, cytokeratin, and inhibin [139,143], and may focally stain for S-100 [165] and calretinin. A few cases have been reported as showing positivity for epithelial membrane antigen (EMA) and NSE. There is no staining with antibodies to placental alkaline phosphatase (PLAP), excluding seminoma, which may be a diagnostic problem in some cases [166]. Antibodies against human chorionic gonadotrophin (HCG) and α-fetoprotein are also negative. Ultrastructurally, features of steroid-secreting cells are usually seen in SCT including abundant cisternae of smooth endoplasmic reticulum. Charcot-Bottcher filaments (perinuclear bundles of fine filaments) are considered to be pathognomonic of Sertoli cells [167].

Variants of Sertoli Cell Tumor

Large Cell Calcifying SCT

This is a rare variant of SCT, characterized by large cells with abundant eosinophilic cytoplasm and calcification [162,163,168]. These tumors are commonly seen in the context of Peutz-Jeghers or Carney's syndromes and affect mostly young children and adolescents, with a mean age 17 years [169]. Most are solitary and benign, but up to 40% may be bilateral [170]. Tumor cells are large and polygonal, with vesicular nuclei and prominent nucleoli. Mitoses are scarce. The stroma is hyalinized, with a prominent neutrophilic infiltrate and characteristic large areas of microcalcification and/or ossification (Fig. 26.4). Although few cases behave in a malignant manner, possible morphological indicators of aggressive behavior include large size, necrosis, marked nuclear atypia, lymphovascular permeation, and mitotic rate greater than three mitoses per 10 high power fields [171–173].

Sclerosing SCT

This is a rare variant seen in young adults (commonly 25 to 35 years age) with tubules composed of neoplastic Sertoli cells entrapped in a dense sclerotic stroma. Usually these tumors have a benign outcome [174,175].

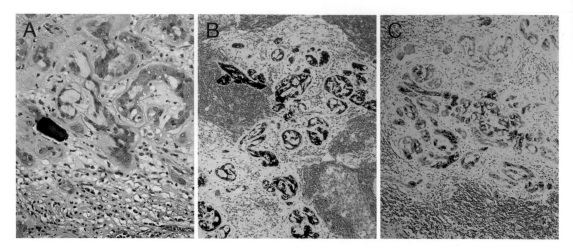

Fig. 26.4. A large cell calcifying Sertoli cell tumor (A, H&E) showing strong cytoplasmic immunohistochemical staining for inhibin (B) and weaker staining for calretinin (C). Original magnification: A, 400×; B and C, 200×.

Malignant SCT

Although rare (<10% of cases), a malignant form of SCT does occur. The following are clinical and morphological features that correlate with an increased risk of malignant behavior: large tumor size (>5 cm), marked nuclear pleomorphism, increased mitotic activity (>5 per 10 high power fields), necrosis, infiltrative margins, and the presence of lymphovascular invasion [161]. Malignant cases may arise at any age, including childhood (unlike LCT), and more commonly present with gynecomastia than benign tumors.

Biology and Genetics

The majority of SCTs are sporadic, and their etiology remains unknown. In patients at increased risk of SCT, including those with androgen insensitivity syndrome, there are individual case reports of patients whose tumors show activating point mutations of the androgen receptor (AR) gene [176,177]. However, whether these findings can be extrapolated to a larger group of sporadic SCTs, in patients without androgen insensitivity syndrome, remains to be elucidated.

Treatment and Outcome

The majority of SCTs are benign and thus potentially curable by complete local excision of the primary tumor mass. The minority of SCTs that

behave in a malignant fashion are usually very aggressive, resulting in a poor prognosis with median survival of around 1 year. In these, a combination of retroperitoneal lymph node dissection, chemotherapy, and radiotherapy appears to offer the best palliative treatment [178]. In the large cell calcifying variant of Sertoli cell tumor (LCCSCT), the prognosis is good in the majority of cases, particularly in younger children, and some authors advocate conservative treatment with testis-sparing surgery for cases identified as LCCSCT by ultrasonographic criteria [179].

References

1. Freeman C, Berg JW, Cutler SJ. Occurrence and prognosis of extranodal lymphomas. Cancer 1972;29:252–260.
2. Colevas AD, Kantoff PW, DeWolf WC, et al. Malignant lymphoma of the genitourinary tract. In: Vogelzanf NJ, Shipley WU, Scardino PT, et al., eds. Comprehensive Textbook of Genitourinary Oncology, 2nd ed. Philadelphia: Lippincott Williams & Wilkins, 2000:1120–1132.
3. Jaffe ES, Harris NL, Stein H, et al., eds. World Health Organization Classification of Tumours. Pathology and Genetics of Tumours of Haematopoietic and Lymphoid Tissues. Lyon: IARC Press, 2001.
4. Shahab N, Doll DC. Testicular lymphoma. Semin Oncol 1999;26:259–269.

5. Moller MB, d'Amore F, Christensen BE. Testicular lymphoma: a population-based study of incidence, clinicopathological correlations and prognosis. Eur J Cancer 1994;30A:1760–1764.

6. Zucca E, Conconi A, Mughal TI, et al. Patterns of outcome and prognostic factors in primary large-cell lymphoma of the testis in a survey by the international extranodal lymphoma study group. J Clin Oncol 2003;21:20–27.

7. Visco C, Medeiros LJ, Mesina OM, et al. Non-Hodgkin's lymphoma affecting the testis: Is it curable with doxorubicin-based therapy? Clin Lymphoma 2001;2:40–46.

8. Seymour JF, Solomon B, Wolf MM, et al. Primary large-cell non-Hodgkin's lymphoma of the testis: a retrospective analysis of patterns of failure and prognostic factors. Clin Lymphoma 2001;2:109–115.

9. Linassier C, Desablens B, Lefrancq T, et al. Stage I-IIe primary non-Hodgkin's lymphoma of the testis: results of a prospective trial by the GOELAMS study group. Clin Lymphoma 2002;3:167–172.

10. Ferry JA, Harris NL, Young RH, et al. Malignant lymphoma of the testis, epididymis, and spermatic cord. A clinicopathologic study of 69 cases with immunophenotypic analysis. Am J Surg Pathol 1994;18:376–390.

11. Wilkins BS, Williamson JM, O'Brien CJ. Morphological and immunohistological study of testicular lymphomas. Histopathology 1989;15:147–156.

12. Lagrange JL, Ramaioli A, Theodore CH, et al. Non-Hodgkin's lymphoma of the testis: a retrospective study of 84 patients treated in the French anticancer centres. Ann Oncol 2001;12:1313–1319.

13. Fonseca R, Habermann TM, Colgan JP, et al. Testicular lymphoma is associated with a high incidence of extranodal recurrence. Cancer 2000;88:154–161.

14. Dogan A, Bagdi E, Munson P, et al. CD10 and bcl-6 expression in paraffin sections of normal lymphoid tissue and B-cell lymphomas. Am J Surg Pathol 2000;24:846–852.

15. Hyland J, Lasota J, Jasinski M, et al. Molecular pathological analysis of testicular diffuse large cell lymphomas. Hum Pathol 1998;29:1231–1239.

16. Lossos IS, Okada CY, Tibshirani R, et al. Molecular analysis of immunoglobulin genes in diffuse large B-cell lymphomas. Blood 2000;95:1797–1803.

17. Pasqualucci L, Neumeister P, Goossens T, et al. Hypermutation of multiple proto-oncogenes in B-cell diffuse large-cell lymphomas. Nature 2001;412:341–346.

18. Alizadeh AA, Eisen MB, Davis RE, et al. Distinct types of diffuse large B-cell lymphoma identified by gene expression profiling. Nature 2000;403:503–511.

19. Rosenwald A, Wright G, Chan WC, et al. The use of molecular profiling to predict survival after chemotherapy for diffuse large-B-cell lymphoma. N Engl J Med 2002;346:1937–1947.

20. Shipp MA, Ross KN, Tamayo P, et al. Diffuse large B-cell lymphoma outcome prediction by gene-expression profiling and supervised machine learning. Nat Med 2002;8:68–74.

21. de Leval L, Harris NL. Variability in immunophenotype in diffuse large B-cell lymphoma and its clinical relevance. Histopathology 2003;43:509–528.

22. Colomo L, Lopez-Guillermo A, Perales M, et al. Clinical impact of the differentiation profile assessed by immunophenotyping in patients with diffuse large B-cell lymphoma. Blood 2003;101:78–84.

23. Barrans SL, Carter I, Owen RG, et al. Germinal center phenotype and bcl-2 expression combined with the international prognostic index improves patient risk stratification in diffuse large b-cell lymphoma. Blood 2002;99:1136–1143.

24. Hans CP, Weisenburger DD, Greiner TC, et al. Confirmation of the molecular classification of diffuse large B-cell lymphoma by immunohistochemistry using a tissue microarray. Blood 2004;103:275–282.

25. Kramer MH, Hermans J, Wijburg E, et al. Clinical relevance of bcl-2, bcl-6, and myc rearrangements in diffuse large B-cell lymphoma. Blood 1998;92:3152–3162.

26. Gascoyne RD, Adomat SA, Krajewski S, et al. Prognostic significance of bcl-2 protein expression and bcl-2 gene rearrangement in diffuse aggressive non-Hodgkin's lymphoma. Blood 1997;90:244–251.

27. Barrans SL, Evans PA, O'Connor SJ, et al. The t(14;18) is associated with germinal center-derived diffuse large B-cell lymphoma and is a strong predictor of outcome. Clin Cancer Res 2003;9:2133–2139.

28. Huang JZ, Sanger WG, Greiner TC, et al. The t(14;18) defines a unique subset of diffuse large B-cell lymphoma with a germinal center B-cell gene expression profile. Blood 2002;99:2285–2290.

29. Monni O, Joensuu H, Franssila K, et al. Bcl-2 overexpression associated with chromosomal amplification in diffuse large B-cell lymphoma. Blood 1997;90:1168–1174.

30. Lambrechts AC, Looijenga LH, van't Veer MB, et al. Lymphomas with testicular localisation show a consistent bcl-2 expression without a translo-

cation (14;18): a molecular and immunohisto-chemical study. Br J Cancer 1995;71:73–77.

31. Ye BH, Chaganti S, Chang CC, et al. Chromosomal translocations cause deregulated bcl-6 expression by promoter substitution in B cell lymphoma. EMBO J 1995;14:6209–6217.

32. Pasqualucci L, Migliazza A, Basso K, et al. Mutations of the bcl-6 proto-oncogene disrupt its negative autoregulation in diffuse large B-cell lymphoma. Blood 2003;101:2914–2923.

33. Ichikawa A, Kinoshita T, Watanabe T, et al. Mutations of the p53 gene as a prognostic factor in aggressive B-cell lymphoma. N Engl J Med 1997; 337:529–534.

34. Houldsworth J, Mathew S, Rao PH, et al. Rel proto-oncogene is frequently amplified in extranodal diffuse large cell lymphoma. Blood 1996; 87:25–29.

35. Davis RE, Brown KD, Siebenlist U, et al. Constitutive nuclear factor kappaB activity is required for survival of activated B cell-like diffuse large B cell lymphoma cells. J Exp Med 2001;194:1861–1874.

36. Riemersma SA, Jordanova ES, Schop RF, et al. Extensive genetic alterations of the HLA region, including homozygous deletions of HLA class II genes in B-cell lymphomas arising in immune-privileged sites. Blood 2000;96:3569–3577.

37. Jordanova ES, Riemersma SA, Philippo K, et al. Beta 2–microglobulin aberrations in diffuse large B-cell lymphoma of the testis and the central nervous system. Int J Cancer 2003;103: 393–398.

38. Horstmann WG, Timens W. Lack of adhesion molecules in testicular diffuse centroblastic and immunoblastic B cell lymphomas as a contributory factor in malignant behaviour. Virchows Arch 1996;429:83–90.

39. Zouhair A, Weber D, Belkacemi Y, et al. Outcome and patterns of failure in testicular lymphoma: a multicenter rare cancer network study. Int J Radiat Oncol Biol Phys 2002;52:652–656.

40. Moller MB, Pedersen NT, Christensen BE. Diffuse large B-cell lymphoma: clinical implications of extranodal versus nodal presentation—a population-based study of 1575 cases. Br J Haematol 2004;124:151–159.

41. Connors JM, Klimo P, Voss N, et al. Testicular lymphoma: improved outcome with early brief chemotherapy. J Clin Oncol 1988;6:776–781.

42. Coiffier B, Lepage E, Briere J, et al. CHOP chemotherapy plus Rituximab compared with CHOP alone in elderly patients with diffuse large-B-cell lymphoma. N Engl J Med 2002;346: 235–242.

43. Dalle JH, Mechinaud F, Michon J, et al. Testicular disease in childhood B-cell non-Hodgkin's lymphoma: the French society of pediatric oncology experience. J Clin Oncol 2001;19:2397–2403.

44. Kim TH, Hargreaves HK, Chan WC, et al. Sequential testicular biopsies in childhood acute lymphocytic leukemia. Cancer 1986;57:1038–1041.

45. Grundy RG, Leiper AD, Stanhope R, et al. Survival and endocrine outcome after testicular relapse in acute lymphoblastic leukaemia. Arch Dis Child 1997;76:190–196.

46. Pileri SA, Sabattini E, Rosito P, et al. Primary follicular lymphoma of the testis in childhood: an entity with peculiar clinical and molecular characteristics. J Clin Pathol 2002;55:684–688.

47. Ferry JA, Young RH, Scully RE. Testicular and epididymal plasmacytoma: a report of 7 cases, including three that were the initial manifestation of plasma cell myeloma. Am J Surg Pathol 1997;21:590–598.

48. Anghel G, Petti N, Remotti D, et al. Testicular plasmacytoma: report of a case and review of the literature. Am J Hematol 2002;71:98–104.

49. Kim YB, Chang SK, Yang WI, et al. Primary NK/T cell lymphoma of the testis. A case report and review of the literature. Acta Haematol 2003;109: 95–100.

50. Henley JD, Ferry J, Ulbright TM. Miscellaneous rare paratesticular tumors. Semin Diagn Pathol 2000;17:319–339.

51. Vega F, Medeiros LJ, Abruzzo LV. Primary paratesticular lymphoma: a report of 2 cases and review of literature. Arch Pathol Lab Med 2001; 125:428–432.

52. Givler RL. Involvement of the bladder in leukemia and lymphoma. J Urol 1971;105:667–670.

53. Kempton CL, Kurtin PJ, Inwards DJ, et al. Malignant lymphoma of the bladder: evidence from 36 cases that low-grade lymphoma of the MALT-type is the most common primary bladder lymphoma. Am J Surg Pathol 1997;21:1324–1333.

54. Ohsawa M, Aozasa K, Horiuchi K, et al. Malignant lymphoma of bladder. Report of three cases and review of the literature. Cancer 1993;72:1969–1974.

55. Bates AW, Norton AJ, Baithun SI. Malignant lymphoma of the urinary bladder: a clinicopathological study of 11 cases. J Clin Pathol 2000;53: 458–461.

56. Al-Maghrabi J, Kamel-Reid S, Jewett M, et al. Primary low-grade B-cell lymphoma of mucosa-associated lymphoid tissue type arising in the urinary bladder: report of 4 cases with molecular genetic analysis. Arch Pathol Lab Med 2001; 125:332–336.

57. Pawade J, Banerjee SS, Harris M, et al. Lymphomas of mucosa-associated lymphoid tissue arising in the urinary bladder. Histopathology 1993;23:147–151.

58. Du MQ, Isaccson PG. Gastric MALT lymphoma: From aetiology to treatment. Lancet Oncol 2002; 3:97–104.

59. Krober SM, Aepinus C, Ruck P, et al. Extranodal marginal zone B cell lymphoma of MALT type involving the mucosa of both the urinary bladder and stomach. J Clin Pathol 2002;55:554–557.

60. Streubel B, Lamprecht A, Dierlamm J, et al. T(14;18)(q32;q21) involving IgH and MALT1 is a frequent chromosomal aberration in MALT lymphoma. Blood 2003;101:2335–2339.

61. Tsang RW, Gospodarowicz MK, Pintilie M, et al. Stage I and II MALT lymphoma: results of treatment with radiotherapy. Int J Radiat Oncol Biol Phys 2001;50:1258–1264.

62. van den Bosch J, Kropman RF, Blok P, et al. Disappearance of a mucosa-associated lymphoid tissue (MALT) lymphoma of the urinary bladder after treatment for Helicobacter pylori. Eur J Haematol 2002;68:187–188.

63. Oscier D, Bramble J, Hodges E, et al. Regression of mucosa-associated lymphoid tissue lymphoma of the bladder after antibiotic therapy. J Clin Oncol 2002;20:882.

64. Patel DR, Gomez GA, Henderson ES, et al. Primary prostatic involvement in non-Hodgkin lymphoma. Urology 1988;32:96–98.

65. Sarris A, Dimopoulos M, Pugh W, et al. Primary lymphoma of the prostate: good outcome with doxorubicin-based combination chemotherapy. J Urol 1995;153:1852–1854.

66. Zein TA, Huben R, Lane W, et al. Secondary tumors of the prostate. J Urol 1985;133:615–616.

67. Bostwick DG, Iczkowski KA, Amin MB, et al. Malignant lymphoma involving the prostate: report of 62 cases. Cancer 1998;83:732–738.

68. Winstanley AM, Sandison A, Bott SR, et al. Incidental findings in pelvic lymph nodes at radical prostatectomy. J Clin Pathol 2002;55:623–626.

69. Weir EG, Epstein JI. Incidental small lymphocytic lymphoma/chronic lymphocytic leukemia in pelvic lymph nodes excised at radical prostatectomy. Arch Pathol Lab Med 2003;127:567–572.

70. Tomaru U, Ishikura H, Kon S, et al. Primary lymphoma of the prostate with features of low grade B-cell lymphoma of mucosa associated lymphoid tissue: a rare cause of urinary obstruction. J Urol 1999;162:496–497.

71. Bogdan CA, Alexander AA, Gorny MK, et al. Chronic lymphocytic leukemia with prostate infiltration mediated by specific clonal membrane-bound IgM. Cancer Res 2003;63:2067–2071.

72. Leung TW, Tung SY, Sze WK, et al. Primary non-Hodgkin's lymphoma of the prostate. Clin Oncol (R Coll Radiol) 1997;9:264–266.

73. Entz-Werle N, Marcellin L, Becmeur F, et al. The urinary bladder: an extremely rare location of pediatric neuroblastoma. J Pediatr Surg 2003;38: E10–12.

74. Yokoyama S, Hirakawa H, Ueno S, et al. Neuroblastoma of the urinary bladder, preclinically detected by mass screening. Pediatrics 1999;103: e67.

75. Kruger S, Schmidt H, Kausch I, et al. Primitive neuroectodermal tumor (PNET) of the urinary bladder. Pathol Res Pract 2003;199:751–754.

76. Ijiri R, Tanaka Y, Kou K, et al. Bladder origin neuroblastoma detected by mass screening. Urology 1998;52:1139–1141.

77. Gupta A, Menon P, Rao KL, et al. Wilms' tumor: Transureteral intravesical extension and presentation as urinary retention. J Pediatr Surg 2003; 38:E4–5.

78. Mitchell CS, Yeo TA. Noninvasive botryoid extension of Wilms' tumor into the bladder. Pediatr Radiol 1997;27:818–820.

79. Williams DH, Hua VN, Chowdhry AA, et al. Synovial sarcoma of the prostate. J Urol 2004;171: 2376.

80. Iwasaki H, Ishiguro M, Ohjimi Y, et al. Synovial sarcoma of the prostate with t(x;18)(p11.2; q11.2). Am J Surg Pathol 1999;23:220–226.

81. Cunningham JA, Fendler JP, Nichols PJ, et al. Metastatic malignant melanoma: an unusual case presentation. Urology 1994;44:924–926.

82. Demirkesen O, Yaycioglu O, Uygun N, et al. A case of metastatic malignant melanoma presenting with hematuria. Urol Int 2000;64:118–120.

83. Lee CS, Komenaka IK, Hurst-Wicker KS, et al. Management of metastatic malignant melanoma of the bladder. Urology 2003;62:351.

84. Nesi G, Vezzosi V, Amorosi A, et al. Paraganglioma of the urinary bladder. Urol Int 1996;56: 250–253.

85. Cramer SF, Aikawa M, Cebelin M. Neurosecretory granules in small cell invasive carcinoma of the urinary bladder. Cancer 1981;47:724–730.

86. Fujita K, Nishimura K, Nonomura N, et al. Early stage small cell carcinoma of the urinary bladder. Int J Urol 2001;8:643–644.

87. Grignon DJ, Ro JY, Ayala AG, et al. Small cell carcinoma of the urinary bladder. A clinicopathologic analysis of 22 cases. Cancer 1992;69:527–536.

88. Trias I, Algaba F, Condom E, et al. Small cell carcinoma of the urinary bladder. Presentation of 23 cases and review of 134 published cases. Eur Urol 2001;39:85–90.

89. Partanen S, Asikainen U. Oat cell carcinoma of the urinary bladder with ectopic adrenocorticotropic hormone production. Hum Pathol 1985; 16:313–315.

90. Reyes CV, Soneru I. Small cell carcinoma of the urinary bladder with hypercalcemia. Cancer 1985; 56:2530–2533.

91. Kim JC, Kim KH, Jung S. Small cell carcinoma of the urinary bladder: CT and MR imaging findings. Korean J Radiol 2003;4:130–135.

92. Kim JC. CT features of bladder small cell carcinoma. Clin Imaging 2004;28:201–205.

93. Yamaguchi T, Imamura Y, Shimamoto T, et al. Small cell carcinoma of the bladder. Two cases diagnosed by urinary cytology. Acta Cytol 2000; 44:403–409.

94. Ali SZ, Reuter VE, Zakowski MF. Small cell neuroendocrine carcinoma of the urinary bladder. A clinicopathologic study with emphasis on cytologic features. Cancer 1997;79:356–361.

95. Algaba F, Sauter G, Schoenberg MP. Small cell carcinoma. In: Eble JN, Sauter G, Epstein JI, et al., eds. Pathology and Genetics of Tumours of the Urinary System and Male Genital Organs. Lyon: IARC Press, 2004:135–136.

96. Chuang CK, Liao SK. A retrospective immunohistochemical and clinicopathological study of small cell carcinomas of the urinary tract. Chang Gung Med J 2003;26:26–33.

97. Kaufmann O, Georgi T, Dietel M. Utility of 123C3 monoclonal antibody against CD56 (NCAM) for the diagnosis of small cell carcinoma on paraffin sections. Hum Pathol 1997;28:1373–1378.

98. Iczkowski KA, Shanks JH, Allsbrook WC, et al. Small cell carcinoma of urinary bladder is differentiated from urothelial carcinoma by chromogranin expression, absence of CD44 variant 6 expression, a unique pattern of cytokeratin expression, and more intense gamma-enolase expression. Histopathology 1999;35: 150–156.

99. Blomjous CE, Vos W, De Voogt HJ, et al. Small cell carcinoma of the urinary bladder. A clinicopathologic, morphometric, immunohistochemical, and ultrastructural study of 18 cases. Cancer 1989;64:1347–1357.

100. Terracciano L, Richter J, Tornillo L, et al. Chromosomal imbalances in small cell carcinomas of the urinary bladder. J Pathol 1999;189:230–235.

101. Selli C, Gelmini S, Scott CA, et al. Evidence for elevated telomerase activity in small cell carcinoma of the bladder. Urology 2000;56:331.

102. Abbas F, Civantos F, Benedetto P, et al. Small cell carcinoma of the bladder and prostate. Urology 1995;46:617–630.

103. Mackey JR, Au HJ, Hugh J, et al. Genitourinary small cell carcinoma: determination of clinical and therapeutic factors associated with survival. J Urol 1998;159:1624–1629.

104. Lohrisch C, Murray N, Pickles T, et al. Small cell carcinoma of the bladder: long term outcome with integrated chemoradiation. Cancer 1999;86: 2346–2352.

105. Nejat RJ, Purohit R, Goluboff ET, et al. Cure of undifferentiated small cell carcinoma of the urinary bladder with M-VAC chemotherapy. 2001; 6:53–55.

106. Lopez Cubillana P, Martinez Barba E, Prieto A, et al. Oat-cell carcinoma of the prostate. Diagnosis, prognosis and therapeutic implications. Urol Int 2001;67:209–212.

107. Helpap B, Kollermann J. Undifferentiated carcinoma of the prostate with small cell features: immunohistochemical subtyping and reflections on histogenesis. Virchows Arch 1999;434:385–391.

108. Abrahamsson PA. Neuroendocrine differentiation in prostatic carcinoma. Prostate 1999;39: 135–148.

109. diSant'Agnese PA, Egevad L, Epstein JI, et al. Neuroendocrine tumours. In: Eble JN, Sauter G, Epstein JI, et al., eds. Pathology and Genetics of Tumours of the Urinary System and Male Genital Organs. Lyon: IARC Press, 2004:207–208.

110. Spieth ME, Lin YG, Nguyen TT. Diagnosing and treating small-cell carcinomas of prostatic origin. Clin Nucl Med 2002;27:11–17.

111. Agoff SN, Lamps LW, Philip AT, et al. Thyroid. transcription factor-1 is expressed in extrapulmonary small cell carcinomas but not in other extrapulmonary neuroendocrine tumors. Mod Pathol 2000;13:238–242.

112. Ordonez NG. Value of thyroid transcription factor-1 immunostaining in distinguishing small cell lung carcinomas from other small cell carcinomas. Am J Surg Pathol 2000;24:1217–1223.

113. Ito T, Yamamoto S, Ohno Y, et al. Up-regulation of neuroendocrine differentiation in prostate cancer after androgen deprivation therapy, degree and androgen independence. Oncol Rep 2001;8:1221–1224.

114. Amato RJ, Logothetis CJ, Hallinan R, et al. Chemotherapy for small cell carcinoma of prostatic origin. J Urol 1992;147:935–937.

115. El-Sherbiny MT, El-Mekresh MH, El-Baz MA, et al. Paediatric lower urinary tract rhabdomyosarcoma: a single-centre experience of 30 patients. BJU Int 2000;86:260–267.

116. Konety BR, Schneck FX. Botryoid rhabdomyosarcoma of the bladder. Urology 1997;50: 604–605.

117. Poggiani C, Teani M, Auriemma A, et al. Sonographic detection of rhabdomyosarcoma of the urinary bladder. Eur J Ultrasound 2001;13:35–39.

118. Kumar S, Perlman E, Harris CA, et al. Myogenin is a specific marker for rhabdomyosarcoma: an immunohistochemical study in paraffin-embedded tissues. Mod Pathol 2000;13:988–993.

119. Lee W, Han K, Harris CP, et al. Detection of aneuploidy and possible deletion in paraffin-embedded rhabdomyosarcoma cells with FISH. Cancer Genet Cytogenet 1993;68:99–103.

120. Bridge JA, Liu J, Weibolt V, et al. Novel genomic imbalances in embryonal rhabdomyosarcoma revealed by comparative genomic hybridization

and fluorescence in situ hybridization: an intergroup rhabdomyosarcoma study. Genes Chromosomes Cancer 2000;27:337–344.

121. Raney B Jr, Heyn R, Hays DM, et al. Sequelae of treatment in 109 patients followed for 5 to 15 years after diagnosis of sarcoma of the bladder and prostate. A report from the Intergroup Rhabdomyosarcoma Study Committee. Cancer 1993;71:2387–2394.

122. Kaefer M, Rink RC. Genitourinary rhabdomyosarcoma. Treatment options. Urol Clin North Am 2000;27:471–487.

123. Ashlock R, Johnstone PA. Treatment modalities of bladder/prostate rhabdomyosarcoma: a review. Prostate Cancer Prostatic Dis 2003;6:112–120.

124. Leuschner I, Harms D, Mattke A, et al. Rhabdomyosarcoma of the urinary bladder and vagina: a clinicopathologic study with emphasis on recurrent disease: a report from the Kiel Pediatric Tumor Registry and the German CWS Study. Am J Surg Pathol 2001;25:856–864.

125. Ulbright TM, Srigley JR, Reuter VE, et al. Sex cord-stromal tumors of the testis with entrapped germ cells: a lesion mimicking unclassified mixed germ cell sex cord-stromal tumors. Am J Surg Pathol 2000;24:535–542.

126. Mikuz G, Schwarz S, Hopfel-Kreiner I, et al. Leydig cell tumor of the testis. Morphological and endocrinological investigations in two cases. Eur Urol 1980;6:293–300.

127. Kim I, Young RH, Scully RE. Leydig cell tumors of the testis. A clinicopathological analysis of 40 cases and review of the literature. Am J Surg Pathol 1985;9:177–192.

128. Shimp WS, Schultz AL, Hastings JR, et al. Leydig-cell tumor of the testis with gynecomastia and elevated estrogen levels. Am J Clin Pathol 1977;67:562–566.

129. Caldamone AA, Altebarmakian V, Frank IN, et al. Leydig cell tumor of testis. Urology 1979;14:39–43.

130. Akman H, Ege G, Yildiz S, et al. Incidental bilateral Leydig cell tumor of the testes. Urol Int 2003;71:316–318.

131. Mahon FB, Jr., Gosset F, Trinity RG, et al. Malignant interstitial cell testicular tumor. Cancer 1973;31:1208–1212.

132. Grem JL, Robins HI, Wilson KS, et al. Metastatic Leydig cell tumor of the testis. Report of three cases and review of the literature. Cancer 1986;58:2116–2119.

133. De Kretser DM. Crystals of Reinke in the nuclei of human testicular interstitial cells. Experientia 1968;24:587–588.

134. Ulbright TM, Srigley JR, Hatzianastassiou DK, et al. Leydig cell tumors of the testis with unusual features: Adipose differentiation, calcification with ossification, and spindle-shaped tumor cells. Am J Surg Pathol 2002;26:1424–1433.

135. McCluggage WG, Shanks JH, Arthur K, et al. Cellular proliferation and nuclear ploidy assessments augment established prognostic factors in predicting malignancy in testicular Leydig cell tumours. Histopathology 1998;33:361–368.

136. Palazzo JP, Petersen RO, Young RH, et al. Deoxyribonucleic acid flow cytometry of testicular Leydig cell tumors. J Urol 1994;152:415–417.

137. Cheville JC, Sebo TJ, Lager DJ, et al. Leydig cell tumor of the testis: a clinicopathologic, DNA content, and MIB-1 comparison of nonmetastasizing and metastasizing tumors. Am J Surg Pathol 1998;22:1361–1367.

138. Hekimgil M, Altay B, Yakut BD, et al. Leydig cell tumor of the testis: comparison of histopathological and immunohistochemical features of three azoospermic cases and one malignant case. Pathol Int 2001;51:792–796.

139. Iczkowski KA, Bostwick DG, Roche PC, et al. Inhibin A is a sensitive and specific marker for testicular sex cord-stromal tumors. Mod Pathol 1998;11:774–779.

140. Augusto D, Leteurtre E, De La Taille A, et al. Calretinin: a valuable marker of normal and neoplastic Leydig cells of the testis. Appl Immunohistochem Mol Morphol 2002;10:159–162.

141. Stewart CJ, Nandini CL, Richmond JA. Value of A103 (Melan-A) immunostaining in the differential diagnosis of ovarian sex cord stromal tumours. J Clin Pathol 2000;53:206–211.

142. Yao DX, Soslow RA, Hedvat CV, et al. Melan-A (A103) and inhibin expression in ovarian neoplasms. Appl Immunohistochem Mol Morphol 2003;11:244–249.

143. McCluggage WG, Shanks JH, Whiteside C, et al. Immunohistochemical study of testicular sex cord-stromal tumors, including staining with anti-inhibin antibody. Am J Surg Pathol 1998;22:615–619.

144. Wilson PO, Barber PC, Hamid QA, et al. The immunolocalization of protein gene product 9.5 using rabbit polyclonal and mouse monoclonal antibodies. Br J Exp Pathol 1988;69:91–104.

145. Wu SM, Leschek EW, Rennert OM, et al. Luteinizing hormone receptor mutations in disorders of sexual development and cancer. Front Biosci 2000;5:D343–352.

146. Liu G, Duranteau L, Carel JC, et al. Leydig-cell tumors caused by an activating mutation of the gene encoding the luteinizing hormone receptor. N Engl J Med 1999;341:1731–1736.

147. Canto P, Soderlund D, Ramon G, et al. Mutational analysis of the luteinizing hormone receptor gene in two individuals with Leydig cell tumors. Am J Med Genet 2002;108:148–152.

148. Vieira TC, Cerutti JM, Dias da Silva MR, et al. Absence of activating mutations in the hot spots of the LH receptor and Gs-alpha genes in Leydig cell tumors. J Endocrinol Invest 2002;25:598–602.

149. Wegner HE, Herbst H, Andresen R, et al. Leydig cell tumor recurrence after enucleation. J Urol 1996;156:1443–1444.

150. Wegner HE, Dieckmann KP, Herbst H, et al. Leydig cell tumor—comparison of results of radical and testis-sparing surgery in a single center. Urol Int 1997;59:170–173.

151. Masoudi JF, Van Arsdalen K, Rovner ES. Organ-sparing surgery for bilateral Leydig cell tumor of the testis. Urology 1999;54:744.

152. Merlini E, Seymandi PL, Betta PG, et al. Testis sparing enucleation of a Leydig-cell tumour in a boy. Pediatr Med Chir 2003;25:63–65.

153. Farkas LM, Szekely JG, Pusztai C, et al. High frequency of metastatic Leydig cell testicular tumours. Oncology 2000;59:118–121.

154. Mosharafa AA, Foster RS, Bihrle R, et al. Does retroperitoneal lymph node dissection have a curative role for patients with sex cord-stromal testicular tumors? Cancer 2003;98:753–757.

155. Bertram KA, Bratloff B, Hodges GF, et al. Treatment of malignant Leydig cell tumor. Cancer 1991;68:2324–2329.

156. Dieckmann KP, Loy V. Response of metastasized sex cord gonadal stromal tumor of the testis to cisplatin-based chemotherapy. J Urol 1994;151:1024–1026.

157. Wysocka B, Serkies K, Debniak J, et al. Sertoli cell tumor in androgen insensitivity syndrome—a case report. Gynecol Oncol 1999;75:480–483.

158. Rodewald A, Kittner T, Hahn G. The Carney complex: a rare differential diagnosis in cases with pituitary adenoma and testicular Sertoli cell tumour. Clin Radiol 2001;56:993–996.

159. Liu P, Thorner P. Sonographic appearance of Sertoli cell tumour: with pathologic correlation. Pediatr Radiol 1993;23:127–128.

160. Gierke CL, King BF, Bostwick DG, et al. Large-cell calcifying Sertoli cell tumor of the testis: appearance at sonography. AJR Am J Roentgenol 1994;163:373–375.

161. Young RH, Koelliker DD, Scully RE. Sertoli cell tumors of the testis, not otherwise specified: a clinicopathologic analysis of 60 cases. Am J Surg Pathol 1998;22:709–721.

162. Chang B, Borer JG, Tan PE, et al. Large-cell calcifying Sertoli cell tumor of the testis: case report and review of the literature. Urology 1998;52:520–522; discussion 522–523.

163. Giglio M, Medica M, De Rose AF, et al. Testicular Sertoli cell tumours and relative sub-types. Analysis of clinical and prognostic features. Urol Int 2003;70:205–210.

164. Terayama K, Hirokawa M, Shimizu M, et al. Sertoli cell tumor of the testis. Report of a case with imprint cytology findings. Acta Cytol 1998;42:1458–1460.

165. McLaren K, Thomson D. Localization of S-100 protein in a Leydig and Sertoli cell tumour of testis. Histopathology 1989;15:649–652.

166. Henley JD, Young RH, Ulbright TM. Malignant Sertoli cell tumors of the testis: a study of 13 examples of a neoplasm frequently misinterpreted as seminoma. Am J Surg Pathol 2002;26:541–550.

167. Tetu B, Ro JY, Ayala AG. Large cell calcifying Sertoli cell tumor of the testis. A clinicopathologic, immunohistochemical, and ultrastructural study of two cases. Am J Clin Pathol 1991;96:717–722.

168. Proppe KH, Scully RE. Large-cell calcifying Sertoli cell tumor of the testis. Am J Clin Pathol 1980;74:607–619.

169. Kratzer SS, Ulbright TM, Talerman A, et al. Large cell calcifying Sertoli cell tumor of the testis: contrasting features of six malignant and six benign tumors and a review of the literature. Am J Surg Pathol 1997;21:1271–1280.

170. Cano-Valdez AM, Chanona-Vilchis J, Dominguez-Malagon H. Large cell calcifying Sertoli cell tumor of the testis: a clinicopathological, immunohistochemical, and ultrastructural study of two cases. Ultrastruct Pathol 1999;23:259–265.

171. Nogales FF, Andujar M, Zuluaga A, et al. Malignant large cell calcifying Sertoli cell tumor of the testis. J Urol 1995;153:1935–1937.

172. Bufo P, Pennella A, Serio G, et al. Malignant large cell calcifying Sertoli cell tumor of the testis (LCCSCTT). Report of a case in an elderly man and review of the literature. Pathologica 1999;91:107–114.

173. De Raeve H, Schoonooghe P, Wibowo R, et al. Malignant large cell calcifying Sertoli cell tumor of the testis. Pathol Res Pract 2003;199:113–117.

174. Anderson GA. Sclerosing Sertoli cell tumor of the testis: a distinct histological subtype. J Urol 1995;154:1756–1758.

175. Gravas S, Papadimitriou K, Kyriakidis A. Sclerosing Sertoli cell tumor of the testis—a case report and review of the literature. Scand J Urol Nephrol 1999;33:197–199.

176. Knoke I, Jakubiczka S, Ottersen T, et al. A(870)E mutation of the androgen receptor gene in a patient with complete androgen insensitivity syndrome and Sertoli cell tumor. Cancer Genet Cytogenet 1997;98:139–141.

177. Ko HM, Chung JH, Lee JH, et al. Androgen receptor gene mutation associated with complete

androgen insensitivity syndrome and Sertoli cell adenoma. Int J Gynecol Pathol 2001;20:196–199.

178. Mene MP, Finkelstein LH, Manfrey SJ, et al. Metastatic Sertoli cell carcinoma of the testis. J Am Osteopath Assoc 1996;96:612–614.

179. Nonomura K, Koyama T, Kakizaki H, et al. Testicular-sparing surgery for the prepubertal testicular tumor. Experience of two cases with large cell calcifying Sertoli cell tumors. Eur Urol 2001;40:699–704.

Index

A

ACTANE. *See* Anglo-Canadian-Texan-Australian-Norwegian-European Union Biomed group
Adenosine triphosphate (ATP)-binding cassette (ABC) transporter drugs, 206
Adenoviruses, 105–106
  viral delivery systems, for gene therapy, 105–106
Adjuvant radiotherapy, 56–57
Adjuvant therapy, 195
AFP. *See* α-Fetoprotein
Age, prostate cancer and, 3
AMACR. *See* α-Methylacyl-coenzyme (CoA) racemase
Androgen receptor (AR), 22
  androgen synthesis and, 7, 8
  erb-B2/HER-2/neu, 9
  interleukin-6, 9
  prostate cancer etiology and, 9–10
  treatment resistance, 7–9
  trinucleotide repeats, 9
Angiogenesis inhibitors, 195–196
  renal cell carcinoma and, 196–198
Anglo-Canadian-Texan-Australian-Norwegian-European Union Biomed (ACTANE) group, 21
Antigen-presenting cell (APC), 91

APC. *See* Antigen-presenting cell
Apoptosis, inhibitors of, 6
AR. *See* Androgen receptor
aTL. *See* Autologous tumor lysate
Autologous tumor lysate (aTL), 212
Azzopardi phenomenon, 318

B

Balanitis xerotica obliterans (BXO), penile tumors and, 276
Bcl-2, 6
BCLC. *See* Breast Cancer Linkage Consortium
BCRP. *See* Breast cancer resistance protein
Beckwith-Wiedemann syndrome, 177
Bellini's tumor, 176
BEP. *See* Bleomycin, etoposide, platinol (cisplatin)
Biochemotherapy, 193–195
Biopsies, 34
  contralateral testicular, 245
Birt-Hogg-Dube syndrome, 169, 175, 301
Bladder
  lymphoma of, 314–316
    biology of, 315
    clinical features of, 315
    genetics of, 315
    outcome of, 316

    pathology of, 315
    treatment of, 316
  rhabdomyosarcoma of, 319–320
    biology of, 320
    clinical features of, 319–320
    genetics of, 320
    immunohistochemical profile of, 320
    outcome of, 320
    pathology of, 320
    treatment of, 320
  small cell tumors of, 317–318
    biology of, 318
    clinical features of, 317–318
    genetics of, 318
    immunohistochemical profile of, 318
    outcome of, 318
    pathology of, 318
    radiological features of, 317–318
    treatment of, 318
    ultrastructure of, 318
Bladder cancer
  genetic model, 123–124
  microarray-based technologies, 124
  pathogenesis of, 115–116
  strategies, 158–159
    corrective, 159–161
Bladder cancer, superficial
  carcinoma in situ, 132–133
  classification of, 131–132
  grade, 132

Bladder cancer, superficial (*cont.*)
  molecular markers, 134
  multifocality, 132
  natural history of, 132–133
  prognostic factors of, 132–133
    risks of clinical, 133–135
  recurrence/frequency, 132
  stage, 132, 133
  transurethral resection, 135
  tumor size, 132
  tumor surveillance, 135
Bleomycin, 232–233
Bleomycin, etoposide, platinol
    (cisplatin) (BEP), testicular
    cancer and, 230–231,
    234–235
Bloom syndrome, 177
Bowenoid papulosis, 275
Bowen's disease, 275, 283
Breast Cancer Linkage
    Consortium (BCLC), 20
Breast cancer resistance protein
    (BCRP), 206
Burkitt lymphoma, 312, 313
Buschke-Löwenstein (GCBL), 275,
    283
BXO. *See* Balanitis xerotica
    obliterans

C
CALGB. *See* Cancer and Leukemia
    Group B
Cancer, prostate, and brain
    (CAPB), 4
Cancer and Leukemia Group B
    (CALGB), 85–86, 205
CAPB. *See* Cancer, prostate, and
    brain
Capecitabine, 205
CAR. *See* Coxsackie and
    adenovirus receptor
Carboplatin, 87
  cisplatin v., 231–232
  paclitaxel and, 148, 149
  paclitaxel and gemcitabine and,
    148
Cardiovascular disease (CVD),
    germ cell tumors and, 238
Carotenoids, 43–44
CCI-779, 207–208, 213
CD44, 13
CGH. *See* Comparative genomic
    hybridization

Chemoprevention, 24–25, 33
Chemoresistance
  biologic basis of, 226–227
  genetic basis of, 226–227
Chemotherapy
  hormone-refractory prostate
    cancer, 83–84
  in hormone-sensitive disease,
    88–92
    adjuvant, 89, 90
    angiogenesis inhibitors,
      90–91
    epidermal growth factor
      receptor inhibitors, 90
    immunotherapy, 91
    neoadjuvant, 88–89
    suramin, 90
    targeted therapies, 89, 91–92
  response to, 84–87
    carboplatin, 87
    docetaxel, 86–87
    estramustine phosphate,
      86–87
    mitoxantrone, 85–86
    paclitaxel, 86
    prednisone, 85–86
    vinblastine, 86
CHG. *See* Comparative genomic
    hybridization
Children/young adults, renal cell
    carcinoma in, 306–307
Chromophobe tumors, 175
Chromosome 9, 117–119
Circumcision, penile tumors and,
    276
Cisplatin, 145
  docetaxel/paclitaxel and, 147
  gemcitabine and, 146–147
  paclitaxel and iosfamide and,
    147–148
Clear cell renal carcinoma,
    169–170
  hereditary, 173
  sporadic, 172–173
Collecting duct carcinoma, 176
Comparative genomic
    hybridization (CGH), 4,
    318
Computed tomography (CT) scan,
    treatment planning and,
    49, 50
Connecticut Tumor Registry,
    33–34

Coxsackie and adenovirus
    receptor (CAR), 157
CpG island promoter methylation,
    6
CT. *See* Computed tomography
    scan
CVD. *See* Cardiovascular
    disease
Cyclooxygenase-2 (COX-2), 33
Cytokine therapy, 186–187
  nephrectomy before, 187–188

D
Dehydroxymethylepoxyquinomici
    n (DHMEQ), 12
Denys-Drash syndrome, 177
DHMEQ. *See*
    Dehydroxymethylepoxyqui
    nomicin
Diet, prostate cancer and
  fat, 42–43
  modification of, 44–45
  plant steroids, 44
  trace elements, 44
  vitamins, 43–44
Dietary calcium, 43
Diffuse large B cell lymphoma
    (DLBCL), testicular,
    310–312
  biology of, 310–311
  clinical features of, 310
  genetics of, 310–311
  outcome of, 311–312
  pathology of, 310
  treatment of, 311–312
Digital rectal examination (DRE),
    24, 34
DLBCL. *See* Diffuse large B cell
    lymphoma, testicular
Docetaxel/paclitaxel, 86–87
  cisplatin and, 147
DRE. *See* Digital rectal
    examination
Drug therapy, targeted, 206–208

E
E2F3 expression, 23
Eastern Cooperative Oncology
    Group (ECOG), 206
EBR. *See* External beam
    radiotherapy
EBRT. *See* Standard external beam
    radiotherapy

EC. *See* Embryonal carcinoma
ECOG. *See* Eastern Cooperative
   Oncology Group
EGF. *See* Epidermal growth factor
Elements, trace, 44
EMA. *See* Epithelial membrane
   antigen
Embryonal carcinoma (EC), 221
Endothelin-1 (ET-1), 13
Environment, tumor interaction
   and, 10
EORTC. *See* European
   Organization for Research
   and Treatment of Cancer
Epidermal growth factor (EGF), 7,
   10, 11
Epidermal growth factor receptor
   (EGFR) inhibitors, 90, 207
Epithelial membrane antigen
   (EMA), 303
Erectile function, surgical
   treatment and, 72–73
ERSPC. *See* European
   Randomized Study of
   Screening for Prostate
   Cancer
Erythroplasia of Queyrat, 275, 283
Estramustine phosphate, 86–87
European Organization for
   Research and Treatment of
   Cancer (EORTC), 78, 79
European Randomized Study of
   Screening for Prostate
   Cancer (ERSPC), 34
External beam radiotherapy
   (EBR), penile cancer and,
   288–289

F
Familial prostate cancer (FPC),
   clinical management of,
   22–25
  biochemical failure, 23
  biological aggressiveness, 22–23
  chemoprevention role, 24–25
  definitive treatment outcome
   in, 23
  genetic counseling, 25
  sporadic and, 23
  survival differences, 23
  targeted screening, 25
  testing/research, 25
  treatment *v.* observation, 23–24

Family history, prostate cancer
   and, 3
Fat, prostate cancer and
  clinical studies, 42–43
  epidemiologic studies, 42–43
  lab studies, 42
Fertility, germ cell tumors and,
   238
α-Fetoprotein (AFP), 221
FGFR3. *See* Fibroblast growth
   factor receptor gene
Fibroblast growth factor receptor
   gene (FGFR3), 119
Fine needle aspiration cytology
   (FNAC), penile cancer and,
   285
5-Fluorouracil (5-FU), 205
Follicle-stimulating hormone
   (FSH), 79
FSH. *See* Follicle-stimulating
   hormone
5-FU. *See* 5-Fluorouracil

G
G3pT1, treatment of, 138–140
GCBL. *See* Buschke-Löwenstein
GCTs. *See* Germ cell tumors
Gemcitabine
  capecitabine and, 205
  cisplatin and, 146–147
  paclitaxel and carboplatin,
   148
Gene analysis, candidate, 20–21
Gene therapy
  cytotoxic approaches to
   selective tumor cell killing,
   162–163
   suicide gene therapy,
   161–162
  delivery systems for, 104–106
   nonviral, 106, 157
   viral, 105, 157–158
  immunologic
   tumor vaccines, 163
   in vivo cytokine transfection,
   163–164
  strategies, 106–110
   enhancing apoptosis,
   106–107
   immunological response
   enhancement, 107–108
   oncolytic viruses, 110
   suicide gene therapy, 108–110

Genetics
  inherited changes, 4
  somatic changes, 4, 5
Genome-wide search (GWS),
   21–22
  CAPB, 22
  hereditary prostate cancer
   1, 21
  low-penetrance genes, 22
  PCaP, 22
  RNASEL, 21
Germ cell tumors (GCTs)
  carcinoma in situ
   diagnosis of, 254–256
   treatment of, 254–256
  differentiation
   biologic basis of, 225–226
   genetic basis of, 225–226
  extragonadal
   biologic basis of, 225
   genetic basis of, 225
  germ cell origin of, 224–225
  invasive, treatment of, 256–264
   base excision repair, 261
   biological basis for, 256–259
   biological basis of drug
   response, 259–260
   chemotherapy efficacy, 263
   DNA binding, 260
   DNA repair pathways,
   261–262
   drug efflux, 260
   drug influx, 260
   drug sensitivity, 260
   execution of apoptosis,
   262–263
   histopathology of, 256–258
   mismatch repair, 261–262
   nucleotide excision repair,
   261
   relapses, 258–259
   teratomas, 263–264
   TP53, role of, 262
   tumor localization, 258
  long-term toxicities of, 238–239
   cardiovascular morbidity,
   238
   fertility, 238
   gonadal function, 238
   neuropathy, 239
   pulmonary function, 238
   secondary malignancies,
   238–239

Germ cell tumors (GCTs) (*cont.*)
  malignant transformation,
    genetic basis of, 227
  pathobiology of, 221–222,
    252–253
  retroperitoneal lymph node
    dissection for, 246
  seminomatous, 221
  transformation, genetic basis
    of, 222–224
GnRH. *See* Gondotropin-releasing
  hormone
Gonad, function of, germ cell
  tumors and, 238
Gondotropin-releasing hormone
  (GnRH), 79
Green tea, 44
Growth factors, 10–12
GSTP1, 22
GWS. *See* Genome-wide search

H
HCG. *See* Human chorionic
  gonadotropin
HDR. *See* High dose rate
  brachytherapy
Hereditary prostate cancer
  (HPC1/2), 4, 17
Herpes viruses, viral delivery
  systems, for gene therapy,
  106
High dose rate (HDR)
  brachytherapy, 55
Hormone-refractory prostate
  cancer (HRPC), 83–84
Hormone therapy
  with combined antiandrogen
    treatment, 79
  intermittent, 79–80
  localized disease, 77–78
  locally advanced disease, 78–79
  metastatic disease, 78–79
  radiotherapy combined with,
    55–56
  recurrent prostate cancer, 80, 81
  side effects of, 80–81
HPC1/2. *See* Hereditary prostate
  cancer
HPV. *See* Human papillomavirus
  (HPV)
HRE. *See* Hypoxia response
  element
HRPC. *See* Hormone-refractory
  prostate cancer

Human chorionic gonadotropin
  (HCG), 222
Human papillomavirus (HPV)
  high-risk, 277
  low-risk, 277
  oncogenic effect of, 277–279
  penile tumors and, 276–277
  telomerase, activation of, 278
Hypoxia response element (HRE),
  207

I
ICPCG. *See* International
  Consortium for Prostate
  Cancer Genetics
Ifosfamide, paclitaxel and
  cisplatin and, 147–148
IGCCCG. *See* International Germ
  Cell Consensus Cancer
  Group
IGF-1. *See* Insulin-like growth
  factor-1
IL-2. *See* Inteleukin-2
Ilioinguinal nodes, management
  of
  cytologically
    confirmed/clinically
    significant, 292–293
  complications of, 292–293
  lymphadenectomy extent,
    292
  impalpable/clinically
    insignificant, 290–292
  occult metastases surgical
    identification, 291
  prophylactic
    lymphadenectomy,
    291–292
  sentinel node biopsy, 291
  surveillance, 290–291
Immunotherapy, 185–186
IMRT. *See* Intensity-modulated
  radiotherapy
INFs. *See* Interferons
Insulin-like growth factor-1 (IGF-
  1), 7, 11, 12, 33
Inteleukin-2 (IL-2), 190–192
Intensity-modulated radiotherapy
  (IMRT), 53
Interferon-α (IFN-α), interleukin-
  2 and, 192–193
Interferons (INFs), 140, 188–190
Interleukin-2 (IL-2), interferon-α
  and, 192–193

Interleukin-6, 9
International Consortium for
  Prostate Cancer Genetics
  (ICPCG), 22
International Germ Cell
  Consensus Cancer Group
  (IGCCCG), 226, 230
Intratubular germ cell neoplasia
  (ITGCN), 221
Intratubular germ cell neoplasia
  unclassified (ITGCNU)
  diagnosis of, 254–26
  treatment of, 254–26
Intravesical therapy, in tumor
  prophylaxis
  chemotherapy, 136
  dose scheduling and, 137–138
  immunotherapy, 136–137
In vivo cytokine transfection,
  163–164
ITGCN. *See* Intratubular germ cell
  neoplasia
Ixabepilone, 206

K
KA11, 13
Keratinocyte growth factor (KGF),
  7, 11
KGF. *See* Keratinocyte growth
  factor
Kidney, primitive
  neuroectodermal tumors
  of, 304
Kidney cancer. *See* Clear cell renal
  carcinoma
KLF6, tumor suppressor, 5
Kulchitsky-type neuroendocrine
  cells, 318

L
Laparoscopic prostatectomy, 70–71
LCTs. *See* Leydig cell tumors
Lentiviruses, viral delivery
  systems, for gene therapy,
  105
Leydig cell tumors (LCTs)
  biology of, 322
  clinical features of, 321
  genetics of, 322
  immunophenotype, 322
  malignant, 322
  outcome of, 322
  pathology of, 321–322
  treatment of, 322

LHRH. *See* Luteinizing hormone-releasing hormone
Linkage analysis, 20
LOD. *See* Logarithm of odds
Logarithm of odds (LOD), 22
LOH. *See* Loss of heterozygosity
Loss of heterozygosity (LOH), 4
Low-penetrance genes, 22
Luteinizing hormone-releasing hormone (LHRH), 54, 61, 79
Lymphoma
  of bladder, 314–316
    biology of, 315
    clinical features of, 315
    genetics of, 315
    outcome of, 316
    pathology of, 315
    treatment of, 316
   Burkitt, 312, 313
  diffuse large B cell, testicular, 310–312
    biology of, 310–311
    clinical features of, 310
    genetics of, 310–311
    outcome of, 311–312
    pathology of, 310
    treatment of, 311–312
  of prostate, 316–317
    biology of, 316–317
    clinical features of, 316
    outcome of, 317
    pathology of, 316–317
    treatment of, 317
  of testis, 309–314
    Burkitt, 312, 313
    childhood disorders, 312, 313
    diffuse large B cell, 310–312
    mature T/NK, 313
    paratesticular tissues, 313–314
    plasma cell neoplasia, 313

M
Mass spectrometry, to identify proteins, 96–97
Matrix metalloproteinases (MMPs), 13
M-CAV. *See* Methotrexate and carboplatin and vinblastine
Medullary carcinoma, renal, 176

Methotrexate, vinblastine, Adriamycin (doxorubicin), and cisplatin (MVAC)
  development of, 145
  improvement of, 146
  limitations of, 145–146
Methotrexate and carboplatin and vinblastine (M-CAV), 148
α-Methylacyl-coenzyme (CoA) racemase (AMACR), 7
Microarray-based technology, 124
Mitoxantrone, 85–86
Mixed epithelial and stromal tumor, renal, 302–303
MLCs. *See* Multileaf collimators
Mohs' micrographic surgery, penile cancer and, 287
Molecular markers, 176
MRP. *See* Multidrug resistance-related protein
Mucinous tubular spindle cell carcinoma, 304–306
Multidrug resistance-related protein (MRP), 206
Multileaf collimators (MLCs), 51, 52
MVAC. *See* Methotrexate, vinblastine, Adriamycin (doxorubicin), and cisplatin

N
Navartis epothilone EPO906, 206
NBS. *See* Nijmegen breakage syndrome
Nephrectomy, before cytokine therapy, 187–188
Neuropathy, germ cell tumors and, 239
Nijmegen breakage syndrome (NBS), 20–21
NKX3-1, tumor suppressor, 5–6
Nuclear factor KB (NF-KB), 12

O
Oncocytoma, 301, 302
Oncogenes, 121
  inhibition/destruction of, 161
  myc, 6
  ras, 6
Oncophage™ product, 211
Orchidectomy
  inguinal
    complications with, 244

    surgical approach and, 243–244
    testicular prostheses and, 244
    timing of, 243
  partial, 245
Osteocalcin, 13
Osteopontin, 13

P
P53, tumor suppressor, 5
Paclitaxel, 86
  carboplatin and, 148, 149
  carboplatin and gemcitabine and, 148
  ifosfamide and cisplatin and, 147–148
Papillary renal cell carcinoma, 173–175
PCaP. *See* Predisposing for prostate cancer
PDGFR. *See* Platelet-derived growth factor receptor
Penile cancer. *See also* Penile tumors
  biopsy, 286
  carcinoma in situ, prevalence in, 277
  chemotherapy for, 293–294
  clinical presentation of, 283–284
  epidemiology of, 283
  etiology of, 283
  histology of, 283–284
  ilioinguinal node management, 290–293
    clinically insignificant, 290–292
    clinically significant, 292–293
    cytologically confirmed, 292–293
    impalpable, 290–292
  local spread of, 284
  management of primary tumor, 286–290
    amputation, 289–290
    conservative therapy, 287–290
    laser therapy, 287–288
    Mohs' micrographic surgery, 287
    radiation therapy, 288–289
    wide excision, 287
  natural history of, 283–284
  nodal metastasis of, 284

Penile cancer (*cont.*)
  pretreatment evaluation,
    285–286
  prevalence in, 276–277
  prognosis of, 294
  psychosexual issues, 294
  quality of life and, 294
  staging pitfalls, 285–286
  techniques for, 286
  treatment for, 286
Penile intraepithelial neoplasia
    (PIN), 275
Penile tumors, etiology of,
    275–277
  balanitis xerotica obliterans,
    276
  circumcision, 276
  human papillomavirus, 276–277
  hygiene, 276
  phimosis, 276
  smoking, 276
Penis
  amputation of, 289–290
  squamous cell carcinoma of,
    279–280
Perineal prostatectomy, 70
Perlman syndrome, 177
PGCs. *See* Primordial germ
    cells
P-glycoprotein (Pgp), 206
Pgp. *See* P-glycoprotein
Phimosis, penile tumors and,
    276
PIN. *See* Penile intraepithelial
    neoplasia
PIN. *See* Prostatic intraepithelial
    neoplasia
PIVOT. *See* Prostate Cancer
    Intervention Versus
    Observation Trial
Plasma cell neoplasia, 313
Platelet-derived growth factor
    receptor (PDGFR), 80
PLOC. *See* Prostate, Lung, Colon,
    and Ovary cancer trial
PNETs. *See* Primitive
    neuroectodermal tumors
Pox viruses, 158
PPI. *See* Present Pain Intensity
Predisposing for prostate cancer
    (PCaP), 4
Prednisone, 85–86
Present Pain Intensity (PPI), 85

Primitive neuroectodermal
    tumors (PNETs), 227, 304,
    305
Primordial germ cells (PGCs),
    252
PROSQOLI. *See* Prostate Cancer-
    Specific Quality of Life
    Instrument
Prostate
  lymphoma of, 316–317
    biology of, 316–317
    clinical features of, 316
    outcome of, 317
    pathology of, 316–317
    treatment of, 317
  small cell carcinoma of,
    318–319
    biology of, 319
    clinical features of, 319
    immunohistochemical profile
      of, 319
    outcome of, 319
    pathology of, 319
    treatment of, 319
Prostate, Lung, Colon, and Ovary
    (PLOC) cancer trial,
    36–37
Prostate brachytherapy, 53–54
  high-dose rate, 55
  permanent implants, 54–55
Prostate cancer (PCa). *See also*
    Familial prostate cancer
  autopsy detected, 3
  chemotherapy, hormone-
    refractory for, 83–84
  diet for, 42–45
  epidemiology evidence of,
    18–20
    case-control studies, 18–19
    cohort studies, 19
    segregation analyses, 20
    twin studies, 19–20
  epidemiology of, 3–4
  fat and, 42–43
  genetic etiology evidence of,
    17–18
  genome searches in, 21–22
  hormone therapy and, 80–81
  inherited genetic changes and,
    4
  mortality rate of, 78
  natural history of, 33–34
  risk factors for, 3, 4

  somatic genetic changes and,
    4, 5
  surgical treatment of, 69–74
Prostate Cancer Intervention
    Versus Observation Trial
    (PIVOT), 35, 49
Prostate Cancer-Specific Quality
    of Life Instrument
    (PROSQOLI), 85
Prostatectomy
  laparoscopic, 70–71
  perineal, 70
  radical, 71
  retropubic, 69–70
Prostatic intraepithelial neoplasia
    (PIN), 32–33
Prostatic-specific antigen (PSA),
    21, 31
Protect (Prostate testing for
    cancer and treatment), 35
Proteomics
  androgen receptor and, 99–100
  diagnostic markers, 100–102
    cell surface, 100–101
    serum, 101–102
  functional, 100
  studies, 97–100
    biopsy, 98
    laser capture microscopy,
      98–99
    normal/cancerous prostate
      proteins, 97
    second-line, 99
    tissue culture, 97–98
  technique in, 95–97
    protein detection and
      analysis, 96
    protein identifying mass
      spectrometry, 96–97
    surface-enhanced laser
      description, 97
    two-dimensional gel
      electrophoresis, 95–96
PSA. *See* Prostate-specific antigen
PTEN/PI$_3$K/AKT, tumor
    suppressor, 5
pVHL. *See* Von Hippel-Lindau
    protein

R
Radiation Therapy Oncology
    Group (RTOG), 77–78
Radical prostatectomy, 71

Radical radiotherapy
  adjuvant/salvage, 56–57
  hormone therapy combined
    with, 55–56
  intensity modulated, 53
  prostate brachytherapy, 53–55
  role of, 48–49
  standard external beam, 49–51
  three-dimensional conformal,
    51–53
Rb, tumor suppressor, 5
Relative risks (RR), in first-degree
  relatives, 18–19
Renal, primary, synovial
  sarcomas, 303–304
Renal cell carcinoma. See also
    Clear cell renal carcinoma
  angiogenesis inhibitors and,
    196–198
  in children/young adults,
    306–307
  prognostic factors of, 184–185
  therapies for, 205
    angiogenic targeting, 212
    conventional cytotoxics,
      205–206
    immunity, 208–210
    leukocyte products, 210–211
    targeted drugs, 206–208
    tumor products, 211–212
    vascular targeting, 212–213
Renal oncocytoma, 175
Renal tumors, mixed epithelial
  and stromal, 302–303
Restriction fragment length
    polymorphism (RFLP),
    170
Retroperitoneal lymph node
    dissection (RPLND), 244
  complications of, 249
  for germ cell tumors, 246
  postchemotherapy, 247–248
  seminoma and, 248
  for Stage I, 246
  for Stage II, 246–247
  stromal tumors and, 248
  surgical technique and, 248–249
Retropubic prostatectomy, 69–70
Retroviruses, 158
  viral delivery systems, for gene
    therapy, 105
RFLP. See Restriction fragment
    length polymorphism

Rhabdomyosarcoma, of bladder,
    319–320
  biology of, 320
  clinical features of, 319–320
  genetics of, 320
  immunohistochemical profile
    of, 320
  outcome of, 320
  pathology of, 320
  treatment of, 320
RNASEL, 4
RPLND. See Retroperitoneal
    lymph node dissection
RR. See Relative risks
RTOG. See Radiation Therapy
    Oncology Group

S
Salvage radiotherapy, 56–57
Screening, for prostate cancer
  instrument for, 34–35
  mortality and, 36
  policies on, 37–38
  program establishment,
    31–36
  public perception of, 37
  study of, 36–37
SCSTs. See Sex-cord-stromal
    tumors, of testis
SCTs. See Sertoli cell tumors
SDS-PAGE. See Standard sodium
    dodecyl sulfate-
    polyacrylamide gel
    electrophoresis
SEER. See Surveillance,
    Epidemiology, and End
    Results database
SELDI. See Surface-enhanced laser
    desorption
SELECT. See Selenium and
    Vitamin E Cancer
    Prevention Trial
Selenium, 44
Selenium and Vitamin E Cancer
    Prevention Trial (SELECT),
    24
Seminoma
  adjuvant chemotherapy for,
    237–238
  carboplatin versus cisplatin,
    231–232
  retroperitoneal lymph node
    dissection and, 248

Sertoli cell tumors (SCTs),
    323–324
  biology of, 324
  clinical features of, 323
  electron microscopy of, 323–324
  genetics of, 324
  immunophenotype of, 323–324
  large cell calcifying, 324
  malignant, 324
  outcome of, 324
  pathology of, 323
  sclerosing, 324
  treatment of, 324
  variants of, 324
Sex-cord-stromal tumors (SCSTs),
    of testis, 320–324
  Leydig cell tumors, 321–322
    biology of, 322
    clinical features of, 321
    genetics of, 322
    immunophenotype, 322
    malignant, 322
    outcome of, 322
    pathology of, 321–322
    treatment of, 322
  sertoli cell tumors, 323–324
    biology of, 324
    clinical features of, 323
    electron microscopy of,
      323–324
    genetics of, 324
    immunophenotype of,
      323–324
    large cell calcifying, 324
    malignant, 324
    outcome of, 324
    pathology of, 323
    sclerosing, 324
    treatment of, 324
    variants of, 324
Small cell carcinoma
  of bladder, 317–318
    biology of, 318
    clinical features of, 317–318
    genetics of, 318
    immunohistochemical profile
      of, 318
    outcome of, 318
    pathology of, 318
    radiological features of,
      317–318
    treatment of, 318
    ultrastructure of, 318

Small cell carcinoma (*cont.*)
   of prostate, 318–319
      biology of, 319
      clinical features of, 319
      immunohistochemical profile
         of, 319
      outcome of, 319
      pathology of, 319
      treatment of, 319
Smoking, penile tumors and, 276
Sorangium cellulosum, 206
Southwest Oncology Group
      (SWOG), 57
Soy-derived products, 44
SRD5A2, 22
Standard external beam
      radiotherapy (EBRT)
   dose and fractionation, 50–51
   efficacy, 51
   pretreatment assessment, 49
   technique, 50
   toxicity, 51
   treatment planning, 49–50
Standard sodium dodecyl sulfate-
      polyacrylamide gel
      electrophoresis (SDS-
      PAGE), 95–96
Steroids, plant, 44
Suicide gene therapy, 108–110
Surface-enhanced laser
      desorption (SELDI), 97
Surgical treatment, for prostate
      cancer
   cancer control with, 71–72
   complications, 72
   erectile function, 72–73
   laparoscopic prostatectomy,
      70–71
   outcomes, 74
   perineal prostatectomy, 70
   quality of life, 73
   radical prostatectomy,
      principles of, 71
   retropubic prostatectomy,
      69–70
   urinary continence, 73
Surveillance, Epidemiology, and
      End Results (SEER)
      database, 33, 34, 36
SWOG. *See* Southwest Oncology
      Group
Synovial sarcomas, primary renal,
      303–304

T
TCC. *See* Transitional cell
      carcinoma
Telomerase protein (TERT), 210
Telomeres, length of, 7
Teratomas, 221, 263–264
TERT. *See* Telomerase protein
Testicular cancer
   contralateral testicular biopsy,
      245
   orchidectomy
      inguinal, 243–244
      partial, 245
   retroperitoneal lymph node
         dissection, 244, 245–248
      complications of, 249
      germ cell tumors, 246
      postchemotherapy, 247–248
      for Stage I, 246
      for Stage II, 246–247
      surgical technique and,
         248–249
Testicular cancer, metastatic
   adjuvant chemotherapy,
      237–238
      nonseminomatous germ cell
         cancer, 237
      testicular seminoma, 237–238
   bleomycin, etoposide, platinol
      (cisplatin), 230–231
   prognostic factors of, 230
   treatment of, 231–237
      bleomycin, 232–233
      carboplatin *versus* cisplatin,
         231–232
      comparative bleomycin,
         etoposide, cisplatin,
         234–235
      good prognosis disease,
         231–235
      intermediate prognosis
         disease, 235
      number of cycles, 233–234
      poor prognosis disease,
         235–237
Testicular intratubular neoplasia
      (TIN)
   diagnosis of, 254–256
   treatment of, 254–256
Testis, lymphoma of, 309–314
   Burkitt, 312, 313
   childhood disorders, 312, 313
   diffuse large B cell, 310–312

   mature T/NK, 313
   paratesticular tissues, 313–314
   plasma cell neoplasia, 313
TGF-α. *See* Transforming growth
      factor-α
Thalidomide, 198–199
3D-CRT. *See* Three-dimensional
      conformal radiotherapy
Three-dimensional conformal
      radiotherapy (3D-CRT)
   dose escalation, 51–53
   toxicity reduction and, 51
TP53, role of, germ cell tumors
      and, 262
Transforming growth factor-α
      (TGF-α), 10, 11
Transforming growth factor-B
      (TGF-B), 10, 11
Transitional cell carcinoma (TCC)
   cisplatin for, 145
   docetaxel/paclitaxel and
      cisplatin, 147
   gemcitabine and cisplatin,
      146–147
   ifosfamide, paclitaxel and
      cisplatin, 147–148
   invasive, molecular alterations
      in, 120–123
      carcinoma in situ, 123
      oncogenes, 121
      prognostic markers in, 123
      tumor-suppressor genes,
         121–122
   locally advanced, treatment of,
      152
   metastatic
      postchemotherapy surgery
         in, 150
      therapeutic strategies in, 149
      treatment of, 150
   methotrexate, carboplatin,
      vinblastine, 148
   methotrexate, vinblastine,
      Adriamycin (doxorubicin),
      and cisplatin, 145
   nonplatinum combinations, 149
   paclitaxel, carboplatin,
      gemcitabine, 148
   paclitaxel and carboplatin, 148,
      149
   perioperative chemotherapy
      for, 150–152
      adjuvant, 152

neoadjuvant, 150–152
superficial, molecular
    alterations in, 116–120
  chromosome 9, 117–119
  fibroblast growth factor
    receptor gene, 119
  progression of, 120
  recurrence of, 120
Transrectal ultrasound (TRUS),
    34, 49
Transurethral resection of the
    prostate (TURP), 54, 60
Treatment, immediate *vs.*
    deferred, 60–67
  clinical trials, 61–65
    localized disease, 62–64
    locally advanced disease,
      64–65
    metastatic disease, 65
TRUS. *See* Transrectal ultrasound
TS. *See* Tuberous sclerosis
Tuberous sclerosis (TS), 173
Tumors
  Bellini's, 176
  chromophobe, 175
  Leydig cell
    biology of, 322
    clinical features of, 321
    genetics of, 322
    immunophenotype, 322
    malignant, 322
    outcome of, 322
    pathology of, 321–322
    treatment of, 322
  penile tumors, 275–277
    balanitis xerotica obliterans,
      276
    circumcision, 276
    human papillomavirus,
      276–277
    hygiene, 276
    phimosis, 276
    smoking, 276
  sertoli cell, 323–324
    biology of, 324
    clinical features of, 323
    electron microscopy of,
      323–324
    genetics of, 324
    immunophenotype of,
      323–324
    large cell calcifying, 324
    malignant, 324

outcome of, 324
pathology of, 323
sclerosing, 324
treatment of, 324
variants of, 324
small cell bladder, 317–318
  biology of, 318
  clinical features of, 317–318
  genetics of, 318
  immunohistochemical profile
    of, 318
  outcome of, 318
  pathology of, 318
  radiological features of,
    317–318
  treatment of, 318
  ultrastructure of, 318
stromal, retroperitoneal lymph
    node dissection and, 248
superficial bladder cancer, 132,
    135
Wilms', 176–178
Tumors, germ cell
  carcinoma in situ
    diagnosis of, 254–256
    treatment of, 254–256
  differentiation
    biologic basis of, 225–226
    genetic basis of, 225–226
  extragonadal
    biologic basis of, 225
    genetic basis of, 225
  germ cell origin of, 224–225
  invasive, treatment of, 256–264
    base excision repair, 261
    biological basis for, 256–259
    biological basis of drug
      response, 259–260
    chemotherapy efficacy, 263
    DNA binding, 260
    DNA repair pathways,
      261–262
    drug efflux, 260
    drug influx, 260
    drug sensitivity, 260
    execution of apoptosis,
      262–263
    histopathology of, 256–258
    mismatch repair, 261–262
    nucleotide excision repair,
      261
    relapses, 258–259
    teratomas, 263–264

TP53, role of, 262
  tumor localization, 258
long-term toxicities of, 238–239
  cardiovascular morbidity, 238
  fertility, 238
  gonadal function, 238
  neuropathy, 239
  pulmonary function, 238
  secondary malignancies,
    238–239
malignant transformation,
    genetic basis of, 227
pathobiology of, 221–222,
    252–253
retroperitoneal lymph node
    dissection for, 246
seminomatous, 221
transformation, genetic basis
    of, 222–224
Tumor-suppressor genes, 121–122
  CpG island promoter
    methylation, 6
  KLF6, 5
  NKX3-1, 5–6
  p53, 5, 121–122
  phosphate and tensin
    homologue deleted
    onchromosome, 122
  PTEN/PI₃K/AKT, 5
  RB, 121–122
  Rb, 5
  restoration/overexpression of,
    159–161
    gelsolin, 161
    p21, 160
    p53, 159–160
    retinoblastoma, 160
TURP. *See* Transurethral resection
    of the prostate
Twins
  prostate cancer and, 3
  relative risk studies in, 19–20
2DGE. *See* Two-dimensional gel
    electrophoresis
Two-dimensional gel
    electrophoresis (2DGE),
    95–96

U
UICC. *See* Union International
    Contre le Cancer tumor,
    node, metastasis (TNM)
    staging, 285

Union International Contre le
    Cancer (UICC) tumor,
    node, metastasis (TNM)
    staging, 285
Urinary continence, surgical
    treatment and, 73

V
Vaccinia virus, viral delivery
    systems, for gene therapy,
    106
VACURG. *See* Veterans
    Administration
    Cooperative Research
    Group
Vascular endothelial growth
    factor (VEGF), 7, 207
VEGF. *See* Vascular endothelial
    growth factor

Veterans Administration
    Cooperative Research
    Group (VACURG), 61
VHL. *See* Von Hippel-Lindau
    disease
Vinblastine, 86, 145–146, 148
Viral delivery systems, for gene
    therapy
    adenoviruses, 105–106
    herpes viruses, 106
    lentiviruses, 105
    retroviruses, 105
    vaccinia virus, 106
Vitamins, prostate cancer and,
    43–44
Von Hippel-Lindau (VHL)
    disease, 169, 170–172

Von Hippel-Lindau protein
    (pVHL), 206

W
WAGR (Wilms' tumor, aniridia,
    genitourinary
    abnormalities, and mental
    retardation) syndrome, 177
Wilms' tumor, 176–178
Wilms' tumor, aniridia,
    genitourinary
    abnormalities, and mental
    retardation (WAGR)
    syndrome, 177

Young adults/children, renal cell
    carcinoma in, 306–307